Veterinary Science: Animal Pathology and Disease Management

Edited by Connor Jenkins

hayle
medical

New York

Hayle Medical,
750 Third Avenue, 9ᵗʰ Floor,
New York, NY 10017, USA

Visit us on the World Wide Web at:
www.haylemedical.com

ISBN: 978-1-63241-801-2

Trademark Notice: Registered trademark of products or corporate names are used only for explanation and identification without intent to infringe.

Cataloging-in-Publication Data

Veterinary science : animal pathology and disease management / edited by Connor Jenkins.
    p. cm.
Includes bibliographical references and index.
ISBN 978-1-63241-801-2
1. Veterinary medicine. 2. Animals--Diseases. 3. Animals--Diseases--Treatment.
4. Animal health. I. Jenkins, Connor.
SF745 .V483 2019
636.089--dc23

Table of Contents

Permissions

List of Contributors

Index

Preface

The purpose of the book is to provide a glimpse into the dynamics and to present opinions and studies of some of the scientists engaged in the development of new ideas in the field from very different standpoints. This book will prove useful to students and researchers owing to its high content quality.

Veterinary medicine is concerned with animal health. A wide range of diseases and conditions occur in animals, such as biliary fever, epilepsy, leucosis, pneumonia, myopia, obesity, subvalvular aortic stenosis, hip dislocation, impaction, etc. Animals are also susceptible to a number of parasitic diseases, such as feline zoonoses, fasciolosis, filariasis, proliferative kidney disease, whirled disease, etc. Animals may be vaccinated to prevent the occurrence of many of these diseases, using anthrax vaccine, brucellosis vaccine, rabies vaccine, DA2PPC vaccine, clostridium vaccine, etc. Veterinarians use several diagnostic tools such as ultrasound, X-ray, ECG, pulse oximeter, etc. They also use novel therapeutic techniques to improve the health of animals. Animal drugs such as sedatives, antiemetics, analgesics, bronchodilators, antibiotics, anti-inflammatory drugs, corticosteroids, histamine blockers, etc. may be prescribed by veterinarians depending on the underlying pathology. Orthopedic surgery, soft tissue surgery and neurosurgery may also be performed on an animal. They may include advanced procedures such as joint replacement, transplantation, complex wound management and minimally invasive procedures. This book contains some path-breaking studies in the field of veterinary science. It unravels the recent studies in the pathology and disease management in animals. It is a resource guide for experts as well as students.

At the end, I would like to appreciate all the efforts made by the authors in completing their chapters professionally. I express my deepest gratitude to all of them for contributing to this book by sharing their valuable works. A special thanks to my family and friends for their constant support in this journey.

Editor

Stride-related rein tension patterns in walk and trot in the ridden horse

Agneta Egenvall[1*], Lars Roepstorff[2], Marie Eisersiö[1], Marie Rhodin[1] and René van Weeren[3]

Abstract

Background: The use of tack (equipment such as saddles and reins) and especially of bits because of rein tension resulting in pressure in the mouth is questioned because of welfare concerns. We hypothesised that rein tension patterns in walk and trot reflect general gait kinematics, but are also determined by individual horse and rider effects. Six professional riders rode three familiar horses in walk and trot. Horses were equipped with rein tension meters logged by inertial measurement unit technique. Left and right rein tension data were synchronized with the gait.

Results: Stride split data (0–100 %) were analysed using mixed models technique to elucidate the left/right rein and stride percentage interaction, in relation to the exercises performed. In walk, rein tension was highest at hindlimb stance. Rein tension was highest in the suspension phase at trot, and lowest during the stance phase. In rising trot there was a significant difference between the two midstance phases, but not in sitting trot. When turning in trot there was a significant statistical association with the gait pattern with the tension being highest in the inside rein when the horse was on the outer fore-inner hindlimb diagonal.

Conclusions: Substantial between-rider variation was demonstrated in walk and trot and between-horse variation in walk. Biphasic rein tensions patterns during the stride were found mainly in trot.

Keywords: Inertial measurement unit, Rein tension, Trot, Walk, Variation

Background

For most of the time since the domestication of the horse, more than five millennia ago, mankind has used the horse mainly for the capabilities of its locomotor system. It is therefore not surprising that the majority of the physical problems of the horse are orthopaedic in nature [1–3] and that the rider/trainer has an influence on the occurrence and manifestation of locomotor problems in the horse [1, 2]. It is likely that at least part of this influence is due to riding technique [1, 2].

Over time, different kinds of tack have been developed to facilitate the use of the horse, tack being equipment used on the horse to facilitate the use of it, such as saddles and reins. In many riding disciplines, reins are attached to a piece of metal that sits in the horse's

mouth—the bit. The rider uses the reins to act on the bit to provide cues to the horse to indicate desired direction, acceleration or deceleration and carriage of the head. Recently scientific interest in the use of tack and the bit in particular has surged, principally related to animal welfare. The use of bits is regularly questioned [4]. Scientific research has been made possible by the development of tools that can measure the specific effects of various elements of the tack of a horse. Rein tension has a strong influence on the effects of the bit on the sensitive tissues of the horse's mouth and can now be measured reliably. It has recently been shown that riders influence rein tension to a large degree [5, 6].

Average rein tensions have been reported as 5.1 N at the walk, 6.3 N at the trot [7] and around 15 N at the canter [8]. Rein tension measurements at trot in unmounted horses or horses ridden with a free head and neck position showed peaks with maximal tension occurring in the second half of each diagonal stance phase [9, 10]. In sitting trot with the horse's nose line on the vertical the largest rein tension peaks were found in the suspension

*Correspondence: agneta.egenvall@slu.se
[1] Department of Clinical Sciences, Faculty of Veterinary Medicine and Animal Husbandry, Swedish University of Agricultural Sciences, Box 7054, 750 07 Uppsala, Sweden
Full list of author information is available at the end of the article

phase. It should be mentioned that the latter conclusions were based on the appraisal of visual differences in a study of three horses and not on statistical analysis [10]. In a study comprising more horses, rein tension in canter was maximal just before the beginning of vertical stance, the release was closer to the suspension phase and also more marked on the outside rein (the rein facing the outside of an arena or a circle) [6]. On average, tension in the outside rein was 7 N less than in the inside rein close to the suspension phase, while at midstance tension in both reins was just over 30 N [6].

Riders are subjected to substantially different locomotion patterns in each of the three main gaits of the horse: walk trot and canter. Of these, walk and trot are symmetrical whereas canter is an asymmetrical gait. It has been shown in a treadmill study that at the slower four-beat walk the extra-sagittal movements of the saddle (i.e. yaw and roll) the rider has to accommodate are several degrees larger than at trot, as fore and hindquarter movements are not synchronous [11]. In another treadmill study it was demonstrated that in the two-beat trot there is less lateroflexion of the equine spine, leaving the sitting rider mainly subjected to vertical and longitudinal forces as the withers and croup move vertically simultaneously [12]. However, the rider can also choose to rise at trot, alternating sitting and rising on the two diagonals.

The aim of the current study was to quantify and analyse stride phase related rein tension at walk and trot. We further hypothesised that rein tension patterns would not only be influenced by the gait, but that individual horse and rider effects would exist and that the latter thus may be a contributing element to the more general rider effects as described earlier [1, 2].

Methods
Ethical permission
According to the Swedish legislation ethical permit was not necessary for this study.

Riders and horses
Data were collected from six professional riders (mean ± STD height 172 ± 8 cm and weight 68 ± 12 kg), each riding three horses that were familiar to them (n = 18). The riders had regularly trained their 'own' horses for between 1 month and 22 years, median 24 months. All horses wore their own correctly fitting saddle and bridle with their ordinary snaffle bit. Fifteen of the snaffles had three parts, two were straight (of these one had rigid rings and one rubber ones); seven had two parts. Two of the fifteen 3-part snaffles had fixed rings, one had a small port and two of the 2-part snaffles were full-cheek. Further information on the horses

and riders can be found in the study by Eisersiö et al. [13], which used the same group of riders and horses with the exception of riders 3 and 5. When asked, one rider stated left-handedness, the others said they were right-handed. Horse laterality was assessed by asking the riders to which side the horses used to bend most easily. Five horses were found to be easier to bend to the left, 11 horses were easier to bend to the right, one horse was equally easy to bend in left and right direction, and one horse was easier to bend to the right at the trot and to the left at the canter. The educational level of the horses was reported by the riders as: basic (n = 6), young horse (n = 3), medium (n = 5) and advanced (n = 4). Advanced horses had competed at Prix St. George, Intermediaire or Grand Prix level (these competition levels include several exercises of great difficulty, such as piaffe, passage and canter pirouettes that are not or rarely performed by basic horses); basic horses had entered low-level competitions only and medium horses were in between. Young horses had been ridden for less than a year and had not competed.

Equipment
Data collection took place at each horse's current stable in an indoor arena (n = 3 riders, 1 sand-fibre arena and two sand-wood chip arenas, the smallest 20 × 50 m and the largest 23 × 62 m), or outdoor arena (n = 3 riders, gravel-based, the smallest 23 × 62 m and the largest 40 × 80 m), depending on weather conditions. Each horse was fitted with a custom-made rein tension meter (128 Hz), measuring range 0–500 N, resolution 0.11 N, fastened on leather reins. A cable from each tension meter ran forwards along the rein and up along the side piece of the bridle (Additional file 1), passing behind the horse's ear and ending at an Inertial Measurement Unit (IMU, x-io Technologies Limited, UK) attached right below the brow band of the bridle using Velcro. The rein tension meters, for each rein separately, were calibrated before the riding sessions started by suspending 13 known weights between 0 and 20 kg. The rein tension meter was also screened in a tensile test machine for stability and repeatability of results (one example see Additional file 2). Further details on the rein tension meter can be found elsewhere [14]. All equipment was fitted on the horse in the riding arena, which took approximately 10 min including synchronization (see below) of the equipment.

Video recordings (Canon Legria HF200, 25 Hz) were made of the entire riding session from the middle of one of the long sides of the arena. All horses were free from lameness according to the clinical judgment of a veterinarian, who visually evaluated the videos of the horses.

Study design

Once the measuring equipment was fitted to the horse, the riders were asked to follow their normal routine with each horse for flatwork/dressage and to ride in all gaits (walk, trot and canter, the latter gait was not analysed within this study). The whole riding arena was used for the exercises and the length of the riding session was determined by the rider. More detail on the content and actual exercises performed during the riding sessions is presented in detail elsewhere [13].

Synchronization of equipment

After the rider had mounted, and before dismounting at the end, the rein tension meter was synchronized with the video recordings by pulling on the right tension meter five times twice in a row while counting out loud in front of the camera. This procedure allowed for processing of the data from the rein tension meter with the corresponding video frames.

Data management

One investigator (ME) scrutinized the videos and categorized the behavioural data. Further detailed information on this protocol can be found elsewhere [13]. In brief, the categories used in this study were rider's position in the saddle (sitting, rising), corners and turns (corner left/right, turn left/right), lateral movements (half-pass to the left/right, shoulder-in left/right, leg-yield left/right) or riding in lengthening (trot with longer strides). The accuracy of the assessment and classification of the video frames by the evaluator (ME) was checked during the data analysis process by comparing to head acceleration and head angle data from the IMUs by a second person (AE). In this process the gait transitions could be traced and confirmed easily, proving correctness of gait classification. Similarly, alterations in head angles were checked and correct synchronization between data and events on video frames could be confirmed. Rein tension data were downloaded to a personal computer and handled in Matlab (MathWorks Inc., USA). Using custom-written scripts, data were split to generate half-strides (e.g. from midstance of the right forelimb to midstance of the left forelimb) based on the most vertical acceleration signal from the poll using the 'peakfinds' function in Matlab. Euler angles of the IMU on the croup (around the horizontal cranio-caudal axis) were used to make sure the split was made on right forelimb midstance, which in trot is the right fore/left hind diagonal and in walk at right forelimb stance. The stride-split was thus in both gaits from right forelimb mid-stance to the next right forelimb midstance. The data were graphically verified before accepting the stride-splits. Using this approach, the suspension phase in trot will start at around 25 and 75 %

of the stride [15]. Time-normalised rein data (0–100 %) were constructed using stride split times. The nose angle range of motion (ROM, defined as the maximal minus the minimal nose angle that was measured) as well as whether the nose was moving backwards (in) or forwards (out) relative to the frame of the horse, was determined from Euler angles, derived from the gyroscopic inertial measurement unit signal from the head.

Statistical modeling

The outcomes were rein tension in the left and right rein during walk and trot separately [both on short reins (long reins were defined as hanging in a loop and the horse having an unrestrained head and neck position; with short reins the rider had contact with the horse's mouth)]. However, for each gait rein tension data on left and right reins were evaluated in the same model. Dependent data were time-normalised stride means (one series in one horse = one normalised stride of 101 data points) that each belonged to a compound category (e.g. sitting trot in half-pass to the right ridden in a turn, with baseline for corners and no lengthening). Rein tension was checked for normality, i.e. means and medians were deemed close (i.e. mean differing from median by preferably not more than 5 % of the median), the standard deviations judged as small, and skewness and kurtosis close to zero; or otherwise suitably transformed. Fixed effects modeled over the stride (i.e. those effects were not constant over a normalised stride) were stride percentage (0–100 %), and whether the nose angle increased or decreased. Fixed effects trial-level (effects that were constant over a normalised stride) variables were nose angle ROM (first tested as a dummy variable to check linearity versus rein tension), whether the horse-rider combination was turning (left/right or baseline not turning), passed through a corner (left/right or baseline not passing through corners), performed lateral movements (shoulder-in left/right direction, half-pass left/right direction, leg-yield left/right direction or baseline no lateral movements) or was riding in lengthening (only trot). The activity was also categorized according to position in saddle (sitting/rising to the trot). Horse level was included as a fixed effect. Left/right rein was forced in as a fixed effect. Random effects were horse-side, rider and horse and category within horse-side, the horse-side effect essentially modeling left/right reins in the random effect. The 2-way interaction between rein and stride percentage was tested. The percentage of the variation contributed by horse and rider was estimated, dividing by the sum of all sources of variation. Horse-specific models were also developed and in these the random effects were reduced to only trial within horse-side for the horse models, and fixed effects with single categories were successively removed. Models were reduced based on the type III sums of squares. The correlation structure was variance component. PROC MIXED (SAS Institute Inc., Cary, NC, 27513, USA) was used for modeling. Variables were retained if $P < 0.05$. In the graphs pair-wise comparisons were considered significant if $P < 0.0001$. Stride data were demonstrated by using the same type of modelled data for position in saddle and left/right turns.

Results

Descriptive data

The 18 horses ridden by the six riders were ridden during 1.5–19 min in walk on short reins and for a period of 4–19 min on short reins in trot. Three riders only used rising trot while trotting, while for the others the proportion of rising trot of all time trotted varied from 43 to 99 %, median 72 %. From these time slots in total 3118 walk strides and 9308 trot strides were selected after stride split. Within-horse, the number of strides per category of defined activity varied from 3 to 500. Figures 1 and 2 demonstrate a sample of raw data for walk and trot respectively, demonstrating the variation in the rein tension signal and the localisation of the stride split. Figures 3 and 4 demonstrate the distribution of the rein tension data by rein (left/right) for the variables turns, corners, position in saddle and lateral movements in walk and trot. Table 1 demonstrates descriptive statistics (rein tension and degrees) related to nose angle direction, nose angle ROM and lengthening in trot.

The models

Rein tension was deemed best as square root transformed in walk and best as logarithm transformed in trot. In walk

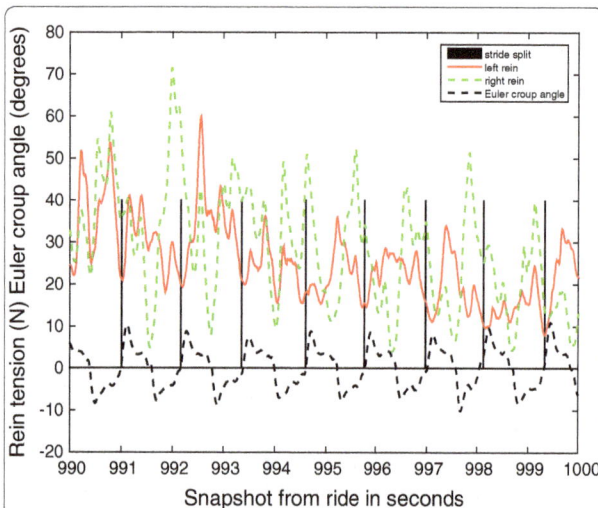

Fig. 1 Graph of raw (calibrated) rein tension data at walk (rider 8, horse 1, riding straight). *Blue bars* indicate the stride split

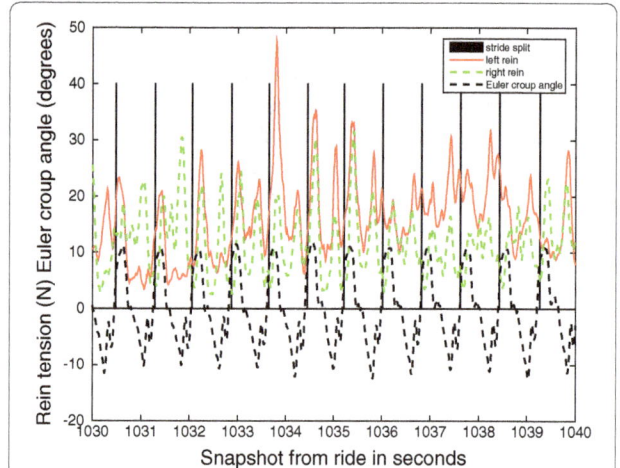

Fig. 2 Graph of raw (calibrated) *left* and *right* rein tension data at rising trot (first straight and then turning *left*, rider 6, horse 1). *Blue bars* Indicate the stride split

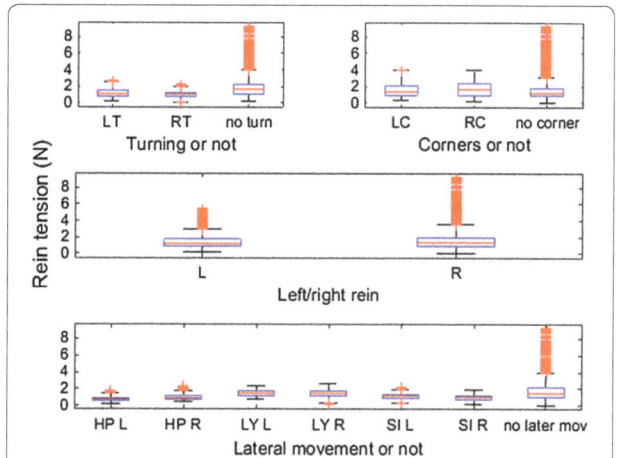

Fig. 3 Boxplot of rein tension in walk by, turns (*LT* turn to the left, *RT* turn to the right and no turn), corners (*LC* corner to the left, *RC* corner to the right and no corner), *left* (L)/*right* (R) rein and lateral movements (HP/LY/SI Left/Right = half-pass/leg-yield/shoulder-into *left* and *right* direction in averaged stride split data from 6 riders and 18 horses, n = 21,008 data points)

the transformed distribution was as follows: mean 3.68; std 0.99; median 3.57; 5th percentile 2.24; 95th percentile 5.38; 21,008 observations/208 normalised strides (101 data points per normalised stride and rein). In trot the transformed distribution was as follows: mean 2.96; std 0.68; median 2.98; 5th percentile 1.92; 95th percentile 3.95; 37,168 observations/368 normalised strides. From the final walk model 29 %/27 % of the variation originated from the rider and horse respectively and these figures in trot were 20 %/7 %.

In the walk model the remaining variables were stride percentage ($P < 0.0001$), the interaction stride percentage

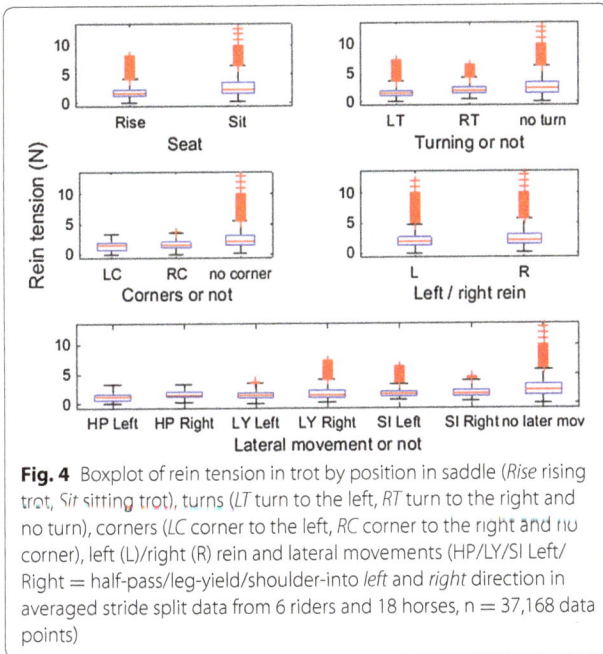

Fig. 4 Boxplot of rein tension in trot by position in saddle (*Rise* rising trot, *Sit* sitting trot), turns (*LT* turn to the left, *RT* turn to the right and no turn), corners (*LC* corner to the left, *RC* corner to the right and no corner), left (L)/right (R) rein and lateral movements (HP/LY/SI Left/Right = half-pass/leg-yield/shoulder-into *left* and *right* direction in averaged stride split data from 6 riders and 18 horses, n = 37,168 data points)

Stride percentage ($P < 0.0001$) and the interaction stride percentage and rein were significant ($P < 0.0001$). Turns ($P < 0.0001$), corners ($P = 0.0003$) and lateral movements ($P = 0.001$) were associated with higher rein tension compared to their baselines. From Table 3 we note that none of the comparisons between specific exercises to the left and right (within corners, turns and lateral movements) were significant. Rising trot was associated with a lower rein tension compared to sitting trot ($P < 0.0001$). Lengthening the stride was associated with a higher rein tension than not lengthening ($P = 0.01$). Also moving out (i.e. towards a position in front of the vertical) of the nose in trot was associated with a higher rein tension than moving inwards ($P < 0.0001$). Horse level was significant ($P = 0.01$). Rein tension decreased among horse categories in the following order: advanced horses/young horses/medium and basic horses, with several significant pairwise comparisons.

Figures 5 and 6 illustrate modelled stride curves for walk overall and for turning left and right. A significantly higher rein tension in the right rein at 50 % of the stride was recorded during rising trot compared to sitting trot (Fig. 7). Given the model, this interaction was controlled for bend orientation of the horse and direction of travel. Comparing sitting to rising trot, in rising trot significantly higher rein tension in the right rein was found at 50 % of the stride (Fig. 7). The inside rein (the rein facing the inside of an arena or a circle) has higher tension than the outside rein when the horse is turning, both left and right, with the horse on the outer fore-inner hind limb diagonal (Fig. 8).

A biphasic pattern corresponding with the two diagonal phases of the trot was found in all 18 horses, and most often for both reins (Additional file 3, Additional

and rein ($P < 0.0001$), whether the nose was moving in or out ($P < 0.0001$) and nose angle ROM ($P = 0.01$). Table 2 shows least square means that are controlled for each of the other variables in the model. The nose going out was associated with a higher value than if the nose was moving towards the horse (i.e. towards a position behind the vertical), and having a small head ROM ($<12°$ and $\geq 12° < 16°$) was associated with higher rein tension, compared to if the ROM was larger.

In the trot model nose angle ROM was not retained in the model, while all other variables remained (Table 3).

Table 1 Descriptive statistics (std- standard deviation; p5, p50, p95- 5th, 50th and 95 % percentiles) for nose direction in both walk and trot and lengthening in trot [rein tension (N)], nose angle range of motion (ROM; degrees)

Gait	Variable	Category (if relevant)	n	Rein tension (N)				
				Mean	std	p5	p50	p95
Walk	Nose direction	In	9906	15	8	5	13	29
		Out	11,102	14	8	5	13	29
Trot	Nose direction	In	16,998	23	14	7	19	50
		Out	20,170	25	16	8	21	56
	Lengthening		606	30	14	10	29	54
Gait	**Variable**	**Category (if relevant)**	**n**	**Degrees**				
				Mean	std	p5	p50	p95
Walk	Nose angle ROM		21,008	17	7	8	17	29
Trot	Nose angle ROM		37,168	8	4	4	8	16

Data on nose angle ROM are presented above and these were analysed multivariably in categorized formats (categories in walk see Table 2) and in trot; $<5°$, $\geq 5°-9°$, $\geq 9°-13°$, $\geq 13°-17°$ and $\geq 17°$

Table 2 Back-transformed least square means from the multivariable modeling of rein tension (N) in walk (data from 6 riders and 18 horses, n = 21,008 data points/208 normalised strides)

Variable	Category	LS mean	Group P value	Significant within-category			
Rein	Left	12.5	0.67				
	Right	12.8					
Nose direction	In	12.3	<0.0001	c			
	Out	12.9		c			
Nose angle ROM (degrees[a])	<12	14.1	0.01	a		b	
	≥12–16	13.8		a			b
	≥16–20	11.8					
	≥20–24	12.9					
	≥24	10.6				b	b

The model also contained the fixed effects of stride percentage (P < 0.0001) and its interaction with rein (P < 0.0001). If pair-wise comparisons within a variable were associated with P < 0.0001 this is marked with 'c', if 0.01 < P ≥ 0.0001 then 'b' and if P < 0.01 then 'a', these letters are indicated in both categories

[a] The nose angle categories contained from top to bottom: 4747; 3939; 6666; 3434 and 2222 observations. Rein tension was modelled square root transformed, hence confidence intervals could not be produced on the back-transformed scale

Table 3 Back-transformed least square means (LS means) for rein tension in trot (logarithm transformation, in N) from multivariable modeling (data from 6 riders and 18 horses, n = 37,168 data points/368 normalised strides)

Variable	Category	LS mean 95 % CI	Group P value	Significant within-category			
Turn	Turn L	37 (27, 51)	<0.0001	c			
	Turn R	29 (22, 38)			b		
	BL	36 (26, 50)		c	b		
Corner	Corner L	39 (28, 54)	0.0003	c			
	Corner R	34 (24, 48)			b		
	BL	29 (22, 38)		c	b		
Lateral movements	Leg-yield L	28 (21, 37)	0.001	a			
	Leg-yield R	33 (23, 46)			a		
	Half-pass L	33 (23, 46)					
	Half-pass R	32 (22, 45)				b	
	Shoulder-in L	40 (28, 58)					b
	Shoulder-in R	38 (27, 53)					
	BL	34 (24, 47)		a	a	b	b
Seat	Rising	28 (21, 39)	<0.0001	c			
	Sitting	40 (29, 54)		c			
Lengthening	Lengthening	28 (22, 36)	0.01	a			
	BL	40 (27, 61)		a			
Nose direction	In	32 (23, 43)	0.0001	b			
	Out	36 (26, 49)		b			
Rein	Left	33 (25, 45)	0.01	a			
	Right	34 (25, 46)		a			
Horse level	Advanced	45 (30, 68)	0.01	a	b		
	Medium	28 (20, 41)		a			
	Young horse	38 (26, 56)				b	
	Basic	26 (19, 37)			b	b	

The model also contained the fixed effects of stride percentage (P < 0.0001) and its interaction with rein (P < 0.0001). If pair-wise comparisons within a variable were associated with P < 0.0001 this is marked with 'c', if 0.01 < P ≥ 0.0001 then 'b' and if P < 0.01 then 'a', these letters are indicated in both categories. For lateral movements only comparisons to baseline (B) and within the same type of movements were performed (e.g. half-pass left (L) and right (R) were not significantly different and the comparison is therefore not shown)

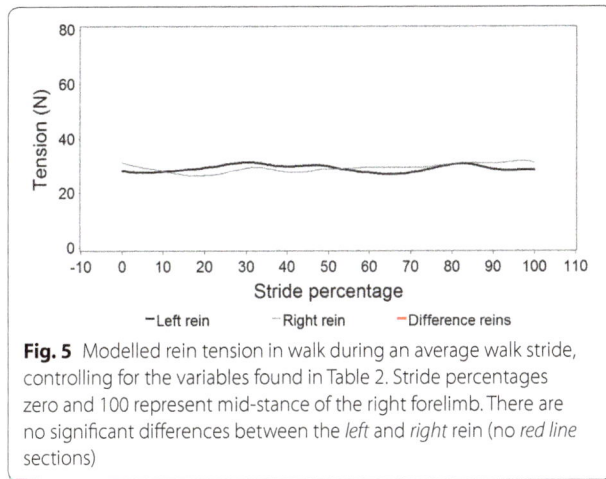

Fig. 5 Modelled rein tension in walk during an average walk stride, controlling for the variables found in Table 2. Stride percentages zero and 100 represent mid-stance of the right forelimb. There are no significant differences between the *left* and *right* rein (no *red line* sections)

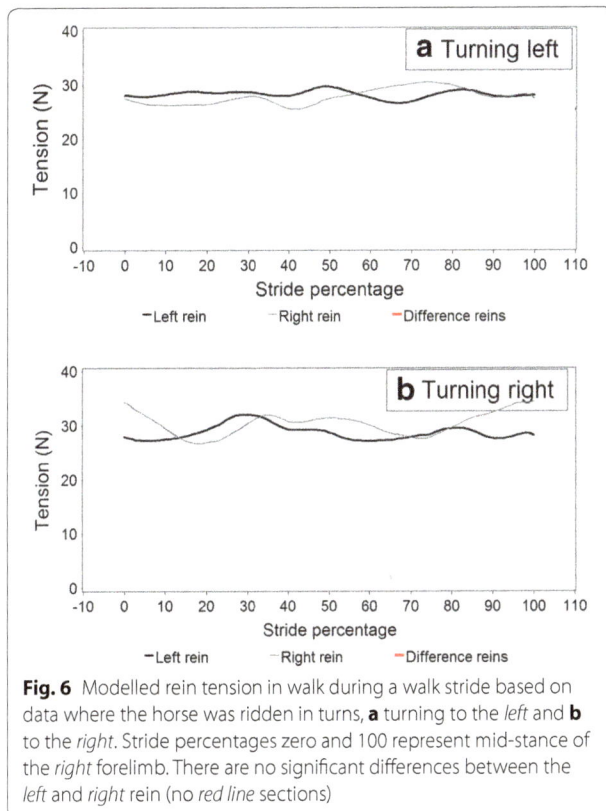

Fig. 6 Modelled rein tension in walk during a walk stride based on data where the horse was ridden in turns, **a** turning to the *left* and **b** to the *right*. Stride percentages zero and 100 represent mid-stance of the *right* forelimb. There are no significant differences between the *left* and *right* rein (no *red line* sections)

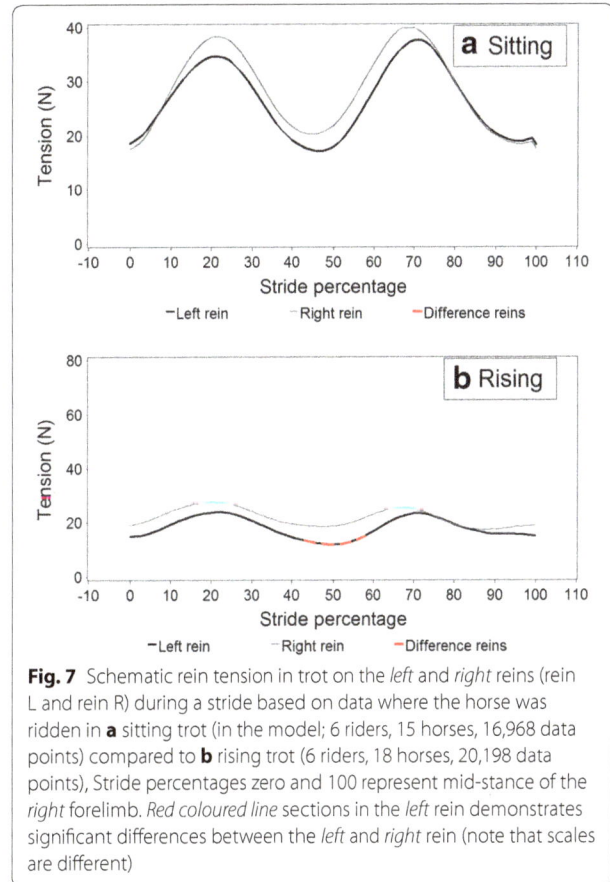

Fig. 7 Schematic rein tension in trot on the *left* and *right* reins (rein L and rein R) during a stride based on data where the horse was ridden in **a** sitting trot (in the model; 6 riders, 15 horses, 16,968 data points) compared to **b** rising trot (6 riders, 18 horses, 20,198 data points), Stride percentages zero and 100 represent mid-stance of the *right* forelimb. *Red coloured line* sections in the *left* rein demonstrates significant differences between the *left* and *right* rein (note that scales are different)

file 4). The maxima were most commonly found at around 10–30 and 60–80 % of the stride, coinciding with the suspension phase. One rider demonstrated a biphasic pattern in the walk (rider 4 in 2 horses) with the left rein showing a more pronounced biphasic pattern compared to the right rein, which showed a flatter signal and there were also statistically significant differences between the reins in this rider (statistically significant differences in walk were found in two riders and four horses). At trot, riders 4, 6 and 7 presented with significant, but

non-systematic, within-horse differences between the left and right rein. These differences were non-systematic, as they were not found in the same parts of the stride cycle; some differences were found closer to the minimum rein tension and some closer to the maximum rein tension. For example in rider 4, horse 1 in trot (Additional file 4) the left rein has significantly higher rein tension around 5–20 % of the stride and in horse 3 the right rein is associated with the highest rein tension, but around 30–50 and 75–100 % of the stride.

Discussion

Between-gait, rider and horse variation

Both rider and horse variations were substantial at walk, while rider variation was relatively higher than horse variation at trot. This may have to do with the very regular character of the latter gait, which is characterized by low ranges of motion of the equine thoracolumbar column [16]. In trot the pattern in each rider was similar but the significant differences that were seen were not consistently found in the same phases of the stride cycle. Additional files 3 and 4 also suggest within-rider differences, both related to timing and the level of rein tension.

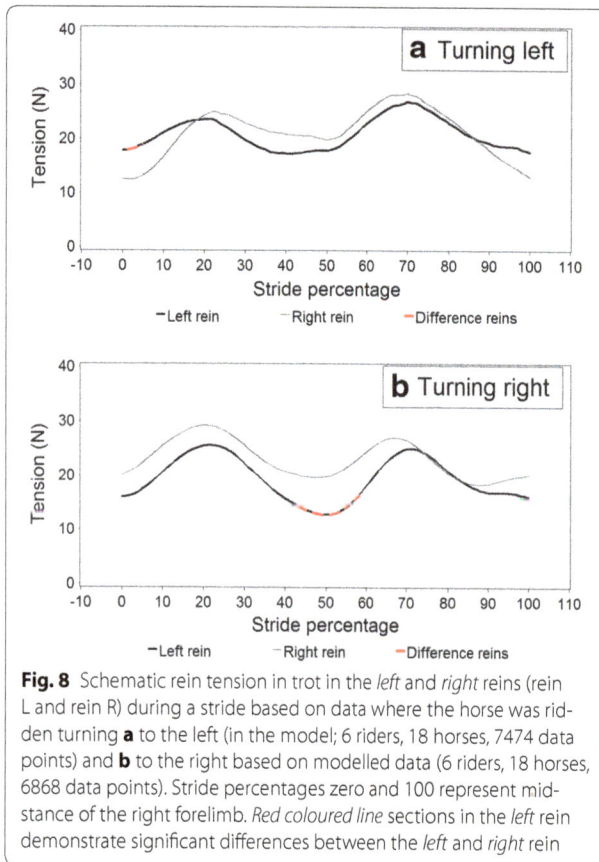

Fig. 8 Schematic rein tension in trot in the *left* and *right* reins (rein L and rein R) during a stride based on data where the horse was ridden turning **a** to the left (in the model; 6 riders, 18 horses, 7474 data points) and **b** to the right based on modelled data (6 riders, 18 horses, 6868 data points). Stride percentages zero and 100 represent midstance of the right forelimb. *Red coloured line* sections in the *left* rein demonstrate significant differences between the *left* and *right* rein

Reins, turns and position within saddle

Figure 5 and Additional file 3 demonstrate that the average pattern in walk does not have a biphasic nature. The graphs for turning left and right in walk (Fig. 6) suggest a phase shift between the reins. The data were stride split on right forelimb midstance and turning right the left rein had its maxima at 30 and 80 %, which is at left and right hindlimb midstance, while the right rein had the maxima at 95 and 35 %, at the beginning of right and left forelimb stance. At turning left, the maxima of the left rein were at 50 and 85 % (left forelimb midstance and initiation of right forelimb stance), and those of the right rein at 35 and 70 % (left and right hindlimb midstance). The between-graph differences are likely to be due to the fact that the various individual differences preclude a stable common pattern, but the reasons for the individual differences (as reflected by the large shares of rider and horse variation) are likely locomotory habits and laterality issues in the riders and the horses. Several differences between the two reins have been demonstrated [8]. The authors' interpretation of these findings was that this is most likely related to laterality in horses and riders, but this cannot be substantiated based on the current data.

In trot the right rein is associated with slightly higher rein tension, which was shown to be significant in rising trot between 42 and 58 % of the stride, i.e. during left forelimb stance. The riders actually managed to ride during equal time periods rising trot in left and right directions, and were in general rising to the 'recommended' diagonal, namely rising on the inside forelimb, outside hindlimb [17]. At the trot, when the horses were turning left and right respectively and when the horses were using the outer fore- inner hindlimb diagonal the inner rein was acting more intensively. This was likely because the rider strived at taking the turn with the longitudinal axis of the horse in a regularly bent position. It is possible that riders were applying greater tension on the inner rein in order to achieve slight lateral bending of the horses' head in the direction of the turn, following standard recommendations from riding manuals [17]. Additionally, turns and corners to the right were associated with lower rein tension than turns and corners to the left and the general baseline (Table 3), which is likely a function of rider- and or horse laterality. Ideally, the rider should be able to manage both the rider's laterality and that of the horse to the degree that right and left corners would be associated with the same rein tension levels. Previous research has demonstrated that this may not always be the case [8]. Left rein tension has been found to be more stable and generally higher than the tension in the right rein when subjects simulated halts on a model horse. This was interpreted as being in agreement with the fact that the left hand/rein acts more based on *postural input*, while the actions and reactions of the right hand, featuring both high and low tension spikes, is more dependent on *visual input* [19].

The results from the multivariable models

At walk, in general nose angle ROM had lower values when rein tension was higher (Table 2). Rein tension was likely lower when horses were walked in a less restrained (restraining being normally effectuated by being held back by the rider or moving slowly) way, i.e. principally at higher speed and with a greater pendulum movement of the head. Nose angle ROM was not significant in trot, which is possibly caused by the more limited ROM of the head in this gait that is, as alluded to earlier, characterized by a low range of motion of all parts of the axial skeleton [16], including the cervical part and thus the head that is attached to this.

Rein tension was higher when the nose was moving forwards or 'out' (moving towards a position in front of the vertical) in relation to the body in both gaits (in both gaits this is from 0 to 25 and 50 to 75 % of the stride, data not shown). Either the rider was not 'following' as well as they intended (because of the motion of the head of the horse the riders need to adjust hand-position in every stride), or the riders were actively trying to interact, either trying to bring the horse's head closer to the chest or trying to make it slow down and/or increase collection. In that latter case the cue might not have been working well, as the tension was found to be significantly higher when the nose was moving forwards. While riding in trot, the maximal distance from the riders hand to the mouth of the horse is found at midstance [10], which perhaps indicates that 'following' the horse's movement by the rider is difficult. Terada et al. [18] investigated the timing of activity of rider muscles and found several muscles that were activated during early stance, including the *m. biceps brachii* and the middle deltoid muscle. This may demonstrate a 'taking' mechanism that may either be an active choice, that is the rider is aware of doing it and can choose to perform it or not, or perhaps a more reflex-based activity that may be a posturally elicited mechanism that the rider is more unaware of. The various lateral movements all led to rein tensions differing from baselines. Magnitude and direction of these changes were variable, however, and require additional work to be fully understood. As found previously, sitting trot and lengthening were associated with higher rein tension than their counterparts, rising and no lengthening. The reason is likely that more difficult exercises are performed when sitting/lengthening. Sitting trot and riding a lengthened stride likely means that the rider's body is experiencing a more violent acceleration/deceleration pattern so the increased tension may be an unconscious (or semi-automated) postural anti acceleration response. With regard to horse level advanced and young horses were ridden with higher rein tension, which was almost double compared to basic horses. This may be because both of these groups are asked to perform either absolutely or relatively (given the level of training) difficult and demanding exercises.

Limitations of the study

Since there was a problem with the synchronization of the signals form horse's croup and head in two riders/six horses of the original study population [13], only six riders and 18 horses were included in the data analysis. Despite the set-up with one recording person and riding 'as usual' it is possible that riders were somewhat less relaxed compared to a typical training day, which may have influenced the results. Also, no strides featuring collection could be selected from the walk and trot data [20]. This was likely to be because the acceleration signals became more irregular during collection, precluding optimal stride split from the acceleration signal alone. Furthermore, the discussion on laterality in riders

or horses was not based on measurements, but solely on subjective declarations by the riders.

Conclusions

The gait the horse is ridden in has a clear influence on the rein tension pattern. Biphasic patterns were found mainly in trot. The highest rein tension was found in the suspension phase in trot, and the lowest in the stance phase. In walk, the highest rein tension was found at hindlimb stance. Studies of rein tension should hence take both the gait and the stride cycle phase into account. Further, there was substantial between-rider variation in walk and trot and between-horse variation in walk. These differences are most likely due to the much lower range of motion of the thoracic and lumbar equine vertebral column in trot compared to in walk. Future studies on rein tension should include analyses of detailed temporal relationships with horse kinematics, rider kinematics including the seat (taking into account the rider's posture and relative positioning of all body parts), and of the behavior of the horse.

Additional files

Additional file 1. The rein tension meter used in the study. Earlier published in Eisersiö M, Roepstorff L, Rhodin M, Egenvall A. Rein tension in eight professional riders during regular training sessions. JVB: Clinical applications and research. 2015;10:419-426.

Additional file 2. The graph shows an example where one meter that was tested with increasing tension up to 500 N (several cycles). The curve is almost linear, though slightly upward bent (both offset and this bend are corrected for in the calibration). The hysteresis effect was maximally 8 N, measured as the vertical distance between the lines.

Additional file 3. Rein tension during the stride cycle at the walk for the left (black) and right (grey) rein per horse. Each row indicates one rider. Significant differences (P < 0.0001) between the left and right rein are shown as broken red lines in the inside rein. Stride percentages zero and 100 represent mid-stance of the right forelimb.

Additional file 4. Rein tension during the stride cycle at the trot for the left (black) and right (grey) rein per horse. Each row indicates one rider. Significant differences (P < 0.0001) between the left and right rein are shown as broken red lines in the inside rein. Stride percentages zero and 100 represent mid-stance of the right forelimb.

Authors' contributions
AE initiated the study, and participated in design, coordination, data analysis and performed the statistical analysis and drafted the manuscript. LR participated in study design. ME participated in study design, took primary responsibility for the coordination and participated in the data analysis. MR participated in study design and helped draft the manuscript. RvW helped draft the manuscript. All authors read and approved the final manuscript.

Author details
[1] Department of Clinical Sciences, Faculty of Veterinary Medicine and Animal Husbandry, Swedish University of Agricultural Sciences, Box 7054, 750 07 Uppsala, Sweden. [2] Unit of Equine Studies, Department of Anatomy, Physiology and Biochemistry, Faculty of Veterinary Medicine and Animal Husbandry, Swedish University of Agricultural Sciences, Box 7046, 750 07 Uppsala,

Sweden. [3] Department of Equine Sciences, Faculty of Veterinary Medicine, Utrecht University, Yalelaan 114, 3584 CM Utrecht, The Netherlands.

Acknowledgements
The study was funded by The Swedish Research Council Formas. We thank the riders for their contributions.

Competing interests
The authors declare that they have no competing interests.

References
1. Egenvall A, Tranquille CA, Lönnell AC, Bitschnau C, Oomen A, Hernlund E, Montavon S, Franko MA, Murray RC, Weishaupt MA, van Weeren R, Roepstorff L. Days-lost to training and competition in relation to workload in 263 elite show-jumping horses in four European countries. Prev Vet Med. 2013;112:387–400.
2. Murray RC, Walters JM, Snart H, Dyson SJ, Parkin TDH. Identification of risk factors for lameness in dressage horses. Vet J. 2010;184:27–36.
3. Penell JC, Egenvall A, Bonnett BN, Olson P, Pringle J. Specific causes of morbidity among Swedish horses insured for veterinary care between 1997 and 2000. Vet Rec. 2005;57:470–7.
4. McGreevy PD. The advent of equitation science. Vet J. 2007;174:492–500.
5. von König Borstel U, Glissman C. Alternative to conventional evaluation of rideability in horse performance test: suitability of rein tension and behavioural parameters. PLoS One. 2014;9:1–9.
6. Egenvall A, Eisersiö M, Rhodin M, van Weeren R, Roepstorff L. Rein tension during canter. Comp Exerc Physiol. 2015;11:107–17.
7. Warren-Smith AK, Curtis RA, Greetham L, McGreevy PD. Rein contact between horse and handler during specific equitation movements. Appl Anim Beh Sci. 2007;108:157–69.
8. Kuhnke S, Dumbell L, Gauly M, Johnson JL, McDonald K, von Borstel UK. A comparison of rein tension of the rider's dominant and non-dominant hand and the influence of the horse's laterality. Comp Exerc Physiol. 2010;7:57–63.
9. Clayton HM, Larson B, Kaiser LJ, Lavagnino M. Length and elasticity of side reins affect rein tension at trot. Vet J. 2011;188:291–4.
10. Eisersiö M, Roepstorff L, Weishaupt MA, Egenvall A. Movements of the horse's mouth in relation to the horse-rider kinematic variables. Vet J. 2013;198(Suppl 1):e33–8.
11. Byström A, Rhodin M, von Peinen K, Weishaupt MA, Roepstorff L. Kinematics of saddle and rider in high-level dressage horses performing collected walk on a treadmill. Equine Vet J. 2010;42:340–5.
12. Byström A, Rhodin M, Peinen K, Weishaupt MA, Roepstorff L. Basic kinematics of the saddle and rider in high-level dressage horses trotting on a treadmill. Equine Vet J. 2009;41:280–4.
13. Eisersiö M, Roepstorff L, Rhodin M, Egenvall A. A snapshot of the training schedule for 8 professional riders riding dressage. Comp Exerc Physiol. 2015;11:35–46.
14. Eisersiö M. How to build a rein tension meter. Degree project in Biology, Swedish University of Agricultural Science, 2013. http://stud.epsilon.slu.se. Accessed 4 July 2015.
15. Buchner HNF, Savelberg HHCM, Schamhardt HC, Barneveld A. Head and trunk movement adaptations in horses with experimentally induced fore- or hindlimb lameness. Equine Vet J. 1996;28:71–6.
16. Faber MJ, Johnston C, Schamhardt HC, van Weeren PR, Roepstorff L, Barneveld A. Basic three-dimensional kinematics of the vertebral column of horses trotting on a treadmill. Am J Vet Res. 2001;62:757–64.
17. Anonymous. The principles of riding: the official instruction handbook of the German National Equestrian Federation. Shrewsbury: Kenilworth Press; 1997.
18. Terada K, Mullineaux DR, Lanovaz J, Kato K, Clayton HM. Electromyographic analysis of the rider's muscles at trot. Comp Exerc Physiol. 2004;1:193–8.
19. Hawson LA, Salvin HE, McLean AN, McGreevy PD. Riders' application of rein tension for walk-to-halt transitions on a model horse. J Vet Behav. 2015;9:164–8.
20. Eisersiö M, Roepstorff L, Rhodin M, Egenvall A. Rein tension in eight professional riders during regular training sessions. JVB Clin Appl Res. 2015;10:419–26.

2

Catestatin and vasostatin concentrations in healthy dogs

Thanikul Srithunyarat[1,2]* , Ragnvi Hagman[1], Odd V. Höglund[1], Ulf Olsson[3], Mats Stridsberg[4], Supranee Jitpean[2], Anne-Sofie Lagerstedt[1] and Ann Pettersson[1]

Abstract

Background: The neuroendocrine glycoprotein chromogranin A is a useful biomarker in humans for neuroendocrine tumors and stress. Chromogranin A can be measured in both blood and saliva. The objective of this study was to investigate concentrations of and correlation between the chromogranin A epitopes catestatin and vasostatin in healthy dogs accustomed to the sample collection procedures. Blood and saliva samples were collected from 10 research Beagle dogs twice daily for 5 consecutive days, and from 33 privately-owned blood donor dogs in association with 50 different blood donation occasions. All dogs were familiar with sample collection procedures. During each sampling, stress behavior was scored by the same observer using a visual analog scale (VAS) and serum cortisol concentrations. Catestatin and vasostatin were analyzed using radioimmunoassays for dogs.

Results: The dogs showed minimal stress behavior during both saliva sampling and blood sampling as monitored by VAS scores and serum cortisol concentrations. Few and insufficient saliva volumes were obtained and therefore only catestatin could be analyzed. Catestatin concentrations differed significantly and did not correlate significantly with vasostatin concentrations ($P < 0.0001$). Age, gender, breed, and time of sample collection did not significantly affect concentrations of plasma catestatin, vasostatin, and saliva catestatin.

Conclusions: The normal ranges of plasma catestatin (0.53–0.98 nmol/l), vasostatin (0.11–1.30 nmol/l), and saliva catestatin (0.31–1.03 nmol/l) concentrations in healthy dogs accustomed to the sampling procedures were determined. Separate interpretation of the different chromogranin A epitopes from either saliva or plasma is recommended.

Keywords: Catestatin, Chromogranin A, Healthy dogs, Stress behavior visual analog scale, Vasostatin

Background

Chromogranin A (CgA) is a biomarker that is widely used in human medicine, but few studies of CgA have been reported in dogs [1–6]. Chromogranin A, an acidic glycoprotein that belongs to the Granin family, is stored in chromaffin granules and coreleased with catecholamines and neuroendocrine hormones from the adrenal medulla and sympathetic nerve endings when the sympathoadrenal-medullary system is activated [7, 8]. An active secretion of CgA into saliva in the submandibular gland has been found in humans [9], horses, and rats [10, 11]. Chromogranin A can be measured in saliva and blood in humans, pigs, cows, and dogs [4, 12–15]. Several bioactive peptides are derived from CgA degradation, including vasostatin, pancreastatin, catestatin, and serpinin [16–33]. These CgA bioactive peptides play different critical roles in the endocrine, cardiovascular, neurologic, and immune systems [21, 31, 34–36].

Chromogranin A is a reliable biomarker for diagnosing and monitoring treatment outcome and prognosis in humans suffering from neuroendocrine tumors [8, 37–39]. Chromogranin A has detected in the myocardium in several species and has multiple roles in cardiovascular homeostasis [40–42]. Chromogranin A and its derived peptides have shown promise as biomarkers for cardiovascular diseases such as hypertension, heart failure, myocardial infarction, and coronary syndromes [43–47]. Moreover, saliva CgA has been shown to be a sensitive biomarker for

*Correspondence: thanikul.srithunyarat@slu.se
[1] Department of Clinical Sciences, Swedish University of Agricultural Sciences, Box 7504, 75007 Uppsala, Sweden
Full list of author information is available at the end of the article

stress in humans and pigs [12, 14, 48–53]. Some evidence suggests that CgA could be useful as a biomarker for neuroendocrine tumors and stress also in dogs [1, 2].

In humans, saliva sampling is preferable to blood sampling for monitoring stress because the technique is noninvasive [54, 55] and humans can be informed of the procedure and deliver saliva samples by voluntary spitting into a container. To obtain spontaneous saliva samples in dogs, however, collection swabs must be intraorally placed. Although noninvasive, the saliva sample collection procedure itself may cause a stress reaction in dogs [56, 57]. To date, the stress response to saliva sampling in comparison with the stress response to blood sampling has not been evaluated in dogs. Stress evaluation can be performed by subjective and objective measurements, for example, scoring stress behavior using visual analog scale (VAS) scoring and measuring cortisol concentrations [58, 59].

Even though there are interspecies differences in CgA amino acid sequences, CgA can be measured in dogs [4]. A study on cross-reactivity between humans and dogs against different regions of the CgA molecule showed that CgA 17–38 (vasostatin) and CgA 361–372 (catestatin) could be measured using competitive radioimmunoassay (RIA) in dogs, whereas intact CgA could not [4]. Catestatin (CST) and vasostatin (VS), both CgA derived peptides, are bioactive. CST modulates catecholamine secretion (negative feedback) and has antihypertensive, antimicrobial, and cardiosuppressive effects [21, 22, 36, 60–63]. VS regulates plasma calcium, influences vasodilation, and has antimicrobial, and cardiosuppressive effects [17, 35, 42, 64–66]. Fundamental information concerning concentrations of CST and VS in healthy dogs of various breeds and gender that are accustomed to the sampling procedures is, however, lacking. The aims of this study were to investigate and compare concentrations of CST and VS in healthy dogs familiar with the collection procedures. In addition, we hypothesized that if CST and VS have similar halflives then the concentrations should not differ significantly.

Methods

Study design and ethical approval

This study was designed as a prospective clinical study in two parts; part one included destination bred research dogs, and part two included privately owned dogs admitted for routine blood donation. The study was approved by the Uppsala Ethical Committee (C301/12) and all dog owners were informed and gave their consent prior to participation, in accordance with Swedish legislation.

Part one: research dogs

Three male and seven female research Beagle dogs (4–10 years old) were included. All dogs were determined as healthy by complete physical examination including mental status, general attitude, appetite, mucus membrane appearance, capillary refill time, rectal temperature, body weight, body condition score, hydration status, auscultation of heart and respiratory rate and sounds, abdominal palpation, and musculoskeletal system palpation. Dogs were familiar with being handled and routinely participated in practical teaching in the veterinary education program and were housed at the Research Animal Facility, Department of Clinical Sciences, Swedish University of Agricultural Sciences (SLU), Uppsala, Sweden.

Sampling of saliva and blood

Saliva and blood samples were collected twice daily for 5 consecutive days at the following times: (A) 6:30–7:30 am and (B) 1:00–2:00 pm, this time points were selected based on the results from previous pilot study [67, 68]. Saliva samples were collected using a swab size 10×30 mm (SalivaBio, Salimetrics, PA, USA) placed in the oral cavity for 1 min. The swab was then transferred into a 4.5-ml polypropylene cryotube (CryoPure Tubes, Sarstedt, Nümbrecht, Germany) and centrifuged at 3000 rpm (1401 g) for 15 min. The saliva deposited was stored at −70 °C until analysis of all samples.

Two ml of blood was collected from the distal cephalic vein using butterfly needles (BD Vacutainer, Becton-Dickson, Plymouth, United Kingdom) into lithium heparin tubes and clot activator tubes (Vacuette, Greiner Bio-One, Kremsmünster, Austria) and centrifuged at 3300 rpm (1695 g) for 5 min. The obtained heparinized plasma samples were freeze stored in cryotubes (Low Temperature Freezer Vials, VWR, Stockholm, Sweden) at −70 °C until analysis of all samples within a maximum of 11 months storage time. The saliva sampling was performed within 5 min prior to blood sampling.

Visual analog scale (VAS)

Visual analog scale scoring was performed during each saliva and plasma sampling occasion to score the subjective stress behavior on a plain 100-mm line. The pre-established subjective criteria used in this study to determine stress behaviors during saliva and blood sampling are given in Table 1 [69]. All sampling procedures were performed by the same two veterinarians and the sampling stress behavior VAS scores determined by one observer (TS).

Part two: blood donor dogs and donation routines

In total, thirty-three privately-owned dogs, twenty-four males and nine females, aged from one to eight years, of fourteen different breeds (Boxer, Bernese Mountain Dog, Collie, Dalmatian, Flat Coated Retriever, German Shepherd Dog, Golden Retriever, Great Dane, Greyhound,

Table 1 Pre-established subjective criteria used to determine stress behaviors using visual analog scale

Stress intensity	No stress	Mild stress	Moderate stress	Severe stress
A. Criteria used for saliva sampling				
Criteria		Turns head away Spits Lifts paw Moves away	Turns head away Spits Lifts paw Moves away Avoids sampling Lifts lip Shakes Raises hair Growls	Turns head away Spits Lifts paw Moves away Avoids sampling Lifts lip Shakes Raises hair Growls Not able to sample Not able to touch Bites Attacks
B. Criteria used for blood sampling				
Criteria		Withdraws leg Moves away	Withdraws leg Moves away Avoids sampling Lifts lip Shakes Raises hair Growls	Withdraws leg Moves away Avoids sampling Lifts lip Shakes Raises hair Growls Not able to sample Not able to touch Bites Attacks

This stress behavior criteria are modified from Norling et al. [69]

Labrador Retriever, Leonberger, Shorthaired Pointer, White Shepherd, and Mixed Breed), were included in the study. All dogs that routinely donated blood at the University Animal Hospital (UDS), SLU, Uppsala, Sweden during April 2014, and from September to February 2015 were included. All dogs underwent a complete physical examination (as used for the research dogs) and blood samples were obtained from the distal cephalic vein and evaluated for health control purposes. Hematology and biochemistry (creatinine, alanine aminotransferase (ALT), alkaline phosphatase (ALP), total protein, and albumin) were measured using in-house equipment (IDEXX ProCyte Dx and IDEXX Catalyst Dx, IDEXX Laboratories, Maine, USA). In all dogs, positive and negative DEA 1.1 blood type (Quick Vet, Scandinavian Micro Biodevices ApS, Farum, Denmark) and presence of vector borne diseases including *Anaplasma phagocytophilum, Anaplasma platys, Borrelia burgdorferi, Ehrlichia canis, Ehrlichia ewingii, and Dirofilaria immitis* (Snap 4DX tests, IDEXX Laboratories, Maine, USA) were determined. Dogs with antibodies against *Anaplasma phagocytophilum, Anaplasma platys, Borrelia burgdorferi, Ehrlichia canis, and Ehrlichia ewingii* were considered healthy if no signs of active infection was present when examined, whereas dogs with positive antigens of *Dirofilaria immitis* were considered infected. Only healthy dogs were allowed to donate blood, and

were enrolled for routine donation every 3–4 months. All dogs included in the present study were familiar with the sampling procedures and needed no sedation during collection. Dog owners were present throughout procedures.

Sampling of saliva and blood
Heparinized plasma and serum samples remaining after the routine hematology and biochemistry analysis were used for the study. In total, seventeen dogs donated blood on one occasion whereas fifteen donated twice and one donated three times on different occasions (more than 3 months interval) resulting in fifty separate samplings. All blood samples were collected by the same two certified veterinary nurses. Saliva sampling was performed by TS using the same criteria as in research dogs. In contrast to the sampling in research dogs, for practical reasons, blood and saliva sampling was performed on variable times between 8:00 am–2:00 pm, and the order in which the samples were collected was randomized with an interval between saliva and blood sampling of less than 10 min. All samples were handled and stored in the same manner as described for research dogs.

Visual analog scale (VAS)
Visual analog scale scoring was performed by TS using the same criteria as in research dogs.

Analysis of catestatin and vasostatin

Competitive radioimmunoassay (RIA) was used for measuring CST and VS. All heparinized plasma samples were analyzed in duplicates at the Clinical Chemistry Laboratory, Uppsala University Hospital, Uppsala, Sweden as previously described [4, 70]. This method has been developed for both tissue and circulation and used for measuring CgA in humans. The detection limit is 0.01 nmol/l for plasma CST and VS and 0.04 nmol/l for saliva CST and the total coefficient of variance (CV) was <10%. The overall CV in the present study was <10%. For each analysis, 300 µl saliva and 100 µl plasma were required. The saliva sample volume obtained was insufficient for analysis of saliva VS.

Cortisol analysis

Serum samples were analyzed for cortisol concentrations in duplicate using a solid-phase competitive chemiluminescent enzyme immunoassay (Immulite 2000, Siemens, Erlangen, Germany) at Clinical Chemistry Laboratory, UDS. The intraassay CV was <5%.

Statistical analysis

In all analysis of CST and VS, diagnostic plots were used to assess normality and homoscedasticity. Because the distributions of residuals for CST and VS data appeared skewed, these data were log transformed (natural log) prior to analysis. After transformation, no apparent deviations from normality and homoscedasticity could be detected.

In all analysis, post hoc comparisons of least squares means were adjusted for multiplicity using Tukey's method. Results were considered significant when $P < 0.05$. Most analysis were made using the mixed procedure of the SAS package 2014, but other procedures for basic statistics, Proc Univariate, Proc Corr and Proq Freq, were also used. Normal range was calculated using percentile 2.5–97.5 of log transformed data and back-transformed to the original scale.

Research dog data

Because several measurements were made in each dog, mixed linear models [71, 72] were used for the analysis. The fixed part of the models included the variables "category" with three levels (plasma CST, plasma VS, and saliva CST); day (1–5); gender (male or female); time of day (am or pm), and interactions between these factors. The random part of the model included dog, dog * day and dog * category.

The relations between the three measurements (categories) were modeled by allowing the R-side correlations among them to be an unstructured correlation matrix [71, 73]. This corresponds to using multivariate analysis

of variance (MANOVA) model, but still allows for inclusion of random effects in the model.

Blood donor dog data

For the blood donor dog data, the same categories as for the research dog data were used. Because the same dog could have data for one, two or three donation occasions, mixed models (*ibid*) were also used for these data.

Several models were tried. The fixed part of the models included category as above. Moreover, different background variables for the dogs (gender, age, and breed) and site (plasma and saliva) were tested. The R-side correlations were modeled as for the research dogs. Random effects were dog, dog * site and dog * site * variable.

Comparisons between blood donor dogs and research dogs

The two data sets were collected in different ways. To allow comparisons between the groups, mean values were calculated, for all variables, for each dog. This led to a simple data set where comparisons between groups could be made using one-way ANOVA, or, equivalently, using two-sample t tests. These data sets were also used for calculating correlations between different variables.

Results

The mean ± SD age and body weight was 7.5 ± 2.6 years and 14.3 ± 1.2 kg in research dogs and 3.7 ± 2.0 years and 36.2 ± 9.8 kg in blood donor dogs. From the 50 blood donation occasions, 48 plasma and 40 saliva samples were obtained. Due to insufficient volumes remaining in some cases, plasma CST was analyzed in 39 of the 48 plasma samples, plasma VS in 44 of the 48 plasma samples and saliva CST in 40 of the 40 saliva samples. In the research dogs, plasma CST, plasma VS, and saliva CST could be analyzed in all samples collected (100). Mean ± SD values of serum cortisol were 39.9 ± 6.1 nmol/l in research dogs and 65.8 ± 28.2 nmol/l in blood donor dogs. Mean ± SD values of plasma CST, plasma VS, saliva CST, blood and saliva sampling stress behavior VAS scores from research and blood donor dogs are illustrated in Table 2. No significant differences were found between research and blood donor dogs. The normal ranges of plasma CST, plasma VS, and saliva CST in this study was 0.53–0.98, 0.11–1.30, and 0.31–1.03 nmol/l, respectively.

Plasma CST, plasma VS, and saliva CST concentrations did not correlate significantly in any of the groups of dogs. In research dogs, plasma VS concentrations differed significantly from plasma and saliva CST concentrations ($P < 0.002$). In blood donor dogs, plasma CST, VS, and saliva CST differed significantly ($P < 0.0001$). Plasma CST, plasma VS, and saliva CST concentrations did not differ significantly between different collection times in research dogs. Plasma and saliva CST

Table 2 Mean ± SD of plasma catestatin, vasostatin, and saliva catestatin and sampling stress behavior score

Parameters	Research dogs (n = 10)	Blood donor dogs (n = 33)
Plasma catestatin (nmol/l)	0.81 ± 0.08[a]	0.76 ± 0.10[a]
Plasma vasostatin (nmol/l)	0.57 ± 0.55[b]	0.44 ± 0.39[b]
Saliva catestatin (nmol/l)	0.83 ± 0.12[a]	0.64 ± 0.21[c]
Blood sampling stress behavior VAS score (mm)	8.9 ± 10.5[a]	19.1 ± 17.3[a]
Saliva sampling stress behavior VAS score (mm)	11.1 ± 7.8[a]	21.2 ± 16.7[a]

In research dogs, plasma vasostatin concentrations differed significantly from plasma and saliva catestatin concentrations. In blood donor dogs, plasma catestatin, vasostatin, and saliva catestatin differed significantly. Blood and saliva sampling stress behavior VAS scores did not differ significantly between both dog groups

[a,b,c] Different letters within each column of concentration and stress behavior VAS score indicate significant differences using Tukey's method adjustment ($P < 0.05$)

concentrations did not differ significantly when compared between different days of collection. Plasma CST, plasma VS, and saliva CST concentrations did not differ significantly between ages, genders, and breeds in both dog groups. Stress behavior VAS scores were low in all dogs and did not differ between sampling methods, ages, genders, breeds, collection time or day.

In the blood donor dogs, all hematology and blood chemistry results were deemed acceptable for blood donation. Nineteen dogs were positive for DEA 1.1 and 14 negative for DEA 1.1. Plasma and saliva CST and VS did not differ significantly between blood groups. None of the blood donor dogs had positive antigens of *Dirofilaria immitis*. Six dogs had antibodies against *Borrelia burgdorferi* without clinical signs of disease. Plasma CST, VS, and saliva CST concentrations did not differ significantly between positive and negative *B. burgdorferi*.

Discussion

This is the first study in dogs that investigates concentrations of and correlations between CST and VS in healthy dogs familiarized with a sample collection procedure. The concentration values and ranges reported here can be used as reference ranges for plasma CST, plasma VS, and saliva CST concentrations in healthy dogs when analyzed by RIA. Our findings will be useful in future studies on the role and possibilities of using CST and VS as biomarkers in dogs. In a previous study of dogs with pyometra, using the same RIA as in the current study, the reported serum CST concentrations in healthy control dogs were higher than reported here [5]. This difference between studies could be due to different familiarity to the handling techniques, and sample storage time. Although CgA has been reported to be heat stable and the concentrations are stable through freeze and thaw cycle in humans and pigs [15, 74, 75], studies on CST and VS in dogs are lacking. In contrast to the previous study, the dogs included in our study were all well accustomed to the sampling procedures prior to sample collection, and showed minimal stress behaviors

as monitored by stress behavior VAS scoring and serum cortisol concentrations [76].

Although both CST and VS are derived from CgA, the concentrations of plasma CST and VS in this study reflect both the intact CgA molecule and the two respective degradation derived peptides. The significant differences in concentrations seen in the present study may be because the peptides have different functions and clearance rates. The CgA derived peptides might also be secreted differently into saliva and blood [13] which could contribute to our finding that CST concentrations were different in saliva and plasma in the blood donor dogs. Nevertheless, plasma CST, plasma VS, and saliva CST concentrations did not correlate significantly in both dog groups. The concentrations of plasma CST, plasma VS, and saliva CST also did not vary by age, gender, or breed in either group of dogs. The results of the present study show that it is crucial to evaluate different CgA peptides individually, and with regard to whether measurements were made in plasma or saliva because otherwise the results are not comparable.

Saliva sampling is preferable in humans because it is less invasive than blood sampling [54, 55]. In dogs, however, stress behaviors during saliva and blood sampling have not previously been evaluated and prolonged sampling time could induce stress [56, 57]. All dogs, in the present study were well accustomed to the sampling procedures and exhibit minimal stress levels as shown by stress behavior VAS scores and serum cortisol concentrations. However, in order to avoid inducing stress behavior we limited the time for saliva sampling to 60 s. We also chose not to pharmacologically induce saliva secretion because this may affect the secretion of neuroendocrine peptides. In the present study, there was no significant difference in the dogs' acceptance of blood or saliva sampling as monitored by the stress behavior VAS. Our findings indicate that saliva sampling is unpredictable and that for our research purposes, blood sampling is a better choice.

In human studies, saliva CgA has been used for evaluating stress [12, 49–51]. In humans and pigs, active CgA secretion from the mandibular salivary gland has been found [9, 12, 14], however, little is known about CgA secretion in dogs. If similar active secretion also occurs in dogs, analysis of CST or VS in saliva may still be useful for monitoring stress levels. However, the sampling techniques need to be improved to ensure sufficient sample volumes are obtained without undue stress or pharmacological intervention.

Ten research Beagle dogs were included in the study to investigate whether concentrations of CST and VS varied over time in the same individual. In a previous pilot study, using the same RIA, five research Beagle dogs were sampled four times daily between 6:30 am and 3:00 pm, saliva CST was increased in samples collected between 6:30 and 8:00 am [67, 68]. In addition, CgA in saliva has been found to be increased in early morning samples (7:00 am) in humans [13, 77, 78]. In our study, there was no significant difference in the concentrations of plasma CST, VS and saliva CST between time of day, which is in agreement with a previous study that used an ELISA for human CgA 344–374 amino acid sequence for saliva samples in dogs [3]. On the other hand, a circadian variation in CgA has been found in plasma and saliva in humans [13, 79]. However, as stated previously comparisons between different species and studies on different peptides should be made with caution.

The bioactive peptides of CgA have shown promise as prognostic and diagnostic biomarkers for neuroendocrine tumors, cardiac disease, burn trauma and stress in humans [12, 35, 80–82]. The main focus of this study was to investigate the concentrations of and correlation between CST and VS in healthy dogs familiar with the collection procedures. Further studies are warranted to investigate whether CST and VS can be used as biomarkers for neuroendocrine tumors, cardiovascular diseases, and stress in dogs.

Conclusions

Concentrations of plasma CST (0.53–0.98 nmol/l), plasma VS (0.11–1.30 nmol/l), and saliva CST (0.31–1.03 nmol/l) in healthy dogs accustomed to the sampling procedures were determined. The concentrations of plasma CST, plasma VS, and saliva CST significantly differed and were unaffected by age, gender, breed, and time of sampling. No significant correlation between plasma CST and VS, as well as saliva CST could be found indicating that separate interpretation of the different CgA epitopes from either saliva or plasma is mandatory.

Abbreviations

CgA: chromogranin A; CST: catestatin; ELISA: enzyme-linked immunosorbent assay; RIA: radioimmunoassay; RPM: revolutions per minute; VS: vasostatin; VAS: visual analog scale.

Authors' contributions

TS and AP designed the study. TS and SJ collected the samples. AP, RH, OVH, and MS gave input on the study design and data collections. MS performed CgA analyses and UO performed and drafted statistical analyses. The manuscript was drafted by TS and revised with assistance of AP, RH, OVH, MS, UO, ASL, and SJ. All authors read and approved the final manuscript.

Author details

[1] Department of Clinical Sciences, Swedish University of Agricultural Sciences, Box 7504, 75007 Uppsala, Sweden. [2] Department of Surgery and Theriogenology, Faculty of Veterinary Medicine, Khon Kaen University, Khon Kaen 40002, Thailand. [3] Unit of Applied Statistics and Mathematics, Swedish University of Agricultural Sciences, Box 7032, 75007 Uppsala, Sweden. [4] Department of Medical Sciences, Uppsala University, 75185 Uppsala, Sweden.

Acknowledgements

The authors would like to thank the Clinical Pathology Laboratory, Department of Clinical Sciences, UDS, SLU, for allowing the use of laboratory equipment. Annika Rikberg and Emma Hörnebro are acknowledged for their skillful assistance, Louise Pettersson, Britta Liby, and Kristoffer Dreimanis kindly helped us to collect blood donor dog samples.

Competing interests

The authors declare that they have no competing interests.

Funding

TS Doctoral studies are funded by the Royal Thai Government scholarship and AP is funded by Sveland Animals Insurance Company for sample analysis.

References

1. Myers NC, Andrews GA, Chard-Bergstrom C. Chromogranin A plasma concentration and expression in pancreatic islet cell tumors of dogs and cats. Am J Vet Res. 1997;58:615–20.
2. Akiyoshi H, Aoki M, Shimada T, Noda K, Kumagai D, Saleh N, Sugii S, Ohashi F. Measurement of plasma chromogranin A concentrations for assessment of stress responses in dogs with insulin-induced hypoglycemia. Am J Vet Res. 2005;66:1830–5.
3. Kanai K, Hino M, Hori Y, Nakao R, Hoshi F, Itoh N, Higuchi S. Circadian variations in salivary chromogranin a concentrations during a 24-h period in dogs. J Vet Sci. 2008;9:421–3.
4. Stridsberg M, Pettersson A, Hagman R, Westin C, Höglund O. Chromogranins can be measured in samples from cats and dogs. BMC Res Notes. 2014;7:336.
5. Jitpean S, Stridsberg M, Pettersson A, Höglund OV, Holst BS, Hagman R. Decreased plasma chromogranin A361-372 (Catestatin) but not chromogranin A17-38 (Vasostatin) in female dogs with bacterial uterine infection (pyometra). BMC Vet Res. 2015;11:14.
6. Höglund OV, Hagman R, Stridsberg M. Chromogranin A and cortisol at intraoperative repeated noxious stimuli: surgical stress in a dog model. SAGE Open Med. 2015;3:2050312115576432.
7. Blaschko H, Comline RS, Schneider FH, Silver M, Smith AD. Secretion of a chromaffin granule protein, chromogranin, from the adrenal gland after splanchnic stimulation. Nature. 1967;215:58–9.
8. O'Connor DT, Bernstein KN. Radioimmunoassay of chromogranin A in plasma as a measure of exocytotic sympathoadrenal activity in normal subjects and patients with pheochromocytoma. N Engl J Med. 1984;311:764–70.
9. Saruta J, Tsukinoki K, Sasaguri K, Ishii H, Yasuda M, Osamura YR, Watanabe Y, Sato S. Expression and localization of chromogranin A gene and protein in human submandibular gland. Cells Tissues Organs. 2005;180:237–44.

10. Kanno T, Asada N, Yanase H, Iwanaga T, Ozaki T, Nishikawa Y, Iguchi K, Mochizuki T, Hoshino M, Yanaihara N. Salivary secretion of highly concentrated chromogranin a in response to noradrenaline and acetylcholine in isolated and perfused rat submandibular glands. Exp Physiol. 1999;84:1073–83.

11. Sato F, Kanno T, Nagasawa S, Yanaihara N, Ishida N, Hasegawa T, Iwanaga T. Immunohistochemical localization of chromogranin A in the acinar cells of equine salivary glands contrasts with rodent glands. Cells Tissues Organs. 2002;172:29–36.

12. Nakane H, Asami O, Yamada Y, Harada T, Matsui N, Kanno T, Yanaihara N. Salivary chromogranin A as an index of psychosomatic stress response. Biomed Res. 1998;6:401–6.

13. Den R, Toda M, Nagasawa S, Kitamura K, Morimoto K. Circadian rhythm of human salivary chromogranin A. Biomed Res. 2007;28:57–60.

14. Escribano D, Soler L, Gutierrez AM, Martinez-Subiela S, Ceron JJ. Measurement of chromogranin A in porcine saliva: validation of a time-resolved immunofluorometric assay and evaluation of its application as a marker of acute stress. Animal. 2013;7:640–7.

15. O'Connor DT, Pandian MR, Carlton E, Cervenka JH, Hsiao RJ. Rapid radioimmunoassay of circulating chromogranin a in vitro stability, exploration of the neuroendocrine character of neoplasia, and assessment of the effects of organ failure. Clin Chem. 1989;35:1631–7.

16. Helle KB, Marley PD, Angeletti RH, Aunis D, Galindo E, Small DH, Livett BG. Chromogranin A: secretion of processed products from the stimulated retrogradely perfused bovine adrenal gland. J Neuroendocrinol. 1993;5:413–20.

17. Aardal S, Helle KB, Elsayed S, Reed RK, Serck-Hanssen G. Vasostatins, comprising the N-terminal domain of chromogranin A, suppress tension in isolated human blood vessel segments. J Neuroendocrinol. 1993;5:405–12.

18. Aardal S, Helle KB. The vasoinhibitory activity of bovine chromogranin A fragment (vasostatin) and its independence of extracellular calcium in isolated segments of human blood vessels. Regul Pept. 1992;41:9–18.

19. Corti A, Sanchez LP, Gasparri A, Curnis F, Longhi R, Brandazza A, Siccardi AG, Sidoli A. Production and structure characterisation of recombinant chromogranin AN-terminal fragments (vasostatins)—evidence of dimer-monomer equilibria. Eur J Biochem. 1997;248:692–9.

20. Mahata SK, Mahata M, Wen G, Wong WB, Mahapatra NR, Hamilton BA, O'Connor DT. The catecholamine release-inhibitory "catestatin" fragment of chromogranin a: naturally occurring human variants with different potencies for multiple chromaffin cell nicotinic cholinergic responses. Mol Pharmacol. 2004;66:1180–91.

21. Mahata SK, O'Connor DT, Mahata M, Yoo SH, Taupenot L, Wu H, Gill BM, Parmer RJ. Novel autocrine feedback control of catecholamine release. A discrete chromogranin a fragment is a noncompetitive nicotinic cholinergic antagonist. J Clin Invest. 1997;100:1623–33.

22. Mahata SK, Mahata M, Fung MM, O'Connor DT. Catestatin: a multifunctional peptide from chromogranin A. Regul Pept. 2010;162:33–43.

23. Mahata SK, Mahapatra NR, Mahata M, Wang TC, Kennedy BP, Ziegler MG, O'Connor DT. Catecholamine secretory vesicle stimulus-transcription coupling in vivo. Demonstration by a novel transgenic promoter/photoprotein reporter and inhibition of secretion and transcription by the chromogranin A fragment catestatin. J Biol Chem. 2003;278:32058–67.

24. Wen G, Mahata SK, Cadman P, Mahata M, Ghosh S, Mahapatra NR, Rao FW, Stridsberg M, Smith DW, Mahboubi P, et al. Both rare and common polymorphisms contribute functional variation at CHGA, a regulator of catecholamine physiology. Am J Hum Genet. 2004;74:197–207.

25. Tatemoto K, Efendic S, Mutt V, Makk G, Feistner GJ, Barchas JD. Pancreastatin, a novel pancreatic peptide that inhibits insulin secretion. Nature. 1986;324:476–8.

26. Sanchez-Margalet V, Gonzalez-Yanes C, Najib S, Santos-Alvarez J. Metabolic effects and mechanism of action of the chromogranin A-derived peptide pancreastatin. Regul Pept. 2010;161:8–14.

27. Gayen JR, Saberi M, Schenk S, Biswas N, Vaingankar SM, Cheung WW, Najjar SM, O'Connor DT, Bandyopadhyay G, Mahata SK. A novel pathway of insulin sensitivity in chromogranin A null mice: a crucial role for pancreastatin in glucose homeostasis. J Biol Chem. 2009;284:28498–509.

28. Bandyopadhyay GK, Lu M, Avolio E, Siddiqui JA, Gayen JR, Wollam J, Vu CU, Chi NW, O'Connor DT, Mahata SK. Pancreastatin-dependent inflammatory signaling mediates obesity-induced insulin resistance. Diabetes. 2015;64:104–16.

29. Tota B, Gentile S, Pasqua T, Bassino E, Koshimizu H, Cawley NX, Cerra MC, Loh YP, Angelone T. The novel chromogranin A-derived serpinin and pyroglutaminated serpinin peptides are positive cardiac beta-adrenergic-like inotropes. Faseb J. 2012;26:2888–98.

30. Metz-Boutigue MH, Garcia-Sablone P, Hogue-Angeletti R, Aunis D. Intracellular and extracellular processing of chromogranin A. Determination of cleavage sites. Eur J Biochem. 1993;217:247–57.

31. D'Amico MA, Ghinassi B, Izzicupo P, Manzoli L, Di Baldassarre A. Biological function and clinical relevance of chromogranin A and derived peptides. Endocr Connect. 2014;3:R45–54.

32. Fasciotto BH, Gorr SU, Cohn DV. Autocrine inhibition of parathyroid cell secretion requires proteolytic processing of chromogranin-A. Bone Miner. 1992;17:323–33.

33. Fasciotto BH, Denny JC, Greeley GH, Cohn DV. Processing of chromogranin A in the parathyroid: generation of parastatin-related peptides. Peptides. 2000;21:1389–401.

34. Metz-Boutigue MH, Goumon Y, Lugardon K, Strub JM, Aunis D. Antibacterial peptides are present in chromaffin cell secretory granules. Cell Mol Neurobiol. 1998;18:249–66.

35. Helle KB. The chromogranin A derived peptides vasostatin I and catestatin as regulatory peptides for cardiovascular functions. Cardiovasc Res. 2010;85:9–16.

36. Rangon CM, Haik S, Faucheux BA, Metz-Boutigue MH, Fierville F, Fuchs JP, Hauw JJ, Aunis D. Different chromogranin immunoreactivity between prion and a-beta amyloid plaque. Neuroreport. 2003;14:755–8.

37. Ferrari L, Seregni E, Lucignani G, Bajetta E, Martinetti A, Aliberti G, Pallotti F, Procopio G, Della Torre S, Luksch R, et al. Accuracy and clinical correlates of two different methods for chromogranin A assay in neuroendocrine tumors. Int J Biol Markers. 2004;19:295–304.

38. Ferrari L, Seregni E, Martinetti A, Van Graafeiland B, Nerini-Molteni S, Botti C, Artale S, Cresta S, Bombardieri E. Chromogranin A measurement in neuroendocrine tumors. Int J Biol Markers. 1998;13:3–9.

39. Borglum T, Rehfeld JF, Drivsholm LB, Hilsted L. Processing-independent quantitation of chromogranin a in plasma from patients with neuroendocrine tumors and small-cell lung carcinomas. Clin Chem. 2007;53:438–46.

40. Biswas N, Curello E, O'Connor DT, Mahata SK. Chromogranin/secretogranin proteins in murine heart: myocardial production of chromogranin A fragment catestatin (Chga(364–384)). Cell Tissue Res. 2010;342:353–61.

41. Brar BK, Helgeland E, Mahata SK, Zhang K, O'Connor DT, Helle KB, Jonassen AK. Human catestatin peptides differentially regulate infarct size in the ischemic-reperfused rat heart. Regul Pept. 2010;165:63–70.

42. Corti A, Mannarino C, Mazza R, Colombo B, Longhi R, Tota B. Vasostatins exert negative inotropism in the working heart of the frog. Ann N Y Acad Sci. 2002;971:362–5.

43. Liu L, Ding W, Li R, Ye X, Zhao J, Jiang J, Meng L, Wang J, Chu S, Han X, et al. Plasma levels and diagnostic value of catestatin in patients with heart failure. Peptides. 2013;46:20–5.

44. Liu L, Ding W, Zhao F, Shi L, Pang Y, Tang C. Plasma levels and potential roles of catestatin in patients with coronary heart disease. Scand Cardiovasc J. 2013;47:217–24.

45. Zhu D, Wang F, Yu H, Mi L, Gao W. Catestatin is useful in detecting patients with stage B heart failure. Biomarkers. 2011;16:691–7.

46. Angelone T, Mazza R, Cerra MC. Chromogranin-A: a multifaceted cardiovascular role in health and disease. Curr Med Chem. 2012;19:4042–50.

47. Goetze JP, Alehagen U, Flyvbjerg A, Rehfeld JF. Chromogranin A as a biomarker in cardiovascular disease. Biomark Med. 2014;8:133–40.

48. Reshma AP, Arunachalam R, Pillai JK, Kurra SB, Varkey VK, Prince MJ. Chromogranin A: novel biomarker between periodontal disease and psychosocial stress. J Indian Soc Periodontol. 2013;17:214–8.

49. Toda M, Kusakabe S, Nagasawa S, Kitamura K, Morimoto K. Effect of laughter on salivary endocrinological stress marker chromogranin A. Biomed Res. 2007;28:115–8.

50. Yamakoshi T, Park SB, Jang WC, Kim K, Yamakoshi Y, Hirose H. Relationship between salivary chromogranin-A and stress induced by simulated monotonous driving. Med Biol Eng Comput. 2009;47:449–56.

51. Lee T, Shimizu T, Iijima M, Obinata K, Yamashiro Y, Nagasawa S. Evaluation of psychosomatic stress in children by measuring salivary chromogranin A. Acta Paediatr. 2006;95:935–9.

52. Takatsuji K, Sugimoto Y, Ishizaki S, Ozaki Y, Matsuyama E, Yamaguchi Y. The effects of examination stress on salivary cortisol, immunoglobulin A, and chromogranin A in nursing students. Biomed Res. 2008;29:221–4.

53. Nickel T, Vogeser M, Emslander I, David R, Heilmeier B, Op den Winkel M, Schmidt-Trucksass A, Wilbert-Lampen U, Hanssen H, Halle M. Extreme exercise enhances chromogranin A levels correlating with stress levels but not with cardiac burden. Atherosclerosis. 2012;220:219–22.

54. Pfaffe T, Cooper-White J, Beyerlein P, Kostner K, Punyadeera C. Diagnostic potential of saliva: current state and future applications. Clin Chem. 2011;57:675–87.

55. Symons FJ, ElGhazi I, Reilly BG, Barney CC, Hanson L, Panoskaltsis-Mortari A, Armitage IM, Wilcox GL. Can biomarkers differentiate pain and no pain subgroups of nonverbal children with cerebral palsy? A preliminary investigation based on noninvasive saliva sampling. Pain Med. 2015;16:249–56.

56. Kobelt AJ, Hemsworth PH, Barnett JL, Butler KL. Sources of sampling variation in saliva cortisol in dogs. Res Vet Sci. 2003;75:157–61.

57. Oyama D, Hyodo M, Doi H, Kurachi T, Takata M, Koyama S, Satoh T, Watanabe G. Saliva collection by using filter paper for measuring cortisol levels in dogs. Domest Anim Endocrinol. 2014;46:20–5.

58. Desborough JP. The stress response to trauma and surgery. Br J Anaesth. 2000;85:109–17.

59. Weissman C. The metabolic response to stress: an overview and update. Anesthesiology. 1990;73:308–27.

60. Mahata SK, Mahata M, Parmer RJ, O'Connor DT. Desensitization of catecholamine release. The novel catecholamine release-inhibitory peptide catestatin (chromogranin a344-364) acts at the receptor to prevent nicotinic cholinergic tolerance. J Biol Chem. 1999;274:2920–8.

61. Kennedy BP, Mahata SK, O'Connor DT, Ziegler MG. Mechanism of cardiovascular actions of the chromogranin A fragment catestatin in vivo. Peptides. 1998;19:1241–8.

62. Radek KA, Lopez-Garcia B, Hupe M, Niesman IR, Elias PM, Taupenot L, Mahata SK, O'Connor DT, Gallo RL. The neuroendocrine peptide catestatin is a cutaneous antimicrobial and induced in the skin after injury. J Invest Dermatol. 2008;128:1525–34.

63. Imbrogno S, Garofalo F, Cerra MC, Mahata SK, Tota B. The catecholamine release-inhibitory peptide catestatin (chromogranin A344-363) modulates myocardial function in fish. J Exp Biol. 2010;213:3636–43.

64. Imbrogno S, Angelone T, Corti A, Adamo C, Helle KB, Tota B. Influence of vasostatins, the chromogranin A-derived peptides, on the working heart of the eel (Anguilla anguilla): negative inotropy and mechanism of action. Gen Comp Endocrinol. 2004;139:20–8.

65. Brekke JF, Osol GJ, Helle KB. N-terminal chromogranin-derived peptides as dilators of bovine coronary resistance arteries. Regul Pept. 2002;105:93–100.

66. Zhang D, Shooshtarizadeh P, Laventie BJ, Colin DA, Chich JF, Vidic J, de Barry J, Chasserot-Golaz S, Delalande F, Van Dorsselaer A, et al. Two chromogranin a-derived peptides induce calcium entry in human neutrophils by calmodulin-regulated calcium independent phospholipase A2. Plos ONE. 2009;4:e4501.

67. Byström E. Chromogranin A in blood and saliva in dogs. Uppsala: Swedish University of Agricultural Sciences; 2014.

68. Srithunyarat T, Byström E, Stridsberg M, Olsson U, Pettersson A. The correlation of Chromogranin A in saliva and plasma in healthy dogs. In: Ramsey I, editor. Proceeding of BSAVA congress 2014. 1st ed. Gloucester: BSAVA; 2014. p. 645.

69. Norling Y, Wiss V, Gorjanc G, Keeling L. Body language of dogs responding to different types of stimuli. In: Waiblinge S, Winckler C, Gutmann A, editors. Proceeding of the 46th Congress of the International Society for applied ethology 2012. Wageningen: Wageningen Academic; 2012. p. 199.

70. Stridsberg M, Eriksson B, Oberg K, Janson ET. A panel of 11 region-specific radioimmunoassays for measurements of human chromogranin A. Regul Pept. 2004;117:219–27.

71. Littell RC. SAS for mixed models. 2nd ed. Cary: SAS Institute Inc; 2006.

72. Olsson U. Statistics for life science 2. 1st ed. Lund: Studentlitteratur; 2011.

73. Fitzmaurice GM, Laird NM, Ware JH. Applied longitudinal analysis. Hoboken: Wiley; 2004.

74. Escribano D, Gutierrez AM, Fuentes-Rubio M, Ceron JJ. Saliva chromogranin A in growing pigs: a study of circadian patterns during daytime and stability under different storage conditions. Vet J. 2014;199:355–9.

75. Theurl M, Schgoer W, Albrecht K, Jeschke J, Egger M, Beer AG, Vasiljevic D, Rong S, Wolf AM, Bahlmann FH, et al. The neuropeptide catestatin acts as a novel angiogenic cytokine via a basic fibroblast growth factor-dependent mechanism. Circ Res. 2010;107:1326–35.

76. Perego R, Proverbio D, Spada E. Increases in heart rate and serum cortisol concentrations in healthy dogs are positively correlated with an indoor waiting-room environment. Vet Clin Pathol. 2014;43:67–71.

77. Den R, Toda M, Ohira M, Morimoto K. Levels of awakening salivary CgA in response to stress in healthy subjects. Environ Health Prev Med. 2011;16:155–7.

78. Toda M, Den R, Morimoto K. Basal levels of salivary chromogranin A, but not alpha-amylase, are related to plasma norepinephrine in the morning. Stress Health. 2008;24:323–6.

79. Takiyyuddin MA, Neumann HP, Cervenka JH, Kennedy B, Dinh TQ, Ziegler MG, Baron AD, O'Connor DT. Ultradian variations of chromogranin A in humans. Am J Physiol. 1991;261:R939–44.

80. Campana D, Nori F, Piscitelli L, Morselli-Labate AM, Pezzilli R, Corinaldesi R, Tomassetti P. Chromogranin A: is it a useful marker of neuroendocrine tumors? J Clin Oncol. 2007;25:1967–73.

81. Stefanescu AM, Schipor S, Paun D, Dumitrache C, Badiu C. Plasma versus salivary chromogranin A as selective markers in pheochromocytoma diagnosis. Acta Endocrinol. 2011;7:153–61.

82. Lindahl AE, Low A, Stridsberg M, Sjoberg F, Ekselius L, Gerdin B. Plasma chromogranin A after severe burn trauma. Neuropeptides. 2013;47:207–12.

3

Species distribution and in vitro antimicrobial susceptibility of coagulase-negative staphylococci isolated from bovine mastitic milk

Suvi Taponen[1*], Suvi Nykäsenoja[2], Tarja Pohjanvirta[2], Anna Pitkälä[2] and Satu Pyörälä[1]

Abstract

Background: Coagulase-negative staphylococci (CoNS) are the most common bovine mastitis causing bacteria in many countries. It is known that resistance for antimicrobials is in general more common in CoNS than in *Staphylococcus aureus* but little is known about the antimicrobial resistance of specific CoNS species. In this study, 400 CoNS isolates from bovine mastitic milk samples were identified to species level using ribotyping and MALDI-TOF MS, and their antimicrobial susceptibility was determined using a commercially available microdilution system. The results were interpreted according to the epidemiological cut-off values by the European Committee on Antimicrobial Susceptibility testing.

Results: The most common CoNS species were *S. simulans*, *S. epidermidis*, *S. chromogenes* and *S. haemolyticus*. Penicillin resistance was the most common type of antimicrobial resistance. *Staphylococcus epidermidis* was the most resistant among the four major species. Almost one-third of our *S. epidermidis* isolates were resistant to >2 antimicrobials and close to 7 % were multidrug resistant. The majority of *S. epidermidis* isolates were resistant to benzylpenicillin. On the contrary, only few *S. simulans* isolates were penicillin-resistant. Phenotypic oxacillin resistance was found in all four main species, and 34 % of the isolates were oxacillin resistant. However, only 21 isolates (5 %) were positive for the *mec*A gene. Of these, 20 were *S. epidermidis* and one *S. sciuri*. *mec*C positive isolates were not found.

Conclusion: *Staphylococcus epidermidis* differed from the three other major CoNS species as resistance to the tested antimicrobials was common, several isolates were multidrug resistant, and 19 % of the isolates carried the *mec*A gene encoding methicillin resistance.

Keywords: Coagulase-negative staphylococci, CoNS species, Antimicrobial resistance, Bovine, Cow, MIC, *Staphylococcus epidermidis*, *Staphylococcus chromogenes*, *Staphylococcus haemolyticus*, *Staphylococcus simulans*

Background

Prevalence of mastitis in dairy cows and distribution of mastitis-causing bacteria has regularly been monitored in Finland [1, 2]. These surveys have also reported antimicrobial in vitro susceptibility of different bacterial species, including coagulase-negative staphylococci (CoNS). Coagulase-negative staphylococci have become the most common mastitis causing agents in many countries [3]. They mostly cause subclinical mastitis but have also been isolated from clinical mastitis [3, 4]. It is known that resistance for antimicrobials is in general more common in CoNS than in *S. aureus* [4]. The most common resistance among bovine CoNS is production of β-lactamase which confers resistance to benzylpenicillin and aminopenicillins, but also resistance towards aminoglycosides, tetracyclines, and macrolides has been reported [2, 5, 6]. Methicillin-resistant CoNS have been isolated from bovine mastitis which is of special concern because

*Correspondence: suvi.taponen@helsinki.fi
[1] Department of Production Animal Medicine, Faculty of Veterinary Medicine, University of Helsinki, Paroninkuja 20, 04920 Saarentaus, Finland
Full list of author information is available at the end of the article

of the risk of spreading the *mec* genes [7, 8]. Furthermore, emergence of resistance among CoNS is a concern because resistance determinants may be transferred between staphylococcal species and form a risk for public health [9, 10].

Phenotypic identification methods for bovine CoNS have proven to be unsatisfactory [11–13]. Molecular methods have become available for identification of CoNS to species level, which has made species determination more reliable. Reliable genotypic identification has enabled studying frequency of different CoNS species and species-specific antimicrobial susceptibility. Reports on mastitis causing CoNS species and their antimicrobial susceptibility have since been published by some authors [5, 6, 14]. Unfortunately, only few studies have used epidemiological cut-off values (ECOFF) of the European Committee on Antimicrobial Susceptibility testing to determine proportions of resistant isolates [15], which has made comparisons difficult. Studies on genetic mechanisms for resistance of bovine CoNS species have also been published, with different panels of resistance genes [5, 16, 17]. In Finland, antimicrobial susceptibility of CoNS has been reported for bovine CoNS as a group only [2, 18]. It is likely that in the future CoNS will no more be considered as one homogenous group, but species-specific approaches become possible in mastitis control [3]. Knowledge on the antimicrobial susceptibility of different CoNS species is then also necessary.

The aim of this study was to explore the distribution of CoNS species isolated from mastitic milk samples in Finland and to determine the antimicrobial susceptibility of different CoNS species.

Methods

The material consists of CoNS isolates from two studies, Pitkälä et al. [2] (dataset 1) and Finnish veterinary antimicrobial resistance monitoring program 2010–2012 [18] (dataset 2). The number of CoNS isolates was 312 and 88 in dataset 1 and 2, respectively.

The first study (dataset 1) was a nationwide prevalence study carried out in 2001, in which milk samples were collected from all four quarters of all lactating cows in herds randomly allocated into the study. Conventional microbiological methods were used to identify bacteria isolated from the milk samples [2, 19]. The milk samples were classified as mastitic when the milk somatic cell count, measured with an electric counter (Fossomatic Milk Analysis, Foss Electric, Hillerød, Denmark), exceeded 300 000 cells/ml. Of the total of 2103 CoNS isolated in that study, 335 were randomly chosen for in vitro antimicrobial susceptibility testing [2]. Of these isolates, 318 were successfully identified to species level in the present study. Six isolates appeared to belong to *S. aureus*

species and were withdrawn from this study. In the second study (dataset 2) the samples were routine mastitis samples (based on elevated milk somatic cell count and/ or clinical signs of mastitis) submitted during 2012 to the laboratory of Valio Ltd by veterinarians and dairy farmers. Bacteriological etiology of mastitis was determined by a real-time PCR assay (Thermo Scientific PathoProof™ Mastitis Complete-12 Kit, Thermo Fisher Scientific Ltd.,Vantaa, Finland). During the study, the preservative was left out from the milk tubes. Samples positive for CoNS in the PCR test were selected for culture. From the cultured pure samples the first cultured 88 CoNS isolates, but only one isolate per herd, were selected for determination of antimicrobial susceptibility. *Staphylococcus* species identification was performed during the present study.

The CoNS isolates from both datasets were identified to species level with the 16S and 23S rRNA gene restriction fragment length polymorphism method (ribotyping) as described previously [20]. The CoNS species were determined by comparison in a numerical similarity analysis of the ribotype patterns with a ribotype library using BioNumerics 5.1 software package (Applied Maths, St.-Martens-Latem, Belgium). For some isolates ribotyping failed, and they were later analyzed with MALDI-TOF MS (Microflex LT, Bruker Daltonic Gmbh, Bremen, Germany). The correctness of species identification based on ribotyping was confirmed by analyzing a representative sample of all different ribotype patterns by MALDI-TOF MS [21]. The agreement between the methods was excellent.

Antimicrobial susceptibility of CoNS isolates from both datasets was determined in the previous studies [2, 18] using a commercially available microdilution system (VetMIC™; SVA, Uppsala, Sweden). Minimum inhibitory concentrations (MIC) in both datasets were determined for penicillin, cephalothin, oxacillin, erythromycin, chloramphenicol, clindamycin, tetracycline, gentamicin, neomycin, streptomycin, and trimethoprim/ sulfamethoxazole. In addition, MICs for virginiamycin, vancomycin and avilamycin in dataset 1, and for fusidic acid, kanamycin, ciprofloxacin, trimethoprim, florfenicol, and cefoxitin in dataset 2, were determined. Results from the susceptibility testing were interpreted according to the epidemiological cut-off values (ECOFFs) by the European Committee on Antimicrobial Susceptibility testing (EUCAST) [22] as non-wild type (from now on referred as resistant) or wild type (sensitive). If a specific ECOFF was not available for the specific species or for CoNS as a group, ECOFF of *Staphylococcus aureus* was used. Production of beta-lactamase was tested using nitrocefin discs (dataset 1: AB Biodisk, Solna Sweden; dataset 2: Becton–Dickinson, NJ, USA). The isolates with MIC values for oxacillin >1 mg/l were tested for presence of the *mec*A gene in dataset 1 and for presence of the *mec*A and *mec*C genes in dataset 2, using PCR and primers reported previously [23, 24].

Results

Distribution of CoNS species

The numbers and proportions of isolates of different CoNS species are shown in Table 1. In dataset 1, a total of 14 staphylococcal species were identified. The most common CoNS species were *S. simulans* (25.0 %), *S. epidermidis* (25.0 %), *S. chromogenes* (15.4 %), *S. haemolyticus* (11.9 %), and *S. warneri* (10.3 %). Three isolates could not be identified by ribotyping or by MALDI-TOF MS and were grouped as *Staphylococcus* sp. In dataset 2, similarly as in the dataset 1, *S. simulans* (34.1 %) and *S. epidermidis* (30.7 %) were the most common species. *Staphylococcus chromogenes* was the third most common species (6.8 %). The proportion of both *S. haemolyticus* and *S. cohnii* isolates was 5.7 %. Three isolates could not be identified by ribotyping or MALDI-TOF MS and were grouped as *Staphylococcus* sp. The unidentified isolates may represent a new *Staphylococcus* species or one of the few CoNS species, like *S. devriesei*, which were not included in the ribotype and MALDI-TOF MS comparison databases at the time of the analyses. The four most common CoNS species represented 77.3 % of all 400 isolates.

In vitro antimicrobial susceptibility

The four major CoNS species differed in their in vitro antimicrobial susceptibility. Among them, antimicrobial resistance was most common in *S. epidermidis* (Tables 2 and 3). MIC distributions of the four major CoNS species for the tested antimicrobials in 2001 and 2012 are shown in Tables 2 and 3. The MIC results of all 400 isolates by species are shown in the Additional file 1: Table S1 and as a CoNS group in the Additional file 2: Table S2.

The majority, 74.4 and 74.1 % of *S. epidermidis* isolates in years 2001 and 2012, respectively, were resistant to benzylpenicillin (ECOFF 0.125 mg/l). Resistance to benzylpenicillin was also common in *S. haemolyticus* of which 64.9/40.0 % were resistant. Prevalence of isolates producing betalactamase, i.e. positive in the nitrocefin test, varied between CoNS species, and was lower in *S. chromogenes* (20.8/16.7 %) and *S. simulans* (3.9/6.7 %) than in *S. epidermidis* (59.0/70.4 %) and *S. haemolyticus* (51.4/0.0 %). Combining years 2001 and 2012, a total of 165 of the total of 400 isolates (41.3 %) had a MIC > 0.125 mg/l for benzylpenicillin i.e. were penicillin-resistant. In the nitrocefin test, 137 (34.3 %) isolates out of 400 were positive (penicillin resistant). Out of 165 isolates with MIC for > 0.125 mg/l for benzylpenicillin, 127 (77.0 %) isolates were positive in the nitrocefin test (true positive), and 38 were negative (false negative). Out of 235 isolates with MIC ≤ 0.125 mg/l for benzylpenicillin,

Table 1 Distribution of coagulase-negative *Staphylococcus* species isolated in bovine milk samples in 2001 (dataset 1) and 2012 (dataset 2)

CNS species	2001		2012		In total	
	n	%	n	%	n	%
S. agnetis	7	2.2	3	3.4	10	2.5
S. capitis	1	0.3	1	1.1	2	0.5
S. chromogenes	48	15.4	6	6.8	54	13.5
S. cohnii	7	2.2	5	5.7	12	3.0
S. epidermidis	78	25.0	27	30.7	105	26.3
S. equorum	3	1.0	0	0	3	0.8
S. haemolyticus	37	11.9	5	5.7	42	10.5
S. hyicus	4	1.3	1	1.1	5	1.3
S. kloosii	0	0	3	3.4	3	0.75
S. pasteuri	2	0.6	0	0	2	0.5
S. saprophyticus	2	0.6	1	1.1	3	0.8
S. sciuri	2	0.6	1	1.1	3	0.8
S. simulans	78	25.0	30	34.1	108	27.0
S. warneri	32	10.3	1	1.1	33	8.3
S. xylosus	8	2.6	2	2.3	10	2.5
Staphylococcus sp.	3	1.0	2	2.3	5	1.3
In total	312		88		400	

The material consisted of CoNS isolates from two studies, Pitkälä et al. [2] (dataset 1) and Finnish veterinary antimicrobial resistance monitoring program 2010–2012 [18] (dataset 2). In dataset 1 all quarters of cows were sampled in a mastitis survey, in dataset 2 samples originated from quarters with mastitis

Table 2 In vitro susceptibility to 14 antimicrobials of S. chromogenes, S. epidermidis, S. haemolyticus and S. simulans isolated in bovine milk samples from data-set 1 (2001)

MIC mg/l, % of isolates

Benzylpenicillin (ECOFF[a] = 0.125[b])

Organism	N	N (%) > ECOFF	≤0.06	0.12	0.25	0.5	1	2	4	8	≥16
S. chromogenes	48	14 (29.2)	68.8	2.1	4.2	6.3	12.5	6.3			
S. epidermidis	78	58 (74.4)	23.1	2.6	6.4	9.0	12.8	15.4	9.0	11.5	10.3
S. haemolyticus	37	24 (64.9)	32.4	2.7	16.2	27.0	13.5	5.4	2.7		
S. simulans	78	3 (3.8)	93.6	2.6	2.6			1.3			

Oxacillin (ECOFF[a] = 1.0)

Organism	N	N (%) > ECOFF	≤0.5	1	2	4	≥8
S. chromogenes	48	19 (39.6)	20.8	39.6	37.5	2.1	
S. epidermidis	78	27 (34.6)	38.5	26.9	15.4	6.4	12.8
S. haemolyticus	37	10 (27.0)	32.4	40.5	24.3	2.7	
S. simulans	78	15 (19.2)	38.5	42.3	19.2		

Cephalothin (ECOFF[a] = 1.0[b])

Organism	N	N (%) > ECOFF	≤0.12	0.25	0.5	1	2	4	≥8
S. chromogenes	48		22.9	70.8	6.3				
S. epidermidis	78		21.8	55.1	9.0	14.1			
S. haemolyticus	37		10.8	67.6	21.6				
S. simulans	78		6.4	56.4	37.2				

Streptomycin (ECOFF[a] = 16.0[b])

Organism	N	N (%) > ECOFF	≤2	4	8	16	32	64	128	≥256
S. chromogenes	48		81.3	14.6	4.2					
S. epidermidis	78	17 (21.8)	71.8	2.6	2.6	1.3	2.6	5.1	6.4	7.7
S. haemolyticus	37		97.3	2.7						
S. simulans	78	1 (1.3)	68.2	19.2	5.1	5.1	1.3			

Neomycin (ECOFF[a] = 1.0[b])

Organism	N	N (%) > ECOFF	≤2	4	8	16	32	≥64
S. chromogenes	48		97.9	2.1				
S. epidermidis	78		89.7	1.3	3.8	3.8	1.3	
S. haemolyticus	37		100.0					
S. simulans	78		100.0					

Gentamicin (ECOFF[a] = 0.5)

Organism	N	N (%) > ECOFF	≤0.25	0.5	1	2	4	8	≥16
S. chromogenes	48		95.8	4.2					
S. epidermidis	78		100.0						
S. haemolyticus	37		100.0						
S. simulans	78	2 (2.6)	88.5	9.0	2.6				

Table 2 continued

MIC mg/l, % of isolates. ECOFF[a]

Clindamycin — ECOFF[a] 0.25

Organism	N	N (%) > ECOFF	≤1	2	4	≥8
S. chromogenes	48		100.0			
S. epidermidis	78		100.0			
S. haemolyticus	37		97.3		2.7	
S. simulans	78		100.0			

Erythromycin — ECOFF[a] 1.0

Organism	N	N (%) > ECOFF	≤0.5	1	2	4	≥8
S. chromogenes	48	2 (4.2)	95.8				4.2
S. epidermidis	78	11 (14.1)	84.6	1.3			14.1
S. haemolyticus	37	1 (2.7)	94.6	2.7			2.7
S. simulans	78		100.0				

Chloramphenicol — ECOFF[a] 16.0

Organism	N	N (%) > ECOFF	≤2	4	8	16	≥32
S. chromogenes	48		4.2	77.1	18.8		
S. epidermidis	78	2 (2.6)	1.3	87.2	1.3	7.7	2.6
S. haemolyticus	37		10.8	86.5	2.7		
S. simulans	78		3.8	47.4	46.2	2.6	

Tetracycline — ECOFF[a] 1.0

Organism	N	N (%) > ECOFF	≤0.5	1	2	4	8	16	32	64	≥128
S. chromogenes	48	3 (6.2)	87.5	6.3						2.1	4.2
S. epidermidis	78	36 (46.2)	47.4	6.4	7.7	20.5	2.6		1.3	3.8	10.3
S. haemolyticus	37		75.7	24.3							
S. simulans	78	4 (5.1)	21.8	73.1	2.6	1.3			1.3		

Trimetoprim-sulfamethoxazole — ECOFF[a] 0.5/9.5

Organism	N	N (%) > ECOFF	≤0.25/4.25	0.5/9.5	1/19	2/38	4/76	8/152	≥16/304
S. chromogenes	48	5 (10.4)	75.0	14.6	4.2		2.1	2.1	2.1
S. epidermidis	78	7 (9.0)	73.1	17.9		5.1	2.6	1.3	
S. haemolyticus	37		89.2	10.8					
S. simulans	78	6 (7.7)	29.5	62.8	6.1	2.6			

Vancomycin — ECOFF[a] 4.0

Organism	N	N (%) > ECOFF	≤1	2	4	8	16	32	≥64
S. chromogenes	48		83.3	16.7					
S. epidermidis	78		26.9	73.1					
S. haemolyticus	37		81.1	18.9					
S. simulans	78	1 (1.3)	91.0	6.4	1.3		1.3		

Virginiamycin — ECOFF[a] 1.0[c]

Organism	N	N (%) > ECOFF	≤0.5	1	2	4	≥8
S. chromogenes	48	2 (4.2)	25.0	70.8	4.2		
S. epidermidis	78	1 (1.3)	65.4	33.3	1.3		
S. haemolyticus	37	1 (2.7)	37.8	59.5	2.7		
S. simulans	78	2 (2.6)	15.4	82.1	1.3	1.3	

Table 2 continued

Antimicrobial	Organism	N	N (%) > ECOFF	MIC mg/l, % of isolates							ECOFF[a]
				≤0.5	1	2	4	8	16	32	≥64	
Avilamycin											ND
	S. chromogenes	48				27.1	54.2	18.8			
	S. epidermidis	78					29.5	65.4	5.1		
	S. haemolyticus	37				16.2	59.5	21.6	2.7		
	S. simulans	78			1.3	1.3	11.5	37.2	33.3	15.4	

In this dataset, all quarters of cows were sampled in a mastitis survey [2]

ND not determined

[a] Current (March 2015) EUCAST epidemiological cut-off (ECOFF) values (mg/l) for CNS were used to define resistant isolates. If ECOFF for CNS was not available, the value for *S. aureus* was used. For virginiamycin, ECOFF for *S. intermedius* was used

[b] ECOFF for *S. aureus*

[c] ECOFF for *S. intermedius*

Table 3 In vitro susceptibility to 17 antimicrobials of S. chromogenes, S. epidermidis, S. haemolyticus and S. simulans isolated in bovine milk samples from data-set 2 (2012)

MIC mg/l, % of isolates

Benzylpenicillin

Organism	N	N (%) > ECOFF	≤0.03	0.06	0.12	0.25	0.5	1	2	4	≥8	ECOFF[a]
S. chromogenes	6	1 (16.7)	33.3	50.0				16.7				0.125[b]
S. epidermidis	27	20 (74.1)	18.5	3.7	3.7	11.1	7.4	18.5	7.4	22.2	7.4	
S. haemolyticus	5	2 (40.0)	20.0	40.0				40.0				
S. simulans	30	2 (6.6)	63.3	30.0				3.3	3.3			

Oxacillin

Organism	N	N (%) > ECOFF	≤0.12	0.25	0.5	1	2	4	8	16	≥32	ECOFF[a]
S. chromogenes	6		16.7	16.7	66.7							1.0
S. epidermidis	27	4 (14.8)		3.7	66.7	14.8		3.7	3.7		7.4	
S. haemolyticus	5				80.0	20.0						
S. simulans	30			6.7	36.7	50.0	3.3	3.3				

Cephalothin

Organism	N	N (%) > ECOFF	≤0.06	0.12	0.25	0.5	1	2	4	≥8	ECOFF[a]
S. chromogenes	6			50.0	50.0						1.0[b]
S. epidermidis	27	2 (7.4)	3.7	40.7	37.0	11.1		7.4			
S. haemolyticus	5			20.0	40.0	40.0					
S. simulans	30	2 (6.6)			70.0	23.3		6.7			

Streptomycin

Organism	N	N (%) > ECOFF	≤4	8	16	32	≥64	ECOFF[a]
S. chromogenes	6		83.3		16.7			16.0[b]
S. epidermidis	27	2 (7.4)	81.5	11.1		3.7	3.7	
S. haemolyticus	5		100.0					
S. simulans	30	1 (3.3)	73.3	20.0	3.3	3.3		

Neomycin

Organism	N	N (%) > ECOFF	≤4	8	16	32	≥64	ECOFF[a]
S. chromogenes	6		100.0					1.0[b]
S. epidermidis	27		96.3	3.7				
S. haemolyticus	5		100.0					
S. simulans	30	1 (3.3)	96.7				3.3	

Gentamicin

Organism	N	N (%) > ECOFF	≤0.5	1	2	4	8	≥16	ECOFF[a]
S. chromogenes	6		100.0						0.5
S. epidermidis	27		100.0						
S. haemolyticus	5		100.0						
S. simulans	30	1 (3.3)	96.7	3.3					

Table 3 continued

Clindamycin — ECOFF[a] 0.25

Organism	N	N (%) > ECOFF	≤0.25	0.5	1	2	4	≥8
S. chromogenes	6		100.0					
S. epidermidis	27		100.0					
S. haemolyticus	5		100.0					
S. simulans	30	3 (10.0)	90.0					10.0

Erythromycin — ECOFF[a] 1.0

Organism	N	N (%) > ECOFF	≤0.25	0.5	1	2	4	≥8
S. chromogenes	6			83.3	16.7			
S. epidermidis	27		25.9	70.4	3.7			
S. haemolyticus	5		20.0	80.0				
S. simulans	30		10.0	86.7	3.3			

Chloramphenicol — ECOFF[a] 16.0

Organism	N	N (%) > ECOFF	≤2	4	8	16	≥32
S. chromogenes	6			33.3	66.7		
S. epidermidis	27			92.6	7.4		
S. haemolyticus	5			100.0			
S. simulans	30			76.7	23.3		

Tetracycline — ECOFF[a] 1.0

Organism	N	N (%) > ECOFF	≤0.5	1	2	4	8	16	32	64	≥128
S. chromogenes	6		100.0								
S. epidermidis	27	7 (25.9)	66.7	7.4	18.5				7.4		
S. haemolyticus	5		100.0								
S. simulans	30	2 (6.7)	90.0	3.3				6.7			

Trimetoprim-sulfamethoxazole — ECOFF[a] 0.5/9.5

Organism	N	N (%) > ECOFF	≤0.5/9.5	1/19	2/38	≥4/76
S. chromogenes	6		100.0			
S. epidermidis	27	2 (7.4)	92.6			7.4
S. haemolyticus	5		100.0			
S. simulans	30		100.0			

Cefoxitin — ECOFF[a] 4.0[b]

Organism	N	N (%) > ECOFF	≤0.12	0.25	0.5	1	2	4	8	16	≥32
S. chromogenes	6				83.3	16.7					
S. epidermidis	27	5 (18.5)				3.7	55.6	22.2	7.4	3.7	7.4
S. haemolyticus	5						40.0	60.0			
S. simulans	30				3.3		80.0	16.7			

Kanamycin — ECOFF[a] 8.0[b]

Organism	N	N (%) > ECOFF	≤0.12	0.25	0.5	1	2	4	8	16	32	≥64
S. chromogenes	6				33.3	66.7						
S. epidermidis	27	2 (7.4)		48.1	18.5		25.9			3.7		3.7
S. haemolyticus	5				80.0	20.0						
S. simulans	30				30.0	40.0	30.0					

Table 3 continued

Florphenicol (ECOFF[a] = 8.0[b])

Organism	N	N (%) > ECOFF	≤2	4	8	≥16
S. chromogenes	6		50.0	50.0		
S. epidermidis	27		48.1	51.9		
S. haemolyticus	5		60.0	40.0		
S. simulans	30		10.0	86.7	3.3	

Trimetoprim (ECOFF[a] = 2.0[b])

Organism	N	N (%) > ECOFF	≤0.5	1	2	4	8	16	32	≥64
S. chromogenes	6			50.0	50.0					
S. epidermidis	27	4 (14.8)	11.1	44.4	29.6		3.7	3.7		7.4
S. haemolyticus	5	4 (80.0)			20.0	40.0	40.0			
S. simulans	30	29 (96.7)	3.3			6.7	36.7	50.0	3.3	

Ciprofloxacin (ECOFF[a] = 1.0)

Organism	N	N (%) > ECOFF	≤0.06	0.12	0.25	0.5	≥1
S. chromogenes	6			100.0			
S. epidermidis	27			14.8	81.5	3.7	
S. haemolyticus	5				80.0	20.0	
S. simulans	30			50.0	50.0		

Fusidic acid (ECOFF[a] = 0.5)

Organism	N	N (%) > ECOFF	≤0.06	0.12	0.25	0.5	1	2	4	8	≥16
S. chromogenes	6	1 (16.7)			66.7	16.7	16.7				
S. epidermidis	27	10 (37.0)			3.7	59.3	25.9	3.7			7.4
S. haemolyticus	5					100.0					
S. simulans	30	10 (33.3)			6.7	60.0	33.3				

In this dataset, samples were collected in the Finnish veterinary antimicrobial resistance monitoring program 2010-2012 [18] and they originated from quarters with mastitis

[a] Current (March 2015) EUCAST epidemiological cut-off (ECOFF) values (mg/l) for CNS were used to define resistant isolates. If ECOFF for CNS was not available, the value for S. aureus was used. For virginiamycin, ECOFF for S. intermedius was used

[b] ECOFF for S. aureus

225 isolates (95.7 %) were negative in the nitrocefin test (true negative), and 10 isolates were positive (false positive). The positive predictive value of the nitrocefin test in relation to penicillin resistance determined based on the MIC value of the isolate was 92.7 and the negative predictive value 85.6.

Considerable proportions of *S. epidermidis* were resistant to tetracycline (46.2/25.9 %) and streptomycin (21.8/7.4 %) (years 2001/2012). In the other species this resistance was rare (Tables 1, 2). Oxacillin resistance (conferring resistance also to methicillin), using ECOFF of 1.0 mg/l, was found in all the four main species (Tables 2, 3). Combining years 2001 and 2012, a total of 137 isolates (34.3 %) were oxacillin resistant. The *mec*A gene was detected in 16 *S. epidermidis* isolates (20.5 %) from the year 2001 and in four *S. epidermidis* isolates (14.8 %) from the year 2012, and in the one *S. sciuri* isolate. Isolates harboring *mec*C were not found. Resistance to trimethoprim, measured only in dataset 2, was most common in *S. simulans* and *S. haemolyticus*, but the number of isolates of the latter species was low (Table 3). *Staphylococcus epidermidis* was the only species showing resistance to cefoxitin using the ECOFF of *S. aureus* (4 mg/l) (Table 3). Resistance to fusidic acid was common in all other species but *S. haemolyticus* (Table 3). One *S. simulans* isolate was resistant to vancomycin, using the specific ECOFF (4 mg/l) for that species (Table 2).

Combining datasets 1 and 2, a total of 44.4 % of *S. chromogenes*, 23.8 % of *S. haemolyticus*, 45.4 % of *S. simulans* and 16.2 % of *S. epidermidis* isolates were susceptible to all antimicrobials tested. Resistance to more than one antimicrobial was most common in *S. epidermidis* isolates. Close to one-third (28.6 %) of them were resistant to >2 antimicrobials. Among the other three major species, one *S. chromogenes* isolate, one *S. haemolyticus* isolate, and five *S. simulans* isolates (4.6 %) were resistant to >2 substances. Seven *S. epidermidis* isolates (6.7 %) were multidrug-resistant (MDR = resistant to 3 or more classes of antimicrobials); one isolate was resistant to five different antimicrobial classes. Among the other species, only one MDR *S. simulans* isolate was found.

Discussion

The most common CoNS species in our data, *S. simulans, S. epidermidis, S. chromogenes,* and *S. haemolyticus,* belong to the CoNS species reported most frequently in numerous studies on bovine intramammary infection (IMI) or mastitis. *Staphylococcus chromogenes* has been isolated most commonly in almost all studies [11–13, 25–29]. It is much more common in primiparous than multiparous cows [11, 28, 30], with peak occurrence around the first calving [4]. *Staphylococcus chromogenes* seems to be present in all herds [26–29] and has been frequently

isolated not only from milk but also from bovine teat skin and orifice and from other body sites of heifers and cows [20, 31]. *Staphylococcus simulans* and *S. epidermidis* are common causes of IMI in some herds but not found or only occasionally found in some other herds [26, 27, 29, 30, 32]. Both *S. epidermidis* and *S. simulans* are reported to be more common in IMIs of multiparous than primiparous cows [11, 28, 30]. For some reason, *S. simulans* is common in the Nordic countries [11, 12, 33] but not so much in Middle European countries [12, 25, 26]. *Staphylococcus xylosus* is commonly reported in Dutch and Belgian studies [13, 26, 27] but is rare in Finland, Norway and Sweden [6, 11, 28]. *Staphylococcus haemolyticus* is a fairly common finding in many studies [11, 13, 26–29]. The reasons for variable proportions of CoNS species isolated from dairy cattle in different countries and individual herds are not fully elucidated but are likely related to different environmental conditions and herd management [10, 31].

In the present study, genotypic identification of CoNS species and species-specific or CoNS-specific EUCAST ECOFFs when available were used. In only few other studies species-specific identification and the same cutoffs than here have been used [5, 6]. In a Swedish study, prevalence of resistant isolates in the four major CoNS species was substantially lower than here [6]. Our results agree with them in that the most common resistance was to benzylpenicillin, but proportion of resistant isolates was clearly lower in the Swedish study. Only one out of 34 Swedish *S. epidermidis* isolates was resistant to oxacillin and harboured the *mec*A gene. In a Swiss study [5], oxacillin resistance was the most common resistance phenotype. They found as much as 47.0 % of the isolates (all CoNS together) to be oxacillin resistant, but the cutoff used was two dilutions lower (0.25 mg/l) than the current EUCAST ECOFF, which explains the discrepant results. The *mec*A gene was present in 9.7 % of the isolates classified as oxacillin-resistant. In the study by Frey et al. [5] the total proportion of penicillin-resistant isolates was lower (23.3 %) than in our study, using the same ECOFF, but the selection of CoNS species was different from ours. Results from the nitrocefin test were compared with results based on the penicillin MIC values of the isolates. The nitrocefin test performed better in detecting penicillin susceptible CoNS isolates; of isolates with MIC for benzylpenicillin >0.125 mg/l, considered as resistant, 23 % were negative in the test. These results agree with the study by Pitkälä et al. [34] comparing different betalactamase tests, who found no false positive but some false negative results for *bla*Z positive CoNS using nitrocefin disk test. In testing bovine *S. aureus* isolates, nitrocefin test has been found to be very reliable [34, 35]. Frey et al. [5] carried out in vitro betalactamase testing with pre-incubation with benzylpenicillin but did not report the results, so we cannot compare them with ours. Interpreting results of bovine CoNS isolates from nitrocefin disk assay is challenging, as the color change is sometimes slow and not clear (Suvi Nykäse-noja, Evira, personal communication). The performance of the nitrocefin tests may not be fully satisfactory in detecting penicillin resistance of bovine CoNS. This is of practical importance because nitrocefin tests are widely used to predict betalactamase production of bovine staphylococci.

Staphylococcus epidermidis was the most resistant among the four major species identified. Almost one-third of our *S. epidermidis* isolates were resistant to >2 antimicrobials and close to 7 % were MDR, which were not found among the other species. This agrees with previous studies which also have reported *S. epidermidis* being frequently resistant to several antimicrobials [5, 36]. The most common combination was resistance to penicillin and tetracycline. All *mecA* positive isolates, except one *mecA* positive *S. sciuri* isolate, were *S. epidermidis*. However, phenotypic methicillin (oxacillin) resistance was also common in the other CoNS species. Among the other three major species, MIC values to oxacillin in the methicillin-resistant isolates were mainly only one step higher than ECOFF and did not form a distinctly different population with clearly higher MIC values. According to many studies, methicillin-resistance is much more common in *S. epidermidis* than in other CoNS species [8, 36–38]. Among clinical *S. epidermidis* isolates from humans, 75–90 % are resistant to methicillin (reviewed by Otto [39]). *Staphylococcus epidermidis* differs from other mastitis causing CoNS in many aspects. It is a well-known human pathogen which causes nosocomial infections often associated with medical devices [39, 40]. *Staphylococcus epidermidis* has a selection of virulence characteristics which include biofilm formation and antimicrobial resistance [3, 40]. It has been suggested that bovine *S. epidermidis* may originate from humans [38, 41]. A Finnish study did not find bovine methicillin-resistant *S. epidermidis* strains being closely related to human isolates [8].

Nearly all *S. simulans* isolates were resistant to trimethoprim. No specific ECOFF is available for this antimicrobial, and we used that of *S. aureus*. The MICs of trimethoprim of most *S. simulans* isolates were several steps above the ECOFF used, which indicates true resistance. More than one-third of *S. epidermidis* and *S. simulans* were resistant to fusidic acid according to ECOFF for CoNS. Looking at the MIC distributions of our isolates, this ECOFF seemed not optimal for this group of CoNS. In a Norwegian study, 10 % of bovine CoNS isolates were resistant to fusidic acid using the same ECOFF, but all

isolates classified as resistant had MIC values several steps over the cut-off [42]. In some CoNS species resistance is more common (Table 2). Almost half of *S. epidermidis* isolates of human origin have been resistant to fusidic acid and harbored the same horizontally acquired resistance determinants than reported in *S. aureus* [43].

Antimicrobial resistance among bovine CoNS isolates causes two types of concerns. First, it decreases options for antimicrobial treatment of mastitis as well as response to treatment. Mastitis caused by CoNS is mostly subclinical or mild clinical and routine treatment is not recommended [4]. In cases where treatment is warranted, resistance to benzylpenicillin is an issue at least in countries where penicillin or aminopenicillins are the drugs of choice [4]. Penicillin resistance of three of the four major CoNS species was here at so high level that penicillin can no more be considered as the first treatment option in mastitis caused by these species. Another option could be macrolides to which some degree of resistance was also found, in particular among *S. epidermidis* isolates. Prevalences of oxacillin resistant isolates were alarmingly high in all four major species. Cloxacillin is commonly used to treat mastitis, also mastitis caused by CoNS, so this is of practical relevance. If the causing CoNS strain harbors a *mec* gene, treatment with any betalactam antimicrobial is inefficient and only increases selection pressure.

The second concern is related to public health: cows can pass resistant CoNS to humans via direct contact or indirectly [37]. Bovine CoNS can also act as a reservoir for resistance determinants [3, 44]. The greatest concern is methicillin-resistance which was common in bovine CoNS and presents a relevant risk for public health [38, 40]. There is evidence for transfer of resistance determinants between staphylococcal species and also from CoNS to the more pathogenic species *S. aureus* [9, 44–46]. Regarding critically important antimicrobials [47] included in the present study, the situation was good as only one CoNS isolate (*S. simulans*) was resistant to vancomycin and no isolates to ciprofloxacin.

Unfortunately specific ECOFFs are not yet available for all CoNS species, and we had to use those of *S. aureus* for several antimicrobials. EUCAST ECOFFs are not veterinary specific but isolates originate from multiple sources and perhaps mainly from humans. Most studies on antimicrobial resistance of CoNS have used CLSI (Clinical and Laboratory Standards Institute) [48] breakpoints for veterinary pathogens. CLSI breakpoints are aimed for clinical purposes only [48]. They are derived from animal specific microbiological, pharmacokinetic and pharmacodynamic data, which is not relevant for studies on in vitro susceptibility of epidemiological data sets [15]. Furthermore, animal specific breakpoints are not available for all antimicrobials and those based on human data have been used [48]. CLSI documents do not give specific breakpoints for bovine CoNS, but some breakpoints are available for *S. aureus*. In general, CLSI breakpoints are higher than EUCAST ECOFFs. Studies which have used different breakpoints for resistance cannot be compared. After phenotypic screening of antimicrobial resistance, as done here, the next step would be to study the genetic mechanisms for resistance. For many antimicrobials several genes can code for resistance in staphylococci, and new genes are discovered [44, 45]. Selection of a representative panel of resistance genes for genotypic studies is challenging.

Conclusions

The most common CoNS species were *S. simulans*, *S. epidermidis*, *S. chromogenes*, and *S. haemolyticus*. *Staphylococcus epidermidis* differed from the three other most common CoNS species isolated from mastitic bovine milk samples as resistance to most tested antimicrobials was more common in *S. epidermidis* than in *S. chromogenes*, *S. haemolyticus* or *S. simulans*. Except one *S. sciuri* isolate, all *mec*A gene positive isolates were *S. epidermidis*. Resistance to more than two antimicrobials was also common in *S. epidermidis*.

Authors' contributions
ST and SP planned the study. AP, SN and TP collected the data and performed the in vitro antimicrobial susceptibility analyses. ST performed the *Staphylococcus* species identification and data analysis. ST and SP wrote the manuscript. AP, SN and TP commented on the manuscript. All authors read and approved the final manuscript.

Author details
[1] Department of Production Animal Medicine, Faculty of Veterinary Medicine, University of Helsinki, Paroninkuja 20, 04920 Saarentaus, Finland. [2] Finnish Food Safety Authority Evira, Mustialankatu 3, 00790 Helsinki, Finland.

Acknowledgements
Taina Lehto is thanked for excellent laboratory assistance in ribotyping of the isolates. Walter Ehrström Foundation is acknowledged for financial support for ribotyping.

Competing interests
The authors declare that they have no competing interests.

References
1. Myllys V, Asplund K, Brofeldt E, Hirvelä-Koski V, Honkanen-Buzalski T, Junttila J, et al. Bovine mastitis in Finland in 1988 and 1995—changes in prevalence and antimicrobial resistance. Acta Vet Scand. 1998;39:119–26.
2. Pitkälä A, Haveri M, Pyörälä S, Myllys V, Honkanen-Buzalski T. Bovine mastitis in Finland 2001—prevalence, distribution of bacteria, and antimicrobial resistance. J Dairy Sci. 2004;87:2433–41.
3. Vanderhaeghen W, Piepers S, Leroy F, Van Coillie E, Haesebrouck F, De Vliegher S. Invited review: effect, persistence, and virulence of coagulase-negative *Staphylococcus* species associated with ruminant udder health. J Dairy Sci. 2014;97:5275–93.
4. Pyörälä S, Taponen S. Coagulase-negative staphylococci—emerging mastitis pathogens. Vet Microbiol. 2009;134:3–8.
5. Frey Y, Rodriguez JP, Thomann A, Schwendener S, Perreten V. Genetic characterization of antimicrobial resistance in coagulase-negative staphylococci from bovine mastitis milk. J Dairy Sci. 2013;96:2247–57.
6. Persson Waller K, Aspán A, Nyman A, Persson Y, Grönlund Andersson U. CNS species and antimicrobial resistance in clinical and subclinical bovine mastitis. Vet Microbiol. 2011;152:112–6.
7. Huber H, Ziegler D, Pflüger V, Vogel G, Zweifel C, Stephan R. Prevalence and characteristics of methicillin resistant coagulase-negative staphylococci from livestock, chicken carcasses, bulk tank milk, minced meat, and contact persons. BMC Vet Res. 2011;7:6.
8. Gindonis V, Taponen S, Myllyniemi A-M, Pyörälä S, Nykäsenoja S, Salmenlinna S, et al. Occurrence and characterization of methicillin-resistant staphylococci from bovine mastitis milk samples in Finland. Acta Vet Scand. 2013;55:61.
9. Juuti K, Ibrahem S, Virolainen-Julkunen A, Vuopio-Varkila J, Kuusela P. The pls gene found in methicillin-resistant *Staphylococcus aureus* strains is common in clinical isolates of *Staphylococcus sciuri*. J Clin Microbiol. 2005;43:1415–9.
10. Vanderhaeghen W, Vandendriessche S, Crombé F, Nemeghaire S, Dispas M, Denis O, et al. Characterization of methicillin-resistant non-*Staphylococcus aureus* staphylococci carriage isolates from different bovine populations. J Antimicrob Chemother. 2013;68:300–7.
11. Taponen S, Simojoki H, Haveri M, Larsen HD, Pyörälä S. Clinical characteristics and persistence of bovine mastitis caused by different species of coagulase-negative staphylococci identified with API or AFLP. Vet Microbiol. 2006;115:199–207.
12. Capurro A, Artursson K, Persson Waller K, Bengtsson B, Ericsson-Unnerstad H, Aspán A. Comparison of a commercialized phenotyping system, antimicrobial susceptibility testing, and a *tuf* gene sequence-based genotyping for species-level identification of coagulase-negative staphylococci isolated from cases of bovine mastitis. Vet Microbiol. 2009;134:327–33.
13. Sampimon OC, Zadoks RN, De Vliegher S, Supré K, Haesebrouck F, Barkema HW, et al. Performance of API Staph ID 32 and Staph-Zym for identification of coagulase-negative staphylococci isolated from bovine milk samples. Vet Microbiol. 2009;136:300–5.
14. Moser A, Stephan R, Ziegler D, Johler S. Species distribution and resistance profiles of coagulase-negative staphylococci isolated from bovine mastitis in Switzerland. Schweiz Arch Tierheilkd. 2013;155:333–8.
15. Schwarz S, Silleya P, Simjee S, Woodford N, van Duijkeren E, Johnson AP, et al. Editorial: assessing the antimicrobial susceptibility of bacteria obtained from animals. Vet Microbiol. 2010;141:1–4.
16. Ruegg PL, Oliveira L, Jin W, Okwumabua O. Phenotypic antimicrobial susceptibility and occurrence of selected resistance genes in grampositive mastitis pathogens isolated from Wisconsin dairy cows. J Dairy Sci. 2015;98:1–14.
17. Wendlandt S, Kadlec K, Feßler AT, Schwarz S. Identification of ABC transporter genes conferring combined pleuromutilin–lincosamide–streptogramin A resistance in bovine methicillin-resistant *Staphylococcus aureus* and coagulase-negative staphylococci. Vet Microbiol. 2015;177:353–8.
18. FINRES-Vet 2010–2012. Finnish Veterinary Antimicrobial Resistance Monitoring and Consumption of Antimicrobial Agents. Evira publications 2/2015. Finnish Food Safety Authority Evira, Helsinki, Finland. ISSN 1797-299X, ISBN 978-952-225-143-5 (pdf). http://www.evira.fi/portal/fi/tietoa+evirasta/julkaisut/?a=view&productId=412 .
19. Honkanen-Buzalski T, Seuna E. Isolation and identification of pathogens from milk. In: Sandholm M, Honkanen-Buzalski T, Kaartinen L, Pyörälä S, editors. The bovine udder and mastitis. Gummerus, Jyväskylä, Finland; 1995. p. 121–41.
20. Taponen S, Björkroth J, Pyörälä S. Coagulase-negative staphylococci isolated from bovine extramammary sites and intramammary infections in a single dairy herd. J Dairy Res. 2008;75:422–9.
21. Dubois D, Leyssene D, Chacornac JP, Kostrzewa M, Schmit PO, Talon R, et al. Identification of a variety of *Staphylococcus* species by matrix-assisted laser desorption ionization-time of flight mass spectrometry. J Clin Microbiol. 2010;48:941–5.
22. EUCAST: European Committee on Antimicrobial Susceptibility testing. European Society of Clinical Microbiology and Infectious Diseases. http://www.eucast.org/.

23. Murakami K, Minamide W, Wada K, Nakamura E, Teraoka H, Watanabe S. Identification of methicillin-resistant strains of staphylococci by polynerase chain reaction. J Clin Microbiol. 1991;29:2240–4.

24. Stegger M, Andersen PS, Kearns A, Pichon B, Holmes MA, Edwards G, et al. Rapid detection, differentiation and typing of methicillin-resistant *Staphylococcus aureus* harbouring either *mecA* or the new *mecA* homologue *mecA* (LGA251). Clin Microbiol Infect. 2012;18:395–400.

25. Rajala-Schultz PJ, Torres AH, DeGraves FJ, Gebreyes WA, Patchanee P. Antimicrobial resistance and genotypic characterization of coagulase-negative staphylococci over the dry period. Vet Microbiol. 2009;134:55–64.

26. Piessens V, Van Coillie E, Verbist B, Supré K, Braem G, Van Nuffel A, et al. Distribution of coagulase-negative *Staphylococcus* species from milk and environment of dairy cows differs between herds. J Dairy Sci. 2011;94:2933–44.

27. Supré K, Haesebrouck F, Zadoks RN, Vaneechoutte M, Piepers S, De Vliegher S. Some coagulase-negative *Staphylococcus* species affect udder health more than others. J Dairy Sci. 2011;94:2329–40.

28. Mørk T, Jørgensen HJ, Sunde M, Kvitle B, Sviland S, Waage S, et al. Persistence of staphylococcal species and genotypes in the bovine udder. Vet Microbiol. 2012;159:171–80.

29. Bexiga R, Rato MG, Lemsaddek A, Semedo-Lemsaddek T, Carneiro C, Pereira H, et al. Dynamics of bovine intramammary infections due to coagulase-negative staphylococci on four farms. J Dairy Res. 2014;81:208–14.

30. Thorberg BM, Danielsson-Tham ML, Emanuelson U. Persson Waller K. Bovine subclinical mastitis caused by different types of coagulase-negative staphylococci. J Dairy Sci. 2009;92:4962–70.

31. De Visscher A, Piepers S, Haesebrouck F, De Vliegher S. Teat apex colonization with coagulase-negative *Staphylococcus* species before parturition: distribution and species-specific risk factors. J Dairy Sci. 2016;99:1–13.

32. Gillespie BE, Headrick SI, Boonyayatra S, Oliver SP. Prevalence and persistence of coagulase-negative *Staphylococcus* species in three dairy research herds. Vet Microbiol. 2009;134:65–72.

33. Waage S, Mørk T, Røros A, Aasland D, Hunshamar A, Ødegaard SA. Bacteria associated with clinical mastitis in dairy heifers. J Dairy Sci. 1999;1999(82):712–9.

34. Pitkälä A, Salmikivi L, Bredbacka P, Myllyniemi A-L, Koskinen MT. Comparison of tests for detection of ß-lactamase-producing Staphylococci. J Clin Microbiol. 2007;45:2031–3.

35. Haveri M, Suominen S, Rantala L, Honkanen-Buzalski T, Pyörälä S. Comparison of phenotypic and genotypic detection of penicillin G resistance of *Staphylococcus aureus* isolated from bovine intramammary infection. Vet Microbiol. 2005;106:97–102.

36. Sampimon OC, Lam TJ, Mevius DJ, Schukken YH, Zadoks RN. Antimicrobial susceptibility of coagulase-negative staphylococci isolated from bovine milk samples. Vet Microbiol. 2011;150:173–9.

37. Feßler AT, Billerbeck C, Kadlec K, Schwarz S. Identification and characterization of methicillin-resistant coagulase-negative staphylococci from bovine mastitis. J Antimicrob Chemother. 2010;65:1576–82.

38. Jaglic Z, Michu E, Holasova M, Vlkova H, Babak V, Kolar M, et al. Epidemiology and characterization of *Staphylococcus epidermidis* isolates from humans, raw bovine milk and a dairy plant. Epidemiol Infect. 2010;138:772–82.

39. Otto M. *Staphylococcus epidermidis*—the "accidental" pathogen. Nat Rev Microbiol. 2009;7:555–67.

40. Schoenfelder SMK, Langea C, Eckart M, Hennig S, Kozytska S, Ziebuhr W. Success through diversity—how *Staphylococcus epidermidis* establishes as a nosocomial pathogen. Int J Med Microbiol. 2010;300:380–6.

41. Thorberg B-M, Kühn I, Aarestrup FM, Brändström B, Jonsson P, Danielsson-Tham M-L. Pheno- and genotyping of *Staphylococcus epidermidis* isolated from bovine milk and human skin. Vet Microbiol. 2006;115:163–72.

42. Yazdankdhah SP, Åsli AW, Sørum H, Oppegaard H, Sunde M. Fusidic acid resistance, mediated by fusB, in bovine coagulase-negative staphylococci. J Antimicrob Chemother. 2006;58:1254–6.

43. McLaws F, Chopra I, O'Neill AJ. High prevalence of resistance to fusidic acid in clinical isolates of *Staphylococcus epidermidis*. J Antimicrob Chemother. 2008;61:1040–3.

44. Nemeghaire S, Argudín MA, Feßler AT, Hauschild T, Schwarz S, Butaye P. The ecological importance of the *Staphylococcus sciuri* species group as a reservoir for resistance and virulence genes. Vet Microbiol. 2014;171:342–56.

45. Wendlandt S, Feßler AT, Monecke S, Ehricht R, Schwarz S, Kadlec K. The diversity of antimicrobial resistance genes among staphylococci of animal origin. Int J Med Microbiol. 2013;303:338–49.

46. Zhang Y, Agidi S, LeJeune JT. Diversity of staphylococcal cassette chromosome in coagulase-negative staphylococci from animal sources. J Appl Microbiol. 2009;107:1375–83.

47. Collignon P, Powers J, Chiller T, Aidara-Kane A, Aarestrup F. World Health Organization ranking of antimicrobials according to their importance in human medicine: a critical step for developing risk management strategies for the use of antimicrobials in food production animals. Clin Inf Dis. 2009;49:132–41.

48. CLSI. VET01-S2. Performance standards for Antimicrobial disk and dilution susceptibility test for bacteria isolated from animals; Second Informational Supplement. Clinical and Laboratory Standards Institute, 950 West Valley Road, Suite 2500, Wayne; 2013.

4

Heritability of hypothyroidism in the Finnish Hovawart population

Johanna Åhlgren and Pekka Uimari[*]

Abstract

Background: The Hovawart is a working and companion dog breed of German origin. A few hundred Hovawart dogs are registered annually in Finland. The most common disease with a proposed genetic background in Hovawarts is hypothyroidism. The disease is usually caused by lymphocytic thyroiditis, an autoimmune disorder which destroys the thyroid gland. Hypothyroidism can be treated medically with hormone replacement. Its overall incidence could also be reduced through selection, provided that the trait shows an adequate genetic basis. The aim of this study was to estimate the heritability of hypothyroidism in the Finnish Hovawart population.

Results: The pedigree data for the study were provided by the Finnish Kennel Club and the hypothyroidism data by the Finnish Hovawart Club. The data included 4953 dogs born between 1990 and 2010, of which 107 had hypothyroidism and 4846 were unaffected. Prior to the estimation of heritability, we studied the effects of gender, birth year, birth month, and inbreeding on susceptibility to hypothyroidism. Heritability was estimated with the probit model both via restricted maximum likelihood (REML) and Gibbs sampling, using litter and sire of the dog as random effects. None of the studied systematic effects or level of inbreeding had a significant effect on susceptibility to hypothyroidism. The estimated heritability of hypothyroidism varied from 0.47 (SE = 0.18) using REML to 0.62 (SD = 0.21) using Gibbs sampling.

Conclusions: Based on our analysis, the heritability of hypothyroidism is moderate to high, suggesting that its prevalence could be decreased through selection. Thus, breeders should notify the breed association of any affected dogs, and their use for breeding should be avoided.

Keywords: Dog, Gibbs sampling, Heritability, Hovawart, Hypothyroidism, Probit model

Background

Hypothyroidism is one of the most common hereditary diseases in Finnish Hovawart dogs, and actually the most common endocrine disease in all dogs [1]. The prevalence of hypothyroidism between different breeds varies from 0.2 to 0.9 % [2–4]. In some breeds considerable higher prevalence have been reported e.g. 2.7 % for a cohort of 8 year old Gordon setters [5], 13 % for Swedish Hovawarts [6], and as high as 16 % for Giant Schnauzers [6] and for Beagles [7]. The disease is rarely diagnosed in dogs under the ages of 2–4 years [8]. Hypothyroidism is mainly caused by lymphocytic thyroiditis or idiopathic thyroid atrophy [6]. Lymphocytic thyroiditis is

considered as an autoimmune disorder [9, 10] and has a hereditary predisposition [2, 7, 11]. It also has been suggested that the disease may be influenced by a major gene [11]. Lymphocytic thyroiditis is known to be associated with the major histocompatibility complex (MHC) or dog leukocyte antigen (DLA) system class II allele [5, 12–14]. Several DLA haplotypes which increase the risk to acquire hypothyroidism have been identified in different breeds [5, 12, 14]. However, the recent whole genome association study with SNP (single nucleotide polymorphism) markers indicated that a separate region in the vicinity of DLA is also associated with hypothyroidism in dogs [15]. The association between certain DLA haplotypes and the risk of hypothyroidism together with the immune-mediated nature of this disease [16, 17] leads to the hypothesis that inbreeding increases its incidence.

*Correspondence: pekka.uimari@helsinki.fi
Department of Agricultural Sciences, University of Helsinki, Helsinki, Finland

Gender and neutering may also raise the incidence of hypothyroidism: a higher incidence of hypothyroidism has been observed for castrated males and females than for uncastrated males and females [2, 3] and a higher incidence for females than for males [3]. However, the genetic background of hypothyroidism has not been studied extensively, and only a few heritability estimates have been reported. Benjamin et al. [7] obtained a moderate estimate of heritability (0.3) based on 276 laboratory Beagle dogs with 16 % diagnosed as hypothyroid, and a slightly smaller estimate (0.2) based on over 1000 laboratory Beagles in an experiment designed to study the effect of radiation on the risk of hypothyroidism [11]. The heredity estimates presented here for hypothyroidism in the Finnish Hovawart population are based on a pedigree analysis of 107 dogs affected with hypothyroidism and 4846 unaffected dogs. We also tested the effects of gender, birth year, birth month, and level of inbreeding on the dogs' susceptibility to hypothyroidism.

Methods

The list of dogs diagnosed with hypothyroidism was provided by the Finnish Hovawart Club. Only dogs born between 1990 and 2010 were used in this study resulting to 107 affected dogs in the data. The prevalence of hypothyroidism in Finnish Hovawart dogs by birth year is presented in Fig. 1. The dogs with hypothyroidism were self-reported by the breeders or the owners of the dogs to the breed association and were based on diagnoses made by different veterinarians using clinical signs and laboratory tests [see e.g. 18]. The upper birth year of 2010 was selected so that the youngest dogs were at

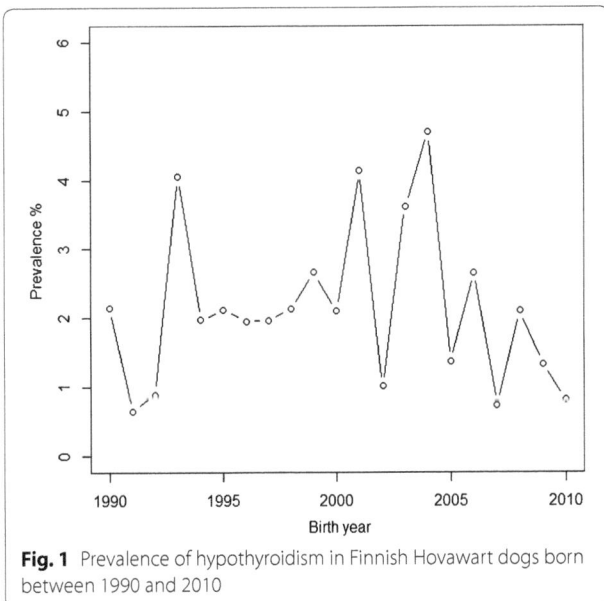

Fig. 1 Prevalence of hypothyroidism in Finnish Hovawart dogs born between 1990 and 2010

least 2–4 years-of-age at the time the affection status data were received from the breed association in September 2014. Some of these dogs may have developed hypothyroidism at older age after that. The pedigree data were obtained from the Finnish Kennel Club and included 7178 animals. Dogs not included in the list of dogs with hypothyroidism and born between 1990 and 2010 were extracted from the pedigree file, a total of 4846 dogs, and treated as unaffected. Based on the phenotypic data, the prevalence of hypothyroidism was 2.2 %. Eight sires had two affected progeny, three sires had three affected progeny, four sires had four affected progeny, and one sire had seven affected progeny in multiple litters. Of the dams, seven had two affected progeny, four dams had three affected progeny, three dams had four affected progeny, and one dam had five affected progeny.

Prior to genetic analysis, we studied the influence of gender, birth year, birth month, and level of inbreeding on hypothyroidism susceptibility using the generalized linear model in IBM SPSS Statistics v.21. Birth months were classified into four seasons: December to February, March to May, June to August, and September to November. The effect of inbreeding on susceptibility to hypothyroidism was tested by logistic regression, only including individuals born between 1990 and 2010 and having a pedigree completeness value [19] of over 90 % based on five ancestral generations. This criterion was met by 4115 dogs.

Variance components were estimated via the restricted maximum likelihood (REML) method [20] with a probit link function assuming an underlying, unobservable, normally distributed liability [21]. The following linear model was used for the variance component estimation:

$$\text{probit}(p_{ijk}) = \mu + \text{birthy}_i + \text{litter}_j + \text{sire}_k,$$

where $\text{probit}(p_{ijk}) = \Phi^{-1} \times P(y_{ijk} = 1)$. $P(y_{ijk} = 1)$ is the probability that the dog has hypothyroidism given that its sire is k and it was born in litter j during year (birthy) i. Φ is the cumulative density function of the underlying normal distribution. The random sire effect was assumed to have a normal distribution with mean 0 and a variance–covariance structure of $A\sigma_s^2$, where A is the additive relationship matrix between the sires and maternal grandsires and σ_s^2 is the sire variance. The litter effect was also a random effect with a normal distribution with mean 0 and a variance structure of $I\sigma_l^2$, where I is the identity matrix with diagonal elements of σ_l^2 (litter variance). Residual variance (σ_e^2) was fixed at 1. The heritability of the underlying liability was estimated as:

$$h^2 = \frac{4\sigma_s^2}{\sigma_l^2 + \sigma_s^2 + 1} \qquad (1)$$

Additionally, we estimated the variance components using a Bayesian analysis via Gibbs sampling. The theoretical basis of the Gibbs sampling approach for mixed linear models is presented by Wang et al. [22] and is not repeated here. The length of the Gibbs chain was set to 205,000, where the first 5000 realizations of the parameter estimates were discarded (burn-in period). The final posterior mean, standard deviation, and distribution were based on every 50th iteration of the chain (thinning). An uninformative prior was used for the birth year effect, and a scaled inverted Chi square distribution with v = 6 as a degree of belief parameter and variance component estimates from the REML method as a prior values for the variance components σ_l^2 and σ_s^2, respectively [22]. A probit link function was used to link the observed binary trait (hypothyroidism status) to the unobserved normally distributed liability. Residual variance (σ_e^2) was fixed at 1, as with the generalized linear mixed model approach. The variance components were estimated using the DMU program package [23].

Results and discussion

The prevalence of hypothyroidism in the Finnish Hovawart population was similar than observed previously for other breeds [2–5]. However, because the affection status was based on self-reporting by the dog owners we can expect that the true prevalence of hypothyroidism in Finnish Hovawart population is in fact higher than reported here. To obtain reliable estimates of the prevalence, the diagnostic criteria for hypothyroidism should remain the same throughout the years. In addition, a specific cohort or cross-sectional study where all the dogs fulfilling e.g. a minimum age of 4 years are diagnosed for hypothyroidism and followed-up later in their life would have also improved the quality of the data. This view is supported by the Swedish study by Ferm et al. [6] where the proportion of affected dogs increased from 6 to 13 % after all dogs that had no clinical signs nor were medically treated for hypothyroidism were tested for TgAA and THS-levels.

With our data, the gender of the dog had no effect on its susceptibility to hypothyroidism (P value = 0.78); the incidence of hypothyroidism in males and females was 2.1 and 2.2 %, respectively. This is contrary to the findings of Panciera [3] but in line with the results of Dixon [4] and Benjamin [7]. Neutering status was not available in our data and was not considered here. The dog's birth year was significant with a 10 % error level (P value = 0.08) and was included in the final mixed model, whereas birth season was not significantly associated with hypothyroidism (P value = 0.21).

The average inbreeding of Hovawart dogs born between 1990 and 2010 is presented in Fig. 2. The average

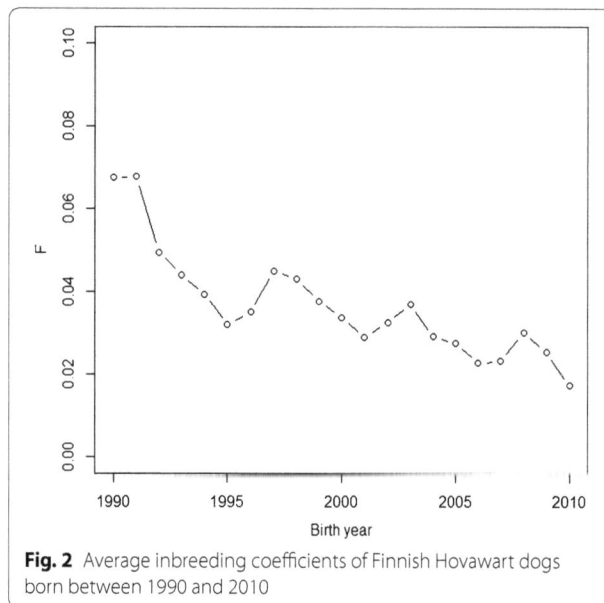

Fig. 2 Average inbreeding coefficients of Finnish Hovawart dogs born between 1990 and 2010

level of inbreeding has generally been on the decline during the last two decades, decreasing from 6.7 % in dogs born in 1990 to less than 2 % in dogs born in 2010. Dogs diagnosed with hypothyroidism had an average inbreeding level of 3.2 %, which is lower than for dogs treated as healthy in this study (3.5 %). The regression coefficient of inbreeding from the logistic regression model was not significant (b = 1.04; SE = 2.08); thus, there was no indication that inbreeding increases the dogs' susceptibility to hypothyroidism, at least with the inbreeding levels typical of the Finnish Hovawart population. Benjamin et al. [11] also found no effect of inbreeding on susceptibility to hypothyroidism.

The REML method with the probit model gave an estimated variance of 0.07 (SE = 0.07) for the litter effect and of 0.14 (SE = 0.06) for the sire effect. The estimated heritability of the underlying liability, thus, was 0.47 (SE = 0.18) [Eq. 1]. The smaller estimates for litter effect than for the sire effect is somewhat unexpected because part of the variance related to dams should be accounted by the litter effect. Given the size of the data the REML method may not have been able correctly distribute the underlying phenotypic variance between the sire and litter effects. The marginal posterior densities based on Gibbs sampling for the litter and sire variances and for heritability are presented in Fig. 3. A high value for the mean of the marginal posterior distribution was obtained for heritability ($h^2 = 0.62$, SD = 0.21). The corresponding posterior means for the sire and litter variances were 0.23 (SD = 0.09) and 0.26 (SD = 0.14), respectively. The difference in heritability estimates between the two methods (REML and Gibbs sampling) is relatively large but not

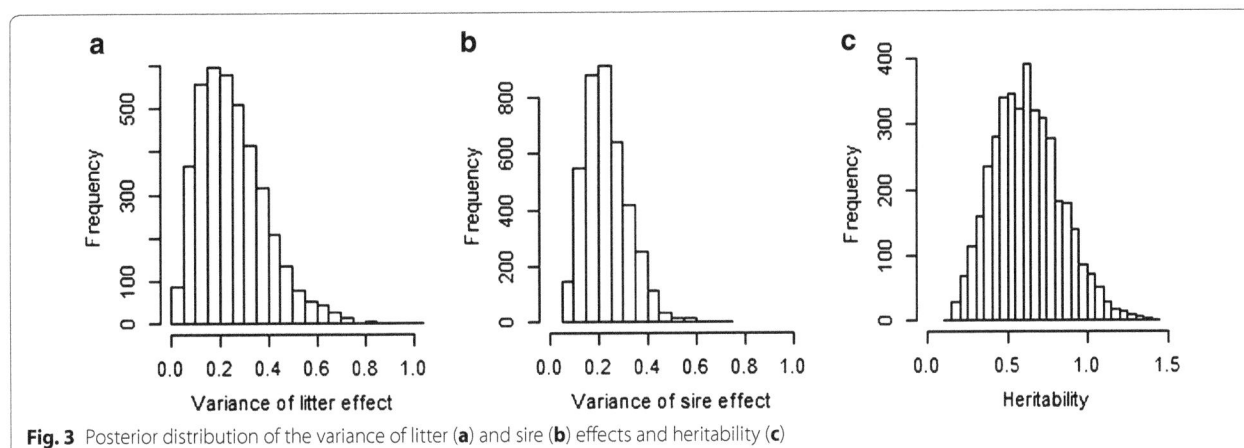

Fig. 3 Posterior distribution of the variance of litter (**a**) and sire (**b**) effects and heritability (**c**)

significant, considering the standard error and standard deviation of the estimates. Also the generalized linear mixed model approach tend to over shrink random effects and their corresponding variances [21]. Thus, the smaller estimates of heritability from the REML method compared to one from Gibbs sampling is expected. Use of a different prior distribution for the variance components ($v = 3$ or $v = 4$ instead of $v = 6$ for the degree of belief of the scaled inverted Chi square distributions) had no effect on the heritability estimates.

The diagnosis of hypothyroidism is challenging, because all affected dogs do not show clinical signs and not all may have been tested in a laboratory. Moreover, notification to the breed club about the disorder is on a voluntary basis, which means that the list of hypothyroid dogs maintained by the Finnish Hovawart Club may be incomplete. Our study data can therefore include dogs given a healthy status although they were, in fact, affected. Also, the data only contained information that is routinely recorded for registration purposes: parents, gender, birth date, color, and breeder, most of which had no influence on susceptibility to hypothyroidism. On the other hand, the data did not enable us to study the effects of other, perhaps more important factors that might increase the risk to acquire hypothyroidism, such as the dogs' nutritional status or exercise level.

Despite the limitations of the data, our results offer clear evidence that hypothyroidism involves a genetic component. The analysis did not allow to determine whether the genetic component is due to only one or just a few risk genes, or whether the genetic background is more polygenic in nature. Based on the immune-mediated character of hypothyroidism it can be postulated that the variation in the DLA area probably explains at least some of the obtained heritability [5, 12–14]. The high heritability of the disease suggests that a reasonable reduction in its incidence could be obtained by avoiding

the use of dogs diagnosed with hypothyroidism and their close relatives in breeding. However, since hypothyroidism can in practice be diagnosed only later in life, it is not possible to exclude all affected dogs from breeding.

Conclusions
The prevalence of hypothyroidism in the Finnish Hovawart population is relatively high. Our pedigree analysis gave moderate to high heritability estimates for this trait, depending on the method applied. The high heritability of hypothyroidism suggests that selection against it should be effective by using only healthy dogs for breeding.

Authors' contributions
Both JÅ and PU performed the statistical analysis and drafted the manuscript. Both authors read and approved the final manuscript.

Competing interests
The authors declare that they have no competing interests.

References
1. Egenvall A, Bonnett BN, Olson P, Hedhammar A. Gender, age and breed pattern of diagnoses for veterinary care in insured dogs in Sweden during 1996. Vet Rec. 2000;146:551–7.
2. Milne KL, Hayes HM. Epidemiologic features of canine hypothyroidism. 1981. http://babel.hathitrust.org/cgi/pt?id=uc1.b4179407;view=1up;seq=11. Accessed 20 Oct 2015.
3. Panciera DL. Hypothyroidism in dogs: 66 cases (1987–1992). J Am Vet Med Assoc. 1994;204:761–7.
4. Dixon RM, Reid SW, Mooney CT. Epidemiological, clinical, haematological and biochemical characteristics of canine hypothyroidism. Vet Rec. 1999;145:481–7.
5. Ziener ML, Dahlgren S, Thoresen SI, Lingaas F. Genetics and epidemiology of hypothyroidism and symmetrical onychomadesis in the Gordon setter and the English setter. Canine Genet Epidemiol. 2015;2:12.
6. Ferm K, Bjornerfeldt S, Karlsson A, Andersson G, Nachreiner R, Hedhammar A. Prevalence of diagnostic characteristics indicating canine autoimmune lymphocytic thyroiditis in giant schnauzer and hovawart dogs. J Small Anim Pract. 2009;50:76–9.

7. Benjamin SA, Stephens LC, Hamilton BF, Saunders WJ, Lee AC, Angleton GM, Mallinckrodt CH. Associations between lymphocytic thyroiditis, hypothyroidism, and thyroid neoplasia in Beagles. Vet Pathol. 1996;33:486–94.

8. Graham PA, Refsal KR, Nachreiner RF. Etiopathologic findings of canine hypothyroidism. Vet Clin North Am Small Anim Pract. 2007;37:617–31.

9. Graham PA, Nachreiner RF, Provencher-Bolliger AL. Lymphocytic thyroiditis. Vet Clin North Am Small Anim Pract. 2001;31:915–33.

10. Ferguson DC. Testing for Hypothyroidism in Dogs. Vet Clin Small Anim. 2007;37:647–69.

11. Benjamin SA, Saunders WJ, Lee AC, Angleton GM, Stephens LC, Mallinckrodt CH. Non-neoplastic and neoplastic thyroid disease in beagles irradiated during prenatal and postnatal development. Radiat Res. 1997;147:422–30.

12. Kennedy LJ, Huson HJ, Leonard J, Angles JM, Fox LE, Wojciechowski JW, Yuncker C, Happ GM. Association of hypothyroid disease in Doberman Pinscher dogs with a rare major histocompatibility complex DLA class II haplotype. Tissue Antigens. 2006;67:53–6.

13. Kennedy LJ, Quarmby S, Happ GM, Barnes A, Ramsey IK, Dixon RM, et al. Association of canine hypothyroidism with a common major histocompatibility complex DLA class II allele. Tissue Antigens. 2006;68:82–6.

14. Wilbe M, Sundberg K, Hansen IR, Strandberg E, Nachreiner RF, Hedhammar A, et al. Increased genetic risk or protection for canine autoimmune lymphocytic thyroiditis in Giant Schnauzers depends on DLA class II genotype. Tissue Antigens. 2010;75:712–9.

15. Bianchi M, Dahlgren S, Massey J, Dietschi E, Kierczak M, Lund-Ziener M, et al. A multi-breed genome-wide association analysis for canine hypothyroidism identifies a shared major risk locus on CFA12. PLoS ONE. 2015;10:e0134720.

16. Beierwaltes WH, Nishiyama RH. Dog thyroiditis: occurrence and similarity to Hashimoto's struma. Endocrinology. 1968;83:501–8.

17. Mizejewski GJ, Baron J, Poissant G. Immunologic investigations of naturally occurring canine thyroiditis. J Immunol. 1971;107:1152–60.

18. Graham P. Canine hypothyroidism: diagnosis and therapy. In Prac. 2009;31:77–82.

19. McCluer J, Boyce A, Dyke B, Weitkamp L, Pfenning W, Parsons J. Inbreeding and Pedigree structure in standardbred horses. J Hered. 1983;74:394–9.

20. Patterson HD, Thompson R. Recovery of inter-block information when block sizes are unequal. Biometrika. 1971;58:545–54.

21. Gilmor AR, Anderson RD, Rae AL. The analysis of binomial data by generalized linear mixed model. Biometrika. 1985;72:593–9.

22. Wang CS, Rutledge JJ, Gianola D. Bayesian analysis of mixed linear models via Gibbs sampling with an application to litter size in Iberian pigs. Genet Sel Evol. 1994;26:91–115.

23. Madsen P, Jensen J. A user's guide to DMU. A package for analyzing multivariate mixed models. V.6, r. 5.2. Center for quantitative genetics and genomics. Dept. of Molecular Biology and Genetics, University of Aarhus. Research Centre Foulum. Denmark. 2013. p. 32.

5

Presence of foodborne pathogens, extended-spectrum β-lactamase -producing *Enterobacteriaceae*, and methicillin-resistant *Staphylococcus aureus* in slaughtered reindeer in northern Finland and Norway

Sauli Laaksonen[1], Antti Oksanen[2], Jérôme Julmi[3], Claudio Zweifel[3], Maria Fredriksson-Ahomaa[4] and Roger Stephan[3*]

Abstract

Background: Various food-producing animals were recognized in recent years as healthy carriers of bacterial pathogens causing human illness. In northern Fennoscandia, the husbandry of semi-domesticated reindeer (*Rangifer tarandus tarandus*) is a traditional livelihood and meat is the main product. This study determined the presence of selected foodborne pathogens, methicillin-resistant *Staphylococcus aureus* (MRSA), and extended-spectrum β-lactamase (ESBL)-producing *Enterobacteriaceae* in healthy semi-domesticated reindeer at slaughter in northern Finland and Norway.

Results: All 470 reindeer fecal samples tested negative for *Salmonella* spp., whereas *L. monocytogenes* was detected in 3%, *Yersinia* spp. in 10%, and Shiga toxins genes (*stx*1 and/or *stx*2) in 33% of the samples. *Listeria monocytogenes* isolates belonged to the serotype 1/2a (14/15) and 4b, *Yersinia* spp. were identified mainly as *Y. kristensenii* (30/46) and *Y. enterocolitica* (8/46), and *stx*2 predominated among the Shiga toxin genes (*stx*2 alone or in combination with *stx*1 was found in 25% of the samples). With regard to the frequency and distribution of *stx*1/*stx*2, striking differences were evident among the 10 different areas of origin. Hence, reindeer could constitute a reservoir for Shiga toxin-producing *E. coli* (STEC), but strain isolation and characterization is required for verification purposes and to assess the potential human pathogenicity of strains. On the other hand, the favorable antibiotic resistance profiles (only 5% of 95 *E. coli* isolates were resistant to one or more of the tested antibiotics) and the absence of MRSA and ESBL-producing *Enterobacteriaceae* (when applying selective methods) suggest only a limited risk of transmission to humans.

Conclusions: Healthy semi-domesticated reindeer in northern Finland and Norway can be carriers of certain bacterial foodborne pathogens. Strict compliance with good hygiene practices during any step of slaughter (in particular during dehiding and evisceration) is therefore of central importance to avoid carcass contamination and to prevent foodborne pathogens from entering the food chain.

Keywords: ESBL-producing *Enterobacteriaceae*, *Listeria monocytogenes*, MRSA, Reindeer fecal samples, *Salmonella*, Shiga toxin genes, *Yersinia*

*Correspondence: roger.stephan@uzh.ch
[3] Institute for Food Safety and Hygiene, Vetsuisse Faculty University of Zurich, Zurich, Switzerland
Full list of author information is available at the end of the article

Background

In northern Finland, the husbandry of Eurasian tundra reindeer (*Rangifer tarandus tarandus*) is a traditional and economically important livelihood [1]. The total area of reindeer husbandry covers approximately 36% (122,936 km^2) of Finland (http://paliskunnat.fi/reindeer/reindeer-herding/). The reindeer (about 192,000 animals in the year 2013 [2]) live as semi-domesticated herds, whereby winter corralling and seasonal or permanent supplementary feeding (leading to close animal contacts) is quite common in certain areas. The main product from reindeer husbandry is meat. In the year 2012/2013, approximately 90,000 reindeer were slaughtered in Finland, producing about 2.0 million kilos of meat (http://paliskunnat.fi/reindeer-herders-association/reindeer-info/). Approximately 74% of the reindeer are slaughtered in 19 EU-approved reindeer slaughterhouses. Responsible for the meat inspection and hygiene control are veterinarians working under the lead of the Regional State Administrative Agencies of Lapland. For private consumption and direct marketing, approximately 26% are slaughtered by traditional methods in the field (Regional State Administrative Agencies of Lapland). The European food hygiene legislation (Reg. [EC] No. 852/2004 and Reg. [EC] No. 853/2004) also covers the slaughter and processing of reindeer.

With regard to food-borne diseases, it must be considered that various food-producing animals were recognized in recent years as healthy carriers of important bacterial pathogens causing human illness [3, 4]. Carriage of such zoonotic pathogens in the intestines or on the hides is correlated with the probability of carcass contamination [5]. Hence, if good hygiene practices are not warranted during slaughter, such zoonotic pathogens might enter the food chain by direct or indirect fecal contamination. The aim of this study was to determine the presence of selected bacterial foodborne pathogens, methicillin-resistant *Staphylococcus aureus* (MRSA) and extended-spectrum β-lactamases (ESBL)-producing *Enterobacteriaceae* in healthy semi-domesticated reindeer at slaughter in northern Finland and Norway.

Methods

Abattoirs and sample collection

The reindeer in Fennoscandia are free ranging on wide pastures during most parts of the year. In Finland, the migration of reindeer is limited by fences between the cooperatives Supplementary feeding is therefore of growing importance. In the Varang area, the reindeer still have the possibility of natural seasonal migration: during the summer to the coast area and during the winter to the lichen rich mountain area. Under normal weather conditions, supplementary feeding is therefore of minor importance. In autumn round-ups, the reindeer are gathered from pastures and slaughter reindeer are separated from breeding reindeer. Slaughter reindeer are transported to slaughterhouses by vans or trailers and, for longer distances, by special reindeer transport trucks.

During one month (October) of the slaughtering period 2015, 470 healthy (approved in ante mortem inspection) semi-domesticated reindeer calves (aged between 6 and 7 months) were sampled at nine reindeer slaughterhouses in Finland and one in Norway. This age group was selected because the majority of reindeer is slaughtered at about this age and we wanted to assess the potential presence of foodborne pathogens in reindeer at slaughter. Finnish abattoirs were owned by local reindeer herding cooperatives and the butcher staff consisted of trained reindeer owners. The Finnish reindeer were slaughtered in the nearest abattoir and the transport distance by vehicle from the round-up site to the abattoir ranged from 0 to 100 km. The Norwegian abattoir is the major reindeer abattoir in Norway, owned by a private company, and staffed with professional butchers. For the herd of Norwegian reindeer, sampled in this study, the transport distance was about 200 km.

The Finnish abattoirs were medium-sized, EU-approved slaughterhouses with a daily slaughter capacity of 200–400 reindeer. The Norwegian, EU-approved abattoir was bigger with a daily slaughter capacity of at least 700 reindeer. The process and hygiene practices of reindeer slaughter are similar to the slaughter of cattle or sheep. Reindeer are first stunned (bolt pistol), followed by immediate bleeding. Before skinning, the head and distal parts of the legs are removed. Skinning is mainly done using a skinning pulley. Afterwards, reindeer are transferred to the clean part of the abattoir, where evisceration is performed. The cooling of the carcasses starts immediately after slaughtering.

Of the sampled reindeer, 410 originated from northern Finland from nine reindeer herding cooperatives and 60 from the northernmost part of Norway (NN) (Fig. 1; Table 1). The ten geographical areas were thereby equivalent to the ten slaughterhouses mentioned before. The complete reindeer herding area was divided in four areas from south to north (1–4) and cooperatives were named according to their east/west location in the numbered area (W = West, M = middle, E = East). These cooperatives were from south to north: 1W (n = 40); 1M (n = 47); 1E (n = 76); 2E (n = 39); 2W (n = 37); 3E (n = 45); 3W (n = 44); 4W (n = 37); 4E (n = 45); and northern Norway (NN, n = 60) (Fig. 1; Table 1).

Sampling comprised a total of 34 sampling-days. From each of the 470 examined reindeer, a fecal sample was collected from the large intestine directly after evisceration.

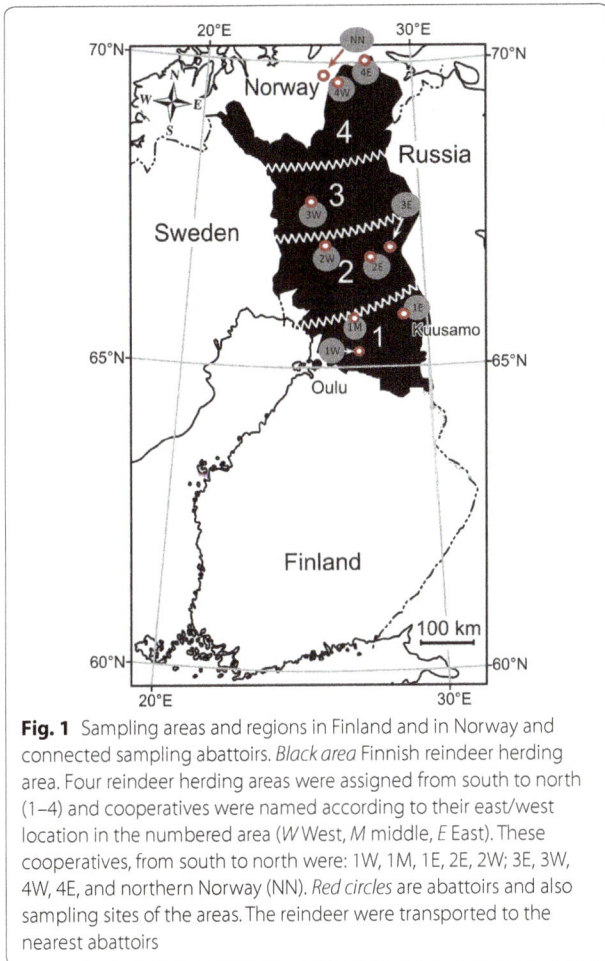

Fig. 1 Sampling areas and regions in Finland and in Norway and connected sampling abattoirs. *Black area* Finnish reindeer herding area. Four reindeer herding areas were assigned from south to north (1–4) and cooperatives were named according to their east/west location in the numbered area (*W* West, *M* middle, *E* East). These cooperatives, from south to north were: 1W, 1M, 1E, 2E, 2W; 3E, 3W, 4W, 4E, and northern Norway (NN). *Red circles* are abattoirs and also sampling sites of the areas. The reindeer were transported to the nearest abattoirs

Fecal samples were packed into sterile stomacher bags and transported chilled to the Regional Office of Finnish Food Safety Authority (Evira) in Oulu. Samples were frozen and stored at −20 °C up to 2 weeks. In the laboratory, fecal samples were analyzed for *Salmonella* spp., *Listeria monocytogenes*, *Yersinia* spp., and Shiga toxin genes (*stx*). In addition, *Escherichia coli* antibiotic resistance profiles and the occurrence of MRSA and ESBL-producing *Enterobacteriaceae* were assessed.

Salmonella spp

Examination for *Salmonella* spp. was done in accordance with ISO 6579:2007-10 with a modification. A subset of each fecal sample (about 1 g) was enriched (24 h, 37 °C) at a 1:10 ratio in buffered peptone water (BPW; Oxoid, Pratteln, Switzerland). From the first enrichment, 0.1 ml were incubated (24 h, 41.5 °C) in 10 ml of Rappaport–Vassiliadis (RV) broth (Oxoid). The enriched samples (one loopful: approx. 10 μl) were subcultured for 24 h at 37 °C on xylose-lysine-desoxycholate (XLD) agar and mannitol lysine crystal violet brilliant green (MLCB) agar (Oxoid). Presumptive colonies (XLD: red colonies, some with black centers; MLCB: large purple-black colonies, atypical salmonellae grow as mauve-grey colonies and may develop a central black area) were tested for the biochemical properties of *Salmonella* (oxidase reaction, acid production from mannitol, o-nitrophenyl-β-D-galactopyranoside (ONPG) test, H_2S and indole production as well as urease and lysin decarboxylase activity).

Table 1 Origin and numbers of sampled reindeer and their transport distances to the abattoirs

Cooperative[a]	No of sampled reindeer	Reindeer density/km2	Transport distance km
Area 1			
1W	40	0.76	50
1M	47	1.18	40
1E	76	1.68	20
Area 2			
2W	37	1.77	60
2E	39	1.25	40
Area 3			
3W	44	1.39	30
3E	45	2.28	100
Area 4			
4W	37	2.44	0
4E	45	2.37	0
NN	60	2.70	200

[a] The reindeer herding area was divided in four areas from south to north (1–4) and studied cooperatives were named according to their east/west location in the numbered area (*W* West, *M* middle, *E* East). *NN*, northern Norway

Listeria monocytogenes

Examination for *L. monocytogenes* was done in accordance with ISO 11290-1:2005-01. A subset of each fecal sample (approx. 1 g) was enriched (24 h, 30 °C) at a 1:10 ratio in Fraser broth with half Fraser supplement (Oxoid). From the first enrichment, 0.1 ml were incubated (24 h, 37 °C) in 10 ml of Fraser broth with Fraser supplement (Oxoid). The enriched samples (one loopful: approx. 10 μl) were subcultured for 48 h at 37 °C on chromogenic Ottaviani Agosti agar (bioMérieux, Marcy l'Etoile, France). Presumptive *L. monocytogenes* colonies (turquoise–blue colonies surrounded by an opaque halo on the chromogenic agar) were streaken (24 h, 37 °C) on sheep blood agar (Difco Columbia blood agar base EH, Becton–Dickinson, Allschwil, Switzerland; 5% sheep blood SB055, Oxoid) for evaluation of hemolysis. Isolated *L. monocytogenes* were serotyped using the commercial set of Listeria O-factor and H-factor antisera from Denka Seiken (Pharma Consulting, Burgdorf, Switzerland).

Yersinia spp

A subset of each fecal sample (approx. 1 g) was enriched (24 h, 30 °C) at a 1:10 ratio in BPW (Oxoid). The enriched samples (one loopful: approx. 10 μl) were subcultured for 24 h at 30 °C on cefsulodinirgasan-novobiosin (CIN) agar (Oxoid). Presumptive *Yersinia* colonies (red bull's-eye surrounded by a transparent border) were streaken (24 h, 37 °C) on sheep blood agar (Difco Columbia blood agar base EH, Becton–Dickinson, Allschwil, Switzerland; 5% sheep blood SB055, Oxoid) and then tested for urease activity. Urease-positive colonies were identified with MALDI-TOF mass spectrometry [6].

Shiga toxin genes

A subset of each fecal sample (about 1 g) was enriched (18–24 h, 37 °C) at a 1:10 ratio in *Enterobacteriaceae* enrichment (EE) broth (Becton–Dickinson). After incubation (24 h, 37 °C) of the enriched samples on sheep blood agar (Difco Columbia blood agar base EH, Becton–Dickinson; 5% sheep blood SB055, Oxoid), the colonies were washed off with 2 ml of 0.85% saline solution. To screen the samples by real-time polymerase chain reaction (PCR) for *stx*1 and *stx*2, the Assurance GDS® Assay MPX ID for Top STEC (Tq 71019-52; Bio Control Systems, Bellevue, WA, USA) was applied [7]. To compare the frequencies of *stx*1, *stx*2, and both *stx*1 and *stx*2 among fecal samples and the occurrence of Shiga toxin genes among fecal samples of reindeer from different areas of origin, contingency tables (Fisher's exact test) were used.

Escherichia coli isolation and antibiotic resistance profiles

To assess antibiotic resistance profiles of *E. coli* isolates, about every fifth of the enrichments prepared for the detection of Shiga toxin genes were selected (EE broth; 18–24 h, 37 °C). The enriched samples (one loopful: approx. 10 μl) were subcultured for 24 h at 37 °C on chromogenic RAPID' *E. coli* 2 agar (Bio-Rad Laboratories, Reinach, Switzerland). One *E. coli* colony (violet to pink on RAPID' *E. coli* 2 agar) from each of the 95 samples was selected and subjected to susceptibility testing against 12 antimicrobial agents by the disc diffusion method according to the Clinical and Laboratory Standards Institute (CLSI) protocols and criteria [8]. The panel included ampicillin (AM, 10 μg), amoxicillin-clavulanic acid (AMC, 30 μg), chloramphenicol (C, 30 μg), cephalothin (CF, 30 μg), ciprofloxacin (CIP, 5 μg), cefotaxime (CTX, 30 μg), gentamicin (GM, 10 μg), kanamycin (K, 30 μg), nalidixic acid (NA, 30 μg), streptomycin (S, 10 μg), tetracycline (TE, 30 μg), and trimethoprim (TMP, 5 μg) (Becton–Dickinson).

Methicillin-resistant *Staphylococcus aureus*

Examination for MRSA was done using a two-step enrichment procedure. A subset of each fecal sample (approx. 1 g) was enriched first (18–24 h, 37 °C) at a 1:10 ratio in Mueller–Hinton broth supplemented with 6.5% NaCl (24 h, 37 °C) and subsequently in 5 ml tryptone soy broth (TSB; Oxoid) supplemented with 75 mg/l aztreonam and 5 mg/l cefoxitin (24 h, 37 °C). The enriched samples (one loopful: approx. 10 μl) were then subcultured for 24 h at 37 °C on chromogenic Brilliance MRSA 2 agar (Oxoid). Denim blue colonies on Brilliance MRSA 2 agar are presumptive positive for MRSA.

ESBL-producing *Enterobacteriaceae*

A subset of each fecal sample (approx. 1 g) was enriched (18–24 h, 37 °C) at a 1:10 ratio in EE broth (Becton–Dickinson). For detection of *Enterobacteriaceae* producing extended-spectrum β-lactamases (ESBLs), the enriched samples (one loopful: approx. 10 μl) were subcultured for 24 h at 37 °C on chromogenic Brilliance ESBL agar (Oxoid).

Results and discussion
Presence of foodborne pathogens

To assess the presence of selected bacterial foodborne pathogens, fecal samples from 470 healthy semi-domesticated reindeer were examined for *Salmonella* spp., *L. monocytogenes*, *Yersinia* spp., and Shiga toxin genes at slaughter. Recent data on the presence of bacterial foodborne pathogens in healthy reindeer are limited to very few surveys, mainly originating from Finland and Norway [9–13].

All 470 fecal samples from reindeer tested negative for *Salmonella* spp. (Table 2). However, it must be considered that freezing of fecal samples for storage might have

Table 2 Presence of foodborne pathogens and detection of Shiga toxin genes in fecal samples collected from reindeer at slaughter

No of fecal samples	No. (%) of fecal samples from reindeer testing positive for			
	Salmonella spp.[a]	Listeria monocytogenes[b]	Yersinia spp.[c]	Shiga toxin genes (stx1 and/or stx2)[d]
470	0 (0%)	15 (3.2%)	46 (9.8%)	153 (32.6%)

[a] Examination according to ISO 6579:2007-10 mod

[b] Examination in accordance with ISO 11290:2005-01, serotyping (serotype 1/2a, n = 14; serotype 4b, n = 1)

[c] Enrichment in BPW, incubation on CIN agar, species identification with MALDI-TOF MS (Y. enterocolitica, n = 8; Y. intermedia, n = 1; Y. kristensenii, n = 30; Yersinia spp., n = 7)

[d] Enrichment in EE broth, screening for stx1 and stx2 by the Assurance GDS® assay for Shiga toxin genes

had an effect on bacterial populations, especially on *Salmonella*. *Salmonella* spp. are still a major cause of foodborne diseases and may colonize the intestinal tract of a large number of mammals and birds [3]. But comparable to our results, *Salmonella* were not detected in other studies examining feces from reindeer [9, 10, 12].

Listeria monocytogenes were detected in 3.2% of the 470 reindeer fecal samples (Table 2). The positive animals originated from six of ten different areas (1W, n = 1; 1M, n = 1; 1E, n = 1; 2E, n = 1; 3W, n = 5; 4W, n = 6). In contrast, Aschfalk et al. [9] did not isolate *Listeria* spp. from Norwegian reindeer, but only 35 fecal samples from cadavers were examined and the isolation procedure was different. *Listeria monocytogenes* as a foodborne pathogen has the potential to cause serious and life-threatening conditions (including septicemia, meningitis, meningoencephalitis, and abortion) in persons with reduced immunity [3, 14]. Of the 15 *L. monocytogenes* isolates from reindeer, 14 belonged to the serotype 1/2a and one to the serotype 4b. Serotype 1/2a strains are frequently found in ready-to-eat food and food-processing environments [15, 16]. Human clinical cases are frequently associated with strains of serotypes 1/2a, 1/2b, and 4b and infections due to serotype 1/2a strains have increased in recent years [15, 17].

Yersinia spp. were detected in 9.8% of the 470 fecal samples from reindeer (Table 2). The positive animals originated from nine of ten different areas (1W, n = 1; 1M, n = 14; 1E, n = 20; 2E, n = 3; 2W, n = 1; 3E, n = 1; 3W, n = 4; 4E, n = 1; NN, n = 1). The species of 39 *Yersinia* isolates was identified by MALDI-TOF mass spectrometry: *Yersinia kristensenii* (n = 30), *Y. enterocolitica* (n = 8), and *Y. intermedia* (n = 1). Similarly, in the survey of Kemper et al. [10], 108 (4.8%) *Yersinia* isolates were obtained from reindeer and *Y. kristensenii* (n = 72) and

Y. enterocolitica (n = 29) predominated. *Yersinia kristensenii* have been isolated from environmental samples, animals, foods, and humans, but their impact on human health remains controversial [18, 19]. On the other hand, although not all *Y. enterocolitica* are considered zoonotic agents and pathogenic for humans, certain strains of *Y. enterocolitica* (some biotypes/serotypes) may cause acute gastroenteritis, reactive arthritis, or mesenteric lymphadenitis and terminal ileitis mimicking appendicitis in humans [3, 20].

Shiga toxin-producing *E. coli* are responsible for a number of human (foodborne) illnesses including diarrhea, hemorrhagic colitis, and the life-threatening hemolytic uremic syndrome (HUS) [3, 21, 22]. The production of one or more Shiga toxins (Stx1, Stx2, and variants) characterizes STEC. However, it must be emphasized that the detection of Shiga toxin genes in fecal samples (without strain isolation and characterization), as performed in the present study, can only be regarded as presumptive presence of STEC. In the examined reindeer fecal samples, genes for Shiga toxins (stx1 and/or stx2) were detected in a remarkable prevalence of 32.6% (Table 2) and stx2 predominated (P < 0.05). Alone or in combination with stx1, stx2 was found in 24.5% of the samples (Table 3). With regard to 10 different areas of origin, striking differences were evident for the frequency and distribution of stx1/stx2 (Table 3). The overall highest frequency was found among samples from 2E (P < 0.05; 100%, mainly stx1), followed by 4W (54%, only stx2) and 2W (46%, only stx2), while the lowest frequencies were detected in samples from 1W (P < 0.05; 5%, only stx2), NN (12%, only stx2), and 3E (13%, only stx2). Moreover, compared to the other areas, the predominance of stx1 in samples from 2E (P < 0.05) and of both stx1 and stx2 in samples from 1E (P < 0.05) was striking.

Reindeer might become colonized with STEC directly from contact with carrier animals or indirectly from contaminated feed or soil. The colonization pressure could thereby be influenced by the husbandry conditions (e.g., animal density of reindeer, supplementary feeding in corrals, duration of transport and of round-up events before slaughter). A high or low animal density of reindeer might have an impact on the colonization pressure (amount of fecal contamination of the pastures). In the present study, area 1W (Fig. 1) showed the lowest animal reindeer density and the lowest stx prevalence.

For most of the sampled reindeer herds, animals are supplementary fed in corrals or on pastures during the winter months. If feeding hygiene is poor and accumulated feces can contaminate the provided fodder, this may increase the colonization pressure. In the areas 1–3 (Fig. 1) reindeer are intensively supplementary fed, mostly in corrals. This may partly explain the high

Table 3 Detection of Shiga toxin genes (*stx*1/*stx*2) in fecal samples from reindeer from different areas of origin in northern Finland and Norway

Area of origin	No. of fecal samples	No. (%) of samples testing positive for			
		*stx*1 (only)	*stx*2 (only)	*stx*1 and *stx*2	*stx* total
1W	40	0 (0%)	2 (5.0%)	0 (0%)	2 (5.0%)
1M	47	1 (2.1%)	13 (27.7%)	2 (4.3%)	16 (34.0%)
1E	76	0 (0%)	7 (9.2%)	18 (23.7%)	25 (32.9%)
1 Total	*163*	*1 (0.6%)*	*22 (13.5%)*	*20 (12.3%)*	*43 (26.4%)*
2E	39	37 (94.9%)	0 (0%)	2 (5.1%)	39 (100%)
2W	37	0 (0%)	17 (45.9%)	0 (0%)	17 (45.9%)
2 Total	*76*	*37 (48.7%)*	*17 (22.4%)*	*2 (2.6%)*	*56 (73.7%)*
3E	45	0 (0%)	6 (13.3%)	0 (0%)	6 (13.3%)
3W	44	0 (0%)	8 (18.2%)	1 (2.3%)	9 (20.5%)
3 Total	*89*	*0 (0%)*	*14 (15.7%)*	*1 (1.1%)*	*15 (16.9%)*
4W	37	0 (0%)	20 (54.1%)	0 (0%)	20 (54.1%)
4E	45	0 (0%)	12 (26.7%)	0 (0%)	12 (26.7%)
4 Total	*82*	*0 (0%)*	*32 (39.0%)*	*0 (0%)*	*32 (39.0%)*
Finland total	410	38 (9.3%)	85 (20.7%)	23 (5.6%)	146 (35.6%)
Northern Norway	60	0 (0%)	7 (11.7%)	0 (0%)	7 (11.7%)
Total	*470*	*38 (8.1%)*	*92 (19.6%)*	*23 (4.9%)*	*153 (32.6%)*

prevalence in some cooperatives. An exemption is the area 3E, where reindeer do not receive any supplementary feeding.

In the area 3E and also in northern Norway (NN) (Fig. 1), the strategy of seasonal translocation between summer and winter pasture is applied. Hence, reindeer are periodically moved to other pastures, on which they have not grazed before. On these pastures, there is less (fresh) fecal contamination pressure. This could partly explain the low *stx* prevalence in the area 3E and NN areas.

Transport distances of reindeer to the abattoirs varied in the present study from zero (reindeer walk from round-up corral to the abattoir; areas 4W and 4E) to about 200 km (NN) (Table 1). Depending on transport distances and durations, reindeer are usually allowed to rest (1–12 h) in fences at the abattoirs before slaughter. Drinking water is freely available and reindeer must be fed if the waiting time exceeds 12 h (Finnish Animal Protection Regulation 7.6.1996/396). In the present study, we did not find any connection between transport distances/durations and the observed *stx* prevalence.

Furthermore, the colonization pressure could be increased by the corralling of large numbers of reindeer before slaughter as well as stressful handling and long durations of round-ups before slaughter (occasionally up to three days). Such aspects could be of particular importance in the areas 4W and 4E.

Although detection of Shiga toxin genes in fecal samples only indicates the presumptive presence of STEC, our results suggest that healthy semi-domesticated reindeer in northern Finland and Norway, as other wild ruminants [23], could probably constitute a reservoir for STEC. However, further investigations (strain isolation and characterization) are required for verification purposes. If reindeer are confirmed as a STEC reservoir, the potential human health risk associated with STEC from reindeer must be evaluated [24]. Further, the risk of STEC transmission from reindeer to humans, by consumption of undercooked meat or other food contaminated by feces, as well as to livestock when sharing pastures with reindeer, must not be neglected. In contrast to our findings, STEC were not or only rarely detected in reindeer in previous studies [9–13] and the few positive *E. coli* isolates harbored *stx*1 [9, 10]. However, direct comparison of our results with the literature is strongly hampered by varying detection procedures applied, and that two surveys [11, 13] focused mainly on *E. coli* O157.

Antibiotic resistance

Disc diffusion tests showed low levels of antibiotic resistances: only five (5.3%) isolates were resistant to one or more of the tested antibiotics. However, it must be considered that clinical breakpoints were used (which could show a lower proportion of resistance than the application of epidemiological cut-offs). One strain showed resistance to ampicillin, amoxicillin with clavulanic acid, cephalothin and cefotaxime, two strains were resistant to streptomycin and tetracycline, while the two remaining strains were resistant to ampicillin or cephalothin. Thereby, the single *E. coli* isolate resistant to cefotaxime could be an ESBL-producer, but this needs further confirmation. Interestingly, Lillehaug et al. [12] reported more resistant *E. coli* in wild reindeer (24%) than in other hunted wild cervids (2.2%).

With regard to antibiotic resistance, methicillin-resistant staphylococci, in particular MRSA, and ESBL-producing *Enterobacteriaceae* are currently of special concern. In recent years, it has been widely recognized that the dissemination of MRSA and ESBL-producing bacteria is an issue no longer restricted to the medical/health care system [25–28]. In our study, applying selective methods, no MRSA or ESBL-producing *Enterobacteriaceae* were detected among the 470 fecal samples from healthy reindeer. Hence, in contrast to livestock, a favorable situation with regards to antimicrobial resistance is present in the reindeer population.

Conclusions
Healthy semi-domesticated reindeer in northern Finland and Norway can be carriers of bacterial foodborne pathogens. In particular, reindeer could constitute a reservoir for STEC, but strain isolation and characterization is required for verification and to assess the potential human pathogenicity. Strict compliance with good hygiene practices during any step of slaughter (in particular during skinning and evisceration) is therefore of central importance to avoid carcass contamination and to prevent foodborne pathogens from entering the food chain.

Authors' contributions
SL, AO, MF and RS designed the study. SL collected the samples. Laboratory work was carried out by JJ and RS. Results were interpreted by RS and CZ. CZ and RS drafted the manuscript. All authors read and approved the final manuscript.

Author details
[1] Department of Veterinary Biosciences, Faculty of Veterinary Medicine, University of Helsinki, Helsinki, Wazama, Finland. [2] Research and Laboratory Department, Production Animal and Wildlife Health Research Unit, Finnish Food Safety Authority Evira, Oulu, Finland. [3] Institute for Food Safety and Hygiene, Vetsuisse Faculty University of Zurich, Zurich, Switzerland. [4] Department of Food Hygiene and Environmental Health, Faculty of Veterinary Medicine, University of Helsinki, Helsinki, Finland.

Acknowledgements
We thank all the reindeer herders and reindeer veterinarians in Finland and Norway for their cooperation in sample collection. The Finnish part of this work was done in the project "Reindeer health in the changing environment 2015–2018" funded by the Finnish Ministry of Agriculture and Forestry (MAKERA).

Competing interests
The authors declare that they have no competing interests.

Ethics statement
Animals used in thus study did not undergo any manipulation prior to stunning for standard slaughter according to the pertinent legislation. For this reason, no specific ethical approval was required.

References
1. Mustonen T, Jones G. Reindeer herding in Finland: a report for Trashumancia y Naturaleza. European Forum on Nature Conservation and Pastoralism and Snowchange. 2015. http://www.snowchange.org/documents-and-files. Accessed 16 July 2016.
2. Erikson B. Rennäringen, en miljardindustri som går mot en kollaps och som idag sysselsätter ca 15,000 årsarbeten i Norrlands inland och i Norra Finland. BENERIK Företagskonsult. 2014. http://www.pajala.se/Documents/PUAB/Rapporter/140601 Rennäringen officiell slutrapport ver 2.0.pdf. Accessed 16 July 2016.
3. EFSA/ECDC. The European Union summary report on trends and sources of zoonoses, zoonotic agents and food-borne outbreaks in 2014. EFSA Journal. 2015;13:4329.
4. Nørrung B, Buncic S. Microbial safety of meat in the European Union. Meat Sci. 2008;78:14–24.
5. Barkocy-Gallagher GA, Arthur TM, Siragusa GR, Keen JE, Elder RO, Laegreid WW, Koohmaraie M. Genotypic analyses of *Escherichia coli* O157:H7 and O157 nonmotile isolates recovered from beef cattle and carcasses at processing plants in the Midwestern States of the United States. Appl Environ Microbiol. 2001;67:3810–8.
6. Stephan R, Cernela N, Ziegler D, Pflüger V, Tonolla M, Ravasi D, Fredriksson-Ahomaa M, Hächler H. Rapid species specific identification and subtyping of *Yersinia enterocolitica* by MALDI-TOF mass spectrometry. J Microbiol Methods. 2011;87:150–3.
7. Margot H, Cernela N, Iversen C, Zweifel C, Stephan R. Evaluation of seven different commercially available real-time PCR assays for detection of Shiga toxin 1 and 2 gene subtypes. J Food Prot. 2013;76:871–3.
8. CLSI, Clinical and Laboratory Standards Institute. Performance standards for antimicrobial susceptibility testing; 23rd informational supplement, CLSI document M100-S23. CLSI, Wayne, PA. 2013.
9. Aschfalk A, Kemper N, Höller C. Bacteria of pathogenic importance in faeces from cadavers of free-ranging or corralled semi-domesticated reindeer in northern Norway. Vet Res Commun. 2003;27:93–100.
10. Kemper N, Aschfalk A, Höller C. *Campylobacter* spp., *Enterococcus* spp., *Escherichia coli*, *Salmonella* spp., *Yersinia* spp., and *Cryptosporidium* oocysts in semi-domesticated reindeer (*Rangifer tarandus tarandus*) in Northern Finland and Norway. Acta Vet Scand. 2006;48:7.
11. Lahti E, Hirvelä-Koski V, Honkanen-Buzalski T. Occurrence of *Escherichia coli* O157 in reindeer (*Rangifer tarandus*). Vet Rec. 2001;148:633–4.
12. Lillehaug A, Bergsjø B, Schau J, Bruheim T, Vikøren T, Handeland K. *Campylobacter* spp., *Salmonella* spp., verocytotoxic *Escherichia coli*, and antibiotic resistance in indicator organisms in wild cervids. Acta Vet Scand. 2005;46:23–32.
13. Wasteson Y, Arnemo JM, Johansen BK, Vold L, Mathiesen SD, Olsen MA, Wiig O, Derocher AE. Analysis of faecal samples from wild animals for verocytotoxin producing *Escherichia coli* and *E coli* O157. Vet Rec. 1999;144:646–7.
14. Allerberger F, Wagner M. Listeriosis: a resurgent foodborne infection. Clin Microbiol Infect. 2010;16:16–23.
15. Gianfranceschi MV, D'Ottavio MC, Gattuso A, Bella A, Aureli P. Distribution of serotypes and pulsotypes of *Listeria monocytogenes* from human, food and environmental isolates (Italy 2002–2005). Food Microbiol. 2009;26:520–6.
16. Martín B, Perich A, Gómez D, Yangüela J, Rodríguez A, Garriga M, Aymerich T. Diversity and distribution of *Listeria monocytogenes* in meat processing plants. Food Microbiol. 2014;44:119–27.
17. Lopez-Valladares G, Tham W, Parihar VS, Helmersson S, Andersson B, Ivarsson S, Johansson C, Ringberg H, Tjernberg I, Henriques-Normark B, Danielsson-Tham M-L. Human isolates of *Listeria monocytogenes* in Sweden during half a century (1958–2010). Epidemiol Infect. 2014;142:2251–60.

18. Loftus CG, Harewood GC, Cockerill FR 3rd, Murray JA. Clinical features of patients with novel *Yersinia* species. Dig Dis Sci. 2002;47:2805–10.

19. Sulakvelidze A. Yersiniae other than *Y. enterocolitica*, *Y. pseudotuberculosis*, and *Y. pestis*: the ignored species. Microbes Infect. 2000;2:497–513.

20. Drummond N, Murphy BP, Ringwood T, Prentice MB, Buckley JF, Fanning S. *Yersinia enterocolitica*: a brief review of the issues relating to the zoonotic pathogen, public health challenges, and the pork production chain. Foodborne Pathog Dis. 2012;9:179–89.

21. Karch HP, Tarr I, Bielaszewska M. Enterohaemorrhagic *Escherichia coli* in human medicine. Int J Med Microbiol. 2005;295:405–18.

22. Brooks JT, Sowers EG, Wells JG, Greene KD, Griffin PM, Hoekstra RM, Strockbine NA. Non-O157 Shiga toxin-producing *Escherichia coli* infections in the United States, 1983–2002. J Infect Dis. 2005;192:1422–9.

23. Obwegeser T, Stephan R, Hofer E, Zweifel C. Shedding of foodborne pathogens and microbial carcass contamination of hunted wild ruminants. Vet Microbiol. 2012;159:149–54.

24. Hofer E, Stephan R, Reist M, Zweifel C. Application of a real-time PCR-based system for monitoring of O26, O103, O111, O145 and O157 Shiga toxin-producing *Escherichia coli* in cattle at slaughter. Zoonoses Public Health. 2012;59:408–15.

25. Guenther S, Ewers C, Wieler LH. Extended-spectrum beta-lactamases producing *E. coli* in wildlife, yet another form of environmental pollution? Front Microbiol. 2011;2:246.

26. Otter JA, French GL. Molecular epidemiology of community-associated meticillin-resistant *Staphylococcus aureus* in Europe. Lancet Infect Dis. 2010;10:227–39.

27. Seiffert SN, Hilty M, Perreten V, Endimiani A. Extended-spectrum cephalosporin-resistant Gram-negative organisms in livestock: an emerging problem for human health? Drug Resist Updat. 2013;16:22–45.

28. Vanderhaeghen W, Hermans K, Haesebrouck F, Butaye P. Methicillin-resistant *Staphylococcus aureus* (MRSA) in food production animals. Epidemiol Infect. 2010;138:606–25.

6

Prevalence of *Yersinia enterocolitica* and *Yersinia pseudotuberculosis* in wild boars in the Basque Country, northern Spain

Maialen Arrausi-Subiza, Xeider Gerrikagoitia, Vega Alvarez, Jose Carlos Ibabe and Marta Barral[*]

Abstract

Background: Yersiniosis is a zoonosis widely distributed in Europe and swine carry different serotypes of *Yersinia enterocolitica* and *Y. pseudotuberculosis*. The aim of this study was to determine the prevalence of *Y. enterocolitica* and *Y. pseudotuberculosis* in wild boars in northern Spain. The blood of wild boars (n = 505) was sampled between 2001 and 2012. Seroprevalence was determined in 490 serum samples with an indirect enzyme-linked immunosorbent assay. Seventy-two of the animals were also examined for the presence of *Y. enterocolitica* or *Y. pseudotuberculosis* in the tonsils with real-time polymerase chain reaction. All the tonsils were analysed twice, directly and after cold enrichment in phosphate-buffered saline supplemented with 1 % mannitol and 0.15 % bile salts.

Results: Antibodies directed against *Y. enterocolitica* and *Y. pseudotuberculosis* were detected in 52.5 % of the animals. *Yersinia enterocolitica* was detected with real-time polymerase chain reaction in 33.3 % of the wild boars and *Y. pseudotuberculosis* in 25 %. Significant differences were observed according to the sampling year, and the highest prevalence was during winter and spring. The highest antibody levels and *Y. enterocolitica* prevalence were observed in mountainous areas at altitudes higher than 600 m, with very cold winters, and with the highest annual rainfall for each dominant climate. Areas with low and medium livestock populations were associated with the highest seroprevalence of *Yersinia* spp. in wild boars, whereas areas with high ovine populations had the highest prevalence of *Y. enterocolitica*.

Conclusions: This study shows that *Y. enterocolitica* and *Y. pseudotuberculosis* are highly prevalent among wild boars in the Basque country, with *Y. enterocolitica* most prevalent. The risk of infection among wild boars is influenced by the season and the area in which they live.

Keywords: *Yersinia enterocolitica*, *Yersinia pseudotuberculosis*, Wild boar, Epidemiology, PCR, ELISA

Background

Yersiniosis is the fourth most frequently reported foodborne zoonosis in humans in Europe, although the number of reported cases of *Yersinia* infection has continued to decrease since 2007 [1]. The genus *Yersinia* is composed of several species, but only *Y. pestis*, *Y. pseudotuberculosis* and some *Y. enterocolitica* strains are human pathogens [1].

Pigs are assumed to be the main reservoir of human pathogenic *Y. enterocolitica*, and serotypes isolated from pig samples, such as 4/O:3, are the same that cause human disease in Europe [1]. *Yersinia pseudotuberculosis* has also been frequently isolated from pigs and these animals might be a source of human 2/O:3 infections [2].

Wild animals constitute a very important factor in the epidemiology of *Yersinia* infection [3, 4], and wild boars (*Sus scrofa*) are considered an important reservoir of enteropathogenic *Yersinia* [5]. A great variety of serotypes, including those that cause human infections, have been isolated from wild boars in Europe [3, 5, 6], although some *Y. enterocolitica* strains differ from those in domestic pigs [2].

*Correspondence: mbarral@neiker.eus
Department of Animal Health, Basque Institute for Agricultural Research and Development-NEIKER, Berreaga 1, 48160 Derio-Bizkaia, Spain

More studies are required to understand the real role of wild boars in the epidemiology of yersiniosis. During the last two decades, the wild boar population has increased significantly in Europe [7], favouring their contact with livestock and the transmission of diseases [8]. Interest in wild boars as a meat source has also increased, thus increasing the risk of the transmission of food-borne diseases [9].

The prevalence of pathogenic *Yersinia* spp. in Spanish wild boars is unknown. Therefore, the aim of this study was to determine the prevalence of *Y. enterocolitica* and *Y. pseudotuberculosis* in wild boars in northern Spain.

Methods

Study area

The Basque country is located in northern Spain, limited by the Cantabrian coastline and distributed in eight regions, defined according to rainfall, temperature, altitude and the dominant vegetation [10, 11]. Climatologically, the Atlantic slope (northern part) is moderate in terms of temperature, but very rainy, whereas the Mediterranean slope (southern part) is less rainy, with warmer summers and colder winters.

Sample collection

Wild boar samples were collected within the context of a wildlife health surveillance program in the Basque Country. In total, 505 wild boars were sampled between 2001 and 2012, during which time 490 serum samples were obtained, and in the last 3 years, 72 tonsils were also collected. Both serum and tonsil samples were obtained from only 57 animals. Most of the animals studied (90 %) had been shot by accredited hunters, and samples were taken in the field in collaboration with competent local authorities, and 8 % were obtained from wildlife rehabilitation centres. The cause of death and the health status of these animals were not recorded. The remaining samples (2 %) were obtained from animals found dead or run over, and necropsies were performed in the laboratory. No significant lesions, except physical trauma, were observed in these animals. The samples were collected in individual containers, properly identified and stored at −20 °C until analysis. The details of each animal, including its sex, age, and the date and geographic location of collection were recorded. The animals were classified into two groups according to age: young, including piglets (<1 year) and yearlings (1–2 years); and adults (>2 years). Details of the animals are given in Tables 1 and 2.

Real-time polymerase chain reaction

The tonsil samples (1–5 g) were weighed and aseptically cut into small pieces. Approximately 150 mg of each tonsil was disrupted and homogenised with 30 chrome–steel beads (1.3 mm) (Biospec Products, Bartlesville, OK, USA) and 750 μL of TE buffer using the TissueLyser system (Qiagen, Hilden, Germany). DNA was extracted from 200 μL of the supernatant for direct real-time polymerase chain reaction (rt-PCR) analysis. The rest of each tonsil sample was mixed with phosphate-buffered saline (PBS) supplemented with 1 % mannitol (Fluka, Seelze, Germany) and 0.15 % bile salts (Fluka, Seelze, Germany) (PBS-MSB), diluted 1:10 and homogenised in a stomacher (Lab-Blender 80, Cole-Parmer, Vernon Hills, IL, USA) until homogeneity. The mixture was incubated for 14 days at 4 °C. DNA was extracted from 200 μL of the supernatant and used as the template for rt-PCR.

DNA extraction was performed with the QIAamp® DNA Blood Mini Kit (Qiagen), according to the manufacturer's instructions, with minor modifications [12], and the DNA was measured with a NanoDrop ND-1000 spectrophotometer (Thermo Scientific, Inc.). DNA (150–200 ng) was used to detect *Yersinia* with the TaqMan rt-PCR assay in three independent reactions, using the Applied Biosystems 7500 Real-Time PCR System and The Express qPCR Supermix, universal kit (Invitrogen™), according to the supplier's recommendations. *Yersinia enterocolitica* was detected with the amplification of the *ail* gene [13], using a previously described procedure [12]. To detect all the *Y. pseudotuberculosis* serotypes, the *wzz* and *ail* genes were amplified in two independent reactions [12, 14, 15]. Amplification of the *ail* gene detects all serotypes but O:11 and O:12, and amplification of the *wzz* gene detects all serotypes but O:6 and O:7 [14, 15]. A sample was considered positive for *Y. enterocolitica* or *Y. pseudotuberculosis* when at least one positive result was obtained in the direct reaction or after enrichment in any of the three rt-PCRs used.

Enzyme-linked immunosorbent assay

The presence of antibodies directed against pathogenic *Yersinia* was determined with a commercial indirect enzyme-linked immunosorbent assay (ELISA) specific for swine (PIGTYPE® YOPSCREEN, Labor Diagnostic, Leipzig, Germany), according to the manufacturer's instructions. The optical density (OD) was measured in an ELISA Multiskan (Thermo Labsystem) spectrophotometer at 450 nm. The ratio between the sample OD and the positive control OD (S/P ratio) was calculated. Samples with an S/P ratio ≥0.3 were considered positive.

Bacteriology

Selective cefsulodin–irgasan–novobiocin (CIN) agar (bioMérieux, Marcy l'Etoile, France) and CHROMagar™ *Y. enterocolitica* (CHROMagar, Paris, France) agar were inoculated with 20 μL of the rt-PCR-positive tonsil mixtures and incubated at 30 °C for 24–48 h to isolate the

Table 1 Seroprevalence of pathogenic *Yersinia* spp. detected in wild boars according to the variables studied

Variables	N	ELISA (%)
Age		
Young	102	42 (41.2)
Adult	98	81 (82.7)
Sex		
Females	104	66 (63.5)
Males	118	72 (61)
Sampling year		
2001	12	7 (58.3)
2002	10	10 (100)
2003	167	74 (44.3)
2004	80	41 (51.3)
2005	67	47 (70.2)
2006	53	39 (73.6)
2010	25	12 (48)
2011	40	15 (37.5)
2012	17	9 (52.9)
Season		
Winter	168	108 (64.3)
Spring	29	19 (65.5)
Summer	5	0
Autumn	269	127 (47. 2)
Natural regions		
1	298	147 (49.3)
2	90	52 (57.8)
3	1	1 (100)
4	17	17 (100)
6	4	4 (100)
Slope		
Atlantic	445	217 (48.8)
Mediterranean	42	37 (88.1)
Porcine census		
Low (10–140)	81	44 (54.3)
Middle (167–426)	219	119 (54.3)
High (580–7332)	162	82 (50.6)
Caprine census		
Low (66–655)	71	53 (74.7)
Middle (909–1056)	234	111 (47.4)
High (1136–2810)	157	81 (51.6)
Ovine census		
Low (1881–6698)	102	60 (58.8)
Middle (8035–15,033)	138	91 (65.9)
High (15,417–32,802)	222	94 (42.3)
Bovine census		
Low (276–4277)	132	77 (58.3)
Middle (4602–6768)	172	103 (59.9)
High (6781–19,109)	158	65 (41.1)

N number of samples analyzed, *ELISA* number and percentage of ELISA positive samples

Table 2 Prevalence of pathogenic *Yersinia* detected with rt-PCR in wild boars according to the variables studied

Variables	N	YE and YP (%)	YE (%)	YP (%)
Age				
Young	25	18 (72)	12 (48)	9 (36)
Adult	20	10 (50)	8 (40)	3 (15)
Sex				
Females	30	19 (63.3)	12 (40)	11 (36.7)
Males	19	12 (63.2)	9 (47.4)	4 (21.1)
Sampling year				
2010	23	18 (78.3)	13 (56.5)	9 (39.1)
2011	32	7 (21.9)	7 (21.9)	0
2012	17	12 (70.6)	4 (23.5)	9 (52.9)
Season				
Winter	8	5 (62.5)	5 (62.5)	1 (12.5)
Spring	9	7 (77.8)	2 (22.2)	6 (66.7)
Summer	10	5 (50)	3 (30)	2 (20)
Autumn	45	20 (44.4)	14 (31.1)	9 (20)
Natural regions				
1	58	26 (44.8)	15 (25.9)	15 (25.9)
2	6	5 (83.3)	5 (83.3)	0
Slope				
Atlantic	72	37 (51.4)	24 (33.3)	18 (25)
Porcine census[a]				
Low	26	12 (46.1)	6 (23.1)	8 (30.8)
Middle	24	11 (45.8)	6 (25)	6 (25)
High	22	14 (63.6)	12 (54.6)	4 (18.2)
Caprine census[b]				
Low	3	0	0	0
Middle	35	19 (54.3)	10 (28.6)	12 (34.3)
High	34	18 (52.9)	14 (41.2)	6 (17.7)
Ovine census[c]				
Low	20	7 (35)	3 (15)	4 (20)
Middle	28	12 (42.9)	6 (21.4)	8 (28.6)
High	24	18 (75)	15 (62.5)	6 (25)
Bovine census[d]				
Low	26	13 (50)	6 (23.1)	9 (34.6)
Middle	17	7 (41.2)	4 (23.5)	3 (17.7)
High	29	17 (58.6)	14 (48.3)	6 (20.7)

N number of samples analyzed, *YE* and *YP* number and percentage of *Y. enterocolitica* and *Y. pseudotuberculosis* positive samples, *YE* number and percentage of *Y. enterocolitica* positive samples, *YP* number and percentage of *Y. pseudotuberculosis* positive samples

[a] Porcine census: low (10–140), middle (167–426), high (580–7332)

[b] Caprine census: low (66–655), middle (909–1056), high (1136–2810)

[c] Ovine census: low (1881–6698), middle (8035–15,033), high (15,417–32,802)

[d] Bovine census: low (276–4277), middle (4602–6768), high (6781–19,109)

Yersinia strains. Red CIN agar "bull's-eye" colonies surrounded with a transparent area of 1 mm and mauve CHROMagar™ colonies were selected. The selected colonies were homogenised in 500 μL of PBS, and 50 μL of this mixture was incubated for 10 min at 100 °C in a water bath and then for 10 min on ice. The mixture was then centrifuged for 10 min at 15,600×*g* and 5 μL of the supernatant was used for *Y. enterocolitica* and *Y. pseudotuberculosis* identification with rt-PCR, with the procedures described above. The colonies were also streaked directly onto triple sugar iron agar (Oxoid Ltd, Basingstoke, England) and onto blood agar (bioMérieux) and identified with the VITEK system (bioMérieux), using a previously reported protocol [12].

The *Yersinia* strains were serotyped with slide agglutination using commercial *Y. enterocolitica* O:1, O:2, O:3, O:5, O:8 and O:9 antisera (Denka Seiken, Coventry, UK), *Y. enterocolitica* O:27 antiserum (SIFIN, Berlin, Germany) and *Y. pseudotuberculosis* O:1–O:6 antisera (Denka Seiken). *Yersinia pseudotuberculosis* was also serotyped with O-genotyping, using a conventional multiplex PCR, according to Bogdanovich et al. [16].

Data analysis

All statistical analyses were performed in the SAS 9.3 software. The official 2009 livestock census data were obtained from the Basque Statistics Institute (http://www.eustat.es) for each region and the PROC RANK Statement was used to classify each region as containing high, medium, or low numbers of each species. The relationships between *Yersinia* prevalence and the different independent variables studied (sex, age, sampling year, season, natural region, slope and livestock numbers) were examined statistically using the χ^2 or Fisher's test. The simple kappa coefficient of agreement was used to determine the degree of agreement between the ELISA and PCR results when applied to the same animal. A *t* test was used to compare the ELISA S/P ratios between the PCR-positive and -negative animals. Differences were considered significant at $P < 0.05$.

Results

Antibodies directed against pathogenic *Yersinia* were detected in 52.5 % (257/490) of the wild boars. The mean S/P ratio was 0.66 (95 % confidence interval [CI] 0.63–0.70) for the ELISA-positive samples and 0.061 (95 % CI 0.05–0.07) for the ELISA-negative samples (Fig. 1).

Yersinia infection was detected with rt-PCR in 51.4 % (37/72) of wild boars. *Yersinia enterocolitica* was present in 33.3 % (24/72) and *Y. pseudotuberculosis* in 25.0 % (18/72) of the animals. Mixed infections of *Y. enterocolitica* and *Y. pseudotuberculosis* were identified in five individuals. Ten of the 18 *Y. pseudotuberculosis*-positive samples were detected with the amplification of both the *ail* and *wzz*

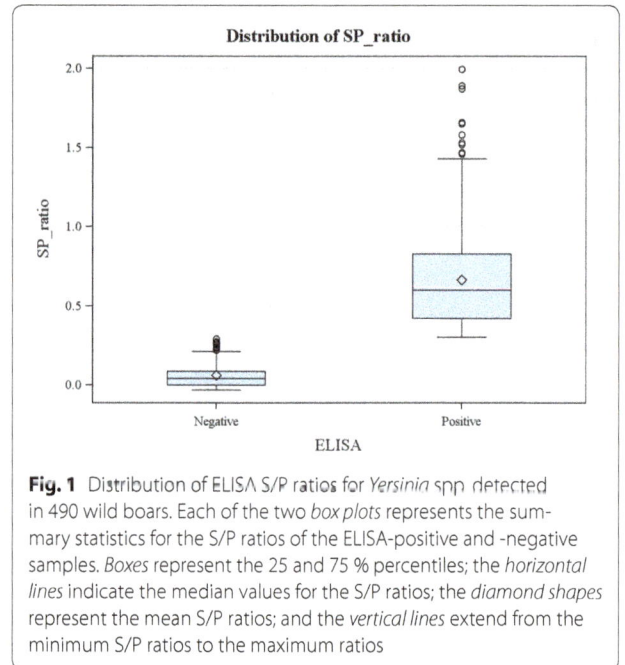

Fig. 1 Distribution of ELISA S/P ratios for *Yersinia* spp. detected in 490 wild boars. Each of the two *box plots* represents the summary statistics for the S/P ratios of the ELISA-positive and -negative samples. *Boxes* represent the 25 and 75 % percentiles; the *horizontal lines* indicate the median values for the S/P ratios; the *diamond shapes* represent the mean S/P ratios; and the *vertical lines* extend from the minimum S/P ratios to the maximum ratios

genes, four with the amplification of only *ail*, and the other four with the amplification of only the *wzz* gene.

Of the 37 rt-PCR-positive samples, 23 were only positive after enrichment and nine were only positive on direct rt-PCR. Eight samples were positive on both direct rt-PCR and after enrichment, but lower cycle threshold (Ct) values were obtained after enrichment (see Additional file 1).

Seroprevalence was higher in the adult animals than in the young animals ($P < 0.0001$; Table 1), but no significant differences were observed according to age with PCR ($P = 0.2157$; Table 2).

Significant differences were observed according to the sampling year. The highest seroprevalence was detected in 2002 and in 2005–2006, although in 2002, only 10 samples were analysed ($P < 0.0001$; Table 1). The prevalence of *Y. enterocolitica* was highest in 2010 ($P = 0.0213$) and that of *Y. pseudotuberculosis* was highest in 2012 ($P < 0.0001$; Table 2).

The overall seroprevalence was highest in winter and spring ($P < 0.0001$; Table 1). The prevalence of *Y. pseudotuberculosis* was highest in spring ($P = 0.0305$), but no significant difference was observed in the prevalence of *Y. enterocolitica* between seasons ($P = 0.3180$; Table 2).

Statistically significant differences were observed in the seroprevalence of *Yersinia* spp. according to the slope and region of habitation ($P < 0.0001$; Table 1). These differences were also significant for *Y. enterocolitica* and regions ($P = 0.0096$; Table 2). The geographic distribution of the positive samples is illustrated in Fig. 2.

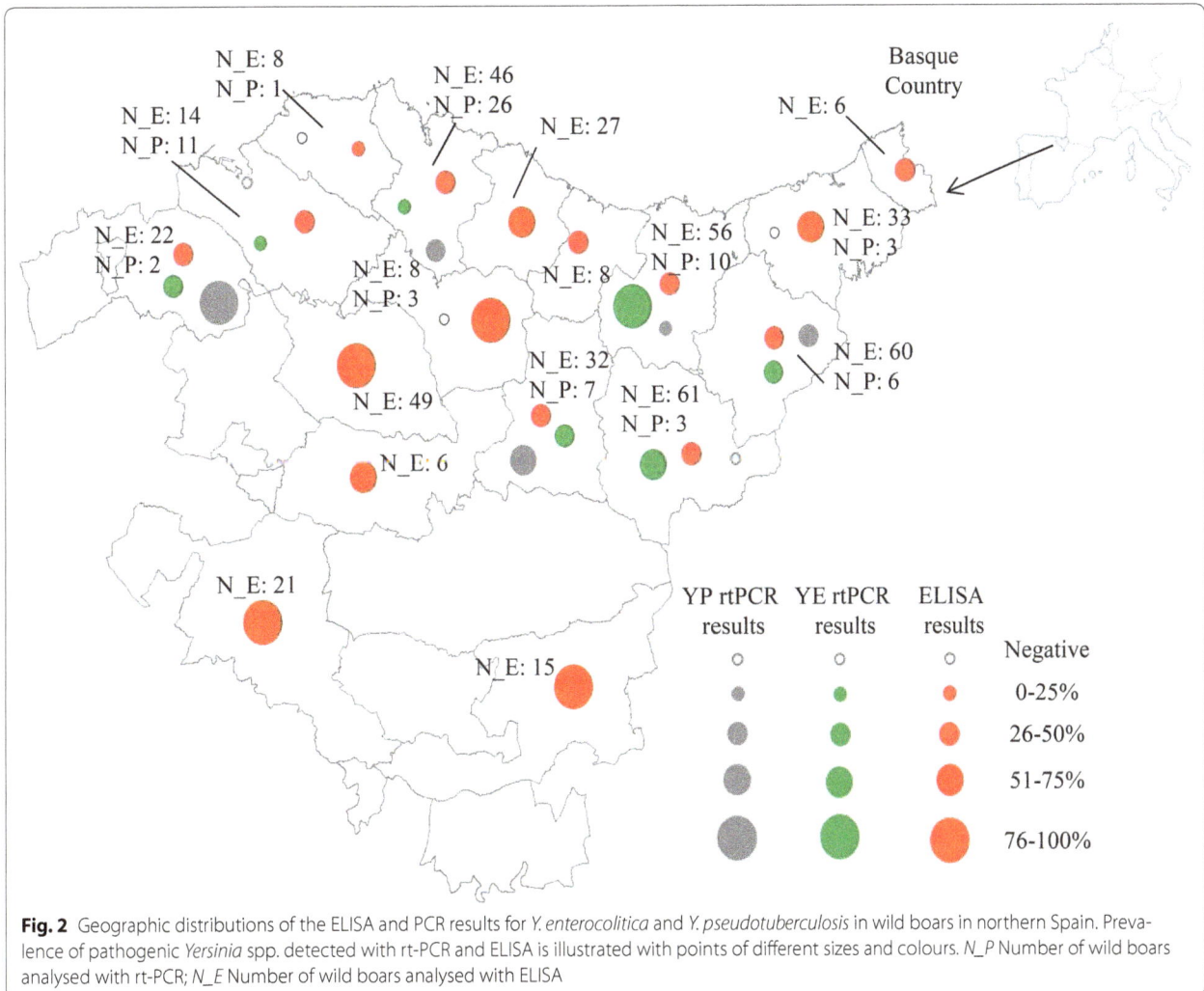

Fig. 2 Geographic distributions of the ELISA and PCR results for *Y. enterocolitica* and *Y. pseudotuberculosis* in wild boars in northern Spain. Prevalence of pathogenic *Yersinia* spp. detected with rt-PCR and ELISA is illustrated with points of different sizes and colours. *N_P* Number of wild boars analysed with rt-PCR; *N_E* Number of wild boars analysed with ELISA

Higher seroprevalence was observed in areas with small livestock populations (caprine, $P < 0.0001$) or medium livestock populations (bovine, $P = 0.0011$; ovine, $P < 0.0001$) (Table 1), whereas *Y. enterocolitica* prevalence was highest in areas with large ovine populations ($P = 0.0012$; Table 2).

Two isolates of *Y. pseudotuberculosis* and two of *Y. enterocolitica* were collected from four different wild boars. The *Y. pseudotuberculosis* isolates were obtained on CIN agar, one with direct plating and the other after enrichment. Both *Y. enterocolitica* isolates were obtained after enrichment, one on CIN agar and the other on CHROMagar™. The identities of *Y. enterocolitica* and *Y. pseudotuberculosis* were confirmed for each isolate with rt-PCR amplification of the *ail* gene. No agglutination was detected when the

Y. pseudotuberculosis isolates were serotyped with the antisera used, but both isolates were identified as serotype O:1c with multiplex O-gene amplification. It was not possible to serotype the *Y. enterocolitica* isolates because of contamination.

Of the 57 wild boars analysed with rt-PCR and ELISA, 13 were positive and 19 were negative with both techniques, seven animals were positive only according to ELISA, and 18 animals were positive only according to rt-PCR (κ index = 0.1452). No differences were observed in the ELISA S/P ratios when the *Y. enterocolitica*-rt-PCR-positive and -negative animals were compared. However, the *Y. pseudotuberculosis*-positive animals had higher S/P ratios (mean 0.53; 95 % CI 0.21–0.86) than the *Y. pseudotuberculosis*-negative animals (mean 0.23; 95 % CI 0.12–0.35; $P = 0.0249$).

Discussion

This study demonstrates that *Y. enterocolitica* and *Y. pseudotuberculosis* infections are widespread among the wild boars in northern Spain. The seroprevalence was high (52.5 %), although slightly lower than those detected in wild boars in Germany and Switzerland (62.6 and 65.0 %, respectively) [5, 17]. The prevalence of *Y. enterocolitica* and *Y. pseudotuberculosis* can also be considered high (33.5 and 25 %, respectively) because their observed prevalence in wild boars in Europe ranges from 4.35 to 35 % for *Y. enterocolitica* and is around 20 % for *Y. pseudotuberculosis* [5, 18, 19]. *Yersinia enterocolitica* was more prevalent than *Y. pseudotuberculosis*, as is usually found in wild boars and pigs [5, 20]. Mixed infections were detected in a proportion of the animals, as previously described [5], but the prevalence of *Y. pseudotuberculosis* (25 %) was higher than expected in wild boars or organically produced pigs, probably because they are in frequent contact with other infected wild species and livestock in extensive grazing systems [4, 21]. The use of two different rt-PCR methods and the higher detection rates recorded when an enrichment step was included before rt-PCR, could also have improved the detection rate for *Y. pseudotuberculosis* [12].

The highest seroprevalence was detected in spring and winter, which is attributable to the highest *Y. pseudotuberculosis* prevalence recorded in spring and the (not significantly) highest *Y. enterocolitica* prevalence recorded in winter. To the best of our knowledge, the seasonality of *Y. enterocolitica* and *Y. pseudotuberculosis* infections has not been reported previously in wild boars. However, in other wildlife species, the disease is usually detected in the coldest months of the year [22] or from November to May, which is related to the birth of newborns [23].

The highest seroprevalence and presence of *Y. enterocolitica* were associated with mountainous areas at altitudes higher than 600 m, very cold winters, and the highest annual rainfall for each dominant climate. A similar trend was observed in pigs slaughtered in China, in which the incidence of *Y. enterocolitica* was higher in cold areas than in warm areas [24].

The highest prevalence of *Y. enterocolitica* was detected in areas with a high ovine presence. Sheep have been described as a reservoir of pathogenic *Y. enterocolitica* and *Y. pseudotuberculosis* [25, 26], but little is known about the infection of sheep in Spain with pathogenic *Yersinia* or their relationship with the *Yersinia* species found in wild boars, although *Yersinia* is reported to cause sporadic abortion in sheep in the area studied [27]. In contrast, the highest *Yersinia* seroprevalence was associated with medium or low numbers of other livestock, suggesting that other wildlife species also contribute to the epidemiology of *Yersinia* infection among wild boars.

However, more studies are required to determine the real impact of pathogenic *Yersinia* on livestock in this area.

The rates of isolation were low, despite the use of two different culture media, including CHROMagar™, which is recommended for the isolation of *Y. enterocolitica* [28]. *Y. enterocolitica* pathogenicity therefore remains unknown, because the *ail* gene is an insufficient marker of virulence, and is also present in some *Y. enterocolitica* biotype 1A strains [29]. The only two *Y. pseudotuberculosis* strains isolated were identified as serotype O:1c. Little is known about the infection of animals or humans by serotype O:1c because the majority of studies have not included this subserotype. However, *Y. pseudotuberculosis* serotype O:1 has been described as one of the most commonly found serotypes infecting wild boars, pigs and humans in Europe [2, 30, 31]. This fact highlights the need for the better characterisation of its pathogenicity.

More efforts are required to isolate and characterise the *Yersinia* strains from infected wild boars in the Basque country to determine their pathogenicity and any potential risk they pose to humans and domestic species.

Conclusions

This study demonstrates that *Y. enterocolitica* and *Y. pseudotuberculosis* are highly prevalent among wild boars in the Basque Country, with *Y. enterocolitica* the most frequently found species. The risk of infection among wild boars is influenced by the season and the area in which the animals live.

Authors' contributions

MA, XG, VA and JCI performed the laboratory analyses. MA and MB performed the statistical analyses and wrote the manuscript. XG and VA participated in writing the manuscript. MA and MB conceived and designed the experiments. MB coordinated and supervised the study. All the authors participated in the interpretation of the results. All authors read and approved the final manuscript.

Acknowledgements

The study was supported by the Spanish National Institute for Agricultural and Food Research and Technology (INIA, RTA2010-00022), the Department of Agriculture and Fisheries (Basque Government) and European Regional Development Fund (ERDF). Maialen Arrausi-Subiza is the recipient of a predoctoral fellowship from "Fundación Candido de Iturriaga y María de Dañobeitia". We would like to thank Zuriñe Pérez and Dr Raquel Atxaerandio for their technical support, Diputaciones Forales and hunters for their collection of samples and Dr Janine Miller for English editing of the manuscript.

Competing interests

The authors declare that they have no competing interests.

Prevalence of Yersinia enterocolitica and Yersinia pseudotuberculosis in wild boars in the Basque...

51

References

1. EFSA (European Food Safety Authority), ECDC (European Centre for Disease Prevention and Control). The European union summary report on trends and sources of zoonoses, zoonotic agents and food-borne outbreaks in 2013. EFSA J. 2015;13:3991. doi:10.2903/j.efsa.2015.3991.
2. Fredriksson-Ahomaa M, Wacheck S, Bonke R, Stephan R. Different enteropathogenic Yersinia strains found in wild boars and domestic pigs. Foodborne Pathog Dis. 2011;8:733–7.
3. Nikolova S, Tzvetkov Y, Najdenski H, Vesselinova A. Isolation of pathogenic Yersiniae from wild animals in Bulgaria. J Vet Med B Infect Dis Vet Public Health. 2001;48:203–9.
4. Fukushima H, Gomyoda M. Intestinal carriage of Yersinia pseudotuberculosis by wild birds and mammals in Japan. Appl Environ Microbiol. 1991;57:1152–5.
5. Fredriksson-Ahomaa M, Wacheck S, Koenig M, Stolle A, Stephan R. Prevalence of pathogenic Yersinia enterocolitica and Yersinia pseudotuberculosis in wild boars in Switzerland. Int J Food Microbiol. 2009;135:199–202.
6. Magistrali CF, Cucco L, Manuali E, Sebastiani C, Farneti S, Ercoli L, Pezzotti G. Atypical Yersinia pseudotuberculosis serotype O:3 isolated from hunted wild boars in Italy. Vet Microbiol. 2014;171:227–31.
7. Acevedo P, Escudero MA, Muñoz R, Gortazar C. Factors affecting wild boar abundance across an environmental gradient in Spain. Acta Theriol. 2006;51:327–36.
8. Köppel C, Knopf L, Ryser MP, Miserez R, Thür B, Stärk KDC. Serosurveillance for selected infectious disease agents in wild boars (Sus scrofa) and outdoor pigs in Switzerland. Eur J Wildl Res. 2006;53:212–20.
9. Sales J, Kotrba J. Meat from wild boar (Sus scrofa L.): a review. Meat Sci. 2013;94:187–201.
10. Barandika JF, Berriatua E, Barral M, Juste RA, Anda P, Garcia-Perez AL. Risk factors associated with ixodid tick species distributions in the Basque region in Spain. Med Vet Entomol. 2006;20:177–88.
11. Gobierno Vasco. Vegetación de la comunidad autónoma del País Vasco. Vitoria: Servicio Central de Publicaciones del Gobierno Vasco; 1989.
12. Arrausi-Subiza M, Ibabe JC, Atxaerandio R, Juste RA, Barral M. Evaluation of different enrichment methods for pathogenic Yersinia species detection by real time PCR. BMC Vet Res. 2014;10:192.
13. Lambertz ST, Nilsson C, Hallanvuo S, Lindblad M. Real-time PCR method for detection of pathogenic Yersinia enterocolitica in food. Appl Environ Microbiol. 2008;74:6060–7.
14. Lambertz ST, Nilsson C, Hallanvuo S. TaqMan-based real-time PCR method for detection of Yersinia pseudotuberculosis in food. Appl Environ Microbiol. 2008;74:6465–9.
15. Matero P, Pasanen T, Laukkanen R, Tissari P, Tarkka E, Vaara M, Skurnik M. Real Time multiplex PCR assay for detection of Yersinia pestis and Yersinia pseudotuberculosis. APMIS. 2009;117:34–44.
16. Bogdanovich T, Carniel E, Fukushima H, Skurnik M. Use of O-antigen gene cluster-specific PCRs for the identification and O-genotyping of Yersinia pseudotuberculosis and Yersinia pestis. J Clin Microbiol. 2003;41:5103–12.
17. Al Dahouk S, Nockler K, Tomaso H, Splettstoesser WD, Jungersen G, Riber U, et al. Seroprevalence of brucellosis, tularemia, and yersiniosis in wild boars (Sus scrofa) from north-eastern Germany. J Vet Med B Infect Dis Vet Public Health. 2005;52:444–55.
18. Bancerz-Kisiel A, Szczerba-Turek A, Platt-Samoraj A, Socha P, Szweda W. Application of multiplex PCR for the evaluation of the occurrence of Ail, Ysta, and Ystb genes in Yersinia enterocolitica strains isolated from wild boars (Sus scrofa). Bull Vet Inst Pulawy. 2009;53:351–5.
19. Sannö A, Aspan A, Hestvik G, Jacobson M. Presence of Salmonella spp., Yersinia enterocolitica, Yersinia pseudotuberculosis and Escherichia coli O157:H7 in wild boars. Epidemiol Infect. 2014;142:2542–7.
20. Ortiz Martínez P, Fredriksson-Ahomaa M, Pallotti A, Rosmini R, Houf K, Korkeala H. Variation in the prevalence of enteropathogenic Yersinia in slaughter pigs from Belgium, Italy, and Spain. Foodborne Pathog Dis. 2011;8:445–50.
21. Laukkanen R, Ortiz Martínez P, Siekkinen KM, Ranta J, Maijala R, Korkeala H. Transmission of Yersinia pseudotuberculosis in the pork production chain from farm to slaughterhouse. Appl Environ Microbiol. 2008;74:5444–50.
22. Mair NS. Yersiniosis in wildlife and its public health implications. J Wildl Dis. 1973;9:64–71.
23. Fukushima H, Gomyoda M, Kaneko S. Mice and moles inhabiting mountainous areas of Shimane Peninsula as sources of infection with Yersinia pseudotuberculosis. J Clin Microbiol. 1990;28:2448–55.
24. Liang J, Wang X, Xiao Y, Cui Z, Xia S, Hao Q, et al. Prevalence of Yersinia enterocolitica in pigs slaughtered in Chinese abattoirs. Appl Environ Microbiol. 2012;78:2949–56.
25. Nikolaou K, Hensel A, Bartling C, Tomaso H, Arnold T, Rosler U, et al. Prevalence of anti-Yersinia outer protein antibodies in goats in lower saxony. J Vet Med B Infect Dis Vet Public Health. 2005;52:17–24.
26. Slee KJ, Skilbeck NW. Epidemiology of Yersinia pseudotuberculosis and Y. enterocolitica infections in sheep in Australia. J Clin Microbiol. 1992;30:712–5.
27. Oporto B, Barandika JF, Hurtado A, Aduriz G, Moreno B, Garcia-Perez AL. Incidence of ovine abortion by Coxiella burnetii in northern Spain. Ann N Y Acad Sci. 2006;1078:498–501.
28. Renaud N, Lecci L, Courcol RJ, Simonet M, Gaillot O. CHROMagar Yersinia, a new chromogenic agar for screening of potentially pathogenic Yersinia enterocolitica isolates in stools. J Clin Microbiol. 2013;51:1184–7.
29. Sihvonen LM, Hallanvuo S, Haukka K, Skurnik M, Siitonen A. The ail gene is present in some Yersinia enterocolitica biotype 1A strains. Foodborne Pathog Dis. 2011;8:455–7.
30. Wacheck S, Fredriksson-Ahomaa M, König M, Stolle A, Stephan R. Wild boars as an important reservoir for foodborne pathogens. Foodborne Pathog Dis. 2010;7:307–12.
31. Rimhanen-Finne R, Niskanen T, Hallanvuo S, Makary P, Haukka K, Pajunen S, et al. Yersinia pseudotuberculosis causing a large outbreak associated with carrots in Finland, 2006. Epidemiol Infect. 2009;137:342–7.

7

The influence of macro- and microelements in seminal plasma on diluted boar sperm quality

Maja Zakošek Pipan[1]* ⓘ, Janko Mrkun[1], Breda Jakovac Strajn[2], Katarina Pavšič Vrtač[2], Janko Kos[3,4], Anja Pišlar[3] and Petra Zrimšek[5]

Abstract

Background: Growing evidence indicates that macro- and microelements in the seminal plasma of humans and various domestic animals are of great importance due to their roles in sperm metabolism, function, survival and oxidative stress. In the present study, we therefore determined the concentrations of macro- and microelements in fresh boar seminal plasma and their relation to sperm quality parameters after 3 days of liquid storage was assessed. Twenty ejaculates from eight boars were collected, and semen volume, concentration, sperm motility, morphology, tail membrane integrity, plasma membrane permeability, mitochondrial membrane potential and DNA fragmentation were determined on the day of collection (day 0) and day 3 (72 h) of storage at 15–17 °C. Seminal plasma was separated and the concentrations of macroelements (Na, K, Ca, and Mg) and microelements (Cu, Fe, Zn and Se) were determined.

Results: After 3 days of storage Se levels correlated significantly with sperm motility, progressive motility and morphology, all of which are routinely used for semen evaluation. On day 3, Se levels also correlated with tail membrane integrity, viability and intact DNA ($P < 0.05$). The correlation coefficients showed that mitochondrial function was better preserved at higher levels of Zn, while higher levels of Cu decreased mitochondrial function, but led to the better preservation of DNA. It was also evident that higher levels of Fe were associated with higher proportions of live spermatozoa and of spermatozoa with normal morphology after 3 days of storage ($P < 0.05$), while higher levels of Ca and Mg in fresh seminal plasma were associated with lower percentages of progressive motile spermatozoa and with a decreased proportion of spermatozoa with intact DNA ($P < 0.05$). Multivariate analysis including microelements showed that Se significantly affected sperm quality parameters, mentioned above, after 3 days of storage.

Conclusions: Macro- and microelements were associated with boar sperm quality and may be important biomarkers of boar sperm quality after liquid storage. Our results demonstrate that the evaluation of Se in fresh boar seminal plasma can serve as an additional tool in predicting sperm quality after storage.

Keywords: Macroelements, Microelements, Boar semen, Liquid storage, Sperm quality

Background

The traditional semen-processing technology used in the swine industry is based on insemination of sows with chilled semen stored at 15–20 °C for 1–5 days after the addition of an appropriate extender [1]. However, the motility and viability of stored boar spermatozoa are diminished and alterations can occur in membrane permeability [2]. To maintain the high quality of semen for insemination, routine assessment based on the concentration and evaluation of motility and morphology is necessary [3]. However, their relation to in vivo fertility remains under discussion [4].

It is well-known that the ionic environment has a great influence on sperm function in humans [5]. The

*Correspondence: maja.zakosekpipan@vf.uni-lj.si
[1] Clinic for Reproduction and Large Animals, Veterinary Faculty, University of Ljubljana, Gerbičeva 60, 1000 Ljubljana, Slovenia
Full list of author information is available at the end of the article

World Health Organization's (WHO) guidance on the assessment of seminal plasma includes analysis of some macro- and microelements, such as Zn and Se, which are associated with sperm quality in humans due to their antioxidant properties [6, 7]. In men with Se deficiency, there is a loss of sperm motility, breakage at spermatozoa mid-piece level and increased incidence of spermatozoa head abnormalities [8]. In boars, the addition of Se to their diet resulted in contradictory results [9, 10]. In a recent study, Se supplementation did not affect sperm quantity or sperm quality [10], but increased levels of the predominant selenoprotein PHGPx, which is responsible for the integrity of mature spermatozoa [11]. Zn is crucial to the quality of spermatozoa and acts as a cofactor for many enzymes. Its deficiency results in disorders of testicular development and in spermatogenic failure [12, 13]. Macro- and microelements in boars have been studied [7, 14], but the nature of the influence of elements on semen characteristics needs further investigation.

The aim of the present study was to determine the concentrations of macro- and microelements in fresh boar seminal plasma and their association with sperm quality characteristics after 3 days of liquid storage.

Methods
Semen samples
Twenty ejaculates (2–3 per boar) obtained from eight mature and healthy boars of various breeds [two Slovenian Landrace line 11, one Slovenian landrace line 55, two Slovenian Large White, two Pietrain, and one Hibride line (54)] aged 12–24 months were included in the study. The boars included were of proven fertility with pregnancy rates of 69.5 ± 7.9% after insemination. Average litter size was 12.1 ± 0.3 piglets; 94.9% of born piglets were alive. The boars were housed in individual pens with straw bedding and received a standard balanced diet. Full ejaculates without the gel fraction were collected by the gloved-hand technique during routine farm operations at a local AI centre. Following collection, the filtered semen of each ejaculate was extended with Beltsville Thawing Solution (BTS, Truadeco, the Netherlands) at a ratio of 1:2.

Sample preparation and basic semen characteristics
After arrival to the laboratory, an initial evaluation was performed of each diluted ejaculate, and those that fulfilled the requirements of >70% total motility, >35% progressive motility, <30% abnormal sperm morphology, and <20% proximal and distal cytoplasmic droplets were included in the study. Motility and progressive motility were determined using assisted semen analysis (Hamilton Thorne IVOS 10.2; Hamilton Thorne Research, MA, USA) with a Makler counting chamber (Sefi Medical Instruments, Haifa, Israel). Before analysis, semen

samples were incubated in a water bath at 37 °C for 8 min. Thereafter, for each sample, 5 µl of diluted semen was mounted on a heated Makler counting chamber. Three randomly selected microscopic fields were scanned three times each, obtaining 9 scans for every semen sample. The mean of the three scans for each microscopic field was used for the statistical analysis. The software settings used in this study are summarized in Table 1.

Concentrations were measured with a photometer (Photometer SDM 5, Minitüb, Germany). The morphology of 200 spermatozoa in diluted semen samples were assessed following eosin-nigrosin staining (Morphology stain, Society for Theriogenology).

Semen analysis was performed on the day of collection (day 0) and on day 3 (72 h) of semen preservation. Semen samples were stored on day 0 for 3 days in closed plastic containers in a thermal box at 15–17 °C with constant gentle agitation.

Additional semen analyses
Hypoosmotic swelling test (HOST)
A HOST was applied to evaluate tail membrane integrity as a test of sperm function. First, 10 µl of the semen sample was mixed gently with 90 µl of hypoosmotic solution (150 mOsm/kg sodium citrate × $2H_2O$ and fructose) at 37 °C. After 1 h of incubation at 37 °C in a warm water tub, 200 spermatozoa per sample were examined under a light microscope at a magnification of 400×. Spermatozoa were considered HOST positive if they showed signs of swelling, as described by Hishinuma and Sekine [15].

Table 1 Software settings for Hamilton Thorne IVOS 10.2 used in this study

Hamilton Thorne settings	
Frames per second	60 Hz
Minimum cell size	10 pixels
Cell intensity	125
Straightness (STR) threshold	80%
Medium VAP cut-off	45 µm/s
Low VSL cut-off	15 µm/s
Low VAP cut-off	25 µm/s
Slow cells motile	No
Static head intensity	0.65–4.90
Static intensity gate	0.50–2.50
Magnification	1.89
Temperature of analysis	37 °C
Type of chamber	Makler

Assessment of membrane modifications using the Yo-Pro-1/PI assay

Staining spermatozoa with Yo-Pro-1/PI was used to detect changes in plasma membrane permeability as described by Idziorek et al. [16]. After staining, different cell populations were distinguished using a flow cytometer (FACS-Calibur, BD Bioscience, San Jose, CA, USA). Channel FL-1 was used to detect green fluorescence (Yo-Pro-1), while channel FL3 was used to detect red fluorescence (PI).

Sheath flow rate was set at 6–24 µl/min, and a minimum of 20,000 events were recorded. The analyser threshold was adjusted on the electronic volume channel to exclude subcellular debris and cell aggregates. Light signals were converted into electrical signals by a photo detector and evaluated by a software programme (Flow Jo, Ashland, USA).

The cell population was separated into three groups: live cells, showing no fluorescence (Yo-Pro-1 −/PI −); (early) apoptotic cells, showing an incrementally higher level of green fluorescence (Yo-Pro-1 +/PI −); and late apoptotic/dead (Yo-Pro-1 +/PI +) and necrotic cells (Yo-Pro-1 −/PI +), showing red fluorescence.

Assessment of mitochondrial membrane potential

Mitochondrial membrane potential (MMP) is an indicator of sperm functionality. MitoTracker Red is a fluorescent probe suitable to differentiate spermatozoa with deteriorated mitochondria (in apoptotic cells) from that of living spermatozoa [17]. A slightly modified protocol was used for this study. Briefly, ten million sperm cells washed in PBS (centrifuged at 400g for 30 min) were added to 1 ml of PBS. Next, 10 µl of stain MitoTracker Red (500 nM) (Invitrogen) was added, and the tubes were gently mixed and incubated for 30 min in the dark at 37 °C. The fluorescence signal was monitored at the FL2 channel of a flow cytometer (FACSCalibur, BD Bioscience, San Jose, CA, USA). Sheath flow rate was set at 6–24 µl/min, and a minimum of 20,000 events were recorded. The analyser threshold was adjusted on the electronic volume channel to exclude subcellular debris and cell aggregates. Spermatozoa incubated in 50 µM carbonyl cyanide *m*-chlorophenyl hydrazone (CCCP), known to reduce mitochondrial membrane potential, were used as a control.

MitoTracker dye positive sperm events indicated cells with active membrane-polarized mitochondria, whereas cells with reduced MitoTracker fluorescence were those whose mitochondria had reduced mitochondrial transmembrane potential.

DNA fragmentation

DNA integrity was evaluated using a commercial test (Sperm Sus-Halomax; Halotech DNA SL, Spain) based on the Sperm Dispersion test and specifically designed for boar spermatozoa. The semen samples were processed according to the manufacturer's instructions and stained with a commercial fluorescence microscopy green staining kit (Halotech DNA, Spain) according to the instructions. The fluorescence stained sample was placed into the well of a slide prior to microscopic assessment. Sperm chromatin dispersion was evaluated using a fluorescence filter (Olympus U-MNIBA3; excitation at 497 nm and emission at 520 nm) with 400× magnification (Olympus BX40). A minimum of 300 spermatozoa were counted per semen sample.

The spermatozoa were classified into three categories according to the shape of the halo effect: (1) normal halo, a clearly visible halo around the head similar to the diameter of the core; (2) a small or absent halo, a small halo spotted around the head or a complete absence of a halo; and (3) a large scattered halo, a very large and scattered halo around the head. Based on the halo effect, spermatozoa were then classified into two categories: spermatozoa with a normal halo effect, denoting intact DNA and spermatozoa with a small, absent or large scattered halo effect, denoting impaired DNA.

Analysis of macro- and microelements

A semen sample was centrifuged at 800g for 10 min at room temperature. The supernatant was removed and centrifuged again at 13,000g for 15 min at 4 °C to separate seminal plasma, which was then aliquoted and frozen at −80 °C until assayed for Na, Mg, Ca, K, Fe, Cu, Zn and Se. Analysis of the elements was performed as described previously [18] with a slight modification. Microwave digestion of the samples was performed using an MARS 5 Microwave Acceleration Reaction System (CEM, Matthews, NC). A total 2 ml of a sample was transferred into a 100 ml Teflon vessel and 3 ml 65% nitric acid, 0.5 ml 30% hydrogen peroxide and 4.5 ml Milli-Q water were added. The samples were digested in a closed 12 vessel microwave system at 200 °C for 30 min. After cooling to room temperature, the solutions were diluted with Milli-Q water and the concentrations of elements were determined by inductively coupled plasma mass spectrometry (Varian 820-MS, Mulgrave, Australia). Argon was used as the carrier gas and the isotopes ^{23}Na, ^{24}Mg, ^{44}Ca, ^{39}K, ^{57}Fe, ^{63}Cu, ^{66}Zn, ^{78}Se were selected as analytical masses in the ICP-MS normal sensitivity mode. A Collision Reaction Interface (CRI) was used for the measurements of Se to reduce common polyatomic interferences.

Statistical analysis

Data are presented as the mean ± standard deviation (SD) and median. The normal distributions of data were tested by the Shapiro–Wilk test. In cases of normal distribution, parametric tests were performed; in case of non-normal distributed data, non-parametric tests were performed. Spearman or Pearson rank correlation coefficients were used to determine the correlation between sperm quality characteristics on days 0 and 3 and to evaluate the association between the concentration of trace elements on day 0 and the sperm quality characteristics on day 3. Statistical analyses were performed using SPSS (IBM SPSS Statistics 22). $P < 0.05$ was considered significant. A multivariate linear regression model was used to assess the association between microelements (Fe, Cu, Zn and Se) and each sperm quality characteristic on day 3 of semen storage. Analyses were performed in R Statistical Software (version 3.1.1).

Results
Characteristics of sperm quality
The mean concentration of spermatozoa in semen ejaculates was $319.5 \pm 116.1 \times 10^6$ ml. Measurement characteristics of sperm quality were made for fresh semen

samples (day 0) and for semen samples after 3 days of storage (day 3) (Table 2). The values of sperm quality characteristics differed significantly between days 0 and 3 for all sperm quality characteristics ($P < 0.05$), except for proximal and distal droplets ($P > 0.05$) (Table 2).

Values of elements measured in seminal plasma on day 0
Values of elements measured in seminal plasma on day 0 are shown in Table 3.

Correlation between sperm quality characteristics on days 0 and 3
Correlation coefficients were determined for sperm characteristics on days 0 and 3 of liquid storage (Table 4).

Intact DNA on day 3 correlated with the highest number of sperm quality characteristics in fresh semen. Significant positive correlations were observed with progressive motility and capacitation ($P < 0.05$), whereas correlations with impaired tail membrane integrity, apoptotic spermatozoa and decreased mitochondrial membrane potential on day 3 were negative ($P < 0.05$). High positive correlation was also observed for intact DNA between day 0 and day 3. Progressive motility on day 3 correlated with four sperm quality characteristics on day 0. Significant positive correlations were observed with motility, the proportion of live spermatozoa and intact DNA ($P < 0.05$), whereas correlation with the proportion of apoptotic spermatozoa was negative ($P < 0.05$). Impaired tail membrane integrity also correlated with motility and intact DNA, but correlations were negative ($P < 0.05$). There was also a negative correlation between impaired tail membrane integrity on day 3 and the proportion of morphologically normal and capacitated spermatozoa on day 0 ($P < 0.05$). Sperm motility and the

Table 2 Values (mean ± SD, median) of boar sperm quality characteristics on day 0 and after 3 days of liquid storage (n = 20)

Semen parameters (%)	Day 0		Day 3	
	Mean ± SD	Median	Mean ± SD	Median
Motility	80.5 ± 4.4	80.1	60.4 ± 11.9	62.6
Progressive motility	47.2 ± 7.7	47.3	30.0 ± 7.8	29.6
Normal sperm morphology	75.6 ± 6.9	76.4	59.8 ± 9.6	57.2
Proximal droplets	4.2 ± 3.5	3.9	4.4 ± 3.4	4.7
Distal droplets	5.5 ± 3.0	4.6	5.6 ± 2.8	4.9
Acrosome reacted spermatozoa	12.3 ± 4.5	11.5	27.2 ± 7.7	25.9
Capacitated spermatozoa	4.1 ± 2.7	3.5	15.3 ± 4.7	15.0
Impaired tail membrane integrity	14.4 ± 3.8	14.7	36.6 ± 9.8	34.9
Membrane potential				
Live spermatozoa	67.3 ± 7.0	66.9	39.1 ± 9.4	40.2
Dead spermatozoa	25.1 ± 6.7	25.6	47.1 ± 9.9	44.9
Apoptotic spermatozoa	7.6 ± 4.6	6.8	13.8 ± 3.5	13.5
Decreased mitochondrial potential	4.8 ± 7.6	3.4	26.1 ± 25.9	21.1
Intact DNA	90.8 ± 6.6	93.3	82.9 ± 6.9	83.8

Table 3 Concentration of elements (mean, median, minimum and maximum) in boar seminal plasma (n = 20)

	Mean	Median	Minimum	Maximum
Na (mmol/l)	96.3	96.4	81.3	106.8
Mg (mmol/l)	2.10	1.78	0.62	4.98
K (mmol/l)	13.2	12.9	11.7	14.8
Ca (µmol/l)	179.4	161.3	76.8	285.9
Fe (µmol/l)	2.71	2.66	1.73	4.58
Cu (µmol/l)	0.94	0.97	0.49	1.35
Zn (µmol/l)	212.4	194.1	59.4	475.7
Se (nmol/l)	78.6	71.5	55.7	150.2

56

Veterinary Science: Animal Pathology and Disease Management

Table 4 Correlations (r value) between sperm quality characteristics on day 0 and sperm quality characteristics after 3 days of storage (n = 20)

Day 0	Day 3							
	Motility	Progressive motility	Normal sperm morphology	Acrosome reacted spermatozoa	Dead spermatozoa	Apoptotic spermatozoa	Intact DNA	Impaired tail membrane integrity
Motility	0.504*	0.466*	0.036	−0.415	−0.357	0.136	0.327	−0.469*
Progressive motility	0.498*	0.384	0.140	−0.147	−0.458*	−0.560*	0.554*	−0.372
Normal sperm morphology	0.325	0.367	0.794*	−0.444*	−0.234	−0.245	0.111	−0.476*
Proximal droplets	−0.212	−0.337	−0.465	−0.166	0.000	0.165	−0.038	0.270
Distal droplets	−0.193	−0.084	−0.153	0.090	0.311	0.099	0.040	0.063
Capacitated spermatozoa	0.138	0.243	0.494*	−0.471*	−0.501*	0.421	0.613*	−0.573*
Impaired tail membrane integrity	−0.027	−0.129	−0.380	0.371	−0.093	0.183	−0.485*	0.242
Live spermatozoa	0.582*	0.502*	−0.011	−0.119	−0.007	−0.322	−0.274	0.150
Apoptotic spermatozoa	−0.392	−0.474*	−0.304	0.072	−0.145	0.494*	−0.652*	−0.284
Decreased mitochondrial potential	−0.027	−0.129	−0.380	0.371	−0.093	0.183	−0.485*	−0.027
Intact DNA	0.342	0.500*	0.199	−0.347	−0.340	−0.571*	0.946*	−0.618*

Only sperm quality characteristics that showed at least one correlation are included in the table

*P values <0.05

proportion of apoptotic spermatozoa on day 3 correlated with three sperm quality characteristics on day 0. Sperm motility on day 3 correlated positively with sperm motility, progressive motility and proportion of live spermatozoa on day 0 (P < 0.05). The proportion of apoptotic spermatozoa on day 3 correlated positively with that of apoptotic spermatozoa on day 0 (P < 0.05), whereas correlations with intact DNA and progressive motility on day 0 were negative (P < 0.05). On day 3, normal sperm morphology correlated positively and acrosome reacted spermatozoa negatively with normal sperm morphology and capacitated spermatozoa on day 0 (P < 0.05). Late apoptotic/dead spermatozoa on day 3 correlated negatively with progressive motility and the proportion of capacitated spermatozoa (P < 0.05).

Capacitated spermatozoa, live spermatozoa and mitochondrial membrane potential on day 3 did not correlate with any sperm quality characteristics on day 0 (P > 0.05).

Correlations between element concentrations in seminal plasma on day 0 and sperm quality characteristics on day 3

Correlations between element concentrations in seminal plasma on day 0 and sperm quality characteristics on day 3 are summarized in Table 5; only correlations with elements that showed at least one significant correlation are presented.

Selenium in the seminal plasma of fresh boar semen correlated with many sperm quality characteristics after 3 days of storage. Significant positive correlations of Se were observed with motility, progressive motility, normal sperm morphology, live spermatozoa and spermatozoa with intact DNA while negative correlations were found for acrosome reacted spermatozoa, dead spermatozoa and spermatozoa with impaired tail membrane integrity on day 3 (all P values <0.05) (Table 5). Iron showed a positive correlation with normal sperm morphology and the proportion of live spermatozoa and a significant negative correlation with the proportion of dead spermatozoa (all P values <0.05), as observed for Se. Ca correlated with three characteristics as for Se, but the correlations were inverse; a positive correlation was observed with impaired tail membrane integrity and a negative correlation with the proportion of progressive motility and DNA fragmentation (all P values <0.05). Magnesium showed the same correlation as did Ca, except for lack of correlation between Mg and impaired tail membrane integrity (P > 0.05).

Table 5 Correlations (r value) between the concentrations of elements in boar seminal plasma measured on day 0 and sperm quality characteristics on day 3 (n = 20)

Semen parameters on day 3	Element concentration in seminal plasma on day 0					
	Mg (mmol/l)	Ca (μmol/l)	Fe (μmol/l)	Cu (μmol/l)	Zn (μmol/l)	Se (nmol/l)
Motility	−0.168	−0.325	0.035	0.042	−0.350	0.674*
Progressive motility	−0.497*	−0.436*	0.177	0.140	−0.087	0.563*
Normal sperm morphology	0.136	0.360	0.555*	−0.126	0.430	0.757*
Proximal droplets	−0.190	−0.231	−0.090	−0.106	0.113	−0.252
Distal droplets	−0.276	−0.157	−0.133	0.225	0.174	−0.045
Acrosome reacted spermatozoa	0.000	0.242	0.208	0.132	−0.007	−0.406*
Capacitated spermatozoa	0.236	−0.144	−0.144	−0.254	−0.117	0.138
Impaired tail membrane integrity	0.147	0.463*	0.119	−0.215	0.187	−0.716*
Live spermatozoa	0.091	0.237	0.496*	−0.323	−0.266	0.467*
Dead spermatozoa	0.022	−0.146	−0.547*	0.207	0.200	−0.455*
Decreased mitochondrial potential	−0.174	−0.438	−0.414	0.582*	−0.625*	−0.303
Intact DNA	−0.475*	−0.567*	0.149	0.506*	0.240	0.473*

*P values <0.05

Copper showed a significant positive correlation while Zn showed a significant negative correlation with decreased mitochondrial membrane potential (P < 0.05). Copper also showed a significant positive correlation with intact DNA (P < 0.05). There was no association of either K or Na with sperm quality characteristics (P > 0.05).

Taken together, DNA fragmentation correlated with the highest number of elements; it negatively correlated with Mg (P < 0.05) and Ca (P < 0.05) and positively correlated with Cu (P < 0.05) and Se (P < 0.05).

Results of multivariate regression model including microelements

Association between microelements in fresh seminal plasma and sperm quality parameters after 3 days of storage was analysed by multivariate linear regression model. Selenium was significantly associated with sperm motility (P = 0.012), progressive motility (P = 0.018), morphology (P = 0.004) and acrosomal reaction of the spermatozoa (P = 0.007). Tail membrane integrity was also affected by Se (P = 0.003) as well as by Fe (P = 0.033), while the proportion of live spermatozoa after storage was significantly associated with Cu (P = 0.032). Moreover, the proportion of live spermatozoa and spermatozoa with intact DNA tended to be higher in semen with higher concentration of Se in fresh seminal plasma (P = 0.056 and P = 0.084, respectively).

Discussion

The results of the present study show correlations between macro- and microelements in fresh boar seminal plasma and sperm quality characteristics after 3 days of liquid storage. Microelement concentrations, especially for Se, were associated with sperm quality characteristics.

The concentrations of macro- and microelements were similar to those in previous studies conducted on fresh boar semen [7, 14]. It has been shown that K helps to preserve sperm motility and is added to several commercial extenders [1] and that Na correlates with normal sperm morphology [14]. In our study, semen was extended with BTS for the purposes of short term storage. BTS contains Na-citrate, Na-bicarbonate, KCl, EDTA, glucose and antibiotics; therefore, no correlations were found between sperm quality characteristics and the concentrations of Na and K. The concentrations of Na and K used were higher in our study than in the study conducted by Lopez Rodriguez et al. [14] because they used fresh boar semen without extenders.

In the male reproductive system, Fe can display either positive or negative roles, depending on its concentration. An increased concentration of Fe in the testes was associated with oxidative damage of lipids, proteins, and DNA [19]. However, Fe deficiency reduced the activity of Fe-containing and Fe-depending enzymes [7]. Massanyi et al. [7] found a strong positive correlation between Fe and Zn in fresh boar semen and it was recently demonstrated in bulls that adding $FeCl_2$ to diluted semen samples at concentrations above 50 μmol/l leads to a significant decrease of sperm motility and mitochondrial activity. However, concentrations below 10 μmol/l $FeCl_2$ stimulated spermatozoa activity, as shown by a significant preservation of motility and viability characteristics in diluted bull spermatozoa [20]. In our study, where the mean Fe concentration in boar seminal plasma was 2.71 μmol/l (minimum, 1.73 μmol/l; maximum,

4.58 μmol/l), higher Fe levels were correlated with a higher level of normal sperm morphology and live spermatozoa after storage. From the multivariate analysis it was found that Fe affected also tail membrane integrity. Because spermatozoa are under increased oxidative stress during storage [2], low levels of Fe, which lead to lower activity of Fe-dependent enzymes such as catalase [7], could lead to increased lipid peroxidation in boar spermatozoa and result in reduced viability.

A significant negative correlation was observed between Zn concentrations on day 0 and decreased mitochondrial membrane potential on day 3, indicating that higher levels of Zn better preserved mitochondrial function. However, the higher levels of Cu decreased mitochondrial function, but better preserved DNA. Copper is essential for many enzymes such as superoxide dismutase, which is involved in protecting cells against oxygen free radicals [21]. This may be the reason for the higher percentage of spermatozoa with intact DNA in our study. Copper is also needed for cytochrome c oxidase, which is responsible for energy supply and for cellular and humoral immunity [21]. However, elevated Cu concentrations reduce glycolysis, which may be the reason for the decreased mitochondrial potential that manifested in the decrease of sperm motility [22]. In our study, among microelements, Cu was found to be significantly associated with the proportion of live spermatozoa. After the addition of Zn to human semen samples, a significantly higher percentage of sperm with intact DNA and normal mitochondrial function was found [23]. We also noted a trend of positive association for Zn with normal sperm morphology after storage, but the correlation was not significant (P = 0.058). A similar correlation was found for fresh human semen [24]. A previous study in boars did not find any correlation between Zn in fresh seminal plasma and sperm quality characteristics, but there was a negative correlation with abnormal tails [14]. It has been suggested that Zn affects sperm quality in different ways, making it difficult to associate it with a single parameter [14]. Zinc is able to protect spermatozoa against oxidative stress [24] and is seen as a better preserver of mitochondrial function since mitochondria are the major site of intracellular formation of reactive oxygen species [25].

Selenium was correlated with most of the sperm quality characteristics. The higher preservation of membrane integrity and normal sperm morphology observed in our study are in agreement with a study conducted on fresh boar semen by Lopez Rodriguez et al. [14], where higher levels of Se were associated with less membrane damage and fewer proximal droplets. Selenium participates in a variety of physiological functions as an integral part of a range of selenoproteins. It is also an important component of the enzyme glutathione peroxidase that protects cell membranes against the adverse effects of lipid peroxides [26], thereby preserving the structural integrity of the spermatozoa plasma membrane [27]. Our study also confirmed these results with correlations between Se and the preservation of membrane integrity, which is also reflected in preservation or increase of ATP in spermatozoa, leading to improved sperm motility and progressive motility [28]. This is again confirmed in our study by the positive correlations between Se and sperm motility and progressive motility. On the basis of multivariate analysis the association between Se in fresh seminal plasma and sperm quality characteristic, mentioned above, was confirmed. Low levels of Se can lead to higher levels of active peroxides during the final stages of spermatogenesis, which can cause oxidative injuries that could accumulate and lead to delayed impairment of viability [29]. Impaired spermatogenesis arising from Se deficiency has been reported in several animal species including boars [28], where changes in mitochondria, decreased sperm ATP concentration and increased percentage of immature spermatozoa were noted in boars fed a low-selenium diet [28]. It was suggested that Se plays a role in establishing the number of spermatozoa reserves and Sertoli cells. Boars fed a low Se diet also possessed spermatozoa with lower motility and increased abnormal morphology [28]. Although in the present study, Se intake was the same in all boars, the content of Se in seminal plasma varied. The same was shown in study conducted on fresh boar semen by Lasota et al. [30]. Even though in our study, semen samples that had a higher content of Se had better preserved sperm quality following 3 days of storage, it was found that when sodium selenite was added directly to the boar extender, sperm motility was reduced [28]. This could be because although Se and Zn can improve sperm quality, they may be harmful above certain levels [31].

Calcium and Mg levels correlated negatively with sperm progressive motility and the increased proportion of spermatozoa with intact DNA. Kasperczyk et al. [32] found a positive correlation between the levels of interleukin-12 and Mg, suggesting that Mg may indirectly promote the development of oxidative stress, thereby leading to impaired DNA and decreased sperm motility. Calcium acts as the trigger of the acrosome reaction in mammalian spermatozoa, and there is substantial evidence that it is differentially involved in sperm motility depending on the stage of sperm maturation, thereby causing decreased sperm motility [33].

The higher levels of Se were consistent with better conserved sperm quality characteristics after 3 days of storage. Infertile men have lower levels of Se in their seminal plasma [34]. Since traditional estimates of sperm quality are not sufficiently sensitive to differentiate between samples that differ in terms of predicting quality following storage [35], measurements of Se in boar seminal plasma could be of value in predicting sperm quality characteristics of semen following storage. Recently, new markers of sperm function that could enable better prediction of fertilizing ability in boars have been sought; the tumour necrosis factor, TNF-α [36], and superoxide dismutase [37], each measured in diluted fresh seminal plasma, were found to be valuable predictors of sperm quality after 3 days of storage. Our study shows that the concentration of Se correlated not only with sperm motility, progressive motility and morphology, which are all used routinely for semen evaluation but also with tail membrane integrity, sperm viability and intact DNA. These methods are also very effective in evaluating semen and can provide additional information about sperm fertility. The results of our study indicate that measuring Se in fresh seminal plasma can be helpful in predicting sperm quality following 3 days of storage.

Although higher concentrations of Se in fresh seminal plasma correlated with improved sperm quality after 3 days of storage in our study, current evidence suggests that optimal levels of Se is needed for good sperm quality [38].

Very high levels of Se could cause an opposite effect and reduce sperm quality. To predict sperm quality after 3 days of storage with Se, reference values should be established on larger numbers of semen samples. Se in fresh seminal plasma must be evaluated as possible predictors of sperm quality after storage. Based on the sperm quality after storage, the highly predictive values of Se could be used in the future as an additional tool in semen evaluation.

Conclusions

An analysis of macro- and microelements in fresh boar seminal plasma demonstrated an association with boar sperm quality and therefore provides additional information about sperm quality after liquid storage. Due to the significant correlations between Se concentrations in fresh seminal plasma and semen parameters after storage, the evaluation of Se in fresh boar seminal plasma could serve as an additional tool in predicting sperm quality after storage.

Authors' contributions

MZP contributed to the study design, interpretation of the results and has been involved in drafting the manuscript; MZP also performed semen analysis. JM coordinated clinical work, was involved in the evaluation of semen data and interpretation of the results. BJS and KPV participated in study design and were involved in macro- and microelements analysis and evaluation of these data. JK was involved in flow-cytometer analysis and helped to draft the manuscript. AP was involved in flow-cytometer analysis and evaluation of

the results from flow-cytometer analysis. PZ was involved in the study design, interpretation of the results and statistical analysis and has been involved in drafting the manuscript. All authors read and approved the final manuscript.

Author details
[1] Clinic for Reproduction and Large Animals, Veterinary Faculty, University of Ljubljana, Gerbičeva 60, 1000 Ljubljana, Slovenia. [2] Department for Environment and Animal Nutrition, Welfare and Hygiene, Veterinary Faculty, University of Ljubljana, Gerbičeva 60, 1000 Ljubljana, Slovenia. [3] Department of Pharmaceutical Biology, Faculty of Pharmacy, University of Ljubljana, Aškerčeva cesta 7, 1000 Ljubljana, Slovenia. [4] Department of Biotechnology, Jožef Štefan Institute, Jamova cesta 39, 1000 Ljubljana, Slovenia. [5] Institute for Preclinical Sciences, Veterinary Faculty, University of Ljubljana, Gerbičeva 60, 1000 Ljubljana, Slovenia.

Acknowledgements
This work was supported by the Slovenian Research Agency and was part of 'Endocrine, immune, nervous and enzyme responses in healthy and sick animals' (P4-0053). The authors are also a member of the Zinc-Net COST Action TD1304. We thank the statistician Mateja Blas, M.Sc. for performing multivariate analysis. The authors also thank American Journal Experts for the English revision of the manuscript.

Competing interests
The authors declare that they have no competing interests.

References
1. Johnson LA, Weitz KF, Fiser P, Maxwell WMC. Storage of boar semen. Anim Reprod Sci. 2000;62:143–72.
2. Kumaresan A, Kadirvel G, Bujarbaruah KM, Bardoloi RK, Das A, Kumar S, et al. Preservation of boar semen at 18 °C induces lipid peroxidation and apoptosis like changes in spermatozoa. Anim Reprod Sci. 2009;110:162–71.
3. Knox R, Levis D, Safranski T, Singleton W. An update on North American boar stud practices. Theriogenology. 2008;70:1202–8.
4. Tsakmakidis IA, Lymberopoulos AG, Khalifa TA. Relationship between sperm quality traits and field-fertility of porcine semen. J Vet Sci. 2010;11:151–4.
5. Hamameh S, Gatti J-L. Role of the ionic environment and internal pH on sperm activity. Hum Reprod. 1998;13(Suppl 4):20–30.
6. Chia SE, Ong CN, Chua LH, Ho LM, Tay SK. Comparison of zinc concentrations in blood and seminal plasma and the various sperm parameters between fertile and infertile men. J Androl. 2000;21:53–7.
7. Massanyi P, Trandzik J, Nad P, Toman R, Skalick M, Kornekov B. Seminal concentrations of trace elements in various animals and their correlations. Asian J Androl. 2003;5:101–4.
8. Agarwal A, Sekhon LH. Oxidative stress and antioxidants for idiopathic oligoasthenoteratospermia: is it justified? Indian J Urol. 2011;27:74–85.
9. López A, Rijsselaere T, Van Soom A, Leroy JL, De Clercq JB, Bols PE, et al. Effect of organic selenium in the diet on sperm quality of boars. Reprod Domest Anim. 2010. doi:10.1111/j.1439-0531.2009.01560.
10. Lovercamp KW, Stewart KR, Lin X, Flowers WL. Effect of dietary selenium on boar sperm quality. Anim Reprod Sci. 2013. doi:10.1016/j.anireprosci.2013.02.016.
11. Martins SM, De Andrade AF, Zaffalon FG, Bressan FF, Pugine SM, Melo MP, et al. Organic selenium supplementation increases PHGPx but does not improve viability in chilled boar semen. Andrologia. 2015;47:85–90.
12. Cigankova V, Mesaros P, Bires J, Ledecky V, Ciganek J, Tomajkova E. Morphological structure of the testes in stallion at zinc deficiency. Slovak Vet J. 1998;23:97–100.
13. Eskenazi B, Kidd SA, Marks AR, Sloter E, Block G, Wyrobek AJ. Antioxidant intake is associated with semen quality in healthy men. Hum Reprod. 2005;20:1006–12.
14. Lopez Rodríguez A, Rijsselaere T, Beek J, Vyt P, Van Soom A, Maes D. Boar seminal plasma components and their relation with semen quality. Syst Biol Reprod Med. 2013;59:5–12.

15. Hishinuma M, Sekine J. Evaluation of membrane integrity of canine epididymal spermatozoa by short hypoosmotic swelling test with ultrapure water. J Vet Med Sci. 2003;65:817–20.

16. Idziorek T, Estaquier J, De Bels F, Ameisen JC. YOPRO-1 permits cytofluoro-metric analysis of programmed cell death (apoptosis) without interfering with cell viability. J Immunol Methods. 1995;185:249–58.

17. Terrell KA, Wildt DE, Anthony NM, Bavister BD, Leibo SP, Penfold LM, et al. Different patterns of metabolic cryo-damage in domestic cat (*Felis catus*) and cheetah (*Acinonyx jubatus*) spermatozoa. Cryobiology. 2012;64(2):110–7.

18. Aguiar GF, Batista BL, Rodrigues JL, Silva LR, Campiglia AD, Barbosa RM, Barbosa F Jr. Determination of trace elements in bovine semen samples by inductively coupled plasma mass spectrometry and data mining techniques for identification of bovine class. J Dairy Sci. 2012;95:7066–73.

19. Marchlewicz M, Wiszniewska B, Gonet B, Baranowska-Bosiacka I, Safranow K, Kolasa A, et al. Increased lipid peroxidation and ascorbic acid utilization in testis and epididymis of rats chronically exposed to lead. Biometals. 2007;20:13–9.

20. Tvrdá E, Lukáč N, Lukáčová J, Jambor T, Massányi P. Dose- and time-dependent in vitro effects of divalent and trivalent Fe on the activity of bovine spermatozoa. Biol Trace Elem Res. 2015;167:36–47.

21. Leonhard-Marek S. Influence of drugs, pollution and trace elements on male fertility. In: Busch W, Holzmann A, editors. Andrology in veterinary medicine. Schattauer: Stuttgart; 2001. p. 474–81.

22. Pesch S, Bergmann M, Bostedt H. Determination of some enzymes and macro- and microelements in stallion seminal plasma and their correlations to semen quality. Theriogenology. 2006;66:307–13.

23. Kotdawala AP, Kumar S, Salian SR, Thankachan P, Govindraj K, Kumar P, et al. Addition of zinc to human ejaculate prior to cryopreservation prevents freeze-thaw-induced DNA damage and preserves sperm function. J Assist Reprod Genet. 2012;29:1447–53.

24. Colagar AH, Marzony ET, Chaichi MJ. Zinc levels in seminal plasma are associated with sperm quality in fertile and infertile men. Nutr Res. 2009;29:82–8.

25. Guthrie HD, Welch GR, Long JA. Mitochondrial function and reactive oxygen species action in relation to boar motility. Theriogenology. 2008;70:1209–15.

26. Pieczyńska J, Grajeta H. The role of selenium in human conception and pregnancy. J Trace Elem Med Biol. 2015;29:31–8.

27. Wu ASH, Oldfield JE, Shull LR, Cheeke PR. Specific effect of selenium deficiency on rat sperm. Biol Reprod. 1979;20:793–8.

28. Marin-Guzman J, Mahan DC, Whitmoyer R. Effect of dietary selenium and vitamin E on the ultrastructure and ATP concentration of boar sperma-tozoa, and the efficacy of added sodium selenite in extended semen on sperm motility. J Anim Sci. 2000;78:1544–50.

29. Foresta C, Flohé L, Garolla A, Roveri A, Ursini F, Maiorino M. Male fertility is linked to the selenoprotein phospholipid hydroperoxide glutathione peroxidase. Biol Reprod. 2002;67:967–71.

30. Lasota B, Błaszczyk B, Seremak B, Udała J. Selenium status and GSH-Px activity in semen and blood of boars at different ages used for artificial insemination. Reprod Dom Anim. 2004;39:309–14.

31. Sağlam HS, Altundağ H, Atik YT, Dündar MŞ, Adsan Ö. Trace elements levels in the serum, urine, and semen of patients with infertility. Turk J Med Sci. 2015;45:443–8.

32. Kasperczyk A, Dobrakowski M, Horak S, Zalejska-Fiolka J, Birkner E. The influence of macro and trace elements on sperm quality. J Trace Elem Med Biol. 2015;30:153–9.

33. Prien SD, Lox CD, Messer RH, DeLeon FD. Seminal concentrations of total and ionized calcium from men with normal and decreased motility. Fertil Steril. 1990;54:171–2.

34. Türk S, Mändar R, Mahlapuu R, Viitak A, Punab M, Kullisaar T. Male infertil-ity: decreased levels of selenium, zinc and antioxidants. J Trace Elem Med Biol. 2014;28:179–85.

35. Rodriguez-Martinez H. Laboratory semen assessment and prediction of fertility: still utopia? Reprod Domest Anim. 2003;38:312–8.

36. Mrkun J, Kosec M, Zrimšek P. Value of semen parameters, with special ref-erence to tnf-α, in predicting the quality of boar semen after short-term storage. Acta Vet Hung. 2013;61:209–19.

37. Zakošek Pipan M, Mrkun J, Kosec M, Svete AN, Zrimšek P. Superoxide dis-mutase: a predicting factor for boar semen characteristics for short-term preservation. Biomed Res Int. 2014. doi:10.1155/2014/105280.

38. Ferguson LR, Karunasinghe N, Zhu S, Wang AH. Selenium and its' role in the maintenance of genomic stability. Mut Res Fundam Mol Mech Mutagen. 2012;733:100–10.

8

Control and eradication of porcine reproductive and respiratory syndrome virus type 2 using a modified-live type 2 vaccine in combination with a load, close, homogenise model: an area elimination study

Poul H. Rathkjen[1]*[ID] and Johannes Dall[2]

Abstract

Background: Porcine reproductive and respiratory syndrome virus (PRRSV) causes significant animal and economic losses worldwide. The infection is difficult to control and PRRSV elimination at local level requires coordinated intervention among multiple farms. This case study describes a successful elimination of PRRSV from all 12 herds on the Horne Peninsula, Denmark, using a combination of load, close, homogenise (LCH) using PRRSV type 2 modified-live vaccine, optimised pig flow, and '10 Golden Rules' (10GR) for biosecurity management. To the authors' knowledge, this is the first successful European PRRSV area elimination project documented in detail. The PRRSV type 2 modified-live vaccine was used as part of the LCH method in breeding herds. Complete or partial depopulation was performed in some infected herds. A simplified biosecurity protocol (10GR) based on the McREBEL™ system of pig flow management, was employed in all herds and at all times throughout the study.

Results: At study commencement, all herds were infected with PRRSV, and most were actively shedding virus. In just over 18 months, all 12 herds on the Horne Peninsula were confirmed to be PRRSV negative by polymerase chain reaction testing and negative for antibodies against PRRSV by enzyme–linked immunosorbent assay testing. All herds were subsequently obtained 'Specific Pathogen Free' status for PRRSV.

Conclusions: This study provides compelling evidence suggesting that an area elimination plan combining LCH with PRRSV type 2 vaccination, optimised pig flow, and 10GR for biosecurity management can effectively eliminate PRRSV from a geographic area. Additionally this study confirms the value of a previously unpublished, simplified alternative to the McREBEL system for controlling PRRSV.

Keywords: Area regional control, Elimination, Modified-live vaccine, Load close homogenise, PRRS

Background

Porcine reproductive and respiratory syndrome (PRRS) is one of the most prevalent viral swine diseases in the world, responsible for substantial economic losses worldwide [1]. In the US, PRRS is estimated to cause annual losses of around $664 million [2]. A 2012 economic analysis in nine Dutch sow herds found that the mean economic loss per sow per 18-week outbreak of PRRSV was €126 [3].

Porcine reproductive and respiratory syndrome is caused by the PRRS virus (PRRSV) and was first reported in the late 1980s [4]. Two PRRSV genotypes have been described: type 1 and type 2, isolated in Europe and North America, respectively. Sequence comparison has

*Correspondence: poul.rathkjen@boehringer-ingelheim.com
[1] Boehringer Ingelheim Vetmedica GmbH, Binger Straße 173, 55216 Ingelheim, Germany
Full list of author information is available at the end of the article

highlighted significant genetic differences between them [5].

Porcine reproductive and respiratory syndrome causes high morbidity and mortality, poor reproductive performance and slow piglet growth rates [1]. The extent of reproductive symptoms varies depending on age, pregnancy status and stage of gestation [6, 7]. In non-pregnant sows, PRRS can develop without symptoms, or cause appetite loss or fever [6]. In pregnant sows, the virus may cross the placenta during late gestation, infect developing foetuses and increase the risk of abortion, early farrowing and foetal death [8, 9]. Neonatal and nursery pigs may experience respiratory distress, listlessness, pneumonia, high fever, anorexia, conjunctivitis and growth retardation [6, 10–12]. In growing and finishing pigs, the severity of PRRS varies from no detectable signs to fatal pneumonia, depending on the viral strain and the presence of opportunistic bacterial or viral coinfections [13].

At both herd and individual level, PRRSV infection is difficult to control for several reasons. PRRSV infection can be completely cleared by the porcine immune system, but considerable gaps remain in our understanding of the immunological response to PRRSV [14]. In the field, the diversity of PRRSV is increasing [15]. Levels of genetic similarity between vaccine and field challenge have often been used as a predictor of vaccine efficacy, but the ability of a vaccine to protect against a certain field virus is not linked to the level of sequence homology it shares with the challenging strain: the degree of genetic similarity does not predict the cross-protective ability of the vaccine [14]. Despite these challenges, vaccination is a popular method of controlling PRRS and reducing losses caused by it. Multiple vaccines are commercially available [11].

Accepted PRRSV control and elimination models for multiple herds include herd closure with either total herd replacement or with normal herd replacement rates, and depopulation/repopulation of infected herds [16, 17]. Herd closure involves preventing entry of new animals, while depopulation/repopulation involves complete removal of PRRSV-positive animals from a herd, cleaning and decontaminating the site, then replacing with PRRSV–negative animals bred elsewhere [17]. Depopulation/repopulation is effective, but expensive because of requirements for large external breeding projects [17] and loss of productivity after depopulation [2]. Alternatively, the load, close, homogenise (LCH) (also known as load, close, expose) model allows the PRRSV status to stabilise in a breeding herd before introduction of new PRRSV-negative animals [18, 19]. Using this model, PRRSV can be completely eliminated from large breeding (sow) herds [14] without incurring substantial losses of productive

time (i.e. time without weaned pigs) for the breeding herd. LCH is accomplished by loading herds with gilts before closing the herds to new animals for minimum of 200 days [14]. Uniform PRRS status must then be achieved either by simultaneous vaccination or by inoculation with serum containing resident virus [19]. The LCH model is inexpensive compared with depopulation/repopulation of a breeding stock [20], and broadly recognised as effective at stabilising PRRSV-positive breeding herds [21, 22], but it requires stringent biosecurity measures to prevent virus transmission within the herd.

The Management Changes to Reduce Exposure to Bacteria to Eliminate Losses™ (McREBEL) system was developed in 1994 to reduce the spread of PRRSV and secondary bacterial infections among farrowing house pigs, and to nursery pigs [22–24]. The McREBEL system helps stabilise PRRSV infection within the breeding herd and reduce mortality among infected nursery pigs [24]. The McREBEL system has several advantages, but the system can be difficult to implement for many reasons. For example, farm staff can be unwilling to abandon cross-fostering and perform piglet euthanasia, and staff incentive plans need to be reviewed to ensure its success [24].

The Horne Peninsula is a region in the southern Danish island of Funen, approximately 50 kilometres southwest of Odense. The peninsula is a naturally limited geographical area; it is surrounded with water on three sides, and spans approximately 6 kilometres North to South, and 10 kilometres East to West. It is an area with intensive pig farming: 12 herds are situated on the peninsula, and include breeding, wean-to-finish and finishing production, but no other herds are situated within 4 km.

Until the current elimination plan started, all farms on the Horne Peninsula repeatedly experienced PRRS outbreaks despite multiple attempts to control the virus. Common problems were periodic outbreaks of abortion, many stillborn piglets, poorly-lactating sows, poorly–performing piglets at weaning, and high mortality in one particular finisher herd. Different attempts to control the PRRSV in the area had already been tried, but with low success. Prior control attempts included depopulation, vaccinating incoming gilts with PRRS modified-live vaccine (MLV) in quarantine and systematically implementing some McREBEL rules to varying degrees. Overall, a systematic approach to control or eliminate PRRSV from the whole area was needed.

The objective of this area elimination case study was to eliminate PRRSV infection as defined by absence of pigs with PRRSV and corresponding antibodies from all herds on the Horne Peninsula, Denmark, using a combination of LCH using PRRS modified-live type 2 vaccine, optimised pig flow, and implementation of '10 Golden Rules' (10GR) for biosecurity management.

Methods

Herds

The study area included all 12 herds on the Horne Peninsula: five finisher herds, four breeding herds, two wean-to-finish herds, and one gilt quarantine (Table 1). Breeding herds contained sows, gilts ready for breeding, and weaned piglets. Wean-to-finish herds received weaned piglets from breeding herds and raised them until slaughter. Finisher herds received piglets at around 11 weeks of age, and raised them until slaughter.

In total, the herds on the peninsula contained approximately 15,000 animals. Movement of animals between the 12 herds was coordinated in two separate pig flows: Flow 1 and Flow 2. All animals in Flow 1 originated from F1B1 and F1B2, and all animals in Flow 2 originated from F2B1 and F2B2. The herds in each flow were controlled by four separate owners who worked closely with each other. PRRSV-negative gilts were imported into F2B1 only after completing 12 weeks in all in, all out (AIAO) quarantine: no other herds received animals from outside of the Horne Peninsula. Animals were exported out of the Horne Peninsula from the nursery of F1B2 only. All other animal movements were within the herds on the peninsula.

Layout of farm buildings

Breeding herds contained separate areas: farrowing rooms and nursery rooms. F1WF1 had four nursery rooms and six finisher rooms: all were separate, but all pigs entered through one nursery room and passed through others whilst in transit. Similarly, pigs moving from nursery to finisher rooms passed through several rooms containing piglets of other ages. At study commencement, F1WF1 operated as continuous flow. F1WF2 comprised two barns: a nursery and a finishing barn, both of which had multiple rooms. AIAO production was observed in all rooms in both the nursery and finishing barns. Finishing herds contained pigs separated into different rooms by age group, and AIAO production was observed. F1Q consisted of two adjacent buildings, connected by corridors. One building housed pregnant sows and finishers that arrived from F1B2, and the other building housed gilts in acclimatisation and quarantine. Separate rooms were entered from the corridor, and rooms did not share airspace and were not connected under the floor slats. Strict AIAO production was observed.

Study timeframe

The study began in the first week of July, 2013.

Week 0

Load close homogenise was commenced at Week 0 in F1B1 and F1B2. At Week 0, F1Q was loaded with gilts 10–32 weeks of age, and sites with sows and gilts were closed for the next 29 weeks. All sows, gilts (existing and newly-introduced), boars and piglets (older than 1 week)

Table 1 Overview of herds included in the study

Herd name	Owner	Type of production	Number and type of animals	Age ranges, weeks	Approximate weight ranges, kg
Flow 1					
F1B1	Owner 1	Breeding	500 sows	Piglets: 0–4	Piglets: 1–7
F1B2	Owner 1	Breeding	300 sows	Piglets: 0–4 Weaned piglets: 4–12	1–7, 5–30
F1Q	Owner 1	Gilt quarantine	200 pregnant sows 550 gilts 1000 finishers	10–32 12–18	30–120 30–110
F1WF1	Owner 2	Wean-to-finish	1220 finishers	4–18	7–110
F1WF2	Owner 3	Wean-to-finish	2000 finishers	4–18	7–110
F1F1	Owner 2	Finishing	1000 finishers	11–18	30–110
F1F2	Owner 4	Finishing	800 finishers	11–18	30–110
Flow 2					
F2B1	Owner 5	Breeding	400 sows 2000 growers	Piglets: 1–4 Weaned piglets: 4–12	1–7 5–30
F2B2	Owner 5	Breeding	320 sows 1300 growers	Piglets 1–4 Weaned piglets: 4–12	1–7 5–30
F2F1	Owner 6	Finishing	1600 finishers	11–18	30–110
F2F2	Owner 7	Finishing	900 finishers	11–18	30–110
F2F3	Owner 5	Finishing	1000 finishers	11–18	30–110

F1B1 Flow 1 Breeding Herd 1, *F1B2* Flow 1 Breeding Herd 2, *F1F1* Flow 1 Finisher Herd 1, *F1F2* Flow 1 Finisher Herd 2, *F1Q* Flow 1 Quarantine, *F1WF1* Flow 1 Wean-Finish 1, *F1WF2* Flow 1 Wean-Finish 2, *F2B1* Flow 2 Breeding Herd 1, *F2B2* Flow 2 Breeding Herd 2, *F2F1* Flow 2 Finisher Herd 1, *F2F2* Flow 2 Finisher Herd 2, *F2F3* Flow 2 Finisher Herd 3

on all sites except F2B1 and F2B2 were homogenised by vaccination with 2 ml PRRSV type 2 MLV (Ingelvac® Boehringer Ingelheim Vetmedica Inc., St. Joseph, MO, USA). F2B1 and F2B2 were already PRRSV positive-stable at study commencement, so homogenisation was deemed unnecessary. From Weeks 0–10, Finisher pigs in F2F1, F2F3 and F2F3 were vaccinated with 2 ml PRRS type 2 MLV upon arrival from F2B1 and F2B2, to avoid introducing naïve pigs. Vaccinations were performed according to the manufacturer's guidelines on dose and administration (Boehringer Ingelheim Vetmedica GmbH, Germany).

Depopulation commenced in F2B1 and F2B2. The nursery rooms containing the two oldest age groups (piglets older than 8 weeks) were depopulated.

Weeks 2–4

All piglets in F1B1 and F1B2 were vaccinated with 2 ml PRRSV type 2 MLV when they reached 7 days of age. Vaccination of sows, boars and gilts was repeated at Week 4. All animals in F2F1, F2F2 and F2F3 that had not been vaccinated previously were also vaccinated at Week 4.

Weeks 6–16

On a rolling basis from Week 6 to 16, all weaned piglets (3 weeks of age) that had not already been vaccinated when entering breeding herd nurseries or wean-to-finish nurseries, were vaccinated with 2 ml PRRSV type 2 MLV upon arrival.

At Week 16, depopulation of nursery rooms in F1B2, and partial depopulation of nursery rooms in F1WF1 commenced.

All times throughout the study

Sampling and diagnostic testing to determine PRRSV shedding and exposure status continued every 5 weeks from study commencement, until all herds were confirmed PRRSV and antibody negative by polymerase chain reaction (PCR) and enzyme-linked immunosorbent assay (ELISA), respectively.

The 10GR for biosecurity and pig flow management were employed in all herds and at all times throughout the study (Table 2). These rules were devised in 2005 by Boehringer Ingelheim, and are based on the principles of the McREBEL system for disease management [23].

10 Golden Rules for biosecurity management

Staff members received training in the 10GR from the responsible veterinarian on each farm. Training emphasised the importance of open and frequent communication among staff members. To ensure optimal compliance with the 10GR, farms were audited by the farm veterinarian at 5-week intervals throughout the study. If the audit found that the 10GR were not being followed, this was communicated to the staff, and corrected.

Sampling and diagnostic testing of PRRSV status

Piglets were randomly selected from among all parity sows. To determine PRRSV status among weaning-age piglets 8 weeks before study commencement, blood samples were taken from 3-week old (pre-wean) piglets, and piglets 2, 3, 4, 6, 7 and 8 weeks after weaning in breeding herd nurseries. Samples were then taken at 5-week intervals throughout the study. Serum was harvested from the blood samples by routine methods.

In breeding and WF herds, blood samples were taken from at least 30 animals at each time point, and comprised samples from a minimum of 5 animals per age group (each week of age). These sample sizes were adequate to detect at least one positive sample with 95% confidence if the prevalence of PRRSV positive pigs was 10% or higher [25], and to meet the sample size requirements needed for declaring of PRRSV free Specific Pathogen Free (SPF) status [26].

In finisher herds, blood samples were taken from at least 20 animals. This sample size was adequate to detect at least one positive sample with 95% confidence if the prevalence of PRRSV positive pigs was 15% or higher. Fewer samples were taken from finisher herds than from breeding and WF herds because it was assumed that if pigs were infected with PRRSV during the early finishing period, the prevalence of infected pigs would be higher. This sample size also met the sample size requirements needed for declaration of PRRS free SPF status in routine monitoring of negative herds.

Individual serum samples were used to evaluate PRRSV exposure status (indicated by the presence of PRRSV antibodies in serum). An ELISA method (IDEXX Herd-Check PRRS X3 ELISA, IDEXX Laboratories Inc., Westbrook, ME, USA) was used to detect PRRSV antibodies. Serum samples from each age group were pooled, and used to determine PRRSV shedding status (indicated by the presence of viral DNA in serum). Reverse transcriptase PCR (rtPCR) was used to detect PRRSV RNA. Combining PCR and ELISA increased the confidence that detection would occur if pigs were exposed to PRRSV.

A herd was declared to have a positive exposure status (ELISA positive; presence of anti-PRRSV antibodies) if one or more individual serum samples was positive (Sample: Positive ratio cut off >0.4). A herd was declared to have a positive shedding status (PCR positive; presence of PRRSV RNA) if one or more pooled serum samples was PCR positive for PRRSV RNA. PRRSV was considered eliminated from a herd

Table 2 The 10 Golden Rules

	Rule	Rationale
1	Minimise cross-fostering and movement of piglets: cross-foster only surplus piglets	The immune system is immature in newborn piglets; immunity depends on passive immunisation transmitted via colostrum [37]. Piglets receive optimal protection from their own mothers so should only be moved if a sow cannot support her whole litter. Furthermore, moving piglets to other sows causes weight loss in both moved piglets and their new litter mates [38]
2	Avoid cross-fostering after 48 h	Maternal immune protection starts to decrease when piglets reach 3 days of age [37]. Cross-fostering before maternal protection decreases is strongly recommended
3	Avoid spreading disease when handling piglets by keeping piglets in pens	Urine, blood, faeces and semen are vehicles for PRRSV transmission; special attention should be paid to the use of equipment (e.g. needles and castration equipment)
4	Change needles between litters	PRRSV is easily transmitted among pigs by needles, so regular replacement of needles (at least between litters) is recommended. Diseased piglets should be treated after healthy piglets
5	Do not move diseased piglets	Diseased piglets often have compromised immunity and comorbidities that increase the likelihood that they are also carrying PRRSV. Their viral load is also likely to be higher, increasing the risk of spreading infection. Therefore diseased piglets should remain with the same sow to limit viral spread: if a piglet is too weak for this, it should be euthanised
6	Wean all piglets from each batch simultaneously, and ban weaned piglets from the farrowing rooms	Holding smaller piglets back in the farrowing rooms for quality before they are weaned can jeopardise PRRS control programmes [39]. Such piglets are more likely to be diseased, and to spread PRRSV to others
7	Maintain strict AIAO batch production at all times from weaning to finishing	After piglets are weaned, batch production should continue, and should be either by site, barn or room. If a batch is not completely removed before placement of new pigs, infection pressure rapidly increases. Do not share needles, equipment, personnel and protective equipment between batches (unless cleaned and disinfected)
8	Avoid contact between age groups	Risk of infection is increased 13-fold if contact is permitted between growing pigs of different ages during restocking of rooms [40]. Mixing PRRSV-positive pigs in one age group with PRRSV-negative, non-vaccinated pigs in other age groups greatly increases PRRSV shedding [41, 42]
9	Avoid contact between sows and piglets (<6 months of age)	Breeding herds and grower/finisher pigs should never be in contact (i.e. when moving pigs and sows around the farm) because cross-contamination between groups can occur
10	Introduce incoming and home-produced gilts via quarantine. Administer PRRSV MLV upon entry to quarantine areas	Natural immunisation of gilts should be avoided because it cannot be monitored or controlled. If natural immunisation occurred just before entering a breeding site, there would be a high risk of introducing wild-type PRRSV to the breeding herd. While in quarantine, gilts should be immunised twice with PRRS MLV (vaccinations should be administered 4 weeks apart)

AIAO all in all out, *MLV* modified-live vaccine, *PRRSV* porcine reproductive and respiratory syndrome virus

after PRRSV RNA or antibodies were not detected after testing at four consecutive time points (taken at 5 week intervals).

PRRS status of herds, and official declaration of PRRSV Specific Pathogen Free status

Throughout the study, overall PRRS status of herds throughout the study was classified according to the American Association of Swine Veterinarians (AASV) terminology, taking into account both PRRSV shedding and exposure status [27]. Herds were classified as either: negative (ELISA negative and PCR negative),

positive-stable (ELISA positive but PCR negative); or positive-unstable (ELISA positive and PCR positive).

In addition, declaration of PRRSV free SPF status was sought, according to the regulations from SPF–SUS, Denmark [26]. PRRSV SPF status can be granted only when PRRSV has been eliminated (proven PCR and ELISA negative) from a herd. To meet the requirements for PRRSV free SPF declaration, 30 PRRSV-negative sentinel gilts were placed into each herd after samples from herds tested both PCR and ELISA negative. PRRSV free SPF status was confirmed if the sentinels remained PCR and ELISA negative after 6 months.

Results

Time taken to eliminate PRRSV from all farms on the Horne Peninsula

The study extended from July 2013 to July 2015. All herds on the Horne Peninsula were initially PRRSV positive-unstable except F2B1 and F2B2, which were positive-stable (Fig. 1; Additional file 1). All herds had confirmed PRRSV free SPF status by April 2015; less than 2 years after study commencement (Table 3).

Elimination in breeding herds

F1B1 and F1B2 were initially weaning PCR and ELISA positive piglets. By September 2013, both were weaning PCR negative, but ELISA positive piglets. Three-week old piglets remained ELISA positive on all sampling points until July 2014 (51 weeks after LCH was implemented). These antibodies were presumed to be maternal because no samples were PCR positive at the same time points.

Virus was detected in 5-week old and 7-week old piglets in the F1B2 nursery in November 2013. The virus was isolated from the ELISA and PCR positive piglets in F1B2, and the virus gene open reading frame 5 (ORF-5) was sequenced (Bioscreen GmBH, Hannover, Germany), and shown to have 99.17% sequence homology to the PRRSV type 2 MLV strain. The nursery was depopulated to prevent the virus spreading to the sows. The oldest pigs (26–32 kg) were exported out of the peninsula, but the youngest pigs (14–26 kg; too small to be sold) were moved to isolation rooms in F1Q, where they were vaccinated and slaughtered at a later time point. Remaining piglets that were considered to be negative were moved to F1WF2. The empty nursery was cleaned and disinfected before repopulation, and no virus was subsequently detected on the site.

In November 2014, two samples (both from F1B2) tested close to the ELISA assay cut-off, and in March 2015, another sample (from F1B2) tested ELISA positive. None of these samples were simultaneously PCR positive so all were assumed to be false-positives (Additional file 2).

PCR testing of samples from 10 week old piglets in F1B1 and F1B2 nurseries revealed that PRRSV remained present until Week 23 (Fig. 2). No virus was detected in any 10-week old piglets from Week 28 onwards.

At study commencement, F2B1 and F2B2 were PRRSV positive-stable, and weaning PRRSV PCR negative piglets. Piglets became PCR positive in the later nursery rooms, so the two rooms containing the oldest age groups were depopulated. F2B1 and F2B2 received PRRSV free SPF status in July 2014.

Elimination in wean-to-finish and finisher herds

F1WF1 was partially depopulated in October 2013, after piglet vaccination (at weaning) stopped, and then all piglets tested PCR negative until February 2014. Up to 20% of piglets continued to test ELISA positive until age 6–7 weeks, probably due to the presence of maternal antibodies (Additional file 3).

F1WF2 received a batch of presumed PCR negative piglets from F1B2 in November 2013, but PCR positive

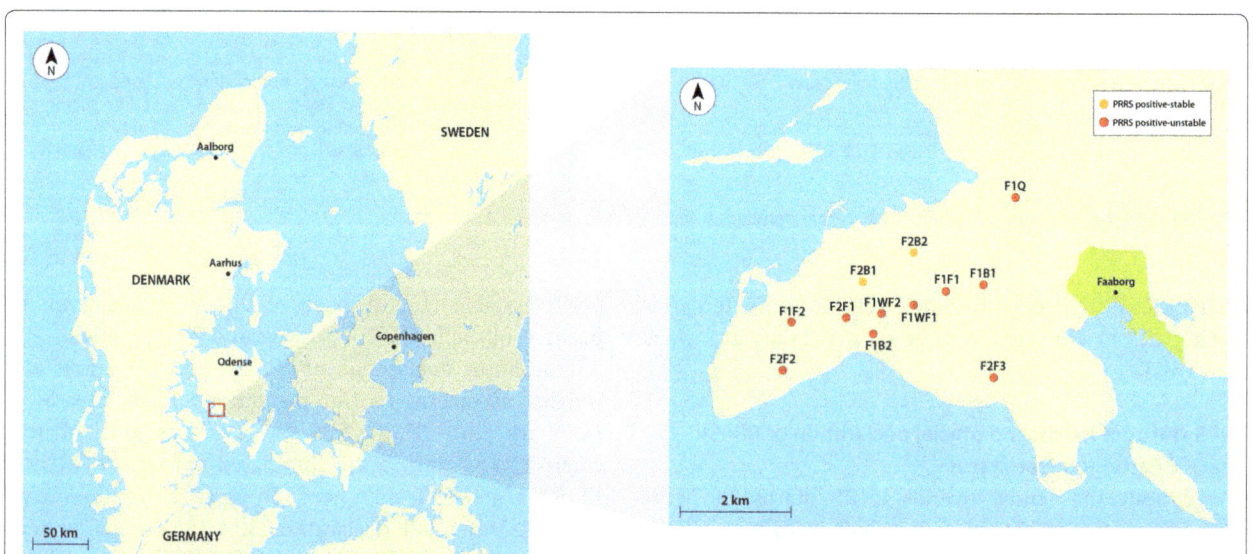

Fig. 1 Locations of herds on the Horne Peninsula, and PRRSV status at study commencement. *F1B1* Flow 1 Breeding Herd 1, *F1B2* Flow 1 Breeding Herd 2, *F1F1* Flow 1 Finisher Herd 1, *F1F2* Flow 1 Finisher Herd 2, *F1Q* Flow 1 Quarantine, *F1WF1* Flow 1 Wean-Finish 1, *F1WF2* Flow 1 Wean-Finish 2, *F2B1* Flow 2 Breeding Herd 1, *F2B2* Flow 2 Breeding Herd 2, *F2F1* Flow 2 Finisher Herd 1, *F2F2* Flow 2 Finisher Herd 2, *F2F3* Flow 2 Finisher Herd 3, *PRRS* porcine reproductive and respiratory syndrome

Table 3 Time for herds to obtain official PRRS free SPF status

Herd	PRRS free SPF status achieved	Notes
F1B1	January 2015	July 2013: weaned ELISA and PCR positive piglets at study commencement September 2013: weaned PCR negative but ELISA positive piglets July 2014: three-week old piglets remained ELISA positive until July 2014
F1B2	January 2015	July 2013: weaned ELISA and PCR positive piglets at study commencement September 2013: weaned PCR negative but ELISA positive piglets November 2013: sentinels were about to be introduced, but two age groups tested PCR positive (5-week old and 7-week old piglets in nursery rooms). Sequencing revealed 99.17% homology to PRRS type 2 MLV The nursery was depopulated to prevent PRRS spreading to the sows: Oldest pigs (26–32 kg) were exported out of the area Younger pigs (14–26 kg) were moved to isolation rooms in F1Q, vaccinated, then eventually slaughtered Piglets considered to be PCR negative were moved to F1WF2. (these were the only extra facilities available) The nursery was cleaned and disinfected before repopulation November 2014: two samples were close to the ELISA assay cut-off (SP > 0.4) March 2015: one sample was ELISA positive, but simultaneously PCR negative. This was assumed to be false positive
F1WF1	Finishers depopulated in February 2015	October 2013: partially depopulated October 2013–February 2014: ≤20% of samples tested from piglets were ELISA positive until age 6–7 weeks. All samples were PCR negative 100% of pigs older than 7 weeks were ELISA and PCR negative February 2014: samples from 17-week old piglets were ELISA positive, but PCR negative March 2014: 16- and 18-week pigs were found to be PCR and ELISA positive April 2014: finisher rooms partially depopulated again. The site then remained PCR and ELISA negative until October 2014 October 2014: samples from 17- to 18-week old piglets were ELISA and PCR positive (possibly from F1WF2) December 2014: samples from 11-week old piglets were ELISA negative, PCR positive. Samples from 13- to 15-week old piglets were both ELISA and PCR positive January 2015: Total depopulation
F1WF2	January 2015	November 2013: received a batch of PCR positive pigs from F1B2 (although these were considered PRRS negative when moved). Lack of compliance with Golden Rule 8 meant the finisher rooms were continuously PCR positive until October 2014 October 2014: finisher barn depopulated, but infection probably spread to nearby F1WF1. Gradual repopulation from nursery. Herd then remained PCR and ELISA negative for the remainder of the study
F1F1	April 2015	October 2013: received depopulated (30 kg) pigs from F1WF1. Samples tested ELISA and PCR positive until March 2015, until the whole herd was depopulated March 2015: repopulated
F1F2	January 2014	November 2013: received PRRS type 2 MLV vaccinated pigs from F1WF1 until October 2013. Partial depopulation. Received pigs from F1WF1 since November 2013 on an AIAO basis.
F1Q	January 2015	July 2013. Mass vaccination of all gilts and sows (two times, 4 weeks apart, according to same schedule as in F1B1 and F1B2). Gilts remained in quarantine for 12 weeks. These gilts had been transferred to breeding herds by December 2013 November 2013: received pigs 14–26 kg from F1B2. These pigs were placed in an isolated room, vaccinated with PRRS type 2 MLV, then later slaughtered to prevent PRRSV from spreading to the rest of the site January 2014: PRRS negative gilts bred elsewhere were introduced to gilt quarantine April 2014: acclimatised (external) gilts were moved to breeding herds
F2B1	July 2014	July 2013: weaned PCR negative piglets at study commencement
F2B2	July 2014	July 2013: weaned PCR negative piglets at study commencement. Nursery rooms containing oldest two age groups were depopulated
F2F1	August 2015 (but no PRRS positive pigs since October 2013)	July 2013: received PCR positive piglets from F2B2 at study commencement. From Weeks 0–10, all finisher pigs were vaccinated after introduction Partially depopulated, and then only received PRRS negative animals October 2013: samples tested PCR negative, and remained negative for the remainder of the study
F2F2	November 2013	July 2013: received PCR positive piglets from F2B2 at study commencement From Weeks 0–10, all finisher pigs were vaccinated after introduction. Partially depopulated, then received only PRRS negative animals November 2013: samples tested PCR negative, and remained negative for the remainder of the study

Table 3 continued

Herd	PRRS free SPF status achieved	Notes
F2F3	November 2013	July 2013: received PCR positive piglets from F2B2 at study commencement. From Weeks 0–10, all finisher pigs were vaccinated after introduction. Partially depopulated, then received only PRRS negative animals
		November 2013: samples tested PCR negative, and remained negative for the remainder of the study

Study commenced in July 2013. Positive-unstable defined as ELISA positive for PRRS antibody, and PCR positive for PRRSV RNA (actively shedding); positive-stable defined as ELISA positive for PRRS antibody in serum but PCR negative (not shedding)

F1B1 Flow 1 Breeding Herd 1, *F1B2* Flow 1 Breeding Herd 2, *F1F1* Flow 1 Finisher Herd 1, *F1F2* Flow 1 Finisher Herd 2, *F1Q* Flow 1 Quarantine, *F1WF1* Flow 1 Wean-Finish 1, *F1WF2* Flow 1 Wean-Finish 2, *F2B1* Flow 2 Breeding Herd 1, *F2B2* Flow 2 Breeding Herd 2, *F2F1* Flow 2 Finisher Herd 1, *F2F2* Flow 2 Finisher Herd 2, *F2F3* Flow 2 Finisher Herd 3, *PRRS* porcine reproductive and respiratory syndrome

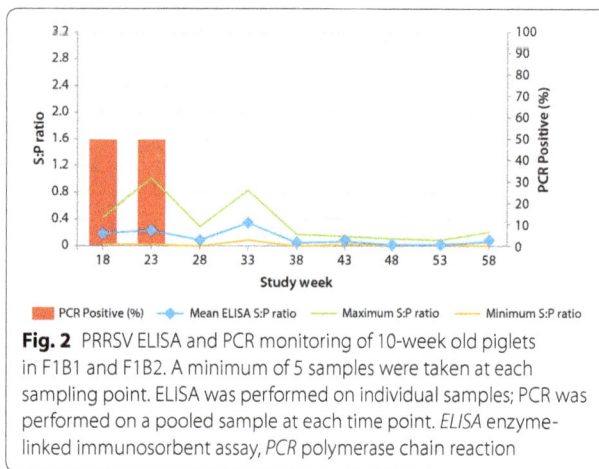

Fig. 2 PRRSV ELISA and PCR monitoring of 10-week old piglets in F1B1 and F1B2. A minimum of 5 samples were taken at each sampling point. ELISA was performed on individual samples; PCR was performed on a pooled sample at each time point. *ELISA* enzyme-linked immunosorbent assay, *PCR* polymerase chain reaction

piglets were detected shortly afterwards. Despite regular auditing of procedures by the veterinarian, staff were not able to comply with Golden Rule 8 (avoid contact between age groups; Table 2). This resulted in finisher rooms remaining continuously PCR positive until they were depopulated in October 2014.

F1F2 remained PCR positive until November 2013; 5 months after study commencement, and received PRRSV free SPF status in April 2014. F2F1 tested PCR negative in October 2013, and F2F2 and F2F3 tested PCR negative one month later, and remained both PCR and ELISA negative for the remainder of the study. PRRSV free SPF status was declared in October 2013 for F2F1, and in November 2013 for F2F2 and F2F3.

Re-infection in F1WF1 and F1F1

In October 2014, just before PRRSV free SPF status was to be declared for F1WF1, and at the same time that the finisher rooms of F1WF2 were depopulated due to reinfection, 20 and 100% of samples from 17- to 18-week old piglets, respectively, tested positive by ELISA, and pooled samples from both age groups were PCR positive

(Additional file 3). Three months later, PRRSV had spread to nearby F1F1, which had also been close to PRRSV elimination. The re-infection prompted full depopulation of both sites, and no new pigs were introduced until March 2015. No further samples tested either ELISA or PCR positive after repopulation. F1F1 was the last on the peninsula to achieve PRRSV free SPF status, in April 2015.

Discussion

The objective of the area elimination case study reported here was to eliminate PRRSV from all herds on the Horne Peninsula, Denmark, using a combination of LCH using PRRSV type 2 MLV, optimised pig flow, and implementation of the 10GR for biosecurity management. This study shows that these techniques, in combination, successfully eliminated PRRSV from all herds on the Horne Peninsula, Denmark, according to Danish SPF-SUS regulations [26]. Eighteen months later (November 2016), all herds still retain PRRSV free SPF status. To the authors' knowledge, this is the first successful European PRRSV area elimination project documented in detail.

Throughout the study, overall PRRS status of herds was classified according to the AASV terminology, and then PRRS was deemed eliminated from a herd when PRRS free SPF status was declared, according to the regulations from SPF–SUS, Denmark [26]. The use of AASV terminology throughout the study enabled herd status to be monitored month by month, thus allowing rapid response to re-infection. PRRS free SPF status was sought to fetch the maximum price when the pigs were sold.

At study commencement, all herds in both flows tested PCR positive for PRRSV infection according to AASV terminology [27], and all except F2B1 and F2B2 were positive-unstable. F2B1 and F2B2 were positive-stable. These initial observations indicated that infection control and pig flow management techniques were sub-optimal, permitting PRRSV transmission among herds and age groups.

To begin eliminating PRRSV, LCH was initiated in F1B1 and F1B2. Herd closure avoided introducing PRRSV from external sites, and decreased the number of susceptible animals in the herds: both limiting viral transmission [17]. Simultaneous vaccination of all animals at both Week 0 and Week 4 increased herd immunity and may have promoted viral elimination by reducing the number of naïve animals. The vaccine used in this study is derived from a type 2 (North American) PRRSV strain, and its efficacy has been clearly demonstrated against both homologous and heterologous strains [28, 29].

The LCH model is a useful tool for PRRSV area elimination programs, and has repeatedly allowed control in individual farms [17, 22]. One of the limitations of LCH is the need for stringent biosecurity measures to prevent virus transmission. In this study, staff reviewed internal and external biosecurity procedures and implemented the 10GR, devised in 2005 by Boehringer Ingelheim, based on 10 years of field experience in controlling PRRSV spread. The 10GR are based on the principles of the McREBEL system for disease management [23], and were developed to simplify the McREBEL procedures and increase the likelihood of implementation. The 10GR are reported here for the first time.

The 10GR involved restricting the movement of pigs to prevent PRRSV transmission between age groups, and quarantining gilts before introducing them to breeding herds to avoid infecting them with PRRSV. F1WF1 was considered the most difficult farm from which to eliminate PRRSV because of its complex pig flow, which made implementing the 10GR difficult. Despite this difficulty, the 10GR were stringently followed in all herds, in both flows, at all times (except in F1WF2, which was unable to comply with rule 8), and this was ensured through regular auditing of all farms. This foundation of good management practice contributed to the success of PRRSV MLV vaccination and the LCH control model in eliminating PRRSV from the study area.

A study on transmission of PRRSV between herds in Ontario concluded that sharing herd ownership and transportation were among the most important factors for the spread of PRRSV between herds [30]. Indeed, sharing of personnel and transportation between F1B1, F1B2 and F1Q (under the same ownership) may have contributed to the endemicity of PRRSV in the Horne Peninsula before this study began. Although shared ownership may cause problems, it can also facilitate communication between producers, which is critical to the success of regional PRRSV control and elimination projects [31]. The naturally limited geographical area, the close relationship between the herd owners, and supervision of all herds by the same veterinarian probably contributed to the successful outcome of this study.

Using a combination of LCH, use of PRRSV type 2 MLV and the 10GR, PRRSV was successfully eliminated from F1B1 and F1B2 by January 2015. PCR positive pigs were detected in the nursery of F1B2 in November 2013, and most animals were exported away from the Horne Peninsula, or to quarantine in F1Q, but some presumed PRRSV negative pigs were moved to F1WF2. Unfortunately, these animals re-introduced PRRSV into F1WF2, and so having an emergency plan to remove infected pigs from the elimination area as soon as they are detected is a key learning from this study. We also suggest that extending the vaccination period of piglets at weaning to span a whole sow cycle (20 weeks) may have avoided the emergence of PRRSV positive pigs in F1B2. Genetic sequencing revealed that the virus strain had over 99% ORF-5 sequence homology to the PRRSV type 2 MLV strain. Although re-infection was disappointing, we were encouraged that field virus was not detected.

F1WF1 tested PRRSV ELISA and PCR negative in four sampling points over 6 months, but became re–infected in October 2014, at the same time that F1WF2 finisher rooms were depopulated following reinfection. F1WF1 and F1WF2 did not share personnel, transportation or equipment, so the infection in in F1WF1 may have been due to airborne transmission of PRRSV from F1WF2, less than 500 m away. Airborne transmission was previously shown under Danish field conditions [32], but no further investigations to confirm this were undertaken in the current study.

Depopulation of the oldest pigs in the nurseries of F2B1 and F2B2 helped to immediately disrupt transmission of PRRSV from nursery to finisher areas, as has been previously shown [33]. Despite depopulation, nurseries in breeding herds remained ELISA positive until September 2013, because piglets born to infected sows had maternal antibodies in serum. This was also the case in nurseries in F1B1 and F1B2, which also remained ELISA positive for several months after becoming PCR negative. A combination of depopulation and strict application of the 10GR led to the rapid elimination of PRRSV (ELISA and PCR negative) in F2B1 and F2B2 in just 2 months after study commencement, and declaration of PRRSV free SPF status 6 months later. Depopulation of the oldest pigs in nursery rooms of breeding herds enabled rapid PRRSV elimination from finisher herds too, by ensuring that no PRRSV positive piglets were introduced to finisher herds.

The authors note some limitations to the current study. To show that PRRSV area elimination is possible using the methods described, the Horne Peninsula was deliberately chosen as a limited geographical area, with few herd owners and simple transportation routes between herds. The breeding herds in this study were comparable in size and production to the Danish average in 2015

(742 sows and 22,077 piglets), while the finisher sites produced about half as many pigs as the Danish average for finisher sites (8008 pigs slaughtered in 2015) [34]. However, the authors acknowledge that elimination would be far more complex in less well defined areas. The current project was driven by a small number of stakeholders who dedicated time to planning and sampling. Extending this project to larger regions with more owners and increased animal transport would require substantially more planning. For example, empty barns would have to be identified so that PRRSV positive pigs could be moved from sites close to achieving PRRSV elimination, to prevent setbacks.

Furthermore, larger projects with more owners may encounter problems with commitment and communication. In this project, six veterinarians were involved with overseeing the study, and ensuring implementation of the 10GR. All but one of these veterinarians were from the same practice (Porcus Pig Practice), making the sharing of information and decisions simple. In larger projects, more stakeholders from different practices (and perhaps with competing interests) may make communication more difficult. Employment of a full-time project coordinator would be recommended, as would involvement of pig producers and representatives from SEGES Danish Pig Research Centre, slaughterhouses and SPF-Denmark.

PRRS is one of the most economically devastating swine diseases, causing substantial animal losses and medication expenses [35, 36]. In Denmark, the costs of PRRS are estimated to be between €4 and €139 per sow, per year [20]. The LCH method is an effective PRRSV elimination strategy when combined with stringent biosecurity measures: this was further confirmed in the present study. A detailed cost-benefit analysis is needed to understand the return on investment for this area PRRSV elimination method.

Conclusions

PRRSV was eliminated from all herds on the Horne Peninsula, Denmark, in just over 18 months, after employing a combination of LCH, vaccination using PRRSV type 2 MLV and the 10GR for biosecurity management. Eighteen months later (November 2016), all herds still have PRRSV free SPF status. Elimination may have been achieved more quickly if the PRRSV positive pigs that were depopulated from F1B2 had been moved out of the area: this would have reduced the risk of area spread. Finally, the 10GR helped improve biosecurity management in all farms on the peninsula, and may offer a simplified alternative to the McREBEL system for controlling PRRSV.

Additional files

Additional file 1. PCR and ELISA results from breeding herds 8 weeks before study commencement. Additional data showing individual PCR and ELISA results from piglets of different age groups in the breeding herds, 8 weeks before study commencement.

Additional file 2. Individual value plot of PRRS ELISA status of pre-wean piglets (3 weeks of age) in LCH breeding herds. Additional data showing ELISA S:P values on all sampling points for up to 90 weeks after implementation of LCH, measured in 3-week old piglets.

Additional file 3. PCR and ELISA results from F1WF1 (receiving piglets from LCH breeding herds) until 60 weeks after LCH commencement. Additional data showing individual PCR and ELISA results from piglets of different age groups on the WF1 site, throughout the entire study duration.

Abbreviations

10GR: 10 Golden Rules; AIAO: all in, all out; ELISA: enzyme-linked immunosorbent assay; LCH: load, close, homogenise; McREBEL: Management Changes to Reduce Exposure to Bacteria to Eliminate Losses; MLV: modified–live vaccine; ORF: open reading frame; PCR: polymerase chain reaction; PRRS: porcine reproductive and respiratory syndrome; PRRSV: porcine reproductive and respiratory syndrome virus; SPF: specific pathogen free.

Authors' contributions

JD was the driver and initiator of this area elimination project. He brought pig producers in the area together and facilitated the decision-making process. He was the daily contact, undertook practical training of staff, and performed diagnostic sampling together with his colleagues from Porcus Pig Practice. JD was directly responsible for the breeding herds in Flow 1. PHR designed the elimination programme outline, the 10GR, and the diagnostic programme. He collected, processed and presented diagnostic information and drafted the manuscript. Both authors have read and approved the final manuscript.

Authors' information

JD is a veterinarian: a specialist in pig health and production, and co-owner of Porcus Pig Practice. PHR is a Veterinarian, Global Technical Manager, PRRS at Boehringer Ingelheim Vetmedica GmbH.

Author details

[1] Boehringer Ingelheim Vetmedica GmbH, Binger Straße 173, 55216 Ingelheim, Germany. [2] PORCUS svinefagdyrlaeger og agronomer, Oerbaekvej 276, 5220 Odense, Denmark.

Acknowledgements

The authors would like to thank the veterinarians in Porcus Pig Practice for providing assistance with diagnostic sampling, and Lars Rasmussen and Jesper Bisgaard Sanden; responsible for WF herds and Flow 2 herds, respectively.

Editorial assistance with this manuscript was provided by InterComm International, Cambridge, UK and this service was funded by Boehringer Ingelheim Vetmedica GmbH.

Competing interests

PHR is currently an employee of Boehringer Ingelheim Vetmedica GmbH (Veterinarian, Global Technical Manager PRRS). In connection with presentations following this study at two meetings for veterinarians and farmers in Denmark, and for symposia in Romania and the UK, JD received fees for consultancy, travel and accommodation from Boehringer Ingelheim Vetmedica Denmark.

Funding

All diagnostic testing of samples from the study farms was funded by Boehringer Ingelheim Denmark. Diagnostic samples were collected by veterinarians from Porcus Pig Practice under normal commercial conditions. Boehringer Ingelheim Animal Health GmbH funded the publication fee for this manuscript.

References

1. Lunney JK, Benfield DA, Rowland RR. Porcine reproductive and respiratory syndrome virus: an update on an emerging and re-emerging viral disease of swine. Virus Res. 2010;154:1–6.
2. Holtkamp DJ, Kliebenstein JB, Neumann EJ, Zimmerman J, Rotto H, Yoder T, et al. Assessment of the economic impact of porcine reproductive and respiratory syndrome virus on United States pork producers. J Swine Health Prod. 2013;21:72–84.
3. Nieuwenhuis N, Duinhof TF, van Nes A. Economic analysis of outbreaks of porcine reproductive and respiratory syndrome virus in nine sow herds. Vet Rec. 2012;170:225.
4. Stevenson GW, Van Alstine WG, Kanitz CL, Keffaber KK. Endemic porcine reproductive and respiratory syndrome virus infection of nursery pigs in two swine herds without current reproductive failure. J Vet Diagn Invest. 1993;5:432–4.
5. Nelsen CJ, Murtaugh MP, Faaberg KS. Porcine reproductive and respiratory syndrome virus comparison: divergent evolution on two continents. J Virol. 1999;73:270–80.
6. Rossow KD. Porcine reproductive and respiratory syndrome. Vet Pathol. 1998;35:1–20.
7. Christianson WT, Collins JE, Benfield DA, Harris L, Gorcyca DE, Chladek DW, et al. Experimental reproduction of swine infertility and respiratory syndrome in pregnant sows. Am J Vet Res. 1992;53:485–8.
8. Karniychuk UU, Nauwynck HJ. Pathogenesis and prevention of placental and transplacental porcine reproductive and respiratory syndrome virus infection. Vet Res. 2013;44:95.
9. Ladinig A, Detmer SE, Clarke K, Ashley C, Rowland RR, Lunney JK, et al. Pathogenicity of three type 2 porcine reproductive and respiratory syndrome virus strains in experimentally inoculated pregnant gilts. Virus Res. 2015;203:24–35.
10. Goyal SM. Porcine reproductive and respiratory syndrome. J Vet Diagn Invest. 1993;5:656–64.
11. Charerntantanakul W. Porcine reproductive and respiratory syndrome virus vaccines: immunogenicity, efficacy and safety aspects. World J Virol. 2012;1:23–30.
12. Li Z, He Y, Xu X, Leng X, Li S, Wen Y, et al. Pathological and immunological characteristics of piglets infected experimentally with a HP-PRRSV TJ strain. BMC Vet Res. 2016;12:230.
13. Dobrescu I, Levast B, Lai K, Delgado-Ortega M, Walker S, Banman S, et al. In vitro and ex vivo analyses of co-infections with swine influenza and porcine reproductive and respiratory syndrome viruses. Vet Microbiol. 2014;169:18–32.
14. Murtaugh MP, Genzow M. Immunological solutions for treatment and prevention of porcine reproductive and respiratory syndrome (PRRS). Vaccine. 2011;29:8192–204.
15. Murtaugh MP, Stadejek T, Abrahante JE, Lam TT, Leung FC. The ever-expanding diversity of porcine reproductive and respiratory syndrome virus. Virus Res. 2010;154:18–30.
16. Perez AM, Davies PR, Goodell CK, Holtkamp DJ, Mondaca-Fernandez E, Poljak Z, et al. Lessons learned and knowledge gaps about the epidemiology and control of porcine reproductive and respiratory syndrome virus in North America. J Am Vet Med Assoc. 2015;246:1304–17.
17. Corzo CA, Mondaca E, Wayne S, Torremorell M, Dee S, Davies P, et al. Control and elimination of porcine reproductive and respiratory syndrome virus. Virus Res. 2010;154:185–92.
18. Linhares D. Evaluation of immune management strategies to control and eliminate porcine reproductive and respiratory syndrome virus (PRRSv) (Doctoral thesis). Minneapolis: University of Minnesota; 2013.
19. Linhares DC, Johnson C, Morrison RB. Economic analysis of immunization strategies for PRRS control [corrected]. PLoS ONE. 2015;10:e0144265.
20. SEGES. Announcement 1032: economic evaluation of the cost of national PRRS elimination [Danish]. http://vsp.lf.dk/~/media/Files/PDF%20-%20Publikationer/Meddelelser%202015/Meddelelse_1032.pdf. Accessed 02 Nov 2016.
21. Desrosiers R, Boutin M. An attempt to eradicate porcine reproductive and respiratory syndrome virus (PRRSV) after an outbreak in a breeding herd: eradication strategy and pesistence of antibody titers in sows. J Swine Health Prod. 2002;10:23–5.
22. Torremorell M, Henry S, Christianson WT. Eradication using herd closure. In: Zimmerman J, Yoon KJ, editors. PRRS compendium. Des Moines: National Pork Board; 2003. p. 157–62.
23. McCaw MB. MCREBEL PRRS: management procedures for PRRS control in large herd nurseries. Proc AD Leman Swine Conf: St. Paul MN; 1995. p. 161–2.
24. AASD Committee on PRRS Members, Dee S, Collins J, Halbur P, Keffaber K, Lautner B, McCaw M, et al. Control of porcine reproductive and respiratory syndrome (PRRS) virus. J Swine Health Prod. 1996;4:95–8.
25. Davies P. Principles of diagnostic testing of animal populations. http://www.ava.com.au/sites/default/files/AVA_website/pdfs/SA_Divison/Davies-Principles%20of%20diagnostic%20testing%20of%20animal%20populations.pdf. Accessed 2 Nov 2016.
26. SPF Sundhedsstyringen. Rules for health control in Blue SPF herds. [in Danish]. In: Blue SPF Folder, SPF-SuS; 2016:4–5.
27. Holtkamp DJ, Polson DD, Torremorell M, Morrison B, Classen DM, Becton L, et al. Terminology for classifying the porcine reproductive and respiratory syndrome virus (PRRSV) status of swine herds. J Swine Health Prod. 2011;39:101–12.
28. Zuckermann FA, Garcia EA, Luque ID, Christopher-Hennings J, Doster A, Brito M, et al. Assessment of the efficacy of commercial porcine reproductive and respiratory syndrome virus (PRRSV) vaccines based on measurement of serologic response, frequency of gamma-IFN-producing cells and virological parameters of protection upon challenge. Vet Microbiol. 2007;123:69–85.
29. Li X, Galliher-Beckley A, Pappan L, Trible B, Kerrigan M, Beck A, et al. Comparison of host immune responses to homologous and heterologous type II porcine reproductive and respiratory syndrome virus (PRRSV) challenge in vaccinated and unvaccinated pigs. BioMed Res Int. 2014;2014:416727.
30. Kwong GP, Poljak Z, Deardon R, Dewey CE. Bayesian analysis of risk factors for infection with a genotype of porcine reproductive and respiratory syndrome virus in Ontario swine herds using monitoring data. Prev Vet Med. 2013;110:405–17.
31. Valdes-Donoso P, Jarvis LS, Wright D, Alvarez J, Perez AM. Measuring progress on the control of porcine reproductive and respiratory syndrome (PRRS) at a regional level: the minnesota N212 regional control project (Rcp) as a working example. PLoS ONE. 2016;11:e0149498.
32. Priebe A, Kvisgaard LK, Rathkjen PH, Larsen LE, Hjulsager CK, Havn K. PRRS type 1 detection in aerosols from three swine herds in Denmark. Proc European Symposium of Porcine Health Management, Nantes; 2015. **(Poster 85)**.
33. Dee SA, Joo HS, Polson DD. Improved performance of a large pig complex after sequential nursery depopulation. The Vet Rec. 1996;138:31–4.
34. SEGES. Announcement 1611: National average for productivity in swine production [Danish]. http://vsp.lf.dk/~/media/Files/PDF%20-%20Publikationer/Notater%202016/Notat_1611.pdf. Accessed 2 Nov 2016.
35. Neumann EJ, Kliebenstein JB, Johnson CD, Mabry JW, Bush EJ, Seitzinger AH, et al. Assessment of the economic impact of porcine reproductive and respiratory syndrome on swine production in the United States. J Am Vet Med Assoc. 2005;227:385–92.
36. Renukaradhya GJ, Meng XJ, Calvert JG, Roof M, Lager KM. Live porcine reproductive and respiratory syndrome virus vaccines: current status and future direction. Vaccine. 2015;33:4069–80.
37. Nechvatalova K, Kudlackova H, Leva L, Babickova K, Faldyna M. Transfer of humoral and cell-mediated immunity via colostrum in pigs. Vet Immunol Immunop. 2011;142:95–100.
38. Thorup F. The importance of litter standardization for litter weight at weaning [Danish]. Copenhagen: Erfaring fra Landsudvalget for Svin; 1998.
39. Linhares D, Torremorell M, Morrison RB. What have we learned using load close expose to produce negative pigs from positive breeding herds?. St. Paul: Proc AD Leman Swine conference; 2013.

9

Preoperative and intraoperative ultrasound aids removal of migrating plant material causing iliopsoas myositis via ventral midline laparotomy

Francesco Birettoni[1†], Domenico Caivano[1†], Mark Rishniw[2,3], Giulia Moretti[1], Francesco Porciello[1*], Maria Elena Giorgi[1], Alberto Crovace[1], Erika Bianchini[1] and Antonello Bufalari[1]

Abstract

Background: Migrating plant material is often suspected clinically to be the underlying cause of iliopsoas myositis in the dog, but cannot always be found pre- or intraoperatively. In most cases, recurrence of clinical signs is related to failure to remove the plant material. Preoperative ultrasonography can be useful to visualize migrating plant material and to determine anatomical landmarks that can assist in planning a surgical approach. The purpose of the present study was to report the role of intraoperative (intra-abdominal) ultrasonography for visualizing and removing the plant material from iliopsoas abscesses using a ventral midline laparotomy approach.

Results: A retrospective case series of 22 dogs with iliopsoas muscle abnormalities and suspected plant material was reported. Preoperative visualization and subsequent retrieval of the plant material was performed during a single hospitalization. In all 22 dogs, the plant material (including complete grass awns, grass awn fragments and a bramble twig) was successfully removed via ventral midline laparotomy in which intraoperative ultrasonography was used to direct the grasping forceps tips to the foreign body and guide its removal. In 11 of these 22 dogs, the plant material was not completely removed during prior surgery performed by the referring veterinarians without pre- or intraoperative ultrasonography. Clinical signs resolved in all dogs and all dogs resumed normal activity after successful surgical removal of the plant material.

Conclusion: Intraoperative ultrasonography is a safe and readily available tool that improves success of surgical removal of plant material within the iliopsoas abscesses via ventral midline laparotomy. Moreover, ultrasonographic findings of unusual plant material can be useful in planning and guiding surgical removal, by providing information about the size and shape of the foreign body.

Keywords: Intraoperative ultrasound, Grass awn, Myositis, Canine

Background

Iliopsoas muscle disease has been well described in canine patients. This pathological process includes traumatic injury [1–3], muscle strain injury [4], primary haemangiosarcoma [5], fibrotic myopathy [6–8] and abscessation [9, 10]. With iliopsoas abscessation, pus accumulates within and around the iliopsoas muscles, often producing a draining cutaneous fistula just cranial to the ileum [10]. Most iliopsoas abscesses result from plant material, such as migrating grass awns, and various diagnostic techniques, including radiology, contrast radiology, ultrasonography, computed tomography (CT), magnetic resonance imaging (MRI), have been used to investigate fistulae associated with iliopsoas abscesses

*Correspondence: francesco.porciello@unipg.it
†Francesco Birettoni and Domenico Caivano contributed equally to this work
[1] Department of Veterinary Medicine, University of Perugia, Via San Costanzo 4, 06126 Perugia, Italy
Full list of author information is available at the end of the article

[10–19]. Additionally, these imaging tools help determine anatomical landmarks that can be used in planning a surgical approach. Ideally, treatment of iliopsoas myositis secondary to migrating plant material requires removal of the foreign body, coupled with antibiotic therapy. Plant material is often suspected clinically to be the underlying cause, but cannot always be found because it can be difficult to identify during an open surgery or it has migrated out of the fistula [11, 13, 18, 19].

To the author's knowledge, no study in the veterinary literature has documented the role of intraoperative ultrasonography for visualizing and removing plant material from iliopsoas abscesses using a ventral midline laparotomy. Therefore, we sought to report a method to routinely investigate and treat dogs with iliopsoas myositis due to migrating plant material.

Methods

Electronic medical records of dogs evaluated at the Veterinary Teaching Hospital of Perugia University between January 2012 and October 2015 were searched to identify those in which ultrasonographic findings of the iliopsoas muscle region were compatible with plant material migration (identification of iliopsoas abscessation/myositis with hyperechoic structures of variable length consistent with a foreign body that cast characteristic shadows through the ultrasonographic image). Dogs with history of trauma to the abdominal cavity were excluded from the study. All dogs required a recorded follow-up >6 months after ultrasonographic exam and surgery. For all cases that satisfied these criteria we reviewed history, signalment, clinical, radiological and CT findings (if available), as well as surgical findings, other treatments, and outcome.

Ultrasonographic examination of the iliopsoas muscle region was performed on awake dogs positioned in left and right lateral recumbency with an ultrasound system[1] equipped with a 5- to 8-MHz microconvex transducer (see footnote 1) after clipping fur over the abdomen and both flanks. Left and right iliopsoas muscle regions were scanned in a cranial to caudal direction with the scan plane held parallel and then perpendicular to the spine. Where possible, the plant material was identified, based on specific, previously described, imaging criteria [15, 17, 20–22]. Subsequently, adjacent anatomical landmarks (e.g., kidneys, aorta, caudal vena cava, renal arteries and their distance from the suspected foreign body) were identified to help the surgeon during intra-abdominal exploration.

In 2 cases, ultrasonography was performed with the dog positioned in dorsal recumbency under deep sedation because these dogs displayed profound abdominal guarding when unsedated (hunched over, unwilling to relax and have the hindlimbs retracted caudally to extend the abdominal musculature), and did not allow an adequate and systematic scan of the sublumbar region and in particular of iliopsoas muscles.

All dogs were hospitalized for 1–2 days after preoperative ultrasonographic visualization of the suspected migrating plant material while awaiting surgical exploration.

Intraoperative (intra-abdominal) ultrasonography was performed by use of a microconvex probe (see footnote 1) encased in a sterile protective cover[2] and positioned directly on the affected region of the iliopsoas muscles (identified by preoperative anatomical landmarks and intraoperative visual inspection) to precisely localize the suspected plant material and guide complete removal.

Anaesthetic and analgesic protocols were determined on an individual basis by the attending anaesthetist. All dogs were positioned in dorsal recumbency for the procedure and a ventral midline laparotomy was performed through a 13–22 cm incision, depending on the size of the dog. The surgical field was isolated with laparotomy gauze and abdominal muscles retracted by a Balfour self-retaining retractor to allow the intraoperative ultrasonographic exploration of the iliopsoas muscles. Once the plant material was identified, an 18 or 20 G spinal needle was introduced through the iliopsoas muscle using ultrasonographic guidance and the bevel was positioned close to the foreign body to act as guide for a #10 scalpel blade. The surgeon then made a small incision (1–2 cm) through the ventral iliopsoas epimysium under ultrasonographic guidance, and introduced grasping forceps through this incision to retrieve the plant material. When a grass awn was identified, the surgeon carefully grasped the tip of the grass awn and gently extracted it through the incision. Because of the harpoon-like shape of grass awns, care was taken not to grasp the grass awn by the barbs, so as to avoid unintentional fragmentation. Various types of grasping forceps were used for the plant material removal, depending on the size of the patient and the surgeon's preference: 7–9 cm Hartmann alligator forceps, 8 cm Kelly curved haemostatic forceps, or 24 cm Kantrowitz thoracic clamps. After plant material removal, intraoperative ultrasonography of the affected region was again performed to confirm its complete removal. The muscle incision was lavaged with sterile saline solution and aspirated, then the incision was sutured with single absorbable sutures. When a minimum amount of fluid was recovered, this approach

---
[1] MyLab 30 Vet Gold, Esaote, Genova, Italy.　　[2] Delta Med Medical Devices, Viadana, Italy.

provided an adequate debridement of the affected region. Omentalization of the abscess cavity was performed in dogs with large amounts of fluid and larger abscess cavities. No cases required extensive debridement or the insertion of a drainage tubes. Postoperative treatment consisted of daily wound and fistula (if present) care, pain management [23] and antibiotic therapy. Cefaxolin (30 mg/kg q12 h) in association with enrofloxacin (5 mg/kg q24 h) were intravenously administrated before the induction and continued in the following days. Antibiotics were changed on the basis of results of microbial culture and susceptibility testing of both the samples collected from the affected region and any retrieved plant material.

Short-term outcome was assessed by reviewing recheck examination records (usually 10 days and 1 months after the surgery), and long-term outcome was reviewed by telephone consultation with the owners or the referring veterinarians. Descriptive data are reported. Statistical analyses were not performed.

Results

Twenty-two dogs with a diagnosis of suspected migrating plant material in the iliopsoas muscle region met the study inclusion criteria. Breeds included English Setter (n = 8), Springer Spaniel (3), Italian Bloodhound (3), Kurzhaar (3), German Shorthaired Pointer (1), Epagneul Breton (1), English Pointer (1), and mixed (3). Of the 22 dogs, 9 were female and 13 were male, with a median age of 4.3 years (range, 1–10 years) and median weight of 19.2 kg (range, 7.5–40 kg). All dogs had been treated with antimicrobial agents and 11 dogs had undergone one to two (n = 4) surgical explorations (via lateral or ventral midline laparotomy) prior to initial evaluation at the Veterinary Teaching Hospital.

In 12/22 dogs, historical findings we considered related to the migration of plant material through the airways towards the iliopsoas muscles, included pyrexia, cough and dyspnea in the previous spring/summer season.

Relevant clinical signs included flank swelling and pain (n = 20), pyrexia (n = 16), depression (n = 16), hindlimb lameness (n = 11) and anorexia (n = 10). Eight dogs had cutaneous fistulae in the dorsal midlumbar region.

Iliopsoas muscle abnormalities were detected within the left (n = 14), right (n = 6) or both (n = 2) iliopsoas muscles with ultrasonographic imaging. In all unilaterally affected dogs the affected muscle appeared swollen with a loss of typical fascicular architecture and in homogeneously hypoechoic with accumulation of flocculent fluid (Fig. 1). A mild to moderate amount of fluid was also present in the subcutaneous tissue in the 8 dogs with a fistula. In 20 dogs, the tissues surrounding the muscle capsule (epimysium) appeared moderately hyperechoic.

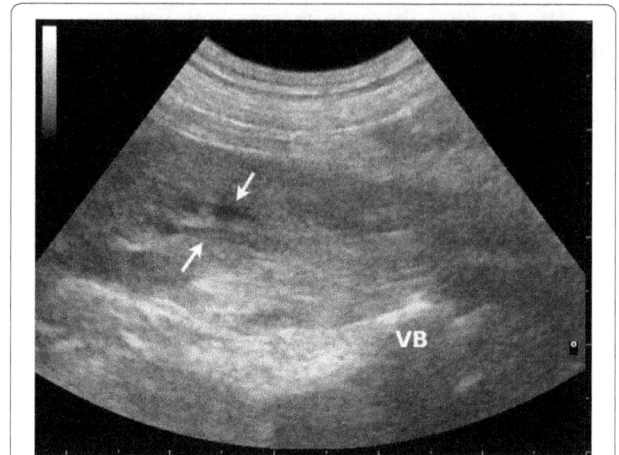

Fig. 1 Ultrasonographic image (longitudinal plane) of an affected iliopsoas muscle. Loss of typical fascicular architecture with inhomogeneously hypoechoic appearance and accumulation of flocculent fluid (*arrows*) is present. *VB* vertebral body

The normal (contralateral) iliopsoas muscle was homogeneously echogenic with low echo intensity and a speckled appearance (in the transverse plane) or linear/pinnate appearance (in the longitudinal plane) because of reflections of perimysial connective tissue (Fig. 2). The suspected plant material, surrounded by a focal hypoechoic zone (consistent with myositis) was preoperatively visualized in all 22 dogs. Plant material was visualized within the affected iliopsoas in dogs with unilateral abnormalities; in the 2 dogs where both iliopsoas muscles showed ultrasonographic abnormalities, the grass awn was observed within the affected iliopsoas (the right iliopsoas in both instances) and within in the medial portion of the left iliopsoas muscle, essentially straddling the midline.

Grass awns typically appeared ultrasonographically as spindle-shaped, shadow casting, hyperechoic structures of variable length (range, 0.5–2.5 cm) (Fig. 3). In 1 dog, the plant material appeared as a 0.3 cm, oval-shaped structure with a small linear hyperechoic projection compatible with a barb (Fig. 4). In 2 dogs that had undergone prior attempts at grass awn removal by the referring veterinarian, fragments of plant material were visualized by preoperative ultrasonography (Fig. 5). In one dog, a 3.5 cm, linear, shadowing, highly hyperechoic foreign body (ultimately identified as a bramble branch) was visualized (Fig. 6).

Two dogs with clinical signs compatible with hind limb paraparesis underwent radiographic and CT studies of the thoracic and lumbar spine before the surgery. Radiographic abnormalities included signs of discospondylitis and osteomyelitis (Fig. 7). On CT, one of these dogs showed mild to moderate irregular bone proliferation in the ventral periosteum of L1–L3 lumbar vertebrae and

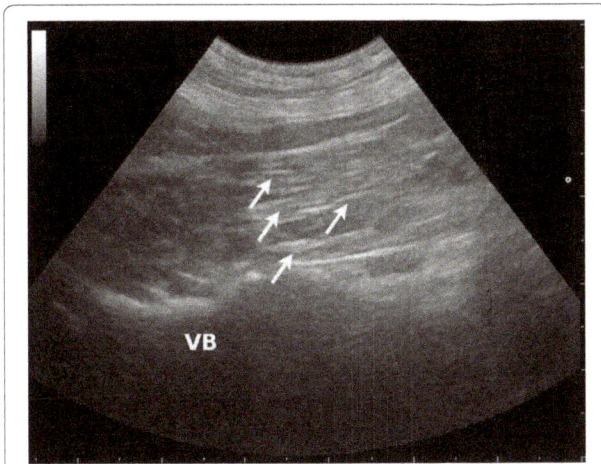

Fig. 2 Ultrasonographic image (longitudinal plane) of a normal iliopsoas muscle. The muscle is homogeneously echogenic with low echo intensity linear appearance (*arrows*) because of reflections of perimysial connective tissue. *VB* vertebral body

the other showed severe ventral spondylosis with lysis and sclerosis of L3 and L4 end plates and vertebral bodies, extensive remodelling and partial collapse of the disc space, osteolytic and osteoproliferative changes including intense periosteal reaction of the vertebral body (Fig. 8). Both dogs showed inhomogeneity of the iliopsoas muscles. Computed tomography did not permit visualization of the plant material but only changes within the surrounding tissue associated with the inflammatory response. Neurological signs in both dogs were considered secondary to the foreign bodies and their impact on the lumbar vertebrae.

In all dogs, the plant material was successfully removed via ventral midline laparotomy in which intraoperative ultrasonography was used to direct the tips of the grasping forceps to the plant material and guide its removal. In 21/22 dogs, the plant material was entirely removed, whereas in one dog occurred fragmentation of the foreign body during the attempt of removing. A fragment was visualized by intraoperative ultrasonography of

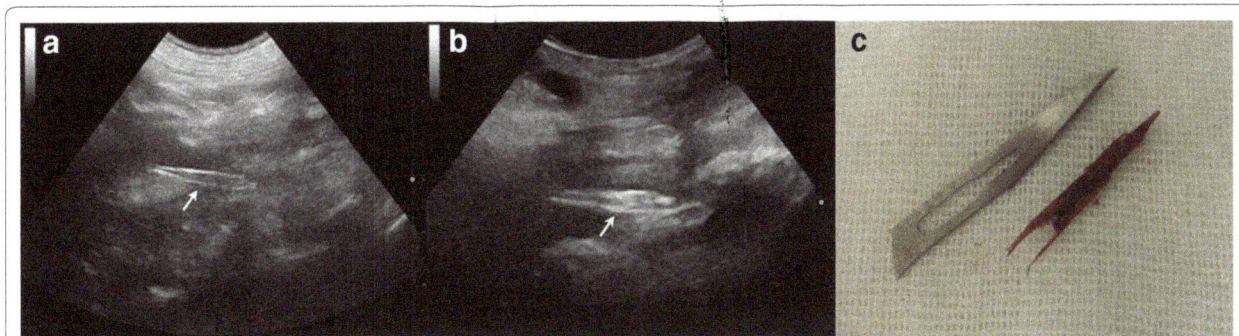

Fig. 3 Ultrasonographic images (**a**, **b**) and intraoperative photograph (**c**) of a 3–year-old German Shorthaired Pointer with a grass awn in the left iliopsoas muscle. **a** Transabdominal ultrasonographic image of a spindle-shaped hyperechoic foreign body consistent with a grass awn (*arrow*). **b** Intraoperative ultrasonographic image of the same awn shown in *panel A* (*arrow*). **c** Photograph of the grass awn after the removal

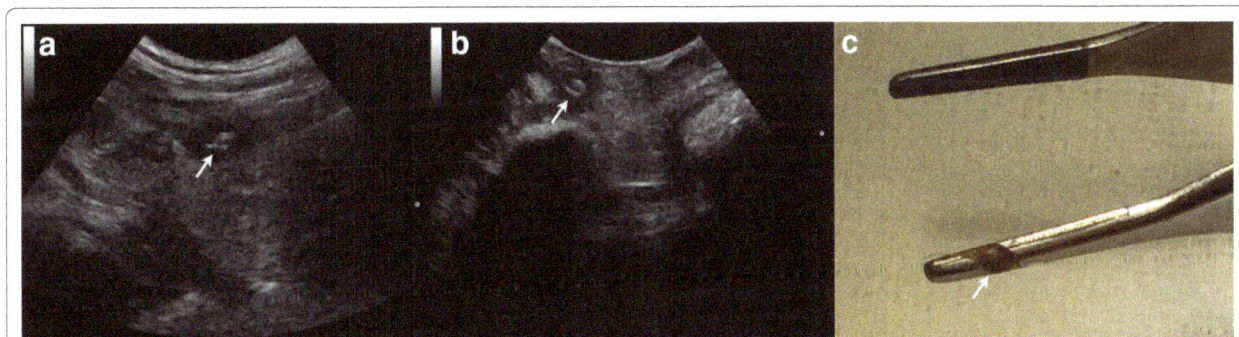

Fig. 4 Ultrasonographic images (**a**, **b**) of a 3–year-old English Setter with an oval plant material in the left iliopsoas muscle and intraoperative photograph of the awn after removal (**c**). **a** Transabdominal ultrasonographic image showing the 0.3-cm-long awn (*arrow*) with a small linear hyperechoic structure compatible with a barb. The foreign body is surrounded by a hypoechoic zone consistent with myositis. **b** Intraoperative ultrasonographic image of the plant material in **a** confirming its presence in the left iliopsoas muscle. **c** The plant material is shown

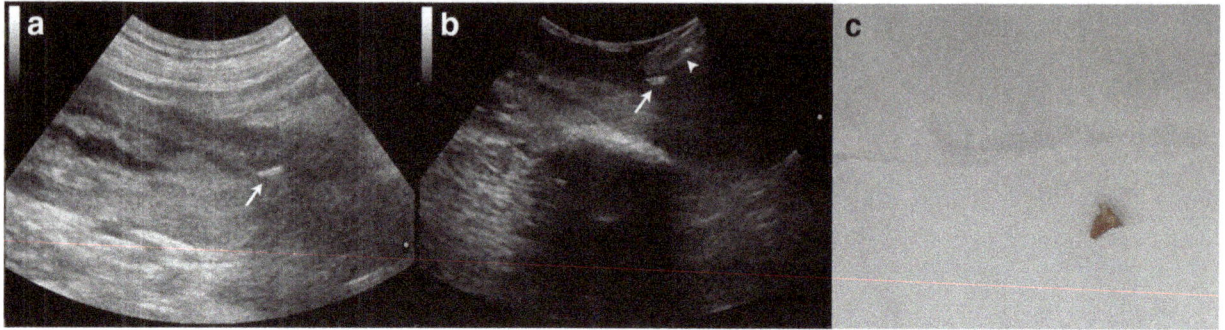

Fig. 5 Ultrasonographic images (**a**, **b**) of a 3–year-old English Setter with a fragment of plant material and intraoperative photograph of the fragment after removal (**c**). **a** Transabdominal ultrasonographic image of a small, linear and hyperechoic foreign body (*arrow*) in the left iliopsoas muscle. **b** Intraoperative ultrasonographic image of the foreign body (*arrow*) in *panel A* confirming its presence. The arm of a Hartmann forceps (*arrowhead*) is visible in proximity to the foreign body. **c** Photograph of the fragment after removal

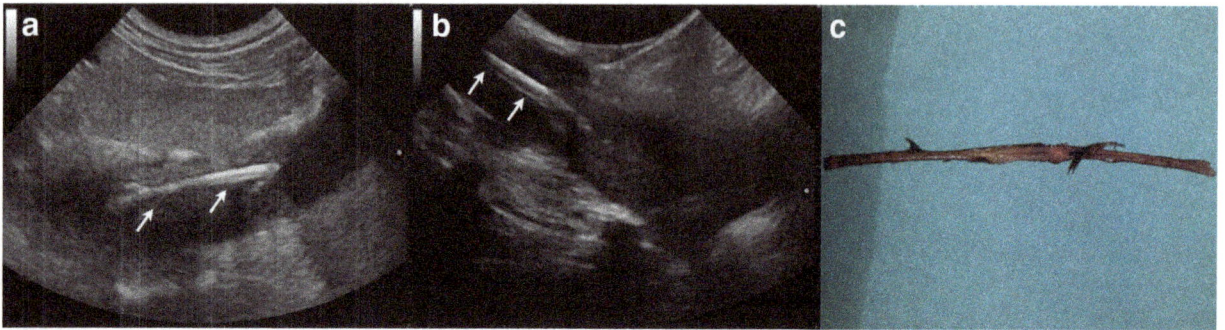

Fig. 6 Ultrasonographic image (**a**, **b**) of a 5–year-old Kurzhaar with a migrating plant material in the right iliopsoas muscle and intraoperative photograph of the foreign body after removal (**c**). **a** Transabdominal ultrasonographic image of a 3.5 cm, linear, shadowing and high hyperechoic foreign body (*arrows*). **b** Intraoperative ultrasonographic image of the foreign body (*arrows*) in *panel A* confirming its presence in the iliopsoas muscle. **c** Photograph of the bramble branch after removal

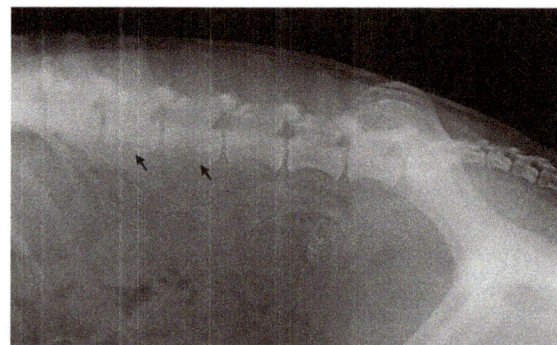

Fig. 7 Lateral projection of the lumbosacral spine of a dog with a foreign body in the iliopsoas muscles; the radiograph shows bone proliferations of the ventral part of the vertebral body of L4 and L3 (*black arrows*), and an irregularity of the periosteum of the ventral profile of L2

affected region and removed during the same surgery. In one dog, the grass awn was intraoperatively visualized more cranially than it had been during preoperative imaging. In 2 dogs with vertebral lesions, the plant material was found straddling the midline of the iliopsoas muscles adjacent to the affected vertebrae. Nevertheless, intraoperative ultrasonographic guidance resulted in successful removal of the migrating plant material. No dog had any intra- or postoperative complications.

All dogs were discharged from the hospital 3–5 days after the surgery with a prescription of antibiotics (cefadroxil 20 mg/kg PO q24 h, enrofloxacin 5 mg/kg PO q24 h, clindamycin 11 mg/kg PO q24 h, prescribed on the basis of microbial culture and susceptibly testing) for 10 days. In 2 dogs, the hospitalization lasted for 2 weeks because vertebral spondylosis and osteolysis secondary to the abscess required physical therapy and prolonged parenteral antibiotic treatment. Bacteriological isolation from the abscess was performed in all dogs. Microorganisms were isolated from abscesses of 12 dogs and included *Streptococcus* spp., *Staphylococcus aureus*, *Pseudomonas* spp., *Escherichia coli*, and *Proteus mirabilis*. None of the isolated microorganisms showed antibiotic

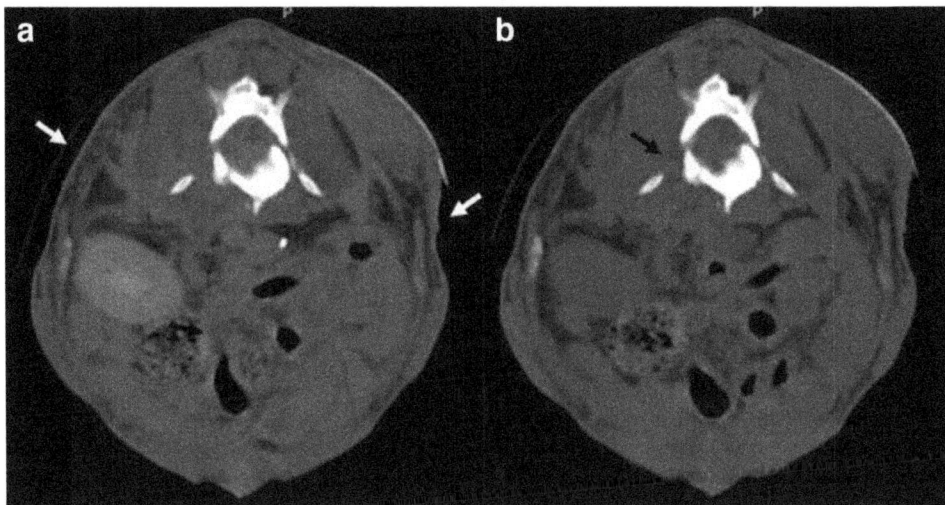

Fig. 8 Intravenous contrast-enhanced (**a**) and non-enhanced (**b**) transverse CT projections. The images are oriented with dorsal at the *top* and the animal's right to the left of the image. Both sections are at the level of L3–L4, and show irregularity and inhomogeneity of the iliopsoas muscles, with severe osteolysis of the vertebral body of the lumbar vertebra (L3) involving the spinal canal (*black arrow*). There is also discontinuity of the soft tissue of both the flanks indicating bilateral subcutaneous fistulae (*white arrows*)

resistance to the panel of antibiotics evaluated, including those isolated from patients receiving long-term antibiotics.

At a 1 month re-evaluation after discharge, the affected iliopsoas muscle in all dogs showed a progressive improvement of the ultrasonographic appearance (homogeneous parenchyma with typical fascicular architecture).

All 22 dogs had complete resolution of the clinical signs and resumed normal activity within 4–5 weeks after successful surgical removal of the plant material. Both dogs with neurological signs and osteomyelitis/discospondylitis recovered completely.

Discussion

Our study provides evidence of the utility of intraoperative ultrasonography for removing plant material from iliopsoas muscles via ventral midline laparotomy. In previous reports of dogs with iliopsoas myositis, migrating plant material was often suspected or visualized by preoperative imaging, but was retrieved during surgical exploration in only some cases. The cause of this retrieval failure can only be speculated upon: it is possible that in these cases, the plant material had migrated from the abscess and exited via the fistula prior to surgical exploration, or that the plant material was not located within the abscess but elsewhere in the musculature or lumbar parenchyma during surgical exploration. In either situation, intraoperative ultrasonography would have likely guided the surgeons to the plant material or conclusively demonstrated its absence, as we have demonstrated in

this study, increasing the rate of successful retrieval of plant material. When a grass awn was ultrasonographically identified, intraoperative ultrasound allowed the surgeon to grasp the tip of the grass awn after making a precise incision through the muscle, minimizing the risk of fragmentation and iatrogenic muscle damage. To the author's knowledge, this is the first report of such a surgical strategy for removing plant material from iliopsoas muscles.

Oronasal ingestion or inhalation of the grass awns, especially in hunting dogs (which represented 100% of our cohort), commonly causes respiratory disease during spring and summer [13, 24, 25]. In our cases, respiratory disease signs and fever were recorded in 12/22 dogs during spring or summer season: these historical findings could be useful for the clinician approaching dogs with this clinical condition. Acute inhalation can go unnoticed by the owner, resulting in subsequent migration through the airways into the lung and then into the pleural space, pericardium, retroperitoneal cavity, iliopsoas muscles, or out through the thoracic/abdominal wall [15, 20, 21, 25–29]. This unidirectional migratory characteristic of grass awns is attributable to their backward-pointing barbs and fusiform shape [15, 20, 21, 25–29]. Grass awns cause severe and septic tissue reactions and variable clinical signs, depending upon their location. Grass awn migration into the iliopsoas muscles commonly causes local inflammation. Grass awns introduce bacteria, incite a foreign body response, interfere with local host defences and provide a nidus for chronic, infections [13]. Similar to previous reports [11, 13, 18], the most relevant clinical signs were flank swelling and pain, pyrexia and depression: these clinical signs are the consequence of septic tissue reaction secondary to the plant material migration, but are not specific for foreign-body-related iliopsoas myositis.

Ultrasonography is a safe, readily available, and non-invasive diagnostic technique that can be used to identify anatomic landmarks for planning and guiding a surgical approach for removing plant material [14, 15, 17, 20–22]. In contrast to CT or MRI, abdominal ultrasonography can be performed without anaesthesia. Moreover, CT and MRI are less frequently available to clinicians and require more advanced training for their use. Ultrasonographic findings in sublumbar migration are characterized by an enlargement of the affected iliopsoas muscles (when compared to the contralateral muscle), and an unstructured hypoechoic appearance with anechoic areas of variable size and number. Hyperechoic structures, typically as spindle-shaped casting an acoustic shadow, are frequently surrounded by this anechoic area and are consistent with a grass awn [13]. Similar to previous reports, identification of the plant material in dogs of the present study was enhanced by a surrounding hypoechoic region of fluid associated with an inflammatory response [15, 20–22].

Studies using CT examinations to characterize iliopsoas abscesses were able to detect plant material in only 38–47% of dogs in which plant material was found at surgery [16, 18]. This low rate of detection was attributed at least in part to local inflammation preventing visualization of the foreign body [18]. Holloway et al. reported hypointense muscle lesions consistent with foreign material on MRI in five patients but foreign material was ultimately identified in only two of these patients [8]. The authors concluded that the specificity of MRI in identifying small foreign objects appears to be low.

In 11 dogs in our study, the plant material was not removed during the initial surgery performed by the referring veterinarians. These dogs had undergone surgical exploration via lateral or ventral midline laparotomy without pre- or intraoperative ultrasonography. This suggests that our approach, utilizing both preoperative and intraoperative ultrasonographic localization and guidance, increases the likelihood of successful plant material removal. In all dogs, the plant material visualized pre- and intraoperatively was removed. Preoperative ultrasonography allowed us to identify the cause of the iliopsoas myositis and provided valuable landmarks for surgical approach. In one dog, immediate, intraoperative, post-removal scanning identified a remnant that was quickly removed before closure—had this not been performed, there is a high probability that clinical signs would have persisted in this dog. Therefore, it can be speculated that intraoperative ultrasonography is important to not only guide the surgical approach, but to confirm complete removal of the foreign body, especially where fragmentation of the plant material is suspected.

Some authors suggest that surgical exploration and debridement of the affected region, after a preoperative CT scan, can successfully resolve the problem, even if the plant material is not identified or removed [11, 18, 19]. In 2 cases we performed CT imaging to better investigate the neurological signs and associated lumbar vertebral abnormalities. In neither case was the foreign body visualized with CT imaging, consistent with findings of previous studies. We found that placing the probe directly on the affected muscle via the laparotomy allowed high-resolution visualization of the plant material without interference from the surrounding tissues (skin, fat, bone etc.). Therefore, we would suggest that even in dogs undergoing surgical exploration for iliopsoas myositis, suspected to be secondary to plant material, on the basis of CT or MRI findings, in which the foreign body is not visualized preoperatively, clinicians should perform intraoperative ultrasonography directly over the affected muscle to increase the probability of detecting plant material. Furthermore, this technique permits a more precise and less traumatic surgical approach to the plant material, and, in the case of grass awns, allows withdrawal of the grass awn in a manner that reduces risk of barb fragmentation.

The variations in grass awn length identified by ultrasonography and confirmed by surgical removal likely reflect the different species of grass awns present in Italy [15, 20, 21, 25]. However, similar species of grasses exist elsewhere, suggesting that our ultrasonographic descriptions are likely to be applied to grass awns in various regions of the world. The authors speculate the unusual plant material consistent with bramble twig behaved similarly to grass awns during its migration through lung to retroperitoneal cavity: thorns on the twig mimicked backward-pointing barbs of grass awns. Both bramble twig and fragments of grass awn, different ultrasonographically from typical spindle-shaped grass awns, were successful identified pre- and intraoperative ultrasonography. Ultrasonographic characteristics of this unusual plant material were useful in planning its surgical removal.

Aortic rupture has been described as a complication of surgical exploration of iliopsoas abscesses [11]. In the present study, intraoperative ultrasonography was useful to guide successfully plant material removal, but also to avoid possible damage of surrounded tissues by real-time monitoring of the surgical instruments (spinal needle, scalpel blade and forceps) as they were introduced into the muscle.

In dogs in the present study, a surgical approach by ventral midline laparotomy permitted excellent exposure and visualization of the affected area, closeness and proximity of the grass awn to the dorsal peritoneum and consequently to the surgeon's hands, cleanliness of the surgical field and an accurate and targeted approach to preserve the iliopsoas muscles. These advantages cannot be always obtained by a lateral, transcutaneous approach to the sublumbar region. Moreover, an ultrasonographic probe can be easily positioned close to the diseased region with fewer imaging artifacts, compared to the lateral approach. In our study, no dogs suffered post-operative complications (e.g. peritonitis or wound dehiscence), and in all patients the clinical signs due to migrating plant material resolved. The Authors believe that an appropriate preparation of the surgical field by using wet laparotomy gauzes, and lavage and suction of the area around the grass awn reduces the incidence of complications. Our cases did not need extensive debridement during the surgical procedure or the establishment of drainage in the postoperative period with drainage tubes, because a limited amount of the fluid was recovered from the affected region. This might have been due, in part, to the long-term antibiotic therapy that most of these dogs had been subjected to before presentation to our institution. However, debridement or the establishment of drainage can be considered when iliopsoas myositis is markedly abscessated.

Our study had several limitations. The study was retrospective, with the limitations inherent in such study designs, although retrospective studies often provide the most suitable means of collecting sufficient data for evaluation of infrequently diagnosed disorders in a timely manner. Also, ultrasonography is a highly operator-dependent technique, and our results might not be readily extrapolated to similar situations where the methods involve other, less experienced, clinicians or different ultrasonography imaging systems or other imaging techniques. However, given the characteristic findings of the plant material we observed, we believe that most clinicians should be able to successfully image the iliopsoas muscles to locate migrating plant material. Finally, the study population was also somewhat small.

Conclusions

Intraoperative ultrasonography is a safe and readily available tool that improves success of surgical removal of plant material within the iliopsoas muscles region via ventral midline laparotomy.

Abbreviations

CT: computed tomography; MRI: magnetic resonance imaging.

Authors' contributions

FB, DC, FP and MEG performed ultrasonography, participated in the design of the study, analyzed the data regarding the ultrasonographic findings and drafted the manuscript. GM, AC, AB and AB performed laparotomy, participated in the design of the study and analyzed the data regarding the radiographic, CT and surgical findings. MR contributed to interpretation of the results, and revised critically the manuscript. All authors read and approved the final manuscript.

Author details

[1] Department of Veterinary Medicine, University of Perugia, Via San Costanzo 4, 06126 Perugia, Italy. [2] Department of Clinical Sciences, Cornell University, Ithaca, NY 14853, USA. [3] Veterinary Information Network, Davis, CA 95616, USA.

Acknowledgements

The Authors thank Dr. Franco Vescera, Dr. Giuseppe De Nicola and Dr. Gualtiero Ercolani for referred cases, and Mattia Tessadori in collecting the data.

Competing interests

The authors declare that they have no competing interests.

References

1. Rossmeisl JH, Rohleder JJ, Hancock R, Lanz OI. Computed tomographic features of suspected traumatic injury to the iliopsoas and pelvic limb musculature of a dog. Vet Radiol Ultrasound. 2004;45:388–92.
2. Breur GJ, Blevins WE. Traumatic injury of the iliopsoas muscle in three dogs. J Am Vet Med Assoc. 1997;210:1631–4.
3. Stepnik MW, Olby N, Thompson RR, Marcellin-Little DJ. Femoral neuropathy in a dog with iliopsoas muscle injury. Vet Surg. 2006;35:186–90.
4. Nielsen C, Pluhar GE. Diagnosis and treatment of hind limb muscle strain injuries in 22 dogs. Vet Comp Orthopaed Traumatol. 2005;18:247–53.
5. Tucker DW, Olsen D, Kraft SL, Andrews GA, Gray AP. Primary hemangiosarcoma of the iliopsoas muscle eliciting a peripheral neuropathy. J Am Anim Hosp Assoc. 2000;36:163–7.
6. Da Silva CA, Bernard F, Bardet JF, Theau V, Krimer PM. Fibroticmyopathy of the iliopsoas muscle in a dog. Vet Comp Orthopaed Traumatol. 2009;22:238–42.
7. Ragetly GR, Griffon DJ, Johnson AL, Blevins WE, Valli VE. Bilateral iliopsoas muscle contracture and spinous process impingement in a German Shepherd Dog. Vet Surg. 2009;38:946–53.
8. Holloway A, Dennis R, McConnell F, Herrtage M. Magnetic resonance imaging features of paraspinal infection in the dog and cat. Vet Radiol Ultrasound. 2009;50:285–91.
9. Laksito MA, Chambers BA, Hodge PJ, Milne ME, Yates GD. Fibrotic myopathy of the iliopsoas muscle in a dog. Aust Vet J. 2011;89:117–21.
10. Grösslinger K, Lorinson D, Hittmair K, Konar M, Weissenböck H. Iliopsoas abscess with iliac and femoral vein thrombosis in an adult Siberian husky. J Small Anim Pract. 2004;45:113–6.
11. Woodbridge N, Martinoli S, Cherubini GB, Caine A, Nelissen P, White R. Omentalisation in the treatment of sublumbar abscessation: long-term outcome in 10 dogs. Vet Rec. 2014;175:20–7.
12. Lamb CR, White RN, Mc Evoy FJ. Sinography in the investigation of draining tracts in small animals: retrospective review of 25 cases. Vet Surg. 1994;23:129–34.
13. Frendin J, Funkquist B, Hansson K, Lönnemark M, Carlsten J. Diagnostic imaging of foreign body reactions in dogs with diffuse back pain. J Small Anim Pract. 1999;40:278–85.
14. Staudte KL, Hopper BJ, Gibson NR, Read RA. Use of ultrasonography to facilitate surgical removal of non enteric foreign bodies in 17 dogs. J Small Anim Pract. 2004;45:395–400.
15. Gnudi G, Volta A, Bonazzi M, Gazzola M, Bertoni G. Ultrasonographic features of grass awn migration in the dog. Vet Radiol Ultrasound. 2005;46:423–6.

16. Jones JC, Ober CP. Computed tomography diagnosis of non gastrointestinal foreign bodies in dogs. J Am Anim Hosp Assoc. 2007;43:99–111.

17. Attanasi G, Laganga P, Rossi F, Terragni R, Vizzardelli G, Cortelli Panini P, Vignoli M. Utilizzo dell'ecografia e della TC nella diagnosi e nel trattamento dei corpi estranei vegetali in 56 cani. Veterinaria. 2011;1:25–30.

18. Bouabdallah R, Moissonnier P, Delisle F, De Fornel P, Manassero M, Maaoui M, Fayolle P, Viateau V. Use of preoperative computed tomography for surgical treatment of recurrent draining tracts. J Small Anim Pract. 2014;55:89–94.

19. Vansteenkiste DP, Lee KC, Lamb CR. Computed tomographic findings in 44 dogs and 10 cats with grass seed foreign bodies. J Small Anim Pract. 2014;55:579–84.

20. Caivano D, Bufalari A, Giorgi ME, Conti MB, Marchesi MC, Angeli G, Porciello F, Birettoni F. Imaging diagnosis—Transesophageal ultrasound-guided removal of a migrating grass awn foreign body in a dog. Vet Radiol Ultrasound. 2014;55:561–4.

21. Caivano D, Birettoni F, Rishniw M, Bufalari A, De Monte V, Proni A, Giorgi ME, Porciello F. Ultrasonographic findings and outcomes of dogs with suspected migrating intrathoracic grass awns: 43 cases (2010–2013). J Am Vet Med Assoc. 2016;240:413 21.

22. Della Santa D, Rossi F, Carlucci F, Vignoli M, Kircher P. Ultrasound-guided retrieval of plant awns. Vet Radiol Ultrasound. 2008;49:484–6.

23. Bufalari A, Adami C, Angeli G. Pain assessment in animals. Vet Res Commun. 2007;31:55–8.

24. Johnston DE, Summers BA. Osteomyelitis of the lumbar vertebrae in dogs caused by grass-seed foreign bodies. Aust Vet J. 1971;47:289–94.

25. Schultz RM, Zwingenberger A. Radiographic, computed tomographic, and ultrasonographic findings with migrating intrathoracic grass awns in dogs and cats. Vet Radiol Ultrasound. 2008;49:249–55.

26. Brennan EK, Ihrke PJ. Grass awn migration in dogs and cats: a retrospective study of 182 cases. J Am Vet Med Assoc. 1983;182:1201–4.

27. Hopper BJ, Lester NV, Irwin PJ, Eger CE, Richardson JL. Imaging diagnosis: pneumothorax and focal peritonitis in a dog due to migration of an inhaled grass awn. Vet Radiol Ultrasound. 2004;45:136–8.

28. Aronson LR, Gregory CR. Infectious pericardial effusion in five dogs. Vet Surg. 1995;24:402–7.

29. Puerto DA, Brockman DJ, Lindquist C, Drobatz K. Surgical and nonsurgical management of and selected risk factors for spontaneous pneumothorax in dogs: 64 cases. J Am Vet Med Assoc. 2002;220:1670–4.

10

Killing of *Gyrodactylus salaris* by heat and chemical disinfection

Perttu Koski[1*], Pasi Anttila[1,2] and Jussi Kuusela[1,3]

Abstract

Background: *Gyrodactylus salaris* is a monogenean, which has collapsed tens of wild Atlantic salmon populations. One of the means of preventing the spread of the parasite is the disinfection of the fishing equipment, which is used in the rivers having susceptible salmon populations. Little is known about the dosage of disinfectants against *G. salaris*. There are not standards for the testing of disinfectants against multicellular parasites. The present investigation developed a method to test disinfectants and examined the effectiveness of heated water and a commercially available disinfectant (Virkon S) in killing *G. salaris*. Individual *G. salaris* worms were followed under the microscope during treatment with heated water or Virkon S disinfectant blend. The logarithm of the time needed to kill the parasite was used as a dependent variable in linear regression. The upper 99.98 % prediction line for the dependent variable was used to obtain a value resembling the time needed for a 4 log reduction of the microbial pathogen, which is commonly used as a criterion for disinfectants. Also 6 log reduction was applied.

Results: Exposure to a relatively low temperature was found to kill the parasite. Even 5–50 min treatment (=10–100 times the 99.98 % upper prediction value) with heated water at 40 °C might be used. This would enable the utilisation of hot tap water in the disinfection of fishing gear. The present practice of 1 % Virkon S for 15 min was also found to kill the parasite.

Conclusions: The follow-up of single parasites of a test population and the use of the calculated upper predictive line in the regression analysis offers a method to analyse the effects of disinfectants on parasites like *G. salaris*. The results of our tests give possibilities for using disinfection methods, which may be more acceptable by the fishermen than the present ones.

Background

Gyrodactylus salaris Malmberg 1957 was first identified on farmed Atlantic salmon (*Salmo salar* L.) at a fish farm in the Baltic Sea catchment area [1]. Since the 1970s, *G. salaris* has collapsed populations of wild Atlantic salmon in tens of Norwegian rivers and one Russian river [2, 3]. The parasite is widespred in the Baltic Sea catchment area [4–8]. Measures to prevent the spread of the parasite include prohibition of the transport of live fish to rivers containing wild Atlantic salmon unless the source of the fish is known to be free of *G. salaris* [9], barriers to stop fish migration upstream from infected river areas to uninfected ones, and eradication of infection in rivers by chemical treatment [3, 10, 11].

Although the risk of the spread of *G. salaris* by fishing equipment was not regarded very big [12], have national authorities in Finland, the United Kingdom and Norway provided guidelines or legal regulations on the disinfection of fishing equipment in order to prevent the spread of *G. salaris* to water systems free of the parasite [13–15]. Temperature (heating of equipment to 60 °C for 1 h) and the use of a commercial disinfectant blend (Virkon S) have been advised in addition to complete drying or freezing of the equipment. The suggested concentration–time combination for Virkon S, when mentioned in these instructions, has been at least 1 %–15 min. Some fishermen, especially anglers, fear that the use of disinfectants will harm their valuable equipment. This might reduce

*Correspondence: perttu.koski@evira.fi
[1] Production Animal and Wildlife Health Research Unit, Finnish Food Safety Authority Evira, Elektroniikkatie 3, 90590 Oulu, Finland
Full list of author information is available at the end of the article

their willingness to undertake proper disinfection and perhaps jeopardise the preventive measures.

To our knowledge there are no international standards for the testing of the effect of disinfection of *G. salaris*. The European Committee for Standardisation has not provided norms for the testing of antiparasitic disinfectants [16]. The guidelines of the German Association of Veterinary Medicine provide advice for parasite eggs and Coccidia oocysts, but not for adult worms [17].

The present investigation examined the effectiveness of heated water and a commercially available disinfectant (Virkon S) in killing *G. salaris*. A simple testing method was developed to examine the lethal effect of disinfection on *G. salaris*. The aim was to examine the time needed to kill the parasite, when lower temperatures and concentrations of Virkon S than the present recommendations are used.

Methods

Fish

All rainbow trout (*Oncorhynchus mykiss* Walbaum) used in our experiments were one summer old, ca. 20–25 cm in length and obtained from a commercial fresh water fish farm in Northern Finland. The fish were transported to the laboratory in hatchery water and were maintained in two 500 l plastic fish tanks before the experiments. The tanks were sited in a thermostat-regulated room with a constant temperature of 10 °C. Before the tests involving increasing temperature, the fish and parasites were acclimated to 6 °C for 1 week. The fish were not fed during their stay in the laboratory. Tanks were aerated and had an internal recirculation of water with a sand filter.

Parasites

Because it was assessed too difficult to get the worms unharmed onto the fishing equipment, *G. salaris* in their natural habitat, on the fish fin, were used. The rainbow trout were infected with rainbow trout type *G. salaris* (GenBank accession number AF479750) at the farm, from where they were transported to the laboratory. The species of *Gyrodactylus* was determined by molecular analysis of the mitochondrial CO1 sequence as described in [18].

The parasite survival was followed in the test system at 10 °C (before acclimatizing the fish and parasites to 6 °C). The parasites were found to live up to 85 h. After 48 h the fin and the parasite were already covered with a thick layer of slime and detached epithelium from the fin, but the parasites remained alive.

Test design

In thermal treatments, each fish was killed with a blow on the head and fins were immediately cut while the fish were submerged in tank water. Parasitized fins were individually placed in a Petri dish in heated water from a tank water container. Parasites (1–3 individuals at a time) were continuously observed and the survival time was recorded with a stopwatch. When the parasite complex (including mother *G. salaris* and daughters in her uterus) stopped moving, the worm was gently irritated with an insect needle. In many cases, the parasites responded to irritation. The stopwatch was halted when the parasite did not move nor react to needle stimulation. The fins were handled similarly in the testing of Virkon S. Parasites were observed and the survival time was measured as in the tests with elevated temperature.

The possible recovery of *G. salaris* after the termination of its movements was tested by transferring the fin and attached parasite to fresh water. The amount of the disinfectants concurrently transferred on the surface of the parasite and fin was found to be negligible, as the median volume of water carried with the moved fin was ca. 37 μl (7 weight measurements). If this volume of 1 % Virkon S solution was mixed with the 65 ml of freshwater used in the test, the resulting concentration of Virkon S would be ca. 5.7×10^{-4} %. Based on the results it was concluded that the worms, which had lost their ability to move, could not recover and were dead.

Tests with elevated temperature

Thermal treatments were performed using a thermostat-regulated heating block (Fig. 1). In addition to the heating block, the desk lamp also heated the water. In the first test, 65 ml of tank water in a Petri dish was quickly heated to the test temperature (25, 30, 35 or 40 °C). The fin with the 1–3 parasites on it was then put to the preheated water and the time for the death of the parasite(s) recorded according to the protocol presented in the paragraph 'Test design'. The water temperature was monitored during the tests, and the water was not aerated.

In the second test the temperature was slowly elevated from 6 °C until each worm ceased moving. This varied between 760 and 2359 s depending on the speed of the elevation of the water temperature. The rate of increase of the temperature was regulated by changing the distance of the desk lamp from the microscope. The time when the worm no longer moved even after the irritation by an insect needle was recorded as the time of death.

Tests with Virkon S

Virkon S is a commercial oxidising disinfectant blend. The product used in the experiments described here (produced by Antec Int. Ltd, UK.) was labelled as containing the following: potassium peroxymonosulphate, sodium hexametaphosphate, sodium alcylbenzenesulphonate, malic acid, sulphamic acid, sodium chloride,

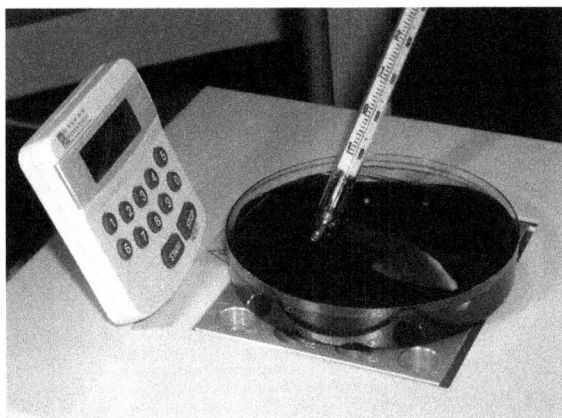

Fig. 1 Test apparatus. *Gyrodactylus salaris* individuals were attached on a rainbow trout fin that was placed in 65 ml of fish tank water. The temperature of the water was maintained (or raised by heating with a desk lamp in the second experiment on heat disinfection) by the heat block under the Petri dish and followed with the thermometer. The survival time of individual parasites was recorded with the stopwatch

fragrance and an indicator dye. Virkon S is widely used in the disinfection of livestock premises and in aquaculture.

All experiments with Virkon S solution were performed at 10 °C. Virkon S concentrations of 0.01, 0.05, 0.1 and 1.0 % were tested. The time until the mother and the daughter parasite did not move even after the irritation with an insect needle was recorded and used as the time of the death of the parasite.

Statistics

Regression analysis was used to test the association between the temperature and survival time and between Virkon S concentrations and survival time. Logarithmic transformations of the original parameters were used, because there appeared to be difficulties in fulfilling the requirement of linearity in regression analysis [19]. The residuals of the logarithmic time variable followed a normal distribution.

The upper 99.98 % prediction line in the regression analysis was used as an estimate for the time needed to

reduce the *G. salaris* population by 4 log. The 6 log reduction was counted on the basis of only 10^{-6} of the normally distributed population lying outside $\pm 5 \times$ standard deviation of the mean.

Statistical analysis was carried out using the analytical software package SPSS for Windows version 22 [20].

Results

Effect of water temperature on the survival time of G. salaris

Gyrodactylus salaris was sensitive to treatment with warm water (Table 1), as the individual worms only survived for 6–18 s in 40 °C. The water temperature and the time until the cessation of movements were found to be associated and the following linear regression formula was obtained ($R^2 = 0.98$, $P < 0.001$):

$$\log \text{TIME} = 8.72 - 0.20 \times \text{TEMPERATURE } (^{\circ}\text{C}).$$

On the basis of this and Fig. 2 it can be concluded that there is a clear killing effect of the increased temperature. Another regression was also tested in which both variables were logarithmically transformed, but R^2 remained the same (0.98).

The higher 99.98 % individual prediction line indicates a survival time of ca. 30 s for *G. salaris* in 40 °C. If the 99.98 % confidence limits for the prediction interval are extrapolated to the temperature at which the predicted survival time of the parasite would be 10 s, 42.5 °C would be sufficient to stop all movement of the parasite. The 1-s treatment temperature would be 47.6 °C. The more critical requirement of 6 log reduction [7]—ca. 5 times the standard deviation from the mean—in 40 °C would be 34 s. This is not very much higher than the 4 log reduction time.

The results of the experiment in which the temperature was gradually raised are illustrated in Fig. 3. It appeared that *G. salaris* had a fairly constant lethal temperature of 30.5–33.5 °C, irrespective of the time taken (13 min 20 s–40 min) to reach this temperature. In the regression analysis the regression coefficient was 0.00 ($R^2 = 0.22$).

Table 1 The survival times of *Gyrodactylus salaris* in heated water and Virkon S

Temperature (°C)	+25	+30	+35	+40
Survival time [median (range)]	119.7 (67.4–209.3) min	12.4 (6.9–21.6) min	50.5 (36–98) s	9 (6–18) s
N	18	36	40	23
Virkon S (%)	0.01	0.05	0.1	1.0
Survival time [median (range)]	11.7 (3.4–34.2) min	3.1 (1.8–4.8) min	2.4 (1.4–4.5) min	14 (8–28) s
N	54	54	55	53

The survival times of single worms in different water temperatures (*upper*) and Virkon S (*below*)

N number of worms tested

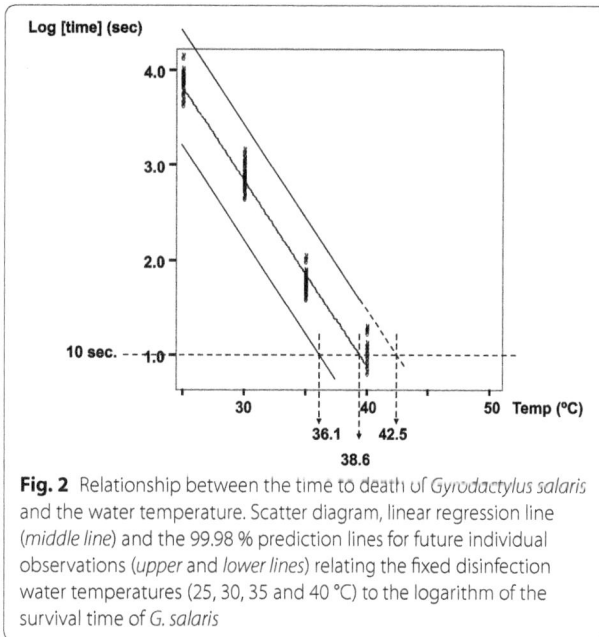

Fig. 2 Relationship between the time to death of *Gyrodactylus salaris* and the water temperature. Scatter diagram, linear regression line (*middle line*) and the 99.98 % prediction lines for future individual observations (*upper* and *lower lines*) relating the fixed disinfection water temperatures (25, 30, 35 and 40 °C) to the logarithm of the survival time of *G. salaris*

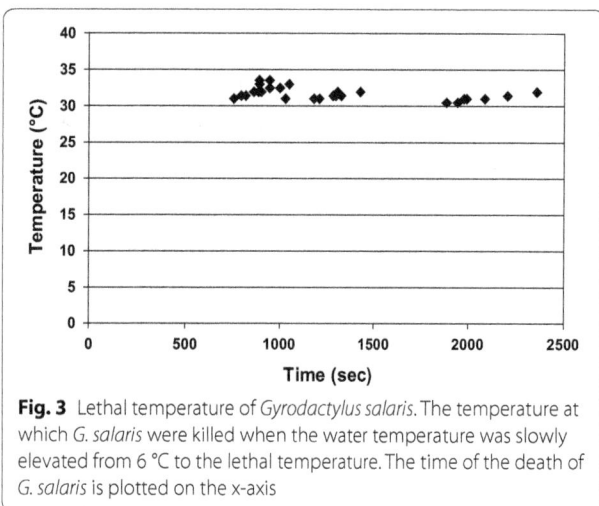

Fig. 3 Lethal temperature of *Gyrodactylus salaris*. The temperature at which *G. salaris* were killed when the water temperature was slowly elevated from 6 °C to the lethal temperature. The time of the death of *G. salaris* is plotted on the x-axis

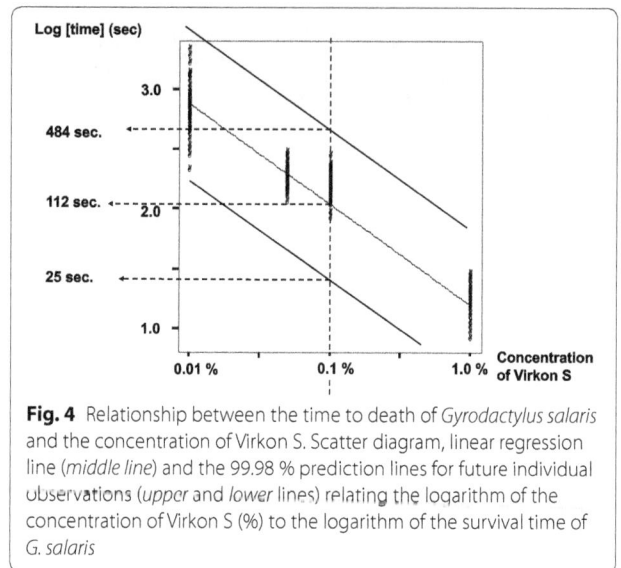

Fig. 4 Relationship between the time to death of *Gyrodactylus salaris* and the concentration of Virkon S. Scatter diagram, linear regression line (*middle line*) and the 99.98 % prediction lines for future individual observations (*upper* and *lower* lines) relating the logarithm of the concentration of Virkon S (%) to the logarithm of the survival time of *G. salaris*

Discussion

Freshly cut rainbow trout fin is most likely a better living environment for *G. salaris* than the surface of fishing equipment. The parasites may tolerate the action of disinfectants, if they thrive well. This may divert the estimations of the survival time of the parasite in a safe direction. On the other hand the presence of extraneous substance like slime may be more probable in the surrounding of the parasite on the fin than on the surface of fishing equipment. The influence of such extraneous material probably divert the estimations to other direction [22], when the applicability of our results to the practical disinfection of fishing gear is considered.

Disinfection that reduces a bacterial, fungal or viral titre by 4–5 logs is commonly regarded as effective [16, 23, 24]. The 6 log reduction is used, when medical devices are designated to be sterile according to [21]. The 99.98 % prediction interval for individual *G. salaris* was used here for counting the 4 log reduction of *G. salaris*. One ten thousandth part of the *G. salaris* population used in the test would stand longer disinfection times than the upper 99.98 % prediction line. Killing times above this line were considered to reduce the *G. salaris* population by 4 log. The basis for selecting the 4 log reduction instead of 5 log was the assumption that relatively low number of *G. salaris* do attach to fishing gear under real conditions.

Effect of water temperature on the survival of *G. salaris*

Study of the biology of *G. salaris* has naturally focused on physiological water temperatures [25]. According to Office International des Epizooties [26], the tolerance of *G. salaris* to temperatures above 25 °C is unknown. The

Survival time in Virkon S

The survival of *G. salaris* in Virkon S is shown in Table 1. The time until the cessation of movement of *G. salaris* and the Virkon S concentration were found to be associated and the following linear regression formula was obtained ($R^2 = 0.93$, $P < 0.001$):

$$\log \text{TIME} = -0.47 - 0.84 \log \text{CONCENTRATION}.$$

The test results are illustrated in Fig. 4. The higher 99.98 % individual prediction line indicates a survival time of 484 s for *G. salaris* in a 0.1 % solution (one tenth of the standard concentration) and 17 s in 1 % solution of Virkon S. The more critical requirement of 6 log reduction [21] in 1 % solution was counted to be ca. 102 s.

temperature and time needed to kill *G. salaris* in this study was much lower than that used for the general disinfection of fish farms [26]. Heat can be used in the disinfection of fishing equipment, but the advice of the [13]—60 °C for 1 h—is very much higher than the time needed to kill the parasite with heated water in this study. The short time of survival (movement) of the parasite at high temperature did not allow temperatures higher than 40 °C to be tested. The extrapolated temperature (42.5 °C, Fig. 2) required to kill the parasite after a 10-s treatment is, however, close to the highest tested temperature and probably a good estimate of the actual lethal temperature in dipping disinfection lasting 10 s, if 4 log reduction would be the goal.

A margin of safety may be applied in the practical disinfection procedures in addition to the 4–5 log reduction of the pathogen. In the review by [27] of the general protocols for effective iodophor disinfection of viral haemorrhagic septicaemia (VHS) virus on salmonid eggs, this margin appeared to increase the treatment time by a factor of ca. 10. The present norm for heat treatment (60 °C for 1 h) could probably be much lowered without jeopardising the efficiency of disinfection. A treatment time as low as 5–50 min (=10–100 times the 99.98 % upper prediction value) with heated water at 40 °C could be used, if a factor of 10–100 was applied.

The results of the second test examining the effect of temperature on *G. salaris* survival supported the use of heated water: the parasite died when the increasing water temperature reached a fairly moderate level.

The killing effect of the temperature treatments might be associated with the decreased oxygen concentrations of the heated water and not the temperature per se. There is ca. 8.1 mg l^{-1} dissolved oxygen (D.O.) in fully saturated water at 25 °C and 6.6 mg l^{-1} at 40 °C. Because the heated water was only kept for a short time in a broad-mouthed vessel (Petri dish), it is unlikely that the saturation would have significantly decreased from the full saturation in the tank water of live fish. We are unaware of the limits for *G. salaris*, but the host fishes do not thrive at D.O. <5 mg l^{-1} [28]. It is unlikely that the requirements of *G. salaris* exceed those of the host fish.

In this study the parasites were, however, treated in warm water, whereas practical disinfection procedures usually involve moist or dry heat, the thermal conductivity of which is much lower. The heated water in this study could therefore be more effective in killing the parasite than disinfection with moist or dry heat. The total energy required to elevate the temperature of the parasite is small due to the small size of the animal.

Effect of low concentrations of Virkon S on the survival of *G. salaris*

Virkon S proved to be efficient in killing *G. salaris*. Even one tenth of the standard concentration of the solution

resulted in death of the parasite in less than 10 min. This would enable the use of Virkon S in lower concentrations than currently recommended. If a similar margin of safety as discussed in the section on heat disinfection (factor 10–100) was applied, the disinfection time for 0.1 % Virkon S would, however, be impractical (1 h 37 min–16 h 8 min).

The present guideline of 1 % Virkon S for 15 min is long enough both on the basis of the evaluation according to 4 log reduction with a safety factor of 10–100 or 6 log reduction.

Conclusions

The demonstrated vulnerability of *G. salaris* to even a moderate heating of the water has practical applications. The lethal temperature to *G. salaris* is unlikely to damage even the most delicate angling equipment such as the line and flies. The short time needed to kill the parasite at temperatures over 40 °C allows the use of routine facilities such as hot tap water to disinfect small fishing equipment. The use of moist or dry heat in sauna or drying cabinet would need more evaluation before the present advice could be safely lowered.

Authors' contributions
All authors participated in the design of the study. PK made the statistical analysis and drafted the manuscript. PA carried out the tests; JK made the species determination of the parasites. All authors read and approved the final manuscript.

Author details
[1] Production Animal and Wildlife Health Research Unit, Finnish Food Safety Authority Evira, Elektroniikkatie 3, 90590 Oulu, Finland. [2] Present Address: Perämeren Kalatalousyhteisöjen Liitto, Piuhatie 8, 90620 Oulu, Finland. [3] Present Address: Lahti University of Applied Sciences, Niemenkatu 73, 15140 Lahti, Finland.

Acknowledgements
We are grateful to Professor Antti Oksanen for constructive criticism of the study during both the performing and writing up of the work. The remarks of the referees greatly improved the original manuscript. The study was financially supported by the Ministry of Agriculture and Forestry of Finland.

Competing interests
The authors declare that they have no competing interests. The authors have not received funding or other financial support from the producer of Virkon S.

References
1 Malmberg G. Om förekomsten av *Gyrodactylus* på svenska fiskar. Skrifter utgivna av Södra Sveriges Fiskeriförening, Årsskrift. 1956;1957:19–76.
2. Kudersky LA, Ieshko EI, Schulman B. Distribution range formation history of the Monogenean *Gyrodactylus salaris*, Malmberg, 1957—a parasite of juvenile Atlantic salmon *Salmo salar* Linnaeus, 1758. In: Veselov AJ, Ieshko EP, Nemova NN, Sterligova OP, Shustov Y, editors. Petrozavodsk: Russian Academy of Sciences, Karelian Research Center, Institute of Biology; 2003. p. 77–83

3. Mo TA. Status of *Gyrodactylus salaris* problems and research in Norway. In: Pike AW, Lewis JW, editors. Parasitic diseases of fish. Dyfed: Samara Publications Ltd; 1994. p. 43–56.

4. Malmberg G, Malmberg M. Species of *Gyrodactylus* (Platyhelminthes, Monogenea) on salmonids in Sweden. Fisheries Res. 1993;17:59–68.

5. Koski P, Malmberg G. Occurrence of *Gyrodactylus* (Monogenea) on salmon and rainbow trout in fish farms in northern Finland. Bull Scand Soc Parasitol. 1995;5(76–88):146.

6. Kuusela J, Zietara MS, Lumme J. Hybrid origin of Baltic salmon-specific parasite *Gyrodactylus salaris*: a model for speciation by host switch for hemiclonal organisms. Mol Ecol. 2007;16:5234–45.

7. Rokicka M, Lumme J, Zietara MS. Identification of *Gyrodactylus* ectoparasites in polish salmonid farms by PCR-RFLP of the nuclear ITS segment of ribosomal DNA (Monogenea, Gyrodactylidae). Acta Parasitol. 2007;. doi:10.2478/s11686-007-0032-1.

8. Anttila P, Romakkaniemi A, Kuusela J, Koski P. Epidemiology of *Gyrodactylus salaris* (Monogenea) in the River Tornionjoki, a Baltic wild salmon river. J Fish Dis. 2008;31:373–82.

9. The Commission of the European Communities: Commission Regulation (EC) No 1251/2008 of 12 December 20008. Off J Eur Union. 2008, L337:41–75.

10. Johnsen BO, Brabrand Å, Jansen PA, Teien H, Bremset G. Evaluering av bekjempelsesmetoder for *Gyrodactylus salaris*. Direktoratet for Naturforvaltning. 2008. http://www.miljodirektoratet.no/old/dirnat/attachment/148/Utredning%202008-7%20Evaluering%20av%20bekjempelses.pdf. Accessed Feb 2 2016.

11. Miljødirektoratet. Handlingsplan mot lakseparasitten *Gyrodatylus salaris* for perioden 2014–2016. Miljødirektoratet. 2014. http://www.miljodirektoratet.no/Documents/publikasjoner/M288/M288.pdf. Accessed Feb 2 2016.

12. Vitenskapskomiteen for mattrygghet. Vurdering av risiko for spredning av *Gyrodactylus salaris* knyttet til ulike potensielle smitteveier. 2005. http://www.vkm.no/dav/9b40351568.pdf. Accessed Feb 2 2016.

13. Finnish Food Safety Authority Evira. Protect the salmon—prevent the spread of salmon parasite *Gyrodactylus salaris*. 2015. http://www.evira.fi/portal/en/about+evira/publications/?a=category&cid=32. Accessed February 2 2016.

14. Scottish Executive Environment and Rural Affairs Department (SEERAD). *Gyrodactylus salaris*—What you need to do. 2011. http://www.gov.scot/Topics/marine/Fish-Shellfish/18364/18610/diseases/notifiableDisease/g-salaris/gsactions. Accessed Feb 2 2016.

15. Norwegian Food Safety Authority. Help us keep our fish healthy. How to stop the spread of *Gyrodactylus salaris*. 2015. http://www.mattilsynet.no/language/english/fish_and_aquaculture/recreationalfishing/how_to_stop_the_spread_of_gyrodactylus_salaris_2015_engelsk.10035/binary/How%20to%20stop%20the%20spread%20of%20Gyrodactylus%20salaris,%202015%20engelsk. Accessed February 2 2016.

16. European Committee for Standardization. Chemical disinfectants and antiseptics. Application of European Standards for chemical disinfectants and antiseptics. 2007, European Standard EN 14885:1–34.

17. Böhm R. Desinfektionsmittelliste der Deutschen Veterinärmedizinischen Gesellschaft (DVG) für die Tierhaltung. Hanover: Schlütersche GmbH & Co; 2003. p. 1–12.

18. Meinilä M, Kuusela J, Zietara MS, Lumme J. Primers for amplifying ~820 bp of highly polymorphic mitochondrial COI gene of *Gyrodactylus salaris*. Hereditas. 2002;137:72–4.

19. Sokal RR, Rohlf FJ. Biometry: the principles and practice of statistics in biological research. New York: W. H. Freeman and Company; 1995.

20. Anonymous SPSS for Windows version 22. 2013.

21. British Standard: Sterilization of medical devices—requirements for medical devices to be designated "STERILE"—Part 1. Requirements for terminally sterilized medical devices. BS EN 556-1: 2001 Incorporating Corrigendum No 1, 2006: p. 1–8.

22. OIE (World Organisation for Animal Health). Aquatic Animal Health Code: general recommendations on disinfection. 2015, http://www.oie.int/index.php?id=171&L=0&htmfile=chapitre_disinfection.htm. Accessed Feb 17 2016.

23. Slavin G. A reproducible surface contamination• method for disinfectant tests. Br Vet J. 1973;129.13=0.

24. Mazzola PG, Penna TC, Martins AM. Determination of decimal reduction time (D value) of chemical agents used in hospitals for disinfection purposes. BMC Infect Dis. 2003;3:24.

25. Bakke TA, Cable J, Harris PD. The biology of gyrodactylid monogeneans: the "Russian Doll-killers". In: Baker JR, Muller R, Rollinson D, editors. Advances of parasitology. 2007. p. 161–376

26. OIE (World Organisation for Animal Health): Aquatic Animal Health Code, Infection with *Gyrodactylus salaris*. 2012. http://www.oie.int/fileadmin/Home/eng/Health_standards/aahm/current/2.3.03_GYRO.pdf. Accessed Feb 28 2016.

27. Bovo G, Hill BJ, Husby A, Håstein T, Midtlyng PJ, Olesen NJ, Storset A: Work package 3 report. Pathogen survival outside the host, and susceptibility to disinfection. 2005, Contract no QLK2-CT-2002-01546 (European Commission). p. 1–41.

28. Rosenthal H, Munro ALS. Der aquatische Lebensraum Umweltbedingungen in natürlichen Gewässern und Aquakulturanlagen. In: Roberts RJ, Schlotfeldt H, editors. Grundlagen der Fischpathologie. Berlin: Verlag Paul Parey; 1985. p. 1–22.

11

Seroprevalence and "Knowledge, Attitudes and Practices" (KAPs) survey of endemic ovine brucellosis in Egypt

Yamen Hegazy[1], Walid Elmonir[2*], Nour Hosny Abdel-Hamid[3] and Essam Mohamed Elbauomy[3]

Abstract

Background: Between February and July 2014, a cross-sectional study to estimate the seroprevalence of brucellosis in sheep in the Kafrelsheikh district of Egypt was carried out, together with a survey of knowledge, attitudes and practices (KAPs) among local shepherds. A total of 273 serum samples were collected from 28 sheep flocks in 10 villages within the study area. These samples were analysed by the Rose Bengal Plate test (RBPT) test, with all positive samples being confirmed by complement fixation test (CFT).

Results: True seroprevalence was 20 % (95 % CI 15.3–24.7 %) with the prevalence of villages with at least one sero-positive sheep estimated at 95.5 % (95 % CI 92.2–100 %); village flock seroprevalence ranged from 0 to 46.8 %. Results of the KAPs survey demonstrated that despite good knowledge regarding brucellosis being potentially present within their flocks, shepherds lacked knowledge regarding routes of livestock to humans disease transmission and the symptoms of brucellosis in humans. This lack of knowledge regarding disease transmission resulted in high-risk practices being widespread—practices such as assisting parturition without protective measures, throwing aborted material into water canals and a reluctance to remove animals that had aborted from the flock.

Conclusions: This study proposes potential measures to reduce seroprevalence of brucellosis in sheep and reduce public health risks from brucellosis such as culling aborted livestock and educational campaigns among shepherds regarding disease risks and modes of transmission.

Keywords: Sheep, Brucellosis, Seroprevalence, Risk factors, Shepherds' KAPs, Control, Egypt

Background

Brucellosis is a major zoonosis affecting public health and economy of many nations throughout the world, particularly in the Middle East, Mediterranean region, Central Asia and Latin America, where insufficient national control programmes has resulted in high endemicity [1, 2]. Brucellosis has however been eradicated from Japan, Canada, Australia, New Zealand and many countries in Northern and Central Europe [3]

Human brucellosis causes acute febrile illness with chronic hepatomegaly, splenomegaly and arthritis and is classified as a risk group III disease due to its ease of airborne transmission [4, 5]. Due to its debilitating nature, the disease has a major economic impact on patients, reducing their ability to work or support a family. The highest recorded incidences of human brucellosis are found in Central Asia and the Middle East [6].

In Egypt, the prevalence of human brucellosis was recently reported to be as high as 8 % in high-risk populations [7]. However, the true incidence of human brucellosis is not easy to known as many patients seek medical treatment in private clinics and not all of these cases are reported to the public health authorities. For instance, Jennings et al. [8] found that in Fayoum governorate, Egypt, hospital-based surveillance identified less than 6 % of the actual human brucellosis cases. Brucellosis in humans is strongly linked to contact with infected animals [9]. Therefore, farmers, shepherds, abattoir workers

*Correspondence: walid.elmonir@gmail.com
[2] Hygiene and Preventive Medicine (Zoonoses) Department, Faculty of Veterinary Medicine, Kafrelsheikh University, Kafrelsheikh 33516, Egypt
Full list of author information is available at the end of the article

and veterinarians are considered as being the highest occupational risk groups [10].

In endemic areas, livestock brucellosis has a severe economic impact through lost productivity due to decreased milk production, abortions and infertility [2]. The high cost of brucellosis surveillance and control programmes is also an economic burden on low-income countries, along with associated impediments to trade [11].

Recent studies carried out in Egypt, particularly those in the area of this study, reported brucellosis to be endemic with high seroprevalence (12.2 % in sheep, 11.3 % in goats and 11 % in cattle) [9, 12]. The national control programme's effectiveness in reducing this prevalence is questionable with brucellosis is still being present in all governorates of Egypt and up to 15 % of all livestock (cattle, buffaloes, sheep and goats) expected to be seropositive in some regions [13–15]. The national control programme was launched in 1985 and consisted of six-monthly serological testing of all female ruminants, with all seropositive livestock slaughtered and compensation provided for owners, together with voluntary vaccination of young female ruminants with either the S19 vaccine for cattle or Rev1 vaccine for sheep and goats [3].

Many factors have however reduced the programme's effectiveness, such as; (1) a lack of reliable information on brucellosis seroprevalence in sheep (2) a lack of adequate communication between the public health authorities, veterinarians and stakeholders, (3) inadequate funding of surveillance and reporting systems, (4) the free movement of small ruminants between the various governorates in Egypt [13, 16].

The aim of this study was to estimate the flock-level seroprevalence of brucellosis among sheep in the Kafrelsheikh district of Egypt and describe the knowledge, attitudes and practices (KAPs) of shepherds, regarding brucellosis, in this district.

Methods

In Egypt, small ruminants are raised mainly either as separate flocks (i.e. either sheep or goats) or as mixed flocks. They are kept in flocks managed by shepherds or by small-scale farmers, who work in growing crops and own small numbers of household reared animals for assistance in farming and for the use of their milk or meat [17, 18]. One shepherd would often keep sheep and goats from a number of different owners; as a result animals from different households are part of the same flock for grazing and breeding during most of the year. Smaller flocks in the same village may be combined together to form a single large village flock managed by a group of shepherds. There is no regulation of animal movement in Egypt and livestock move freely across the country [18].

Study design

A cross-sectional study was conducted between February and July 2014 to estimate the seroprevalence of brucellosis in the sheep population and collect information on KAPs of shepherds towards brucellosis in the Kafrelsheikh district, Egypt.

Sampling

The Kafrelsheikh district has 10 main villages where sheep are managed in flocks by a number of shepherds. Our target population was all the sheep (n = 24,000) in the 10 villages. Each of these villages was assumed to have a similar flock size. The total number of sheep was calculated using a 2010 census and individual sheep were the primary sampling units. The sample size was estimated using Win episcope 2.0 with an expected prevalence of 15 and a 5 % accepted error being 196 animals. We increased this sample size to 270 sheep [9]. This number was divided equally across the main 10 villages. In each of the villages, the total desired sample of 27 sheep was equally divided between the present flocks. Within each flock, sheep were selected by simple random sampling. A total of 273 serum samples were collected from 28 flocks in the 10 villages.

Serological testing

Serum was extracted from whole blood by centrifugation at 3000 rpm for 15 min at 4 °C and stored at −20 °C until examined. The Rose Bengal Plate Test (RBPT) was conducted according to manufacturer's manual (Prionics AG, Schlieren-Zurich, Switzerland) and samples positive by RBPT were subsequently tested by complement fixation test (CFT). Antigen for the CFT was obtained from the NVSL/DBL, USDA, USA. Complement and hemolysin were prepared and preserved according to Alton et al. [19] and were titrated according to Hennager [20]. Sheep erythrocytes were collected on Alsever's solution from an adult healthy ram serologically negative for brucellosis and standardized to 3 % suspension in veronal buffer saline. Results of the CFT were interpreted as positive at a cutoff point of ≥ 20 ICFTU/ml [19].

Epidemiology

The apparent seroprevalence (AP) of brucellosis was estimated as follows [21]:

$$AP = (\text{Number of animals seropositive to both RBPT and CFT} \\ /\text{Number of examined animals}) \times 100$$

The true seroprevalence (TP) of brucellosis was estimated as follows [21]:

$$TP = AP + Se - 1/Se + Sp - 1$$

where TP is the true seroprevalence, Se is the in series combined sensitivity of both of RBPT and CFT (78 %) and Sp is the in series combined specificity of both RBPT and CFT (99 %) [9].

The confidence interval (CI) for the TP was obtained as follows [21]:

$$CI = p \pm Z * \sqrt{\frac{p * (1 - p)}{n}}$$

The village flock true seroprevalence (VFTP) for each of the 10 studied villages was calculated as VFTP = (Village flock AP + Sp − 1)/(Se + Sp − 1). The proportion of villages, which had at least one seropositive sheep after accounting for the village flock combined Se (VFCSe) and Sp (VFCSp) of serological tests was calculated as described by Hegazy et al. [9]. The VFCSe and VFCSp values used were 0.93 and 0.76 respectively [9].

Questionnaire

Data concerning shepherd KAPs was collected using a structured questionnaire, developed in English and translated into Arabic. The questionnaire was piloted in one village, with three shepherds interviewed and the questionnaire subsequently revised. After revision, the questionnaire was then administered to all shepherds (n = 26).

The awareness of shepherds regarding brucellosis was investigated through the use of open questions concerning the main diseases causing abortion in sheep, whether or not these diseases affect humans, the main signs of the disease and potential routes of transmission to humans. Attitudes and practices relating to brucellosis were assessed by asking the shepherds questions regarding the use of hygienic measures in handling aborted material or recently aborted sheep and the role of veterinarians in such cases. The level of collaboration with the national control programme was investigated through questions regarding the number of visits undertaken by the General Organization of Veterinary Services campaigns annually to collect blood samples for serological examination for brucellosis. The questionnaire is shown in Additional file 1.

Ethical approval

Ethical approval was obtained from the Committee of Research, Publication and Ethics of the Faculty of Veterinary Medicine, Kafrelsheikh University. All procedures were explained to flock owners and owners' informed verbal consents were obtained.

Results

Seroprevalence

A total of 273 serum samples were collected from 28 sheep flocks in the 10 villages. The sera were examined by RBPT with agglutination recorded in 47 samples (17.95 %). Positive RBPT serum samples were confirmed by CFT with 16.48 % (45/273) of the samples being positive for both tests (AP). The TP was estimated at 20 % (95 % CI 15.3–24.7 %).

The prevalence of villages with at least one seropositive sheep for brucellosis after adjusting for the VFCSe and VFCSp was estimated at 95.5 % (95 % CI 92.2–100 %) with 9 out of 10 villages having at least one sheep that tested positive. The village flock prevalence ranged from 0 to 46.8 % (Fig. 1).

Shepherds' KAPs

Out of 26 shepherds who responded to the questionnaire, 16 (61 %) declared that brucellosis alone was the main causative agent of abortion in their flocks, while 4 (15 %) stated that Rift Valley Fever virus in combination with *Brucella* spp. were the main causative agents of abortion in their flocks. Six shepherds (23 %) did not give an answer to this question. The shepherds (n = 20), who answered the questions, believed that humans could be infected by *Brucella* spp. while assisting aborting ewes and considered this as the only route for disease transmission to humans. Five of 16 shepherds (31.3 %) described fever as a sign of human brucellosis while the rest were not aware of any signs of the disease in humans.

Out of 18 shepherds, 10 (55.5 %) fed the aborted materials to their dogs while 5 (27.8 %) throw aborted materials into the water canals and only 3 (16.7 %) bury aborted materials. Out of 21 shepherds, 15 (71.4 %) keep aborted animals in their flocks for further breeding seasons. Five shepherds (23.8 %) would sell these animals and only one shepherd said that he slaughtered them. Two of the shepherds, who would keep aborted animals in the flock, reported having suffered from fever and being diagnosed with brucellosis. Assisted parturition, not wearing protective gloves or masks when assisting with the parturition, slaughtering sheep and eating meat of slaughtered sheep were practiced by all shepherds interviewed.

Although all shepherds interviewed were aware of the official test and slaughter program for brucellosis control in Egypt, none of them had ever had their flocks tested by the veterinary authorities. Only one shepherd out of 19 (5.3 %) said that he might call the veterinarian, official or private, for advice regarding aborted animals.

Discussion

Sheep are considered the primary source of *Brucella mellitensis*, which is the most pathogenic *Brucella* sp. in humans and the predominant strain circulating in Middle East, including Egypt [22, 23]. Recent non-governmental studies indicate that brucellosis is highly endemic in ruminants in Egypt, though large discrepancies in

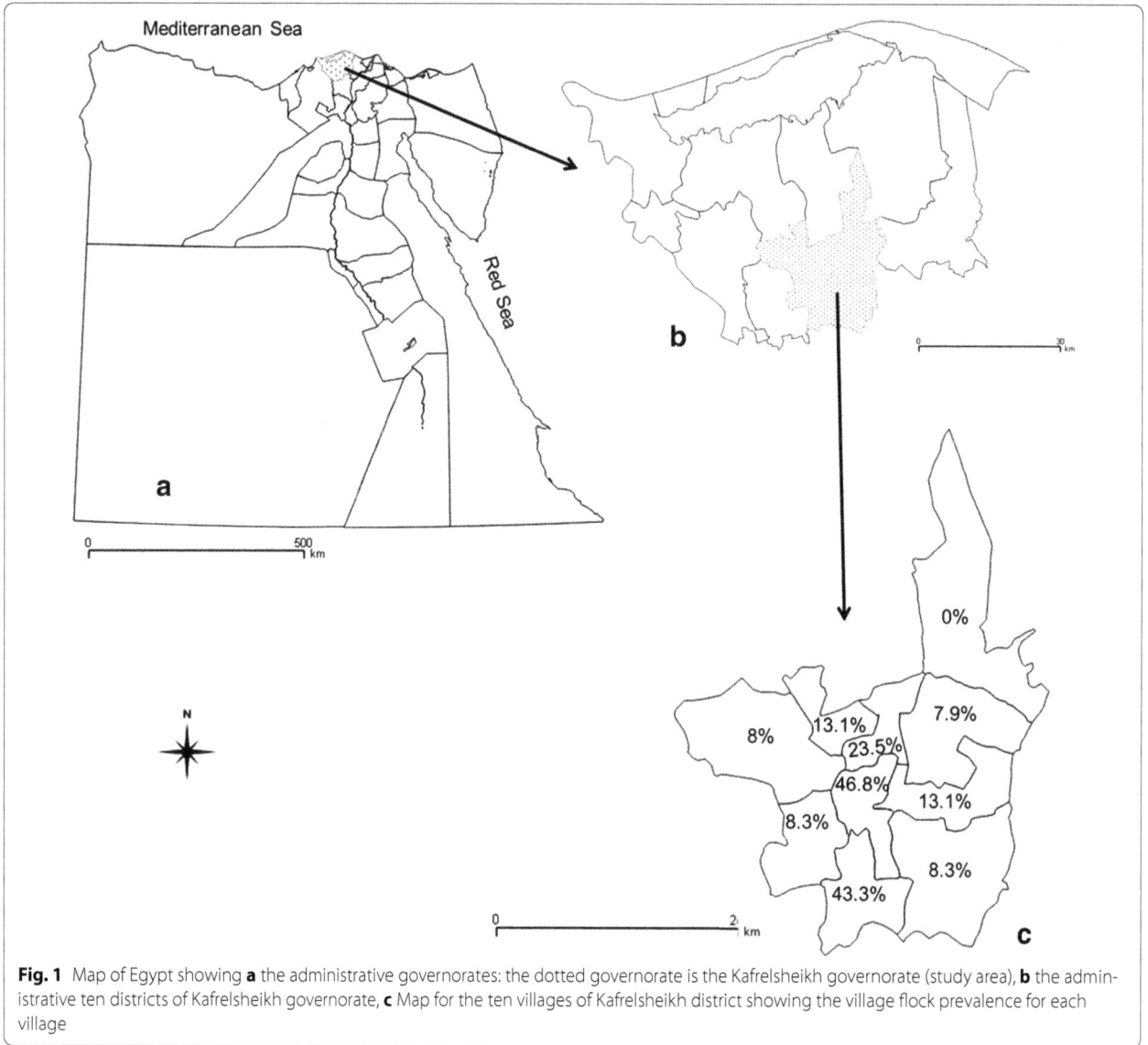

Fig. 1 Map of Egypt showing **a** the administrative governorates: the dotted governorate is the Kafrelsheikh governorate (study area), **b** the administrative ten districts of Kafrelsheikh governorate, **c** Map for the ten villages of Kafrelsheikh district showing the village flock prevalence for each village

seroprevalence exist between peer-reviewed published studies and those reported by the government [9, 12].

The seroprevalence of brucellosis in sheep in the study area was estimated at 20 % (95 % CI 15.3–24.7 %). Official Egyptian government figures nationwide for *Brucella* seroprevalence in sheep between 1999 and 2011 range from 0.5 to 2.5 % [15]. The seroprevalence in this study is slightly higher than that reported by Hegazy et al. [13]. This study agrees with Hegazy et al. [13] stating that brucellosis is endemic in Egypt with a high seroprevalence (around 15 %) despite the current national control programme. This may be due to poor availability of resources, a lack of compliance among livestock owners and the structure of the local production systems. To our knowledge the proportion of villages with at least one

sheep seropositive for brucellosis reported in the current study area is the highest ever reported.

Results from the KAPs survey show that official testing and culling had apparently never been conducted and the majority of shepherds tended to keep aborted animals within their flocks—both of these factors potentially responsible for the persistently high *Brucella* seroprevalence in the study area [13]. Free movement of flocks, lack of livestock identification, open livestock markets, unhygienic parturition measures and the throwing of aborted material into water canals are also significant in the transmission and persistence of the disease.

Results from the shepherd KAPs survey showed that most of the participant shepherds had good awareness of ovine brucellosis. Farmers participating in another study in Egypt also showed similarly high levels of awareness [12]. The high endemicity of livestock brucellosis in Egypt is likely to have increased public awareness, particularly among livestock owners and those working closely with livestock. Furthermore, the high economic impact of the disease and risks of human infection may have also strengthened this knowledge.

All the shepherds who answered the questionnaire identified brucellosis as the main cause of abortion within their flocks and were aware of the risks of human infection. They were not however aware of any potential modes of transmission to humans other than direct contact with aborted ewes and aborted material. As a result of this lack of awareness, shepherds continue high-risk practices including home slaughter of sheep and subsequent meat preparation [24]. None of the participant shepherds drank sheep milk though, due to a lack of awareness about cross-species transmission, they still drink milk from goats, even though their flocks may be suffering abortions in both sheep and goats.

Despite their knowledge of human brucellosis, only a few shepherds described fever as a sign of the disease. A lack of awareness about the signs of the disease may cause the seriousness of the disease to be underestimated, with infected shepherds not seeking immediate medical attention and thus exposing themselves to more severe complications of the disease. This underestimation of disease severity may also play a role in the shepherd's ignorance regarding high-risk practices such as assisting parturition or handling of aborted material from ewes without gloves or masks [25]. This lack of awareness concerning signs of human brucellosis and modes of transmission may be attributed to inadequate communication by the public health authorities, shortage of awareness campaigns usually associated with the underreporting of disease and inadequate surveillance [8].

Most farmers and shepherds infected with brucellosis do not share information about their illness with the public health authorities, veterinarians or even their co-workers for fear of the economic losses caused by governmental tracing and culling of their livestock [12]. Infected shepherds thus fail to add to the knowledge about brucellosis in their community, facilitate underreporting and hinder control programmes. Pappas et al. [6] reported that among brucellosis patients' in Greece this attitude of not allowing veterinary investigation, for fear of an adverse effect on their herd, was associated with an increased incidence of human infections.

The majority of participants reported that they fed aborted fetuses to their dogs and this practice may also increase transmission and persistence of infection in the flock. Dogs play a role in mechanical transmission of the infection when they drag aborted material across the

ground [3]. Some shepherds also throw aborted material into water canals used by sheep and other livestock for drinking or bathing. Shepherds, farmers and other village residents come into contact with this water though daily routines such as bathing, irrigation of fields, washing of utensils, fishing and other activities. The practice of discarding aborted material into watercourses is a likely cause of water contamination and increases the risk of disease transmission to human and livestock populations in the region [26].

Most shepherds kept aborted animals in their flocks, while a few reported they might sell them at market. Only one shepherd mentioned slaughtering as a possible course of action. This is in contrast with Holt et al. [12], who found that most farmers preferred to sell infected animals in the market (80.4 %) or directly to the butcher (50.5 %) and none would keep such animals. These differences in attitude may be attributed to differences in knowledge of the disease, with farmers showing a high degree of brucellosis awareness and accurate knowledge of the disease, its transmission and its effects when compared to shepherds [12]. This knowledge may help in guiding farmers toward selling infected animals rather than keeping them and thus exposing their households to the risk of infection. Shepherds in this study however lacked knowledge regarding the public health risk of keeping infected animals within their flock. Another possibility is the economic benefit, as it seems that keeping mature ewe for production of offspring is more profitable for shepherds than selling them in the market as this may decrease the production capacity of their flocks.

Only one shepherd stated that he had asked for advice from a veterinarian in an abortion case, while the remaining shepherds claimed they never consulted the veterinarian in cases of abortion. Shepherd attitudes were shown to be very different from farmer attitudes in a village in Menufiya Governorate, Egypt, (and elsewhere) as most farmers preferred to consult a veterinarians, while shepherd consider dystocia management as a required skill for their profession and were reluctant to contact veterinarians [12, 27]. This lack of contact with veterinarians reduced their knowledge of risks and modes of infection transmission for brucellosis, as shown in this study. Consulting a veterinarian may be an important factor in improving awareness regarding brucellosis risks for both shepherds and farmers [27].

None of the shepherds were willing to notify the veterinary authorities in cases of abortion. All shepherds stated that no sampling by the veterinary authorities had ever been undertaken in their flocks for brucellosis (or any other disease) though they were aware of the official test and slaughter policy. In their opinion, this policy is economically unfair and potentially devastating to their flocks. Shepherds in this study and farmers in another study shared their dissatisfaction with the official brucellosis control programme in Egypt, particularly the system of compensation [12]. Based on farmers and veterinarians opinions, the official compensation monetary value for sheep was estimated to be less than 20 % of the actual market value [12]. As a result shepherds and farmers usually seek alternative economic choices, such as selling animals to butchers, or in the market, or simply keeping the animal for continued breeding purposes, as reported by many shepherds in this study. These factors are likely to be an on-going problem, hindering effective brucellosis control in Egypt.

Conclusions

The findings of this study demonstrate that brucellosis is widespread in sheep of the Kafrelsheikh district, Egypt, despite a national control programme operating in the region since 1985. This study recommends control measures to decrease the public health risks associated with brucellosis in Egypt and reduce seroprevalence in sheep.

The results of this study show that eliminating aborted sheep from a flock is an economically favorable way of potentially reducing *Brucella* seroprevalence and it is expected that this information will prove useful in changing the reluctance of shepherds to slaughter apparently healthy animals. Educational campaigns to increase awareness of brucellosis among shepherds are urgently required. Such campaigns must also highlight the importance of disposing placentas and aborted fetuses appropriately and avoiding the high risks associated with (1) throwing aborted materials into water canals (2) home slaughtering of aborted animals and unhygienic handling of their meat (3) lack of protective measures during birth-aid with aborted animals as wearing gloves and using of antiseptics.

Abbreviations

AP: apparent seroprevalence; CFT: complement fixation test; CI: confidence interval; KAPs: knowledge, attitudes and practices; RBPT: rose bengal plate test; TP: true seroprevalence; ICFTU: International Complement Fixation Test Units; NVSL/DBL, USDA: National Veterinary Services Laboratories/Diagnostic Bacteriology Laboratory, United States department of Agriculture; VFTP: village flock true seroprevalence; VFCSe: village flock combined sensitivity; VFCSp: village flock combined specificity.

Authors' contributions

YH and WE contributed to the concept, design, data analysis and manuscript writing. WE conducted the shepherd interviews and YH carried out the livestock field sampling. NHA and EME were responsible for all laboratory analysis and contributed to the manuscript regarding serological test methods. All authors read and approved the final manuscript.

Author details

[1] Animal Medicine Department, Faculty of Veterinary Medicine, Kafrelsheikh University, Kafrelsheikh 33516, Egypt. [2] Hygiene and Preventive Medicine (Zoonoses) Department, Faculty of Veterinary Medicine, Kafrelsheikh University, Kafrelsheikh 33516, Egypt. [3] Brucellosis Research Department, Animal Health Research Institute, Nadi El-Seid Street, Dokki, Giza 12618, Egypt.

Acknowledgements

The authors wish to express their gratitude to the veterinarians and shepherds who provided valuable help in this study. The authors are also grateful to Professor Javier Guitian, Professor of Veterinary Public Health, Royal Veterinary College, London, UK, for his remarks and suggestions that improved the manuscript. Also, authors are thankful to Mr Peter Holloway, PhD student in Production and Population Health, Royal Veterinary College, London, UK, for his help with English editing of this manuscript. This study was financially supported by Kafrelsheikh University (Egypt) research fund (Project Code: KFURF-11).

Competing interests

The authors declare that they have no competing interests.

References

1. Refai M. Incidence and control of brucellosis in the Near East region. Vet Microbiol. 2002;90:81–110.
2. McDermott J, Grace D, Zinsstag J. Economics of brucellosis impact and control in low-income countries. Rev Sci Tech Off Int Epiz. 2013;32:249–61.
3. Díaz Aparicio E. Epidemiology of brucellosis in domestic animals caused by *Brucella melitensis, Brucella suis* and *Brucella abortus*. Rev Sci Tech Off Int Epiz. 2013;32:53–60.
4. World Health Organization (WHO), 2006. The control of neglected diseases. A route to poverty alleviation. Report of a Joint WHO/DFID-AHP meeting with the participation of FAO and OIE. [http://www.who.int/zoonoses/Report_Sept06.pdf].
5. Dean AS, Crump L, Greter H, Hattendorf J, Schelling E, Zinsstag J. Clinical manifestations of human brucellosis: a systematic review and meta-analysis. PLoS Negl Trop Dis. 2012;6:e1929.
6. Pappas G, Papadimitriou P, Akritidis N, Christou L, Tsianos EV. The new global map of human brucellosis. Lancet Infect Dis. 2006;62:91–9.
7. Samaha H, Mohamed TR, Khoudair RM, Ashour HM. Sero-diagnosis of brucellosis in cattle and humans in Egypt. Immunobiology. 2009;214:223–6.
8. Jennings GJ, Hajjeh RA, Girgis FY, Fadeel MA, Maksoud MA, Wasfy MO, El-Sayed N, Srikantiah P, Luby SP, Earhart K, Mahoney FJ. Brucellosis as a cause of acute febrile illness in Egypt. Trans R Soc Trop Med Hyg. 2007;101:707–13.
9. Hegazy YM, Moawad A, Osman S, Ridler A, Guitian J. Ruminant brucellosis in the Kafr El Sheikh Governorate of the Nile Delta, Egypt: prevalence of a neglected zoonosis. PLoS Negl Trop Dis. 2011;5:e944.
10. Al-Shamahy HA, Whitty CJM, Wright SG. Risk factors for human brucellosis in Yemen: a case control study. Epidemiol Infect. 2000;125:309–13.
11. Ragan V, Vroegindewey G, Babcock S. International standards for brucellosis prevention and management. Rev Sci Tech Off Int Epiz. 2013;32:189–98.
12. Holt H, Eltholth M, Hegazy Y, El-Tras W, Tayel A, Guitian J. *Brucella* spp. infection in large ruminants in an endemic area of Egypt: cross-sectional study investigating seroprevalence, risk factors and livestock owner's knowledge, attitudes and practices (KAPs). BMC Public Health. 2011;11:341.
13. Hegazy YM, Ridler AL, Guitian FJ. Assessment and simulation of the implementation of brucellosis control programme in an endemic area of the Middle East. Epidemiol Infect. 2009;137:1436–48.

14. Abdel-Hamid NH, Ebeid MH, Arnaout FK, Elgarhy MM, Elbauomy EM, AhmedHanaa A, Sayour AE. Serological and bacteriological monitoring of ruminant brucellosis in seven governorates with control programme follow-up in three cattle farms. Benha Vet Med J. 2012;23:254–63.

15. Wareth G, Hikal A, Refai M, Melzer F, Roesler U, Neubauer H. Animal brucellosis in Egypt. J Infect Dev Ctries. 2014;8:1365–73.

16. Elbauomy EM, Abdel-Hamid NH, Abdel-Haleem MH. Epidemiological situation of brucellosis in five related ovine farms with suggestion of appropriate programmes for disease control. Anim Health Res J. 2014;2:129–42.

17. Ahmed AM, Kandil MH, El-Shaer HM, Metawi HR. Performance of desert black goat under extensive production systems in North Sinai in Egypt. Meeting of the Sub-Network on Production Systems of the FAO-CIHEAM Inter-Regional Cooperative Research and Development Network on Sheep and Goats, Molina de Segura-Murcia Zaragoza, Spain, 2001. p. 213–7.

18. Aidaros H. Global perspectives-the Middle East: Egypt. Revue Scientifique et Technique de l'Office International des Epizooties. 2005;24:589–96

19. Alton GG, Jones LM, Pietz D, Angus RD. Techniques for the Brucellosis Laboratory. France: INRA Publications; 1988.

20. Hennager SG. Reagent Production Protocol—Guinea Pig Complement Preparation for the Complement Fixation Test. USDA, APHIS, National Veterinary Services Laboratories (NVSL), Ames, Iowa, USA, 2004.

21. Thrusfield M. Veterinary epidemiology. Wiley-Blackwell; 2007.

22. Cloeckaert A, Vizcaíno N, Paquet JY, Bowden RA, Elzer PH. Major outer membrane proteins of Brucella spp.: past, present and future. Vet Microbiol. 2002;90:229–47.

23. Benkirane A. Ovine and caprine brucellosis: World distribution andcontrol/eradication strategies in West Asia/North Africa region. Small Rumin Res. 2006;62:19–25.

24. Walshe MJ, Grindle J, Nell A, Bachmann M. Dairy development in sub-Saharan Africa, World Bank Technical Paper 135, Africa Technical Department Series, World Bank, Washington DC; 1991.

25. Kozukeev TB, Ajeilat S, Maes E, Favorov M. Risk factors for brucellosis—Leylek and Kadamjay districts, Batken Oblast, Kyrgyzstan, January–November, 2003. MMWR Morb Mortal Wkly Rep. 2006;28:31–4.

26. El-Tras WF, Tayel AA, Eltholth MM, Guitian J. *Brucella* infection in fresh water fish: Evidence for natural infection of Nile catfish, *Clarias gariepinus*, with *Brucella melitensis*. Vet Microbiol. 2009;141:321–5.

27. Lindahl E, Sattorov N, Boqvist S, Magnusson U. A study of knowledge, attitudes and practices relating to brucellosis among small-scale dairy farmers in an urban and peri-urban area of Tajikistan. PLoS One. 2015;10:e0117318.

12

Ecological niche modeling of rabies in the changing Arctic of Alaska

Falk Huettmann[1], Emily Elizabeth Magnuson[2] and Karsten Hueffer[3*]

Abstract

Background: Rabies is a disease of global significance including in the circumpolar Arctic. In Alaska enzootic rabies persist in northern and western coastal areas. Only sporadic cases have occurred in areas outside of the regions considered enzootic for the virus, such as the interior of the state and urbanized regions.

Results: Here we examine the distribution of diagnosed rabies cases in Alaska, explicit in space and time. We use a geographic information system (GIS), 20 environmental data layers and provide a quantitative non-parsimonious estimate of the predicted ecological niche, based on data mining, machine learning and open access data. We identify ecological correlates and possible drivers that determine the ecological niche of rabies virus in Alaska. More specifically, our models show that rabies cases are closely associated with human infrastructure, and reveal an ecological niche in remote northern wilderness areas. Furthermore a model utilizing climate modeling suggests a reduction of the current ecological niche for detection of rabies virus in Alaska, a state that is disproportionately affected by a changing climate.

Conclusions: Our results may help to better inform public health decisions in the future and guide further studies on individual drivers of rabies distribution in the Arctic.

Keywords: Rabies, Alaska, Ecologic niche, Data mining, Predictions

Background

Rabies is a global zoonotic disease that lacks satisfactory treatment and kills 50,000–70,000 people annually, mostly in developing countries where dog-associated rabies is not well controlled [1]. In developed countries rabies among wild animals poses a threat to human health through direct contact with infected wildlife or through the infection of unvaccinated dogs, and cats [2]. The economic burden of rabies is significant even in areas without large numbers of human rabies cases due to the costs of prevention efforts and required infrastructure [1].

In the circumpolar region the arctic fox (*Vulpes lagopus*) is considered the primary maintenance host for rabies [3]. The arctic fox has been displaced in some regions by the red fox (*Vulpes vulpes*) presumably driven

by anthropogenic change [4–6]. However, this trend is not found in all regions of the Arctic [7].

In Alaska, rabies is of significant concern to public health, particularly in the face of environmental change [8], see also Additional file 1 for detail on human health implications. Enzootic rabies (defined as always being present at a certain level) is believed to be primarily limited to northern and western coastal regions of Alaska that have only limited human development [9]. Occasionally epizootic rabies occurs in interior regions of Alaska [10]. Although the exact extent of enzootic regions is unknown. Large urban settlements such as the cities of Anchorage, Fairbanks and Juneau, are not directly affected by enzootic rabies apart from occasional importation of the disease through translocation of infected dogs from enzootic rural areas (for an example see [11]). The regions of Alaska with the highest burden of rabies cases in both wildlife and domestic dogs, like many other remote arctic communities, generally lack adequate veterinary care and dog vaccination. In addition, the

*Correspondence: khueffer@alaska.edu
[3] Department of Veterinary Medicine, University of Alaska Fairbanks, 901 Koyukuk Drive, PO Box 757750, Fairbanks, AK 99775, USA
Full list of author information is available at the end of the article

true burden of rabies, especially in foxes is not known, because diagnostic testing is generally limited to incidents of possible human exposure and animals suspected of having rabies in regions considered non-enzootic. There is little active surveillance of rabies among wildlife in enzootic regions of Alaska. The majority of rabies testing occurs only in close proximity to human infrastructure. Industrial developments in remote areas are known to enhance invasive species, including diseases (see [12] for invasive species in Alaska) and can provide significant attractions to wildlife through food subsidies, as well as olfactory or light stimuli [13, 14].

Rabies dynamics in Alaska are characterized by cyclical increases in reported cases with 4–5 year intervals [15] (Fig. 1). During the period from 2000 to 2014, 272 animals were reported positive for rabies by the Section of Epidemiology for the State of Alaska in their annual disease reports [16–23]. Ninety-nine percent of these rabies-positive animals originated in Northern and Southwestern Alaska that are considered enzootic for wildlife rabies. In contrast South-central and parts of central interior Alaska did not contribute any cases of

rabies in terrestrial mammals. The spread of arctic variant rabies into areas previously not affected poses a risk even in the more populated areas of Alaska. This can be seen by the spread of arctic variant-rabies into southern Ontario for instance [24].

Both red and arctic foxes are frequently diagnosed with rabies, but red foxes are diagnosed with rabies more often than arctic foxes [15]. Within Alaska the rabies virus is maintained as three distinct genetic variants [25, 26]: Arctic rabies variants 2, 3 and 4. The general spatial distribution of these variants seems to be stable [25–27]. The biogeography and mechanism of maintaining at least three distinct strains over time is not well understood [27]. However, the population structure of arctic foxes appears to be more closely related to the distribution of rabies variants compared to the population structure of red foxes. It suggests that the mesocarnivore arctic fox is the maintenance host, while the red fox serves as a frequent spillover host for this virus. Alternatively, the red and arctic fox provide a dynamic multi-host maintenance system for arctic rabies virus variants in Alaska [27]. The consequences on rabies dynamics of a supposedly

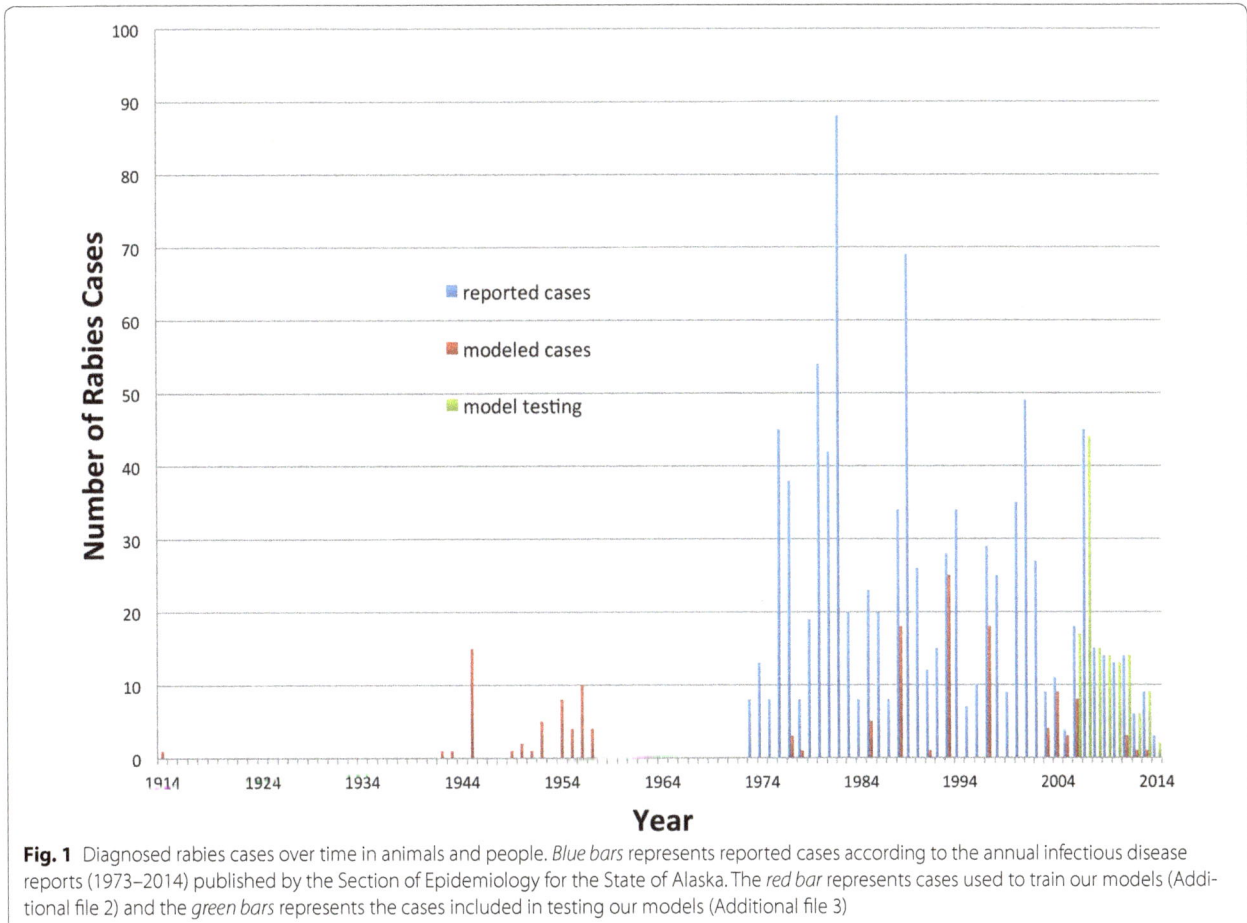

Fig. 1 Diagnosed rabies cases over time in animals and people. *Blue bars* represents reported cases according to the annual infectious disease reports (1973–2014) published by the Section of Epidemiology for the State of Alaska. The *red bar* represents cases used to train our models (Additional file 2) and the *green bars* represents the cases included in testing our models (Additional file 3)

increased displacement of arctic foxes by red foxes is not known [28]. However Kutz provides examples for increased disease in Northern regions, mainly parasitic infections, associated with extreme weather events and warmer temperatures [29]. Similar dynamics could also hold true for rabies at high latitudes.

Some examples of increased disease transmission in the circumpolar North due to a changing climate have been described [30]. With climate change predicted to be more extreme at high latitudes, e.g. 10 or more degrees Celsius temperature increase during the next 100 years [31], it is imperative to base future public health decisions on the best available data and predictions [32]. This should be guided by public access, transparency, repeatability, as well as a thorough and justifiable understanding of the ecological niche occupied by the disease of concern [33].

Because of a sampling effort bias towards human development and under-sampling of animals for rabies diagnostics from remote areas, a complete picture of the presence and prevalence of rabies does not yet exist for Alaska. To overcome such problems, predictive modeling emerged as a powerful method, based on empirical data and best-available science ([34] for rabies; for other examples see [35–38]). Organisms, including pathogens and their hosts, are bound by a certain ecological niche [32, 33, 39]. Describing and predicting the ecological niche of a disease can greatly help to further our understanding of pathogen dynamics, even in the face of limited sampling [40, 41].

Following best practice and state-of-the art methods [33, 34, 38, 41, 42], this investigation tried to define the quantitative envelope of the ecological niche for rabies in the Arctic using Alaska as a test case. We carried out such an analysis with an ecological niche model using machine learning algorithms, based on geographical information systems (GIS) and publicly available environmental data, applied to presence only locations of compiled rabies detections.

Methods

Publically available information on 153 diagnosed rabies cases from 1914 to 2013, in terrestrial mammals was compiled and manually divided into a stratum that occurred in areas considered enzootic by the State of Alaska Section of Epidemiology, and a second stratum diagnosed outside this enzootic area [9] (Additional file 2). The classification of enzootic or non-enzootic greatly influences rabies control measures. An independent set of recent diagnosed rabies cases (Additional file 3) was used to compare different approaches.

Rabies cases were model-predicted with machine learning algorithms comparing them to pseudo-absences (created randomly in GIS for Alaska). Classification and regression trees (CARTs)- based boosting and bagging (TreeNet, RandomForest, SPM7, Salford Systems Ltd) using the 'default' settings for those models because they are specifically designed for presence data, data mining (see Table 1 for details) were used to model the ecological niche of rabies in Alaska. These model settings generalize best for data such as used here (https://www.salford-systems.com/products/treenet) [33, 35]. Because these models employ 'recursive partitioning' the models are

Table 1 Settings and explanations of the TreeNet model run

Metric	Setting	Effect	Justification
Learnrate	AUTO	A detailed but slow model run	Known to provide best results for the algorithm 'learning' data
Subsample fraction	50%	Internal testing while model is grown	Standard approach for balanced tree models
Logistic residual trim fraction	0.10	Fine-tuning	Allows for better fits
Huber-M fraction of error squared	0.90	Accuracy level	A statistical standard threshold for certainty
Optimal logistic model selection	Cross entropy	How to find the optimal model	Usually the best setting for tree-based models
Number of trees to build	1000	Number of trees tried out for the best solution	This number should widely overshot the known optimum
Maximum number of nodes	6	Determines the node depth of trees used	This number determines whether a 'stump' or a fully fit tree is run
Terminal node minimum training cases	10	For most data cases it provides a robust tree	Number of cases for each tree branch split
Maximum number of most-optimal models to save summary results	1	Just 1 most-optimal model is saved	
Regression loss criterion	Huber-M (Blend LS and LAD)	A statistical metric to express gain vs cost of a new rule	Standard approach in trees

rather robust for correlations and interactions, as judged by high AUC ROCs and assessment metrics [33].

The environmental layers used are shown in Table 2. These model layers are known to contribute to the ecological niche, and also act as a proxy to inquire further if deemed relevant in future studies. In addition, these layers are currently 'the best available GIS layers for the state of Alaska [35, 43, 44].

For improved inference and validity, models should be assessed for their predictive performance in order to express their reliability [33, 40]. AUC ROC inherent in Salford Predictive Modeler (SPM) was one performance metric used. Machine learning approaches, as used in this study, express the ecological niche as a relative index of occurrence (RIO) visualized in the figures along a quantitative (color) gradient, red-yellow-green. Red is essentially high RIO, yellow is a mid range value, and green is low RIO.

Finally, in order to better predict the distribution of rabies in Alaska for the future, the climate niche models of rabies was predicted to 2050, using regionalized IPPC climate models for Alaska. Predictors for this model of a possible future rabies niche are limited to climate ones because Alaska still lacks reliable and available planning scenarios for the future explicit in space and time for land cover and its socio-economic features [45, 46]. 2050 was used as a more realistic and testable 'future', and thus having a real-world application.

Results

This study provides for the first time publically available data of 153 confirmed rabies cases from 1914 to 2013 with different degrees of geo-referencing quality. This data set is available in Additional file 2 and from the authors upon request (sensu Zuckerberg [47]). This dataset is an essential part of the result. The cases of terrestrial rabies (excluding 2 bat cases) were divided into two subsets: confirmed animal rabies cases from the area of Alaska considered enzootic for rabies, and areas not considered enzootic (Fig. 2). The latter cases were considered associated with sporadic epizootics. Most of these epizootic associated cases were temporally associated with a large-scale outbreak in interior Alaska during the 1950s [10]. Using these data sets machine learning algorithms were utilized to build the following three ecological niche models each for a test which provides us the best generalization for Alaska: models were informed by (a) only cases from areas considered enzootic for rabies (enzootic cases), (b) only cases from non-enzootic areas (outbreak cases), and (c) all confirmed rabies cases. Utilizing these three approaches models were created and assessed for performance, and then predicted risk maps for rabies detection in Alaska were generated. 'Risk' is defined here as pixels with a relative index of occurrence of rabies, as predicted from the model [35, 41].

These maps of the relative index of occurrence varied somewhat, depending on the capability of the algorithm employed and on the data used to inform the model. However, all models predicted the northern coastal areas as high-risk areas for the detection of rabies, which is even true for models only informed by outbreak-associated samples, which excluded samples from this area. Another area consistently identified among all models is located south of the Brooks Range east of Chandalar Lake (Eastern Yukon River Basin). This area is of interest because cases from that region were not included in the data set that informed the model based on enzootic cases. However, this area was involved in the outbreak in the middle of the twentieth century [10] and it has recently seen isolated cases of rabies at its western most boundary [48].

To better compare the different approaches, the models were confronted with a compiled set of recent rabies cases detected by the Alaska State Public Health Laboratory (Fig. 3). The model based on the TreeNet algorithm and informed by all available rabies cases in our data set performed best (Fig. 4; Additional file 4). The remainder of the result section will therefore focus on this model for inference.

This TreeNet-based model identified large areas north of the Brooks Range and areas south along the coast into the Yukon Kuskokwim Delta as areas at highest risk for rabies detection in the state. Interestingly, while the Eastern Yukon River Basin was identified as a high-risk area

Table 2 Predictors of rabies in Alaska and for assembling the ecological niche

Predictor	Source	Comment
Euclidean distance to Alaska coastline	Alaska GAP data	Obtained with ArcGIS tools
Euclidean distance to Alaska infrastructure	Alaska GAP data	Obtained with ArcGIS tools
Elevation	Alaska GAP data	
Monthly mean temperature	Alaska GAP data (taken from SNAP)	
Monthly mean precipitation	Alaska (taken from SNAP)	

For public data sources see [43, 44]

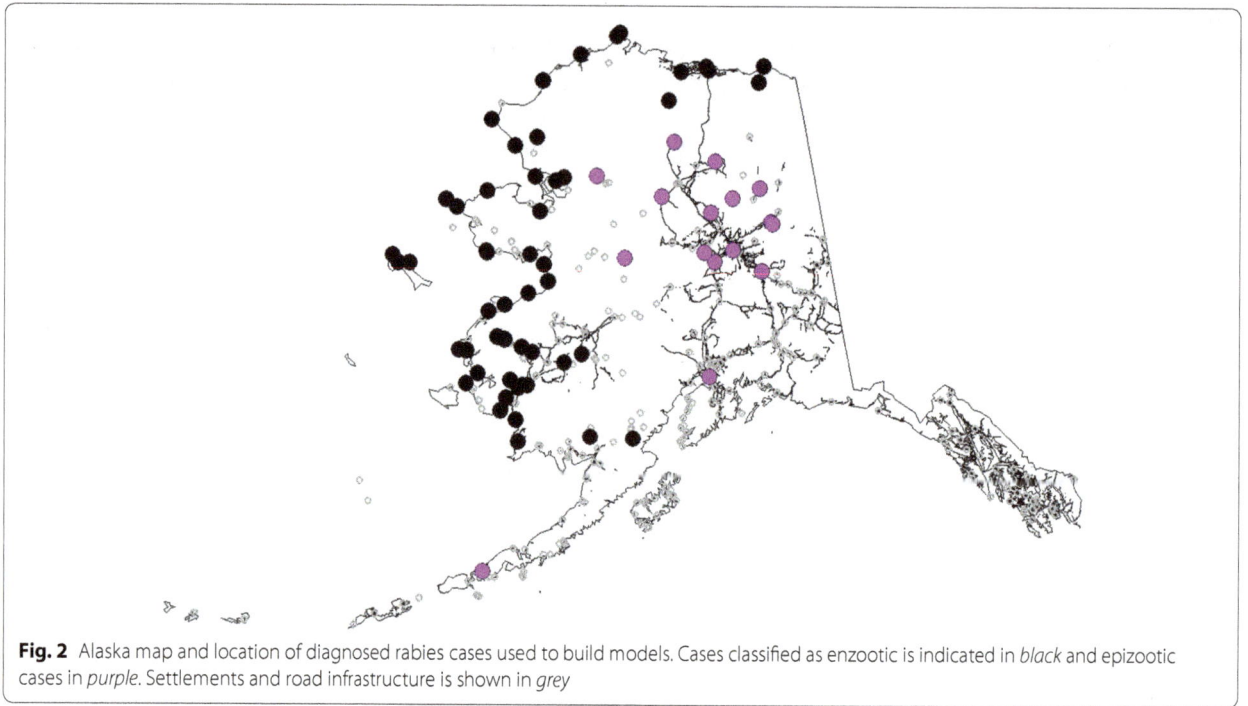

Fig. 2 Alaska map and location of diagnosed rabies cases used to build models. Cases classified as enzootic is indicated in *black* and epizootic cases in *purple*. Settlements and road infrastructure is shown in *grey*

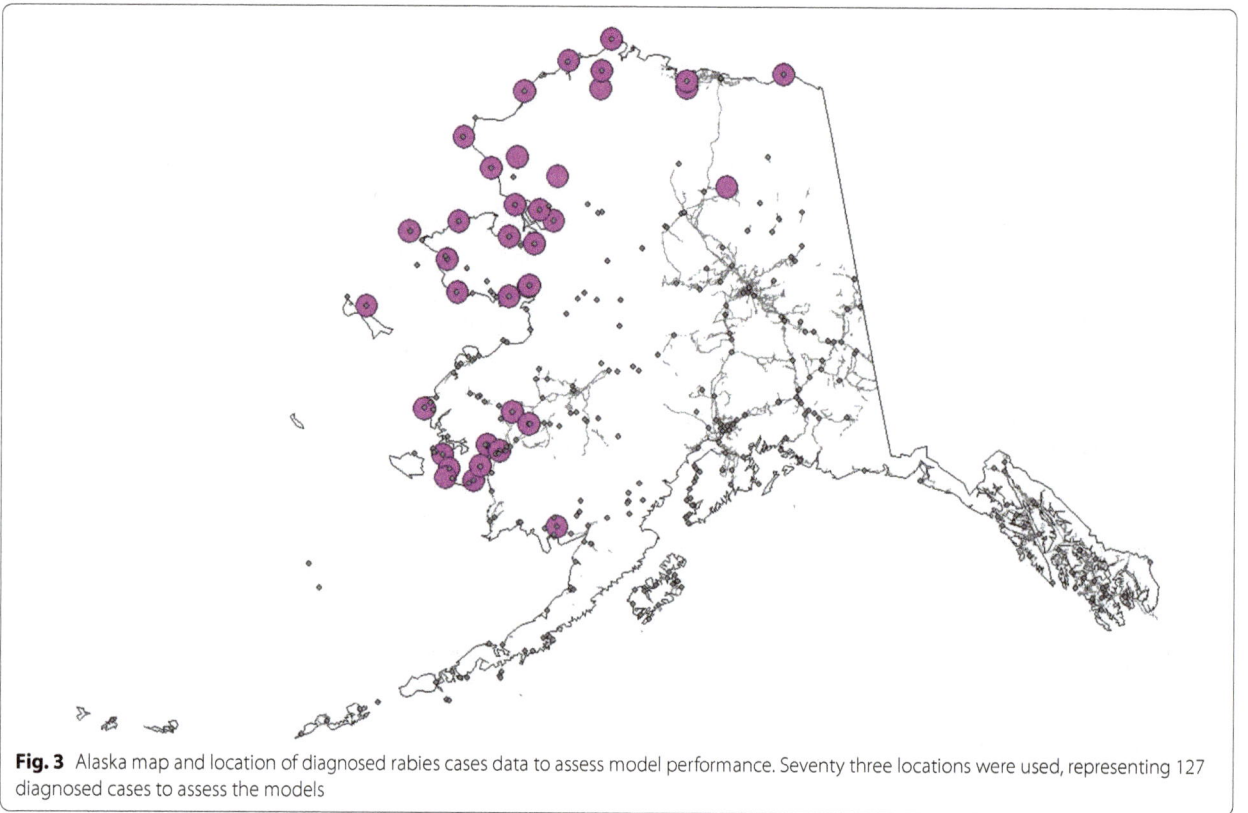

Fig. 3 Alaska map and location of diagnosed rabies cases data to assess model performance. Seventy three locations were used, representing 127 diagnosed cases to assess the models

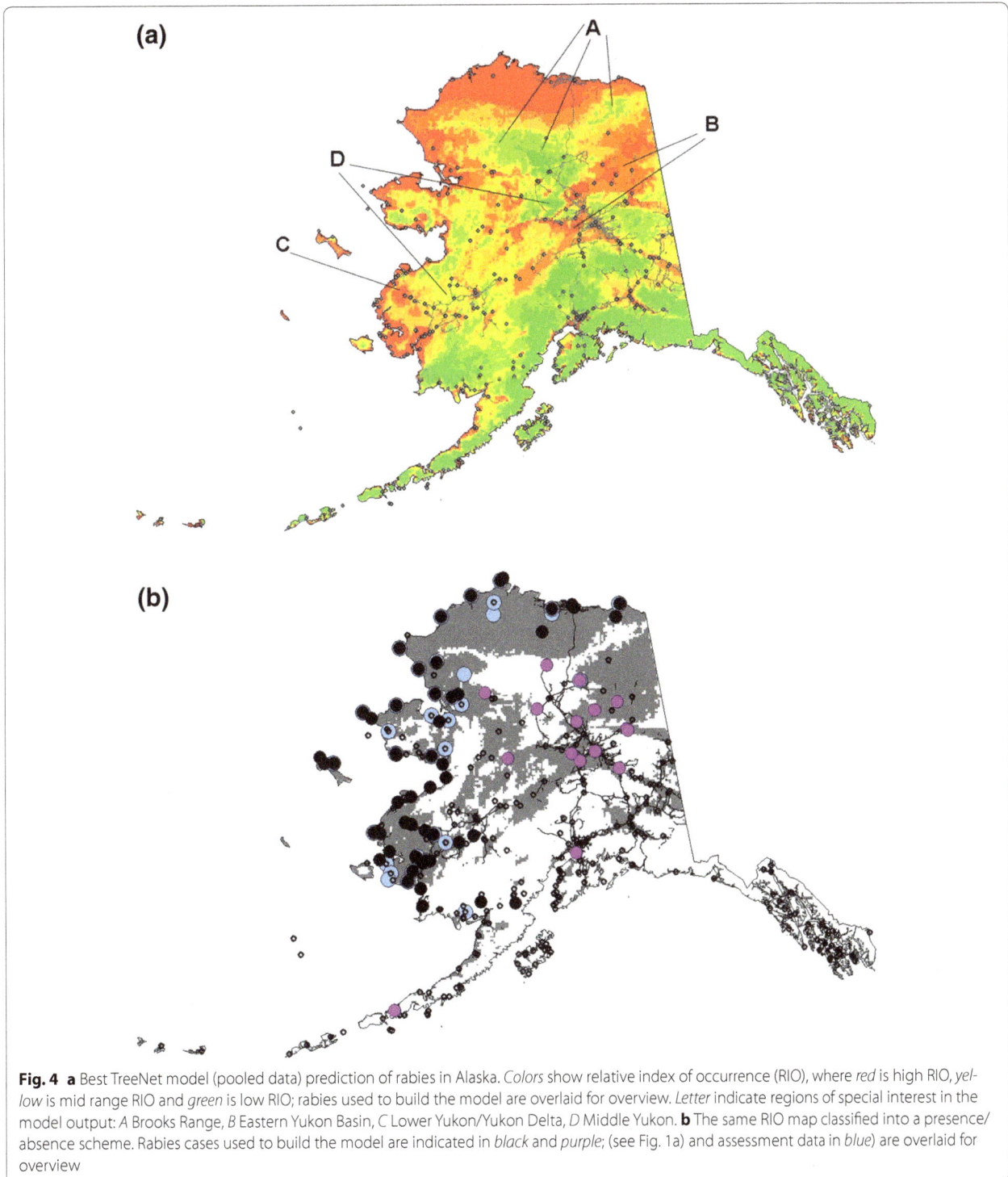

Fig. 4 a Best TreeNet model (pooled data) prediction of rabies in Alaska. *Colors* show relative index of occurrence (RIO), where *red* is high RIO, *yellow* is mid range RIO and *green* is low RIO; rabies used to build the model are overlaid for overview. *Letter* indicate regions of special interest in the model output: *A* Brooks Range, *B* Eastern Yukon Basin, *C* Lower Yukon/Yukon Delta, *D* Middle Yukon. **b** The same RIO map classified into a presence/absence scheme. Rabies cases used to build the model are indicated in *black* and *purple*; (see Fig. 1a) and assessment data in *blue*) are overlaid for overview

for rabies and the mouth of that river is also identified with the high-risk area to the West, the middle section of this major river in Alaska was not identified as an area of high probability for rabies detection. Terrestrial rabies is widely predicted to be absent in southern Alaska, except for the major population center of Anchorage.

The best performing model identified distance to infrastructure, elevation, distance to coast, precipitation in June, and precipitation in February as predictors most important in defining the ecological niche (Table 3).

A model built in TreeNet using only climate variables had a lower performance than the model build on

Table 3 TreeNet variable importance of parameters utilized in best performing model (148 Alaska rabies data locations pooled regardless of outbreak or enzootic locations)

Variable	Score
Distance to infrastructure	100.00
Elevation	56.09
Distance to coast	31.95
Precipitation June	30.63
Precipitation February	21.78
Precipitation October	20.28
Temperature October	20.27
Precipitation March	19.22
Precipitation May	18.64
Temperature April	18.49
Precipitation August	18.29
Temperature December	17.68
Temperature February	17.56
Precipitation April	16.89
Precipitation July	16.77
Precipitation September	16.47
Precipitation December	14.99
Precipitation January	13.40
Temperature August	13.13
Temperature November	12.93
Temperature January	12.50
Temperature May	11.64
Temperature March	10.25
Precipitation November	9.44
Temperature September	8.89
Temperature June	8.64
Temperature July	5.62

The variables are listed by importance together with their relative score in informing the model on the likelihood of rabies occurrence

all predictors (namely the human infrastructure ones). However, it repeated the general results, also identifying similar areas of the state with some extended areas in the Yukon-Kuskokwim Delta compared to a model including non-climate variables.

Unfortunately, we lack any reliable planning and forecast maps and models of infrastructure for Alaska. While those exist for many climate variables [46] they are not available for future development of human infrastructure. We therefore utilized only this climate-based ecological niche model for starting to explore the possible effects of climate change, such as warming in the Arctic and altered precipitation, on the rabies risk distribution in Alaska for the predicted climate scenario in 2050. As done elsewhere [14], we employed an ecological niche model projecting the climate-based niche onto climate data predicted for the year 2050 using the regionalized

IPCC climate model from SNAP (A1B1 scenario). This resulted in a significantly reduced area of predicted future risk of rabies detection, especially in the southern areas of current rabies risk prediction (Fig. 5).

Discussion

Disease prediction is a common effort that can increase understanding of disease ecologies, especially in remote areas [32, 35, 41, 49, 50]. Our approach to better understand rabies dynamics in the circumpolar region becomes possible due to publically available and shared data of confirmed rabies cases, as well as environmental GIS layer predictions and non-parsimonious algorithms. This modeling effort identified several geographic areas of predicted risk for rabies detection. Further, variables were identified by our modeling approach that influenced the distribution of rabies detection throughout the State, specifically the relevance of human infrastructure. A major limitation of our modeling approach was the way most of the data informing the model were collected. Rabies testing in Alaska is largely performed by the public health system with a focus, and consequent bias, towards human exposures. Vast areas in Alaska such as wilderness areas remain largely unstudied for wildlife diseases including rabies. Because of this, knowledge of rabies distribution and ecology Alaska is rather poor and biased through a human-focused detection system. The current pragmatic focus on possible human exposure could skew our model towards ignoring the true role of areas further away from human infrastructure as a variable responsible for majorly influencing the predicted presence of wildlife rabies. However, if one considers our models as an approach to determine possible risk for humans to encounter the rabies virus, this possible bias will still be very reflective of a threat to human health. On the other hand, this bias is likely leading to an underestimation of rabies cases in Alaska. It is still limiting our ability to identify additional variables influencing rabies distribution in remote areas that are relatively unaffected by human activity. Arguably, one wants to know and use as many predictors as possible to test and describe rabies outbreaks, instead of just a parsimonious one.

Our modeling approach provides predictions explicit in space and time and does not attempt to elucidate direct causal relationships between identified predictors and rabies risk. For example, the identified climate variables likely influence rabies occurrence indirectly through effects on wildlife populations rather than direct effect on virus particles or replication of the virus. However, identifying these predictors without detailed knowledge on mechanisms is still important to describe the niche and help focus public health efforts in a spatially explicit form. Large uninhabited areas of Alaska within or

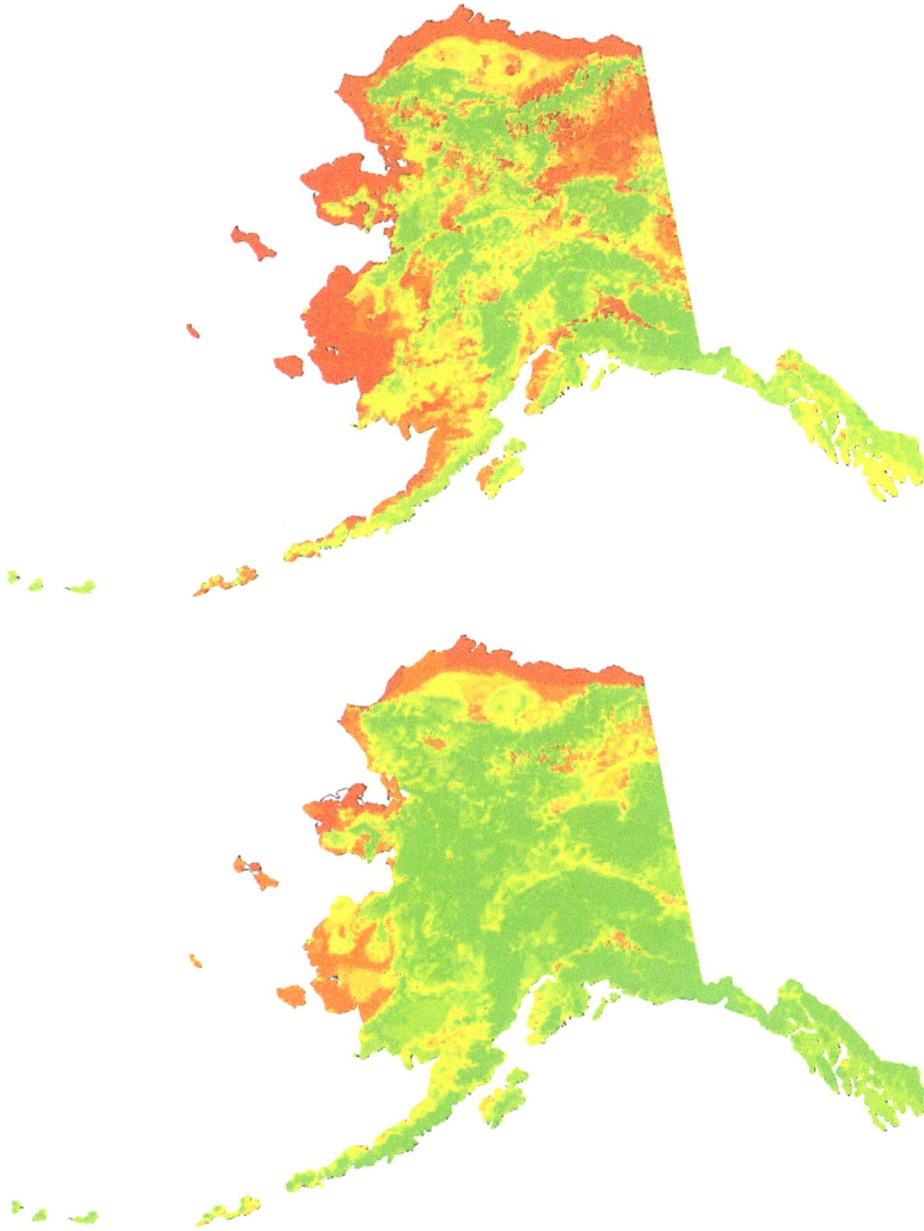

Fig. 5 Climate niche predictions of rabies using Treenet. The *top panel* shows the rabies prediction using the climate niche from 2010 [A1B1 obtained from scenarios network for Alaska + Arctic planning (SNAP)]. The *bottom panel* depicts the rabies prediction using the climate niche from 2050 (A1B1 obtained from SNAP)

adjacent to areas considered enzootic for rabies virus are not systematically surveyed. This limits our ability to fully understand the ecological drivers of this important disease. In addition, information on possible variables at an appropriate landscape level, such as density of reservoir and spillover hosts is needed to better model the ecological drivers of rabies distribution in Alaska. An additional limitation is the possible misdiagnosis of other diseases

(such as canine distemper in foxes) as rabies, especially for cases in the early stages of disease. However, as these cases follow a similar pattern to more recent cases we see this as a minor limitation only.

Our rabies forecast for the state into the future using climate models for 2050 shows a decay of the Arctic rabies niche for the arctic rabies variants. However, we currently lack any information on how rabies variants from the south could enter the state and how they could behave and disperse in a warming Arctic. In addition, the adaptation of the arctic rabies virus variants to a changing environment and host distribution warrants caution in overly relying on our prediction of the extent of the ecological niche for just this rabies virus variant into the future. Our finding that human infrastructure possibly plays a central role, and assuming an increase of infrastructure development, casts doubt on our prediction of reduced rabies risk in a changing Alaska.

Despite the limitations mentioned above, the modeling approach and the results presented can still help public health officials to better focus preventative efforts in the areas most at risk of rabies exposure to humans. Such efforts could include traditional measures such as possible active surveillance efforts in predicted hotspots and coldspots, increased dog vaccinations and population controls and vigilance to detect possible outbreaks or expansion of enzootic areas in the face of a changing Arctic. While currently licensed oral vaccines have been shown to be effective in protecting arctic foxes against infection with virus circulating in Alaska [51], large-scale use of these measures to control rabies are unlikely to be cost effective [51]. However, our methods, open access compilation and results might guide a more limited use of this intervention tool.

Our modeling can especially help target active surveillance efforts in less developed areas of the state. These efforts could test the model presented here and greatly advance our understanding of relevant drivers of rabies maintenance in pristine Arctic areas.

In future work this model and template should be tested and applied further with independent data, ideally data that is less biased and not dependent on human access and human exposure. We also believe that a wider macroecology view and model prediction for rabies overall, and its niche is warranted, assuming that other rabies strains from Canada or more southern regions will enter Alaska sooner or later. This pathogen transport has been seen in other disease system with influenza being a prominent example of pathogen transport to high latitudes [52]. A wider socio-economic perspective to public health and rabies across scales is required. Such an approach will clarify how the findings of our model can be extended beyond the risk of human exposure to start to explain and manage the distribution of rabies in Alaskan wildlife.

Conclusions

I this paper we showed that machine learning approaches and open data sources can help predict the ecological niche of infections disease detection for an important zoonotic disease in the Arctic. These findings can help guide future surveillance efforts as well as inform public health officials in focusing efforts on areas at high risk for rabies virus infections. Future work should test our modeled predictions and lead to further refinement of our predicted ecological niche of rabies virus in Alaska.

Additional files

Additional file 1. Public health impact of rabies in Alaska. This file contains information on the historic public heath impact of rabies in Alaska to put our findings into an appropriate context of One Health.

Additional file 2. Locations of rabies cases in Alaska 1914–2013 used in model development. This file contains the location, dates and vectors of all rabies cases used to build our models. In addition the files indicates if a case was considered part of enzootic rabies or associate with an outbreak in a non-enzootic area.

Additional file 3. Location data of rabies cases used for model assessment. This file lists the location of rabies cases provided by the Alaska Section of Epidemiology in the Department of Health and Social Services of the State of Alaska.

Additional file 4. TreeNet model summary statistics for pooled rabies locations. This file contains summary statistics for the best performing model developed in this studies. It includes partial dependence plots for the three most important predictors in the model (distance to infrastructure, Elevation, and distance to coast), genral Average likelihood statistics and a Gains chart for 104 trees.

Authors' contributions

FH and KH perceived the study. EEM and FH performed the modeling. FH and KH wrote the manuscript. All authors read and approved the final manuscript.

Author details

[1] EWHALE Lab, Institute of Arctic Biology, Department of Wildlife Biology, University of Alaska Fairbanks, 902 N. Koyukuk Dr., P.O. Box 757000, Fairbanks, AK 99775, USA. [2] Department of Biology and Wildlife, University of Alaska Fairbanks, 982 N. Koyukuk Dr., PO Box 756100, Fairbanks, AK 99775, USA. [3] Department of Veterinary Medicine, University of Alaska Fairbanks, 901 Koyukuk Drive, PO Box 757750, Fairbanks, AK 99775, USA.

Acknowledgements

Work reported in this publication was supported by the National Institute of General Medical Sciences of the National Institutes of Health under three linked awards number RL5GM118990. The work is solely the responsibility of the authors and does not necessarily represent the official view of the National Institutes of Health. R. Waltuch kindly provided the first Alaska rabies data compilation for an online UAF eLearning student project (Additional file 2). The Section of Epidemiology, State of Alaska provided data to test our models.

Competing interests

The authors declare that they have no competing interests.

Funding

Work reported in this publication was supported by the National Institute of General Medical Sciences of the National Institutes of Health under three linked awards number RL5GM118990. The work is solely the responsibility of the authors and does not necessarily represent the official view of the National Institutes of Health.

References

1. Hampson K, Coudeville L, Lembo T, Sambo M, Kieffer A, Attlan M, et al. Estimating the global burden of endemic canine rabies. PLoS Negl Trop Dis. 2015. doi:10.1371/journal.pntd.0003709.
2. Rupprecht CE, Hanlon CA, Hemachudha T. Rabies re-examined. Lancet Infect Dis. 2002;2:327–43.
3. Mørk T, Prestrud P. Arctic rabies–a review. Acta Vet Scand. 2004;45:1–9.
4. Macpherson AH. A northward range extension of the red fox in the eastern Canadian Arctic. J Mammal. 1964;45:138–40.
5. Savory G. Foxes and food subsidies: anthropogenic food use by red and Arctic foxes, and effects on Arctic fox survival, on the Arctic Coastal Plain of Alaska. M.Sc. Thesis. University of Alaska.
6. Stickney AA, Obritschkewitsch T, Burgess RM. Shifts in fox den occupancy in the greater Prudhoe Bay area, Alaska. Arctic. 2014;67:196–202.
7. Gallant D, Slough BG, Reid DG, Berteaux D. Arctic fox versus red fox in the warming Arctic: four decades of den surveys in north Yukon. Polar Biol. 2012;35:1421–31.
8. Hueffer K, Parkinson AJ, Gerlach R, Berner J. Zoonotic infections in the US Arctic (Alaska); disease prevalence, potential impact of climate change, and recommended actions for earlier disease detection, research, and prevention and control. Int J Circumpolar Health. 2013. doi:10.3402/ijch.v72i0.19562.
9. Alaska State Section of Epidemiology. http://dhss.alaska.gov/dph/Epi/id/SiteAssets/Pages/Rabies/regions.gif. Accessed Nov 2015.
10. Rausch R. Some observations on rabies in Alaska, with special reference to wild canidae. J Wildl Manag. 1958;22:246–60.
11. Rabies in a dog brought to Anchorage from rural Alaska. In: Bulletin No. 11 2009. Alaska State Section of Epidemiology. 2009. http://epibulletins.dhss.alaska.gov/Document/Display?DocumentId=223 Accessed 14 Oct 2016.
12. Alaska department of fish and game. http://www.adfg.alaska.gov/index.cfm?adfg=invasive.main. Accessed 3 Mar 2017.
13. Weiser EL. Use of anthropogenic foods by glaucous gulls (*Larus hyperboreus*) in Northern Alaska. M.Sc. Thesis. 2010 University of Alaska Fairbanks.
14. Baltensperger AP, Mullet TC, Schmid MS, Humphries GRW, Kövér L, Huettmann F, et al. Seasonal observations and machine-learning-based spatial model predictions for the common raven (*Corvus corax*) in the urban, sub-arctic environment of Fairbanks, Alaska. Polar Biol. 2013;36:1587–99.
15. Kim B, Blanton JD, Gilbert A, Castrodale L, Hueffer K, Slate D, Rupprecht CE, et al. A conceptual model for the impact of climate change on fox rabies in Alaska, 1980–2010. Zoonoses Public Health. 2014;61:72–80.
16. 2001 Annual (January–December) infectious disease report. In: Bulletin No. 8 2002. Alaska State Section of Epidemiology. 2002. http://epibulletins.dhss.alaska.gov/Document/Display?DocumentId=318. Accessed 14 Oct 2016.
17. 2002 Annual (January–December) infectious disease report. In: Bulletin No. 5 2003. Alaska State Section of Epidemiology. 2003. http://epibulletins.dhss.alaska.gov/Document/Display?DocumentId=319. Accessed 14 Oct 2016.
18. 2004 Annual (January–December) infectious disease report. In: Bulletin No. 9 2005. Alaska State Section of Epidemiology. 2005. http://epibulletins.dhss.alaska.gov/Document/Display?DocumentId=321. Accessed 14 Oct 2016.
19. 2006 Annual (January–December) infectious disease report. In: Bulletin No. 8 2007. Alaska State Section of Epidemiology. 2007. http://epibulletins.dhss.alaska.gov/Document/Display?DocumentId=285. Accessed 14 Oct 2016.
20. 2008 Annual (January–December) infectious disease report. In: Bulletin No.14 2009. Alaska State Section of Epidemiology. 2009. http://epibulletins.dhss.alaska.gov/Document/Display?DocumentId=220. Accessed 14 Oct 2016.
21. 2010 Annual (January–December) Infectious Disease Report. In: Bulletin No. 7 2011. Alaska State Section of Epidemiology. 2011. http://epibulletins.dhss.alaska.gov/Document/Display?DocumentId=156. Accessed 14 Oct 2016.
22. 2012 Annual (January–December) infectious disease report. In: Bulletin No. 14 2013. Alaska State Section of Epidemiology. 2013. http://epibulletins.dhss.alaska.gov/Document/Display?DocumentId=92. Accessed 14 Oct 2016.
23. 2014 Annual (January–December) infectious disease report. In: Bulletin No. 12 2015. Alaska State Section of Epidemiology. 2015. http://epibulletins.dhss.alaska.gov/Document/Display?DocumentId=36. Accessed 14 Oct 2016.
24. Nadin-Davis SA, Muldoon F, Wandeler AI. Persistence of genetic variants of the arctic fox strain of Rabies virus in southern Ontario. Can J Vet Res. 2006;70:11–9.
25. Kuzmin LV, Hughes GJ, Botvinkin AD, Gribencha SG, Rupprecht CE. Arctic and Arctic-like rabies viruses: distribution, phylogeny and evolutionary history. Epidemiol Infect. 2008;136:509–19.
26. Nadin-Davis SA, Sheen M, Wandeler AI. Recent emergence of the Arctic rabies virus lineage. Virus Res. 2012. doi:10.1016/j.virusres.2011.10.026.
27. Goldsmith EW, Renshaw B, Clement CJ, Himschoot EA, Hundertmark KJ, Hueffer K, et al. Population structure of two rabies hosts relative to the known distribution of rabies virus variants in Alaska. Mol Ecol. 2016;25:675–88.
28. Hueffer K, O'Hara TM, Follmann EH. Adaptation of mammalian host-pathogen interactions in a changing Arctic environment. Acta Vet Scand. 2011. doi:10.1186/1751-0147-53-17.
29. Kutz S. Polar diseases and parasites: a conservation paradigm shift. In: Huettmann F, editor. Protection of the three poles. Tokyo: Springer; 2012. p. 247–64.
30. Kutz SJ, Hoberg EP, Polley L, Jenkins EJ. Global warming is changing the dynamics of Arctic host–parasite systems. Proc R Soc B Biol Sci. 2005;272:2571–6.
31. Meltofte H, Christensen TR, Elberling B, Forchhammer MC, Rasch M. High-Arctic ecosystem dynamics in a changing climate: ten years of monitoring and research at Zackenberg Research Station, Northeast Greenland. Adv Ecol Res. 2008;40:223–48.
32. Peterson AT, Soberon J, Pearson RG, Anderson RP, Martinez-Meyer E, Nakamura M, et al. Ecological niches and geographic distributions. New Jersey: Princeton University Press; 2011.
33. Drew CA, Wiersma Y, Huettmann F. Predictive species and habitat modeling in landscape ecology. New York: Springer; 2011.
34. Escobar LE, Peterson AT, Papes M, Vogel GM. Ecological approaches in veterinary epidemiology: mapping the risk of bat-borne rabies using vegetation indices and night-time light satellite imagery. Vet Res. 2015. doi:10.1186/s13567-015-0235-7.
35. Herrick KA, Huettmann F, Lindgren MA. A global model of avian influenza prediction in wild birds: the importance of northern regions. Vet Res. 2013. doi:10.1186/1297-9716-44-42.
36. Gomez-Palacio A, Arboleda S, Dumonteil E, Peterson AT. Ecological niche and geographic distribution of the Chagas disease vector, *Triatoma dimidiate* (Reduviidae: Triatominae): evidence for niche differentiation among cryptic species. Infect Genet Evol. 2015. doi:10.1016/j.meegid.2015.08.035.
37. Koch LK, Cunze S, Werblow A, Kochmann J, Doerge DD, Mehlhorn H, Klimpel S. Modeling the habitat suitability for the arbovirus vector *Aedes albopictus* (Diptera: Culicidae) in Germany. Parasitol Res. 2015. doi:10.1007/s00436-015-4822-3.
38. Escobar LE, Qiao H, Peterson AT. Forecasting Chikungunya spread in the Americas via data-driven, empirical approaches. Parasite Vector. 2016. doi:10.1186/s13071-016-1403-y.
39. Cushman S, Huettmann F. Spatial complexity, informatics and wildlife conservation. Tokyo: Springer; 2010.
40. Breiman L. Statistical modeling: the two cultures. Stat Sci. 2001;16:199–231.
41. Peterson AT. Mapping disease transmission risk: enriching models using biology and ecology. Baltimore: Johns Hopkins University Press; 2014.
42. Williams B, Rogers D, Staton G, Ripley B, Booth T. Statistical modelling of georeferenced data: mapping tsetse distributions in Zimbabwe using climate and vegetation data. In: Perry BD, Handsen JW, editors. Modelling vector-borne and other parasitic diseases. Nairobi: ILRAD; 1992. p. 267–80.
43. Baltensperger AP, Huettmann F. Predicted shifts in small mammal distributions and biodiversity in the altered future environment of Alaska: an open access data and machine learning. PLoS ONE. 2015. doi:10.1371/journal.pone.0132054.
44. Ohse B, Huettmann F, Ickert-Bond S, Juday G. Modeling the distribution of white spruce (*Picea glauca*) for Alaska with high accuracy: an open

access role-model for predicting tree species in last remaining wilderness areas. Polar Biol. 2009;32:1717–24.

45. Huettmann F, Franklin SE, Stenhouse GB. Predictive spatial modeling of landscape change in the Foothills Model Forest. For Chron. 2005;8:525–37.

46. Scenarios network for Alaska and Arctic planning SNAP https://www.snap.uaf.edu/. Accessed 3 Mar 2017.

47. Zuckerberg B, Huettmann F, Friar J. Proper data management as a scientific foundation for reliable species distribution modeling. In: Drew CA, Wiersma Y, Huettmann F, editors. Predictive species and habitat modeling in landscape ecology. New York: Springer; 2011. p. 45–70.

48. Second wolf from Chandalar Lake tests positive for rabies. In: Press release May 2 2013. Alaska Department of Fish and Game. 2013. http://www.adfg.alaska.gov/index.cfm?adfg=pressreleases.pr05022013_wolf. Accessed 14 Oct 2016.

49. Caminade C, Kovats S, Rocklov J, Tompkins AM, Morse AP, Colon-Gonzales FJ, et al. Impact of climate change on global malaria distribution. Proc Natl Acad Sci USA. 2014;111:3286–91.

50. Reeves T, Samy AM, Peterson AT. MERS-CoV geography and ecology in the Middle East: analyses of reported camel exposures and a preliminary risk map. BMC Res Notes. 2015. doi:10.1186/s13104-015-1789-1.

51. Follmann EH, Ritter D, Swor R, Hueffer K. Preliminary evaluation of Raboral V-RG® oral rabies vaccine in Arctic foxes (*Vulpes lagopus*). J Wildl Dis. 2011;47:1032–5.

52. Winker K, McCracken KG, Gibson DD, Pruett CL, Meier R, Huettmann F, et al. Movements of birds and avian influenza from Asia into Alaska. Emerg Infect Dis. 2007;13:547–52.

13

Neurological signs in 23 dogs with suspected rostral cerebellar ischaemic stroke

Barbara Thomsen[1*], Laurent Garosi[2], Geoff Skerritt[3], Clare Rusbridge[4,5,6], Tim Sparrow[4], Mette Berendt[1] and Hanne Gredal[1]

Abstract

Background: In dogs with ischaemic stroke, a very common site of infarction is the cerebellum. The aim of this study was to characterise neurological signs in relation to infarct topography in dogs with suspected cerebellar ischaemic stroke and to report short-term outcome confined to the hospitalisation period. A retrospective multicentre study of dogs with suspected cerebellar ischaemic stroke examined from 2010–2015 at five veterinary referral hospitals was performed. Findings from clinical, neurological, and paraclinical investigations including magnetic resonance imaging were assessed.

Results: Twenty-three dogs, 13 females and 10 males with a median age of 8 years and 8 months, were included in the study. The Cavalier King Charles Spaniel ($n = 9$) was a commonly represented breed. All ischaemic strokes were located to the vascular territory of the rostral cerebellar artery including four extensive and 19 limited occlusions. The most prominent neurological deficits were gait abnormalities (ataxia with hypermetria $n = 11$, ataxia without hypermetria $n = 4$, non-ambulatory $n = 6$), head tilt ($n = 13$), nystagmus ($n = 8$), decreased menace response ($n = 7$), postural reaction deficits ($n = 7$), and proprioceptive deficits ($n = 5$). Neurological signs appeared irrespective of the infarct being classified as extensive or limited. All dogs survived and were discharged within 1–10 days of hospitalisation.

Conclusions: Dogs affected by rostral cerebellar ischaemic stroke typically present with a collection of neurological deficits characterised by ataxia, head tilt, and nystagmus irrespective of the specific cerebellar infarct topography. In dogs with peracute to acute onset of these neurological deficits, cerebellar ischaemic stroke should be considered an important differential diagnosis, and neuroimaging investigations are indicated. Although dogs are often severely compromised at presentation, short-term prognosis is excellent and rapid clinical improvement may be observed within the first week following the ischaemic stroke.

Keywords: Canine, Cerebellum, Cerebrovascular accident, Infarct, Ischemic, Occlusion, Rostral cerebellar artery, Syndrome, Vestibular

Background

In dogs affected by ischaemic stroke, one of the most common sites of infarction relate to the cerebellum. The blood supply to the cerebellum is ensured by two paired arteries; the rostral cerebellar artery (RCeA), usually originating from the caudal communicating artery (caudal part of the circle of Willis), and the caudal cerebellar artery (CCeA), originating from the basilar artery. The origin and formation of these vessels are, however, subject to large biological variation [1–3].

Ischaemic stroke is caused by a thrombotic or thromboembolic event, resulting in infarction with loss of neuro-function of the related vascular territory.

*Correspondence: blicher@sund.ku.dk
[1] Department of Veterinary Clinical and Animal Sciences, University Hospital for Companion Animals, University of Copenhagen, Dyrlægevej 16, 1870 Frederiksberg C, Denmark
Full list of author information is available at the end of the article

Neurological signs accordingly reflect infarct topography. The clinical signs are usually sudden, non-progressive, and a gradual improvement is typically seen, although further neurological deterioration may develop within minutes to hours, or rarely up to days, of the acute event due to progressive cell death and a growing brain oedema [4–6].

In dogs, ischaemic stroke is increasingly recognised as a cause of acute neurological deficits. However, the number of publications is still limited, and only a few studies between 2005 and 2014 include a reasonable number of cases (ranging from 12 to 40 dogs) [4, 7–12]. Based on the current literature, it appears that infarcts located to the cerebellum may be particularly frequent in dogs [7, 9, 10, 13–17].

The majority of the reported cases of cerebellar stroke in dogs are related to the area of the RCeA [7, 9, 10, 16, 18–20], whereas CCeA related events seem rare [10, 21].

One of the cerebellum's main functions is to modulate body movement and maintain equilibrium, the latter primarily via the flocculonodular lobe's relation to the vestibular nuclei of the brainstem [22, 23]. These functions may thus be affected with a cerebellar stroke. In humans, the collection of symptoms that occurs with cerebellar infarcts may be referred to as the cerebellar stroke syndrome, which is characterised by vertigo, ataxia, nystagmus, and headache [24–26]. As strokes in dogs and humans compare in many aspects [10], a similar stroke syndrome in dogs might be expected. The possible identification and characterisation of a cerebellar stroke syndrome in dogs might promote the clinician's suspicion of a stroke, which according to previous studies carries a fair to good prognosis, despite a severe clinical onset [4, 6]. This might reduce the risk of any premature decision-making towards euthanasia.

Although previously reported in dogs, new studies on cerebellar stroke are important, not only to confirm previous findings, but also to advance the current understanding of symptomatology and prognosis. The aim of this study was to further characterise neurological signs in relation to infarct topography in dogs with suspected cerebellar ischaemic stroke. Furthermore, short-term outcome for affected dogs was investigated.

Methods
Study design
A retrospective multicentre study was performed, including dogs examined from 2010–2015 at five veterinary referral hospitals (Davies Veterinary Specialists, Herts; Chestergates Veterinary Referral Hospital, Chester; Fitzpatrick Referrals, Surrey; Stone Lion Veterinary Hospital, London, and the University Hospital for Companion Animals, Copenhagen). Dogs with magnetic

resonance imaging (MRI) changes suggestive of a cerebellar ischaemic stroke were eligible for inclusion.

Inclusion criteria were: a full medical record including history, physical and neurological examination, complete blood count, and serum biochemistry. Results of the cerebrospinal fluid analysis were included, when available. Exclusion criteria were: progression of neurological deficits beyond 24 h, any presence of concurrent non-cerebellar strokes, and treatment with immunosuppressive doses of corticosteroids.

All neurological examinations were performed by a DipECVN, a resident working under the supervision of a DipECVN, or by a DVM with a PhD in veterinary neurology.

The study was approved by the Local Administrative and Ethics Committee, Department of Veterinary Clinical and Animal Sciences, Faculty of Health Sciences, University of Copenhagen (Permission no. 1 N/2013).

Diagnostic imaging
The following MRI equipment was used: 0.4T (Aperto Permanent Magnet, Hitachi) at Davies Veterinary Specialists ($n = 10$), 0.35T MRI (Vet-MR Grande, Esaote) at Chestergates Veterinary Referral Hospital ($n = 7$), 1.5T MRI (MAGNETOM Symphony, Siemens Healthcare) at Fitzpatrick Referrals ($n = 3$), and 0.2 T MRI (Vet-MR, Esaote) at Stone Lion Veterinary Hospital ($n = 2$) and the University Hospital for Companion Animals ($n = 1$). Dogs were placed in sternal or dorsal recumbency and scanned under general anaesthesia.

The images were obtained by using, at a minimum, transverse and sagittal T1-weighted (T1W), pre- and postcontrast, and T2-weighted (T2W) images.

Gadolinium dimeglumine (Magnevist, Schering) at a dose of 0.1 mmol/kg IV, gadoteridol (Prohance, Bracco Imaging) at a dose of 0.1 mmol/kg IV, or Gadoteric acid (Dotarem, Guerbet) at a dose of 0.1 mmol/kg IV was used as the paramagnetic contrast medium. Due to the retrospective study setup, fluid attenuated inversion recovery, gradient echo, diffusion weighted imaging or angiography sequences were not available in all cases.

MRI changes were considered compatible with cerebellar ischaemic stroke if a well-defined lesion was seen within the vascular territory of either of the paired RCeA or CCeA and characterised by iso- or hypointense changes in T1W sequences, and hyperintensity in T2W sequences, and with no or little contrast enhancement and no or minimal mass effect.

A DipECVDI or DipACVR and a DipECVN evaluated the MRI scans. The first (BT) and last author (HG) performed the topographical classification. Both were blinded to the specific neurological signs of the dogs.

Infarct topography

Topography of infarcts was classified according to the distribution area of either the RCeA or the CCeA. Lesions were localized to the right, to the left, or to the midline. Occlusions were defined as 'extensive' when the entire supply area of either the RCeA or CCeA was affected, and 'limited' when the affected area represented either a smaller cortical part of the supply area of the RCeA, i.e. the limited area of their arterial branches, or a perforating artery, i.e. lacunar infarcts located in the deep structures of the cerebellum. This classification was based on a subjective evaluation of the infarction visualized on MRI. Further classification of the infarcts into specific distal branches could not be determined due to inconsistency between selected MRI planes and sequences, given the retrospective nature of the data.

Short-term outcome

Short-term outcome was confined to the hospitalisation period and classified as 'good' if dogs with suspected cerebellar ischaemic stroke improved to a stage where they could successfully be discharged and as 'poor' if they either died or were euthanized during the hospitalisation period. Duration of the hospitalisation time was registered according to extensive vs. limited occlusions.

Statistical analysis

The statistics of the present study were mainly descriptive. For the comparison of mean ages between groups a t test was performed on normally distributed data using GraphPad Prism 6 (GraphPad Software, Inc. 7825 Fay Avenue, Suite 230 La Jolla, CA 92037 USA). Results are stated with ±standard error of the mean. P values ≤ 0.05 were considered statistically significant.

Results

Twenty-three dogs were included in the study (ten from Davies Veterinary Specialists, seven from Chestergates Veterinary Referral Hospital, three from Fitzpatrick Referrals, two from Stone Lion Veterinary Hospital, and one from the Copenhagen University Hospital for Companion Animals). All dogs were referral cases, and the study group encompassed thirteen females (11 neutered) and 10 males (five neutered) with a median age of 8 years and 8 months (range 3–12 years). Breeds comprised the Cavalier King Charles Spaniel ($n = 9$), Greyhound ($n = 2$), Labrador Retriever ($n = 2$), Basset Hound, Cairn Terrier, English Cocker Spaniel, German Shepherd, Lurcher, Pointer, Shih Tzu, Tibetan Terrier, Weimaraner, and one medium-sized mixed-breed ($n = 1$). The Cavalier King Charles Spaniel was significantly younger at stroke onset (mean age 7 years ± 9 months) compared

to non-Cavalier King Charles Spaniels (mean age 9 years and 1 month ± 6 months) ($P = 0.03$).

Physical examination was normal in 19 dogs. Twelve dogs had concurrent medical conditions including heart disease ($n = 2$), hyperadrenocorticism ($n = 2$), renal disease ($n = 2$), hypertension ($n = 1$), liver disease ($n = 1$), macrothrombocytopenia ($n = 1$), polyarthritis ($n = 1$), protein-losing enteropathy ($n = 1$), and syringomyelia ($n = 1$).

The most prominent neurological deficits were ataxia with and without hypermetria, head tilt, nystagmus, decreased menace response and postural reaction deficits. The distribution of neurological signs in relation to infarct topography is described in Table 1.

Five dogs had a history of a previous episode (between 2 weeks and 3 years prior to stroke event) of sudden neurological deficits resolving within 24 h suggestive of a possible transient ischaemic attack (TIA) [27].

The median time from onset of clinical signs to MR exam was 1 day. In all dogs, a single cerebellar infarct was identified. All infarcts were located to the rostral and tentorial part of the cerebellum in the territory of the RCeA (right $n = 10$, left $n = 11$, midline $n = 2$), with 19/23 infarcts being territorial and wedge-shaped and 4/23 infarcts being lacunar with a suspected occlusion of a deep penetrating artery from the RCeA resulting in ovoid lesions of the central part of the cerebellum. No significant mass effect or contrast enhancement was seen with any of the lesions (Figs. 1, 2). In addition to conventional MRI, gradient echo imaging, diffusion weighted imaging, and magnetic resonance angiography were performed in 13, 3, and 1 dog, respectively. The lesion appeared hyperintense on gradient echo and diffusion weighted images, and angiography revealed no signs of occlusive disease or vascular malformations. CSF analysis was performed in 10 dogs with unremarkable findings.

All included dogs survived and were discharged within 1–10 days of hospitalisation (median = 1 day). In dogs ($n = 4$) with an extensive occlusion of the RCeA (Fig. 3) the median hospitalisation time was 6.5 days, and in dogs ($n = 20$) with a limited occlusion of the RCeA or a lacunar infarction (Fig. 4) median hospitalisation time was 1 day.

Discussion

The present study describes a cohort of dogs with cerebellar ischaemic stroke, resulting from the thrombotic occlusion of the RCeA or its branches. The clinical presentation was characterised by a peracute to acute onset of non-progressing neurological deficits with an excellent short-term prognosis.

In accordance with previous studies, the most common sign in affected dogs was ataxia [10, 14, 16]. In humans,

Table 1 Neurological signs in relation extensive vs. limited occlusion of the rostral cerebellar artery in 23 dogs with cerebellar ischaemic stroke

Neurological signs	Extensive RCeA occlusion	Limited RCeA occlusion
Mentation ($n = 3$)		
Obtunded ($n = 2$)		2
Depressed ($n = 1$)		1
Posture and body position		
Head tilt ($n = 13$)		
Contralateral ($n = 12$)	3	9
Unclassified ($n = 1$)		1
Tremors ($n = 3$)		
Intention tremors of head ($n = 2$)	1	1
Unclassified ($n = 1$)		1
Increased tone of limbs ($n = 2$)		
Ipsilateral ($n = 1$)		1
Thoracic limbs ($n = 1$)		1
Decerebellate posture ($n = 1$)		1
Opisthotonus ($n = 1$)		1
Torticollis, contralateral ($n = 1$)		1
Gait abnormalities		
Ataxia ($n = 21$)		
Ataxia with hypermetria ($n = 11$)	1	10
Ataxia without hypermetria ($n = 4$)	1	3
Non-ambulatory ($n = 6$)	2	4
Paresis ($n = 1$)		
Non-ambulatory tetraparesis ($n = 1$)		1
Cranial nerve deficits		
Decreased menace response ($n = 7$)		
Ipsilateral ($n = 5$)		5
Bilateral ($n = 2$)	1	1
Anisocoria ($n = 3$)		
Contralateral mydriasis ($n = 2$)	1	1
Miosis ($n = 1$)		1
Nystagmus, positional ($n = 8$)		
Vertical ($n = 4$)	1	3
Horizontal ($n = 2$)	1	1
Rotatory ($n = 2$)	1	1
Strabismus ($n = 3$)		
Positional ($n = 2$)		2
Spontaneous ($n = 1$)	1	
Postural reaction deficits other than proprioceptive deficits ($n = 7$)		
Ipsilateral ($n = 5$)		5
Bilateral ($n = 1$)		1
Unclassified ($n = 1$)		1
Proprioceptive deficits ($n = 5$)		
Ipsilateral ($n = 2$)		2
Contralateral ($n = 1$)		1
Pelvic limbs ($n = 1$)		1
Unclassified ($n = 1$)		1

Table 1 continued

Neurological signs	Extensive RCeA occlusion	Limited RCeA occlusion
Other signs		
Signs of nausea ($n = 4$)		
Vomiting ($n = 2$)	1	1
Salivating ($n = 2$)		2

RCeA rostral cerebellar artery. Occlusions were classified as extensive when affecting the entire vascular territory of the rostral cerebellar artery (RCeA) and as limited when affecting a smaller cortical part of the vascular territory of either the RCeA or a perforating artery

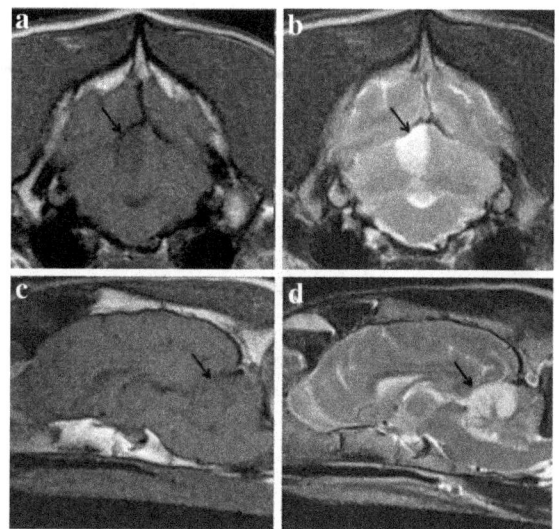

Fig. 1 Territorial infarct classified as limited. Brain magnetic resonance imaging (MRI) from a 10-year-old female neutered Lurcher with an acute right-sided rostral cerebellar artery territorial infarct. *Arrows* indicate the cerebellar region affected by the ischaemic stroke. **a** Transverse plane T_1-weighted (T1W) at the level of the rostral cerebellum, **b** transverse plane T_2-weighted (T2W) at the level of the rostral cerebellum, **c** mid sagittal plane T1W, **d** mid sagittal plane T2W Images obtained by a 1.5T MRI unit (MAGNETOM Symphony, Siemens Healthcare)

the superior cerebellar artery (SCA) corresponds to the RCeA in dogs. The frequent finding of ataxia is in accordance with human studies of infarction of the area supplied by the SCA [28–30]. In the present study, ataxia was commonly accompanied by hypermetria, a sign attributed to uninhibited flexor muscle contraction, which is pathognomonic for a cerebellar or spinocerebellar tract damage [22, 23].

The second most common sign in the dogs was head tilt, a sign that has previously been associated with rostral cerebellar ischaemic stroke [7, 10, 14–16, 18]. In the majority of cases the head tilt was opposite to the lesion representing a so-called paradoxical vestibular syndrome

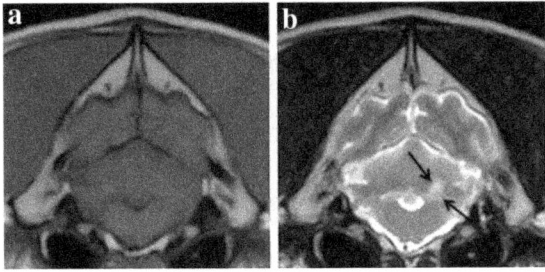

Fig. 2 Lacunar infarct classified as limited. Brain magnetic resonance imaging (MRI) of an 8-year-old female neutered labrador retriever obtained within 48 h after onset of neurological deficits. *Arrows* indicate the cerebellar region affected by the ischaemic stroke. **a** Transverse plane T_1-weighted at the level of the rostral cerebellum, **b** transverse plane T_2-weighted at the level of the rostral cerebellum Images obtained by a 0.4T MRI unit (Aperto Permanent Magnet, Hitachi)

that can be seen with lesions involving the caudal cerebellar peduncle or flocculonodular lobe responsible for the vestibular component of the cerebellum. Damage to these structures and to the fastigial nucleus was presumably also responsible for the nystagmus seen [22, 23]. As the RCeA does not supply these structures [1], this finding is unexpected. Nystagmus has previously been documented to be a frequent sign in dogs affected by rostral cerebellar infarcts [7, 10, 14, 18]. In a study of 293 human

patients with cerebellar infarction, nystagmus was also a common finding irrespective of the vascular territory affected [30], and a recent study further supports the finding that infarcts in the territory of the SCA can cause vestibular signs such as nystagmus [31]. In the present study, the vestibular dysfunction was further reflected by the observed strabismus [32], which has previously been reported in both dogs [14, 18] and humans with cerebellar infarction [33].

Regarding the finding of proprioceptive deficits and paresis in some of the dogs, the most likely aetiology is compression of the brainstem secondary to cerebellar oedema formation [7, 26, 34, 35], but as the SCA has collateral branches to the pons and medulla oblongata [36], it is also possible that the observed proprioceptive deficits and paresis were caused by an infarct in one of these areas that was not visible on MRI, as previously suggested [7]. Paresis has been reported in several other studies of dogs with rostral cerebellar ischaemic stroke [7, 14, 16], and in addition a few studies have described the finding of proprioceptive deficits [14, 18]. Likewise, cerebellar damage as a cause of active proprioceptive deficits in humans was recently documented [37].

One dog in the study appeared depressed, which could possibly be a sign of discomfort or pain and a few dogs of the present study appeared obtunded, which may be due to brain stem compression secondary to cerebellar

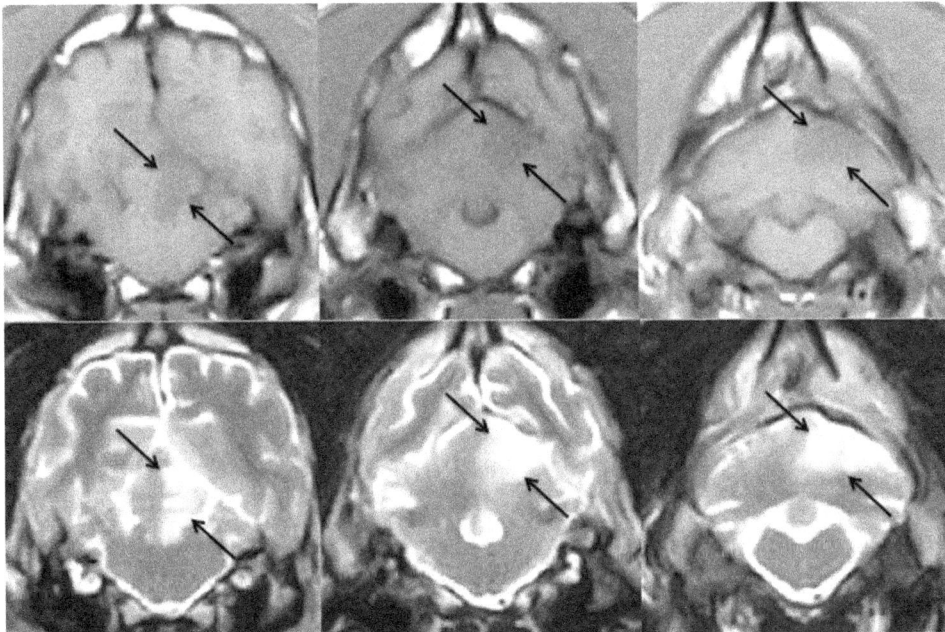

Fig. 3 Territorial infarct classified as extensive. Sequential brain magnetic resonance imaging (MRI) from a 9-year-old female neutered English cocker spaniel with an acute right-sided rostral cerebellar artery territorial infarct. Direction of images: rostral to caudal. *First row*: transverse plane T1-weighted images. *Second row*: transverse plane T2-weighted images. *Arrows* indicate the cerebellar region affected by the ischaemic stroke Images obtained by a 0.4 T MRI unit (Aperto Permanent Magnet, Hitachi)

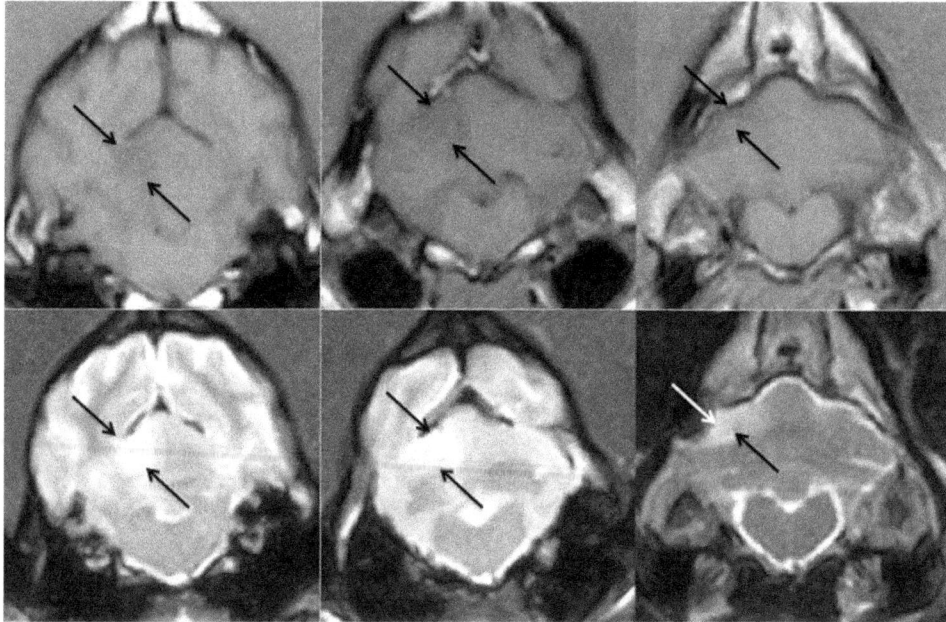

Fig. 4 Territorial infarct classified as limited. Sequential brain magnetic resonance imaging (MRI) from an 11-year-old female neutered mixed-breed with an acute left-sided rostral cerebellar artery territorial infarct. Direction of images: rostral to caudal. *First row*: transverse plane T1-weighted images. *Second row*: transverse plane T2-weighted images. *Arrows* indicate the cerebellar region affected by the ischaemic stroke Images obtained by a 0.4T MRI unit (Aperto Permanent Magnet, Hitachi)

oedema. A few veterinary studies have described dogs affected by rostral cerebellar infarction as being either restless, dull, depressed, or disoriented [10, 14, 18]. Symptoms in humans with SCA infarction such as vertigo, headache and dysarthria [24, 29, 38] may not be identified in dogs. In human patients, the finding of a decreased level of consciousness has been correlated with a worse outcome possibly due to hydrocephalus and brainstem compression [30, 39, 40]. In recent years, research has demonstrated a possible cerebellar impact on cognition [41].

Finally, one dog presented with contralateral torticollis, a sign that is usually considered a consequence of brainstem involvement. Ipsilateral torticollis has previously been reported in one dog with rostral cerebellar infarction [18]. The cause of the observed sign is not known, but recently neuropathological changes specific to the cerebellum were demonstrated in a human post-mortem case-series study from patients with torticollis/cervical dystonia [42]. Although speculative, it is possible that the cerebellar stroke was the direct cause of the observed torticollis.

No immediate cardinal signs justifying the term "syndrome" were identified. However, as dogs did present with a collection of both cerebellar and vestibular signs, dogs showing such neurological characteristics may have suffered a cerebellar ischaemic stroke, and this should alert the clinician of the importance of further diagnostic investigations.

The present study found no obvious association between infarct size, as visualized on MRI, and the observed neurological deficits, i.e. dogs with extensive infarction of the supply area of the RCeA did not show significantly more neurological deficits than the dogs with limited or lacunar ischaemic strokes. For example, when evaluating for some of the most frequently observed neurological signs, a high proportion of all affected dogs exhibited ataxia and/or decreased menace response regardless of whether the infarcts were classified as extensive or limited. A slightly higher proportion of dogs with extensive infarcts presented with head tilt and/or nystagmus, but this was not considered significant due to the small number of dogs in this group. Despite of this lack of association between infarct size and degree of neurological signs observed, a prolonged time of hospitalisation was needed in dogs with extensive occlusion of the RCeA, suggesting that these dogs were actually more seriously affected. This finding is supported by a human study, documenting that large, compared to small, lesions predict a poorer outcome [35], but further studies are needed to investigate this hypothesis in dogs.

A limitation to this study was the low proportion of dogs with extensive infarcts, and it remains unknown whether a higher number of dogs could demonstrate an association between infarct topography and neurological signs. The human cerebellar stroke syndrome may under certain circumstances be further subclassified into three distinct syndromes that describe the signs seen in relation to infarction of the vascular territories of the three major arteries in humans, i.e. the posterior inferior cerebellar artery, the anterior inferior cerebellar artery, and the SCA [26], yet studies have described the difficulty of clinically assessing which part of cerebellum is affected in human patients with ischaemic stroke [25, 30].

Short-term outcome for the dogs included in the present study appeared to be excellent, as all dogs survived and were discharged within 1–10 days. Being referral cases, the results may, however, be biased towards a better outcome, as more severely affected dogs could have been euthanized at the primary practices. Some human studies have reported that cerebellar ischaemic stroke provides a better prognosis than other stroke subtypes [35, 40, 43]. However, disability and death due to complicating oedema formation, subsequent obstructive hydrocephalus and concomitant infarction of the brainstem are known risks in humans [34, 35], and the latter has also been reported in dogs [7]. In one human study of 30 patients suffering from cerebellar infarction, a case fatality rate of 23 % was reported [28], but the relationship between the specific affected cerebellar artery and associated prognosis in humans remains uncertain. Some studies have described superior vs. inferior infarction to be associated with a poorer outcome [30, 40], while another study of 66 human patients with infarction of the SCA vs. infarction of the inferior cerebellar artery territory found that a severe mass effect was only detected in 7 vs. 30 % of the cases [29]. As the RCeA in dogs corresponds to the SCA in humans, this may explain the observed excellent short-term outcome in the dogs of the present study. Importantly, the topographical location of the cerebellum in dogs is different from humans, where the cerebellum is ventral to the cerebrum, and where the human pons has an enlarged conformation [44] in comparison to dogs, which could explain the lack of oedema formation and consequently a better short-term prognosis for dogs with suspected cerebellar ischaemic stroke.

The reason for the high prevalence of rostral cerebellar ischaemic stroke in dogs remains unknown. It is possible that the vascular anatomy of the cerebellum plays an important role where the RCeA usually originates from the caudal communicating artery, thus receiving blood from the carotid arteries, although, in some dogs it originates from the basilar artery [2, 3]. This may predispose dogs to cardiogenic embolism [4]. Furthermore, it has been speculated if the Chiari-like malformation, which is often found in Cavalier King Charles Spaniels,

may cause flow disturbances and predispose affected dogs to rostral cerebellar infarction [4, 8]. The canine cerebellar vascularization contrasts with the cerebellar vascularization of humans, where the SCA originates from the vertebrobasilar system [26], even though the cerebellar vasculature can also be an object of individual variation [45]. Interestingly, a recent study of human patients undergoing carotid artery stenting documented that emboli originating from the carotid arteries in a smaller percentage of the patients did actually reach the posterior circulation causing cerebellar infarcts in the territory of the SCA [46].

All dogs in this report had a cerebellar infarction in the vascular area of the RCeA. This was not surprising, as infarcts of the CCeA territory in dogs seem rare. So far, very few dogs with suspected caudal cerebellar infarction have been described. Neurological signs such as depression, head tilt, generalized ataxia, and unilateral postural reaction deficits were reported, as was also the case in the present study. Dogs with CCeA infarction additionally experienced disorientation, rolling episodes, and hyperextended forelimbs [10, 21]. It is likely that there is an anatomical explanation for the low prevalence of caudal cerebellar infarction, as the CCeA originates from the vertebrobasilar system unlike the RCeA that originates from the circle of Willis [1–3]. Another explanation could be that caudal cerebellar ischaemic stroke in dogs may cause either very mild neurological signs that may go by unnoticed, or they may on the contrary cause very serious neurological deficits resulting in euthanasia, in either case preventing the dogs from being referred for further evaluation.

Similar to the findings from previous studies on canine ischaemic stroke [7, 8], 22 % of the dogs investigated in the present study had previously had short neurological episodes prior to the stroke event suggesting a possible TIA. A TIA is characterised by a short episode of neurological dysfunction, commonly lasting less than 60 min, which is caused by transient focal brain ischaemia, with no evidence of subsequent infarction when investigated by MRI [27]. In a study of 2416 human patients with ischaemic stroke, 23 % of the patients had suffered previous TIA [47]. The findings of the present study thus support the hypothesis that dogs can have episodes of TIA and that such episodes may precede a true stroke.

The present study was subject to certain limitations, e.g. a small population and short follow up. As all dogs recovered from the neurological incidence, results from histopathological evaluations were not available. Unfortunately, MRI does not provide a final diagnosis and previous studies have demonstrated the difficulties of differentiating ischaemic stroke from inflammatory diseases and neoplasia [12, 48]. Finally, given the retrospective data collection, MRI examinations of the included dogs did not follow a standardized MRI protocol, which impeded a detailed description of infarct topography including affection of specific arterial branches of the RCeA and the occurrence of haemorrhagic transformation and due to the relatively low number of cases, statistical analyses were not performed.

Conclusions

Rostral cerebellar ischaemic stroke should be included in the list of possible differential diagnoses in dogs presenting with peracute to acute onset of neurological signs predominated by ataxia and vestibular signs, including contralateral head tilt and nystagmus. Supplementary findings may include mental changes, paresis, proprioceptive deficits, and torticollis, of which paresis and proprioceptive deficits are the most common. The short-term prognosis is excellent, and this encouraging information should be used by clinicians when guiding owners of affected dogs..

Abbreviations
CCeA: caudal cerebellar artery; MRI: magnetic resonance imaging; RCeA: rostral cerebellar artery; SCA: superior cerebellar artery; T1W: T1-weighted; T2W: T2-weighted; TIA: transient ischaemic attack.

Authors' contributions
BT conceived of the study and study design, participated in the coordination of the study, contributed to the acquisition and interpretation of data and drafted the manuscript. LG, GS, CR and TS contributed to the study design and to the acquisition and interpretation of data. MB contributed to study design and the interpretation of data and helped drafting the manuscript. HG conceived of the study and study design, participated in the coordination of the study, contributed to the acquisition and interpretation of data and helped drafting the manuscript. All authors helped editing the final manuscript. All authors read and approved the final manuscript.

Author details
[1] Department of Veterinary Clinical and Animal Sciences, University Hospital for Companion Animals, University of Copenhagen, Dyrlægevej 16, 1870 Frederiksberg C, Denmark. [2] Davies Veterinary Specialists, Manor Farm Business Park, Higham Gobion, Hitchin, England SG5 3HR, UK. [3] Chestergates Veterinary Referral Hospital, Units E & F, Telford Court, Chestergates Road, Chester, Cheshire, England CH1 6LT, UK. [4] Present Address: Fitzpatrick Referrals, Halfway Lane, Eashing, Godalming, Surrey, England GU7 2QQ, UK. [5] Present Address: School of Veterinary Medicine, Faculty of Health and Medical Sciences, University of Surrey, Guildford, Surrey, England GU2 7TE, UK. [6] Stone Lion Veterinary Hospital, 41 High Street, Wimbledon, London SW19 5AU, UK.

Acknowledgements
The study was supported by the Danish Council for Independent Research (Grant number 11-106689/FTP). The authors wish to thank Diplomates of the European College of Veterinary Neurology, Francois-Xavier Liebel, Mark Lowrie, Peter Smith, Ulrike Michal Altay, Luca Motta; Diplomate of the European College of Veterinary Diagnostic Imaging, Virginie De Busscher; resident of the European College of Veterinary Neurology, Anna Tauro; Registered Veterinary Nurse, Sandy Griffith, Mrs. Amanda Luff; and PGDip, BSc, Jelena Jovanovik, for kindly contributing to the collection of material for the present study. Preliminary results were presented as a poster at the 27th Annual Symposium of the ESVN-ECVN, Madrid, 18–20 September 2014.

Competing interests
The authors declare that they have no competing interests.

References
1. Anderson WD, Kubicek W. The vertebral-basilar system of dog in relation to man and other mammals. Am J Anat. 1971;132:179–88.
2. Gillilan LA. Extra- and intra-cranial blood supply to brains of dog and cat. Am J Anat. 1976;146:237–53.
3. DeVos NR, Simeons PJ. Angiologia—arteria. In: Schaller O, editor. Illustrated veterinary anatomical nomenclature. 2nd ed. Stuttgart: Enke Verlag; 2007. p. 272.
4. Garosi L, McConnell JE, Platt SR, Barone G, Baron JC, de Lahunta A, et al. Results of diagnostic investigations and long-term outcome of 33 dogs with brain infarction (2000–2004). J Vet Intern Med. 2005;19:725–31.
5. Hossmann KA. Pathophysiology and therapy of experimental stroke. Cell Mol Neurobiol. 2006;26:1057–83.
6. Gredal H, Toft N, Westrup U, Motta L, Gideon P, Arlien-Soborg P, et al. Survival and clinical outcome of dogs with ischaemic stroke. Vet J. 2013;196:408–13.
7. Garosi L, McConnell JF, Platt SR, Barone G, Baron JC, de Lahunta A, et al. Clinical and topographic magnetic resonance characteristics of suspected brain infarction in 40 dogs. J Vet Intern Med. 2006;20:311–21.
8. McConnell JF, Garosi L, Platt SR. Magnetic resonance imaging findings of presumed cerebellar cerebrovascular accident in 12 dogs. Vet Radiol Ultrasound. 2005;46:1–10.
9. Kent M, Glass EN, Haley AC, March P, Rozanski EA, Galban EM, et al. Ischemic stroke in Greyhounds: 21 cases (2007–2013). J Am Vet Med Assoc. 2014;245:113–7.
10. Gredal H, Skerritt GC, Gideon P, Arlien-Soeborg P, Berendt M. Spontaneous ischaemic stroke in dogs: clinical topographic similarities to humans. Acta Neurol Scand. 2013;128:e11–6.
11. Goncalves R, Carrera I, Garosi L, Smith PM, FraserMcConnell J, Penderis J. Clinical and topographic magnetic resonance imaging characteristics of suspected thalamic infarcts in 16 dogs. Vet J. 2011;188:39–43.
12. Cervera V, Wilfried M, Vite CH, Johnson V, Dayrell-Hart B, Seiler GS. Comparative magnetic resonance imaging findings between gliomas and presumed cerebrovascular accidents in dogs. Vet Radiol Ultrasound. 2011;52:33–40.
13. Joseph RJ, Greenlee PG, Carrilo JM, Kay WJ. Canine cerebrovascular disease: clinical and pathological findings in 17 cases. J Am Anim Hosp Assoc. 1988;24:569–76.
14. Irwin JC, Dewey CW, Stefanacci JD. Suspected cerebellar infarcts in 4 dogs. J Vet Emerg Crit Care. 2007;17:268–74.
15. Cook LB, Coates JR, Dewey CW, Gordon S, Miller MW, Bahr A. Vascular encephalopathy associated with bacterial endocarditis in four dogs. J Am Anim Hosp Assoc. 2005;41:252–8.
16. Paul A, Lenard Z, Mansfield C. Computed tomography diagnosis of eight dogs with brain infarction. Aust Vet J. 2010;88:374–80.
17. Thomas WB, Sorjonen DC, Scheuler RO, Kornegay JN. Magnetic resonance imaging of brain infarction in seven dogs. Vet Radiol Ultrasound. 1996;37:345–50.
18. Berg JM, Joseph RJ. Cerebellar infarcts in two dogs diagnosed with magnetic resonance imaging. J Am Anim Hosp Assoc. 2003;39:203–7.
19. Major AC, Caine A, Rodriguez SB, Cherubini GB. Imaging diagnosis— magnetic resonance imaging findings in a dog with sequential brain infarction. Vet Radiol Ultrasound. 2012;53:576–80.
20. Bagley RS, Anderson WI, de Lahunta A, Kallfelz FA, Bowersox TS. Cerebellar infarction caused by arterial thrombosis in a dog. J Am Vet Med Assoc. 1988;192:785–7.
21. Negrin A, Gaitero L, Anor S. Presumptive caudal cerebellar artery infarct in a dog: clinical and MRI findings. J Small Anim Pract. 2009;50:615–8.
22. Holliday TA. Clinical signs of acute and chronic experimental lesions of the cerebellum. Vet Sci Commun. 1979;3:259–78.
23. de Lahunta A, Glass E. Veterinary neuroanatomy and clinical neurology. 3rd ed. Saint Louis: Saunders Elsevier; 2009. p. 348–88.
24. Warlow C, van Gijn J, Dennis M, Wardlaw JM, Bamford J, Hankey G, et al. Which arterial territory is involved? Stroke practical management. 3rd ed. Singapore: Blackwell Publishing; 2008. p. 131–80.
25. Edlow JA, Newman-Toker DE, Savitz SI. Diagnosis and initial management of cerebellar infarction. Lancet Neurol. 2008;7:951–64.
26. Lee H. Neuro-otological aspects of cerebellar stroke syndrome. J Clin Neurol. 2009;5:65–73.

27. Albers GW, Caplan LR, Easton JD, Fayad PB, Mohr JP, Saver JL, TIA Working Group, et al. Transient ischemic attack—proposal for a new definition. N Engl J Med. 2002;347:1713–6.

28. Macdonell RA, Kalnins RM, Donnan GA. Cerebellar infarction: natural history, prognosis, and pathology. Stroke. 1987;18:849–55.

29. Kase CS, Norrving B, Levine SR, Babikian VL, Chodosh EH, Wolf PA, et al. Cerebellar infarction. Clinical and anatomic observations in 66 cases. Stroke. 1993;24:76–83.

30. Tohgi H, Takahashi S, Chiba K, Hirata Y. Cerebellar infarction. Clinical and neuroimaging analysis in 293 patients. The Tohoku cerebellar infarction study group. Stroke. 1993;24:1697–701.

31. Lee H, Kim HA. Nystagmus in SCA territory cerebellar infarction: pattern and a possible mechanism. J Neurol Neurosurg Psychiatry. 2013;84:446–51.

32. de Lahunta A, Glass E. Vestibular system: special proprioception. Veterinary neuroanatomy and clinical neurology. 3rd ed. Saint Louis: Saunders Elsevier; 2009. p. 319–47.

33. Rowe F, VIS group UK. The profile of strabismus in stroke survivors. Eye. 2010;24:682–5.

34. Cano LM, Cardona P, Quesada H, Mora P, Rubio F. Cerebellar infarction: prognosis and complications of vascular territories. Neurologia. 2012;27:330–5.

35. Ng ZX, Yang WR, Seet E, Koh KM, Teo KJ, Low SW, et al. Cerebellar strokes: a clinical outcome review of 79 cases. Singapore Med J. 2015;56:145–9.

36. Nanda BS. Blood supply to the brain. In: Getty R, editor. Sisson and Grossman's the anatomy of domestic animals. Philadelphia: WB Saunders; 1975. p. 1611–7.

37. Bhanpuri NH, Okamura AM, Bastian AJ. Predictive modeling by the cerebellum improves proprioception. J Neurosci. 2013;33:14301–6.

38. Datar S, Rabinstein AA. Cerebellar infarction. Neurol Clin. 2014;32:979–91.

39. Jauss M, Krieger D, Hornig C, Schramm J, Busse O. Surgical and medical management of patients with massive cerebellar infarctions: results of the German–Austrian cerebellar infarction study. J Neurol. 1999;246:257–64.

40. Kelly PJ, Stein J, Shafqat S, Eskey C, Doherty D, Chang Y, et al. Functional recovery after rehabilitation for cerebellar stroke. Stroke. 2001;32:530–4.

41. Buckner RL. The cerebellum and cognitive function: 25 years of insight from anatomy and neuroimaging. Neuron. 2013;80:807–15.

42. Prudente CN, Pardo CA, Xiao J, Hanfelt J, Hess EJ, Ledoux MS, et al. Neuropathology of cervical dystonia. Exp Neurol. 2013;241:95–104.

43. Ng YS, Stein J, Ning M, Black-Schaffer RM. Comparison of clinical characteristics and functional outcomes of ischemic stroke in different vascular territories. Stroke. 2007;38:2309–14.

44. Felten DL, Shetty AN. Section II: regional neuroscience brain stem and cerebellum. Netter's atlas of neuroscience. 2nd ed. Canada: Saunders Elsevier; 2010. p. 257.

45. Marinkovic S, Kovacevic M, Gibo H, Milisavljevic M, Bumbasirevic L. The anatomical basis for the cerebellar infarcts. Surg Neurol. 1995;44:450–61.

46. Zhu L, Wintermark M, Saloner D, Fandel M, Pan XM, Rapp JH. The distribution and size of ischemic lesions after carotid artery angioplasty and stenting: evidence for microembolization to terminal arteries. J Vasc Surg. 2011;53:971–6.

47. Rothwell PM, Warlow CP. Timing of TIAs preceding stroke: time window for prevention is very short. Neurology. 2005;64:817–20.

48. Young BD, Fosgate GT, Holmes SP, Wolff CA, Chen-Allen AV, Kent M, et al. Evaluation of standard magnetic resonance characteristics used to differentiate neoplastic, inflammatory, and vascular brain lesions in dogs. Vet Radiol Ultrasound. 2014;55:399–406.

14

Testicular length as an indicator of the onset of sperm production in alpacas under Swedish conditions

Maria Celina Abraham[1], Johanna Puhakka[1], Alejandro Ruete[2], Essraa Mohsen Al-Essawe[1], Kerstin de Verdier[3], Jane Margaret Morrell[1*] and Renée Båge[1]

Abstract

Background: The popularity of alpacas (*Vicugna pacos*) is increasing in Sweden as well as in other countries; however, knowledge about optimal management practices under Swedish conditions is still limited. The wide age range reported when the onset of puberty can occur, between 1 and 3 years of age, makes management decisions difficult and may be influenced by the conditions under which the alpacas are kept. The aim of this study was to find out when Swedish alpacas can be expected to start producing sperm, by using testicular length and body condition score as a more precise indirect indicator than age.

Results: This study suggests that animals with a testicular length ≥3.8 cm would be producing sperm; however, if it is crucial to know that there is no sperm production for management purposes, the threshold level for testicular length used to differentiate between sperm-producing and non-sperm producing animals should be ≤1.6 cm instead. If only one variable is considered, testicular length appears to better than age alone to predict sperm production. Body condition score together with testicular length explains the individual onset of puberty and better guide management recommendations.

Conclusions: Using a combination of these parameters (testicular length, body condition score and age) as a tool for decision making for alpaca husbandry under Swedish conditions is suggested.

Keywords: *Vicugna pacos*, Puberty, Animal husbandry, Statistical models, Decision making tools

Background

Alpacas, llamas, guanacos and vicunas are South American camelids and members of the Camelidae family. Alpacas and llamas are domesticated, being kept as production animals (for fibre and meat production, as pack animals, etc.) as well as companion animals. In recent years, the international interest in breeding alpacas has increased together with the demand for more accurate information about their health care and animal husbandry. In Sweden, alpacas have become progressively more popular during the last decade; however, knowledge about optimal management practices and disease

panorama under Swedish conditions is still limited [1, 2]. Alpacas present several physiological peculiarities compared with other domestic species. They are not considered to have a breeding season [3]. Like other camelids they are induced ovulators, with continuous waves of follicular growth throughout the year [4]. However the female may reject the male's attempts to mate depending on the stage of follicular growth [3]. There are no reports of males showing seasonality in their willingness to mate.

It is known that nutritional status could influence the onset of puberty in other species [5] but according to Van Saun [6] studies on nutrition in alpacas and its relationship with reproduction are still lacking. Galloway [7] reported that there is a correlation between body size and testicular size, although the wide variation in testicular size suggests that other factors, probably genetic, are

*Correspondence: jane.morrell@slu.se
[1] Division of Reproduction, Department of Clinical Sciences, Swedish University of Agricultural Sciences, Box 7054, 75007 Uppsala, Sweden
Full list of author information is available at the end of the article

also important. Previous studies have shown that testicular size could be an indicator of sperm production and hence fertility, which is consistent with observations on the bull, ram and stallion [7, 8].

In addition to their physiology, they also have an anatomical difference. The prepuce has adherence to the glans penis until 2 or 3 years of age, making protrusion of the penis impossible in young males [9, 10]. The adherence disappears gradually when the animal matures, apparently in relation to testosterone levels [9, 11].

The detection of sperm production in males is an important factor in managing alpacas for several reasons, among them: (1) owners need to know when young males and females should be separated to avoid undesirable matings, (2) to use good males strategically in breeding programs, (3) to recommend when males should be castrated if they are not going to be used for breeding, (4) for research purposes, to know when it is the best moment to collect samples in order to access useful material, and (5) in a broader perspective, as an indicator of animal welfare.

Research in other countries indicates that male alpacas start producing sperm between 1 and 3 years of age [7, 9]. This wide range is probably influenced by the conditions under which alpacas are kept, and makes management decisions difficult. It is not known if the information generated in other countries, such as Perú, Australia and USA is applicable to Europe. Therefore, the aim of this study was to investigate with higher precision when Swedish alpacas can be expected to start producing sperm, by using the testicular length as an indirect indicator of the onset of sperm production. Two experiments were performed: Experiment 1 (on farm) to measure testicular size and Experiment 2 to determine the presence of sperm post castration or in cadavers. Whether this age could be affected by the body condition of the animal was also investigated.

Methods

Experiment 1
A total of 72 male alpacas, 13–48 months of age (median of 25.5 months), from 11 Swedish farms, were studied during September 2014. Farms were selected for convenience based on geographical distribution and number of animals. The length of the testicles was measured individually with a calliper (Biltema, Sweden) (Fig. 1).

Body condition was scored according to a standardized scale from 1–5, where 1 is emaciated and 5 is obese [12, 13].

Body condition scoring (BCS) was done by palpating over the central backbone near the last ribs. All of the testicle measurements and BCS were performed by the same operator.

Experiment 2
Testicles from routine castrations
Twenty-two pairs of testicles were obtained from on-farm routine castrations of male alpacas on eight Swedish farms. The age of the animals ranged between 11 and 113 months (1–9 years) with a median age of 23 months. The study was conducted from May 2013 to April 2015.

The pairs of testicles were placed in plastic bags with phosphate-buffered saline solution (KV-laboratory, SLU) and were transported to the laboratory in styrofoam boxes containing a cold pack at 4 °C, where they arrived within 24–48 h of surgery.

Testicles from cadavers
Six pairs of testicles were obtained at necropsy from male alpacas originating from five Swedish farms. The age of the animals ranged between 16 and 96 months (1–8 years, median age of 42 months). The post mortem evaluations were conducted at Eurofins in Skara (Sweden) during October 2014–February 2015. The pairs of testicles were placed in plastic bags and were transported to the laboratory, where they arrived within a week of death. None of these animals died because of reproductive diseases.

Procedure: measurement of testicles
After measuring the length of the testicles with a ruler, the tunica albuginea, connective tissues and blood vessels were removed and the epididymides were separated from the testes. The cauda epididymides were isolated, cut into 4–5 pieces and placed in a petri dish, in 1 ml of pre-warmed semen extender AndroMed (Minitüb, Tiefenbach, Germany) or INRA 96 (IMV Technologies, L'Aigle, France) for samples from castrations and in 1 ml of PBS for samples from necropsies. After 10 min of incubation at 37 °C in 5 % CO_2 in an incubator, the presence of spermatozoa was verified using a phase contrast microscope Olympus BX 51 (Olympus, Japan) with 20 and 40× objectives.

Statistical analysis
Testicle size
The relationship between mean testicle length and the individual's age was analysed. We assumed that the mean testicle length follows a normal distribution [$L_i \sim$ Normal (μ_i, σ)] for each individual i and increases over time given by:

$$\mu_i = \frac{\alpha}{1 + e^{-\beta \cdot (Age_i - \gamma)}}$$

where α is the maximum mean testicular length, β and γ are free parameters determining the testicle length increment rate. The parameters where estimated under the

Bayesian framework in JAGS 3.4 [14], because of its flexibility to estimate parameters uncertainty.

For samples obtained from experiment 1, we also tested the effect of body condition (BCS_i) on the mean testicle length increment rate parameters (β, γ) as,

$$\mu_i = \frac{\alpha}{1 + e^{-\beta \cdot (Age_i - \gamma) \cdot BCS_i \cdot \delta}}$$

using the mode of the posterior probability distribution of estimates for parameters β and letting the algorithms estimate α, γ and δ.

The models were evaluated for fit (using the deviance information criteria scores i.e. DIC, Bayesian analogues to the more common Akaike Information Criteria; [15]), and checking the posterior probability distribution.

Sperm presence (logistic models)

We tested for the effect of age and mean testicle length on the presence of sperm in testicles from necropsies using logistic generalized linear models using the glm (family = "Binomial") function on R v3.2 [16]. Model fit was evaluated through each model's R^2, comparing the model's fit through AIC [17] and checking the statistical significance of the estimated parameter.

Results

The distribution of mean testicular length by age groups in Experiment 1 is presented in Table 1. The distribution of mean testicular length by age groups and the presence of sperm in the testicles from castrations and cadavers (Experiment 2) are presented in Table 2.

The testicle length increment model explained the variability in testicular length through time (Table 3). Estimates of increment rate parameters (β and γ) were similar between the experiments and the difference in maximum mean testicle length (α) is coherent with the expected difference in testicle length due to the collection methodology (Fig. 2). There was, however, large variation in maximum mean testicular length in samples from experiment 1 at greater ages, given the lack of data points in animals older than 50 months. The variability in samples from experiment 2 was generally higher than for experiment 1 but consistent throughout the age range (Fig. 2).

The BCS of the animals ranged between 2.5 and 5 with a median value of 4. A large variation between different ages was found. The length increment rate of testicles from experiment 1 was positively affected by BCS, while the maximum mean testicle length remained within the same range (Fig. 3).

There is high variability in mean testicle size 10 and 35 months (Figs. 2, 3). Indeed, the probability of sperm presence is better explained by mean testicular length

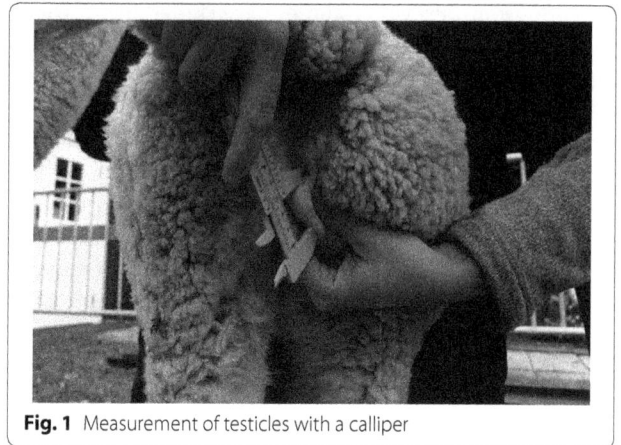

Fig. 1 Measurement of testicles with a calliper

($p = 0.01$; $R^2 = 0.77$; AIC = 14.97; Fig. 4a) than by the animals' age ($p = 0.047$; $R^2 = 0.38$, AIC = 27.87; Fig. 4b).

Discussion

The wide range when the onset of puberty can occur, between 1 and 3 years of age, makes management decisions difficult and may be influenced by the conditions under which the alpacas are kept. The aim of this study was to find out if the same range could be expected in Europe (particularly in Sweden) as in other parts of the world. By using a model of testicular length that accounts for variability in age and BCS (Figs. 2 and 3), we tried to predict when alpacas can be expected to start producing sperm. As expected, we found that if only one parameter is considered, testicular length is better than age alone to estimate sperm production (Fig. 4) but that the inclusion of BCS and age together with testicular length gives better predictability than a single parameter. Therefore, we suggest using a combination of these parameters as a tool for decision making in the selection of potential male sires.

Our results showed a large variation in mean testicular length and the presence of sperm at different ages. These findings are consistent with Galloway [7]. However, the number of observations in the upper end of the range is small; it would be beneficial for our model to include data from more animals at a greater age or with larger testicles (Fig. 2) but such animals were scarce in our study because of the owners' decision when to castrate their alpacas. From our observations (Fig. 4) we would expect that animals with a testicular length ≥ 3.8 cm would be producing sperm (testicular length at which the median probability of sperm presence is ≥ 0.99); however, if it is crucial to know that there is no sperm production for management purposes, the threshold level for testicular length used to differentiate between sperm-producing and non-sperm producing animals should be ≤ 1.6 cm instead (testicular length at which the median probability of sperm presence is ≤0.01).

Measurement of the testicles

Due to the small size of the alpaca testicles, their location very close to the abdomen and the difficulties in restraining the animals, only testicular length was measured in live animals in this study. According to Galloway [7] testicular length is a good measurement of testicle size in alpacas and it is easy to assess accurately. In bulls, measurement of the scrotal circumference is used for evaluating sperm-producing ability, because this is an objective measure, regardless of the operator, and has a strong correlation to the testicle size [18]. However, scrotal circumference is difficult to measure in alpacas due to their anatomical characteristics.

In our study, all the testicle measurements and BCS assessments were done by the same person, to minimize possible methodological errors. It should be noted that the testicular length taken from castrations or cadavers did not include the scrotal layers whereas, of necessity, the measurements on living animals did include the scrotum. Despite this difference in methodology, the measurements followed the same pattern.

Puberty

Puberty is not a single point in time, but an ongoing process requiring endocrinological and behavioural components as well as anatomical and neurological development. In the literature there are different definitions of puberty, including the presence of fully developed genitalia, libido and a minimum concentration of sperm in the ejaculate. Galloway (personal communication, 2014) defines puberty in male alpacas as the moment when, for the first time, a male can mate a female and produce a pregnancy. For this to be possible, sperm production and good libido are necessary, and the penis should be completely free of adhesions. Although young males often begin to show interest in females and can display mounting behaviour around the age of one year, most of them are not able to carry out a mating at this age [19, 20]. Complete erection and intromission is only possible when the preputial attachments to the penis have totally disappeared [10]. The detachment seems to be affected positively by the level of testosterone [21]. Early detachment is a desirable genetic trait in young animals and therefore should be an important parameter in the evaluation of the breeding potential of males, together with large testis size [7, 10, 22] which is assumed to be directly related to sperm production, as in other ruminants [20]. In addition, it is important to know what testicular size should be considered as normal

Table 1 Mean testicular length and number of alpacas by age group (Experiment 1, in vivo measurements)

Mean length (cm)	12–23 months	24–35 months	36–48 months	Total
<3	8	0	0	8
3–3.9	14	8	0	22
>4	8	24	10	42
Total	30	32	10	72

Table 2 Mean testicular length, number of alpacas by age group and sperm presence (Experiment 2, testicles from castration n = 22; testicles from cadavers n = 6)

Mean length (cm)	Age[a] (months)	Sperm presence (%)	
		Castration	Cadavers
<3	12–23	1/6 (17)	0/3 (0)
	24–35	1/4 (25)	–
	>36	1/1 (100)	–
3–3.9	12–23	3/4 (75)	–
	24–35	3/3 (100)	–
	>36	–	–
>4	12–23	–	–
	24–35	–	–
	>36	4/4 (100)	3/3 (100)

[a] Age at castration/necropsy

for the identification of pathological changes, e.g., hypoplasia or degeneration.

According to Tibary [23] the age at puberty varies depending on, among other factors, genetics, nutritional status, climate, and at what time of year the individual was born. Testicular volume may change according to environmental temperature [24]. Therefore, it would be interesting to do additional measurements of testicular length and body condition score in Sweden at different seasons of the year. Although studies suggest that female alpacas may show some seasonality in their willingness to mate, at least in the Peruvian Andes [25], there have not been any reports on the effect of season on male libido, as an indirect indicator of testosterone production. Moreover, if further studies on testicular measurements are to be made, it would be desirable to include a check for the breakdown of the preputial attachments, to provide additional information on the likelihood that mating can take place.

Nutritional status/BCS

Peruvian alpacas have smaller testicles than Australian alpacas probably due to a poorer nutritional status [7]. Our results are in line with Galloway's report,

Table 3 Model fit (DIC and Delta DIC) and parameter estimates for testicle length of Swedish alpacas

Model	DIC	Delta DIC	α	β	γ	δ
Experiment 1						
Null	160.8	0	3.97 (3.8–4.14)			
Increment	117.3	43.5	4.96 (4.33–8.445)	0.078 (0.019–0.26)	5.89 (−0.87–29.77)	
Increment + BCS	116.7	0.6	4.75 (4.32–6.45)	0.078	5.4 (0.56–10.25)	0.35 (0.10–1.02)
Experiment 2						
Null	87.8	0	2.97 (2.55–3.39)			
Increment	66.9	20.9	4.43 (3.67–5.95)	0.069 (0.02–0.16)	15.47 (5.17–31.50)	

Values are (median 95 % CI in brackets). DIC scores are compared to the null model (including only an intercept parameter). For data from experiment 1, the model including body condition score (BCS) is compared to the increment model. Experiment 1, n = 72. Experiment 2, n = 28

a is the maximum mean testicular length

β and γ are free parameters determining the testicle length increment rate

δ BCS effect on increment rate

probably because alpaca husbandry in Sweden is likely to be more similar to Australian conditions than Peruvian conditions, especially in terms of nutrition and thus body weight. In this study, a significant positive effect of body condition on the testicle length increment rate was observed.

Fowler [26] indicates that overweight is probably a more common problem than emaciation in alpacas in the Western world, although a study carried out in Sweden by Björklund [2] found that emaciation can be a problem in weanling alpacas. It is worth mentioning that there are two different systems of production of South American camelids in the world: the traditional Andean herding strategies, in a pastoral economy in the dry highlands, with a high altitude grassland between 3000 and 4800 m above sea level, and the other system under very different and more favourable conditions, at a low altitude of no more than 800 m above sea level [27]. These husbandry conditions are likely to result in differing availability of nutrients and thus possibly the onset of puberty.

It is known that decreased nutrient intake delays the onset of puberty in bulls and that, conversely, a diet with high energy level produce a faster development of the testicles [28, 29]. However, there is little information regarding the effects of diet on reproductive function in male alpacas [6, 30]. It has been shown that certain parameters, including semen volume and sperm concentration

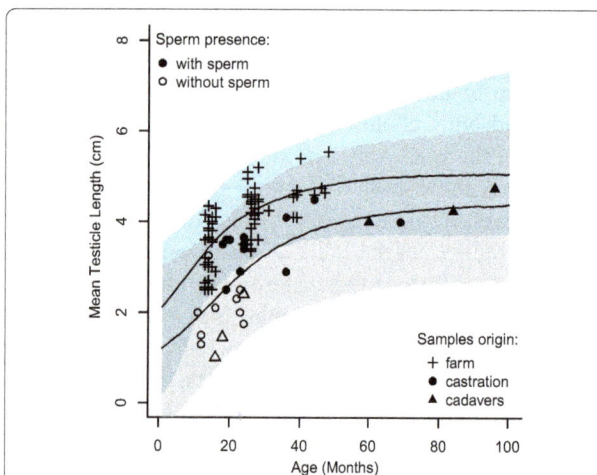

Fig. 2 Length increment model for alpaca testicle length. Experiment 1, "farm", n = 72; *solid line* (mean), and *dark grey polygon* (95 % CI); Experiment 2 (from castrations (n = 22) and cadavers (n = 6); *dashed line* (mean) and *light grey polygon* (95 % CI). Note: the measurements on living animals included the scrotal layers whereas organs obtained after castration or from cadavers did not

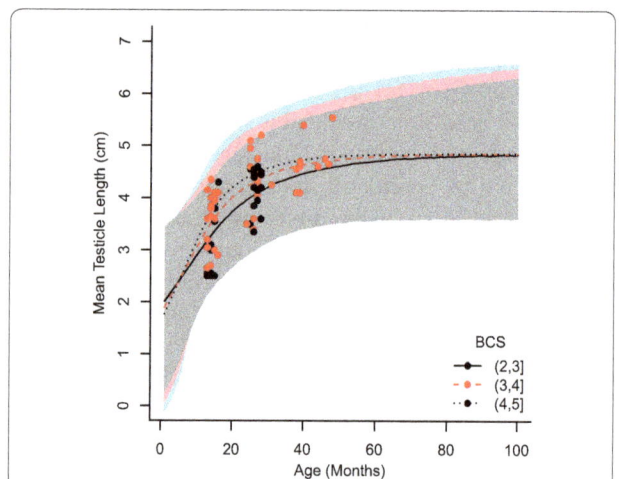

Fig. 3 Length increment model for alpaca testicle length, incorporating age and body condition score (BCS). Testicle length measured in vivo (Experiment 1; n = 72); Circles represent individual values, lines represent means. *Black line and circle* = body condition score range from 2 to 3; *red line and circle* = body condition score range from 3 to 4, *blue line and circle* = body condition score range from 4 to 5. *Shaded area* indicates 95 % confidence interval

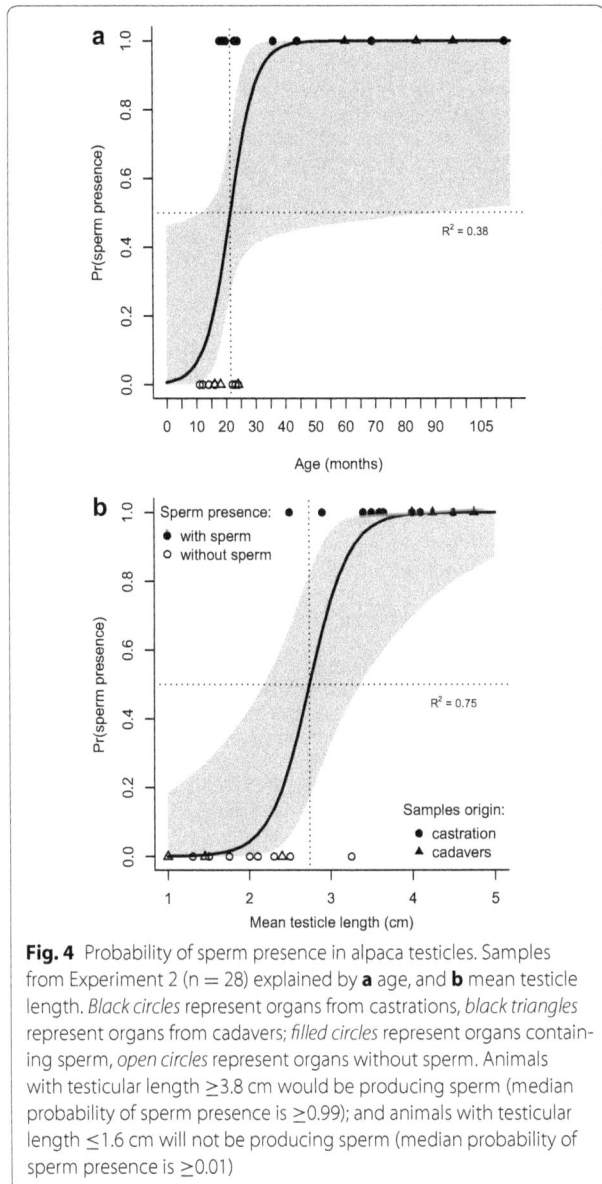

Fig. 4 Probability of sperm presence in alpaca testicles. Samples from Experiment 2 (n = 28) explained by **a** age, and **b** mean testicle length. *Black circles* represent organs from castrations, *black triangles* represent organs from cadavers; *filled circles* represent organs containing sperm, *open circles* represent organs without sperm. Animals with testicular length ≥3.8 cm would be producing sperm (median probability of sperm presence is ≥0.99); and animals with testicular length ≤1.6 cm will not be producing sperm (median probability of sperm presence is ≥0.01)

evaluation of the sexual behavior, BCS and the detachment of preputial adherences, is likely to improve male reproductive efficiency.

Our study supports the recommendations of Vaughan [31]: Breeders/owners are encouraged to measure testicular length and BCS every 6 months, from 12 to 36 months of age, to assist with selection of potential male sires.

Conclusions

If only one parameter is considered, testicular length is better than age alone to predict sperm production. However, the inclusion of BCS and age gives better predictability than a single parameter.

Our results suggests that animals with a testicular length ≥3.8 cm would be producing sperm; however, if it is crucial to know that there is no sperm production for management purposes, the threshold level for testicular length used to differentiate between sperm-producing and non-sperm producing animals should be ≤1.6 cm instead.

A combination of these parameters as a tool for decision making in the selection of potential male sires for animal husbandry under Swedish conditions is suggested.

Authors' contributions
JP, MCA, EMA and JMM were involved in data collection; MCA, JP, KV, JMM, RB participated in the design and coordination of the study and helped to draft the manuscript. AR participated in the design of the study and performed the statistical analysis. All authors read and approved the final manuscript.

Author details
[1] Division of Reproduction, Department of Clinical Sciences, Swedish University of Agricultural Sciences, Box 7054, 75007 Uppsala, Sweden. [2] Department of Ecology, Swedish University of Agricultural Sciences, Box 7044, 75007 Uppsala, Sweden. [3] National Veterinary Institute, 75189 Uppsala, Sweden.

Acknowledgements
MCA is funded by a grant awarded to Professor Jane Morrell by the Veterinary Faculty Swedish University of Agricultural Sciences; Alpaca owners and veterinarians for sending the samples and allowing us to work with their animals; Panisara Kunkitti for help in the laboratory; SVA and Eurofins for the samples from necropsies; Professor emeritus Lennart Söderquist for valuable discussions and critically reading the manuscript.

Competing interests
The authors declare that they have no competing interests.

as well as the biochemical composition of semen may vary depending on the feeding, but it is unclear if this has significance in practice [30].

Breeding management

By detecting puberty in males as early as possible, owners are able to separate females and males to avoid undesirable matings, to use elite males strategically in breeding programs, and to castrate the ones that are not intended to be used as stud males.

When selecting males for breeding, owners should select early maturing males with large testicular size [7, 31]. Selecting for large testicular size, together with an

References
1. de Verdier K, Bornstein S. Alpackor i Sverige—en ny utmaning (in Swedish). (Alpacas in Sweden– a new challenge). Svensk Veterinärtidning. Swed Vet J. 2010;1:19–23.

2. Björklund C. Diseases and causes of death among camelids in Sweden: a retrospective study of necropsy cases 2001–2013. Department of Clinical Sciences, Swedish University of Agricultural Sciences Degree project in Veterinary Medicine. 2014.

3. Vaughan J. Ovarian function in South American camelids (alpacas, llamas, vicunas, guanacos). Anim Reprod Sci. 2011;124:237–43.

4. Vaughan JL, Macmillan KL. D'Occhio MJ. Ovarian follicular wave characteristics in alpacas. Anim Reprod Sci. 2004;80:353–61.

5. Fernandez-Baca S. La alpaca: Reproducción y crianza (in Spanish). (Reproduction and breeding). Centro de Investigación Instituto Veterinario de Investigaciones Tropicales y de Altura (IVITA). Veterinary Research Center for research in tropical and high-altitude areas). Lima, Peru; 1971. 23-27.

6. Van Saun RJ. Effect of nutrition on reproduction in llamas and alpacas. Theriogenology. 2008;70:508–14.

7. Galloway DB. The Development of the testicles in alpacas in Australia. Australian Alpaca Association. Canberra; 2000. p. 21–3.

8. Thompson DL, Pickett BW, Squires EL, Amann RP. Testicular measurements and reproductive characteristics in stallions. J Reprod Fertil. 1979;27:13–7.

9. Sumar J. Studies on reproductive pathology in alpacas. Doctoral Thesis, Department of Clinical Sciences, Swedish University of Agricultural Sciences. 1983.

10. Tibary A, Pearson LK, Anouassi A. Applied andrology in camelids. In: Chenoweth PJ, Lorton SP, editors. Animal andrology: theories and applications. Wallingford: CAB International; 2014. p. 418–49.

11. Bravo PW, Johnson LW. Reproductive physiology of the male camelid. In: Chenoweth PJ, Lorton SP, editors. Applied andrology in camelids animal andrology: theories and applications. Wallingford: CAB International; 2014. p. 418–49.

12. Australian Alpaca Association. Body condition score (BCS) of Alpacas, Alpaca Fact Sheet#4. 2008. https://www.alpaca.asn.au/index.php/resources/alpaca-fact-sheets Accessed June 2015.

13. Swedish Animal Health Service (Svenska Djurhälsovården). Hullbedömning av alpackor (in Swedish). (Alpaca body condition scoring) 2010. http://www.svdhv.org/upload/documents/Artiklar/101207_kamel_hull-bedomning.pdf. Accessed June 2015.

14. Plummer M. JAGS: A program for analysis of Bayesian graphical models using Gibbs sampling. 2012. http://mcmc-jags.sourceforge.net/ Accessed June 2015.

15. Spiegelhalter DJ, Best NG, Carlin BP, van der Linde A. Bayesian measures of model complexity and fit. J R Stat Soc Series B. 2002;64:583–639.

16. R Development Core Team. R: a language and environment for statistical computing. R Foundation for Statistical Computing, Vienna, Austria. 2014.

17. Burnham KP, Anderson DR. Model selection and multimodel inference. Forts Collins: Springer; 2002.

18. Hahn J, Foote RH, Seidel GE Jr. Testicular growth and related sperm output in dairy bulls. J Anim Sci. 1969;29:41–7.

19. Fernandez-Baca S. Manipulation of reproductive functions in male and female New World camelids. Anim Reprod Sci. 1993;33:307–23.

20. Brown BW. A review on reproduction in South American Camelids. Anim Reprod Sci. 2000;58:169–95.

21. San Miguel C, Leyva V, Garcia VW. Administración de testosterona en alpacas con adherencias pene-prepuciales (in Spanish). (Administration of testosterone in alpacas with penile-preputial adhesions). Rev Inv Vet Peru. 2002;13:28–36.

22. Sumar J. Reproduction in llamas and alpacas. Anim Reprod Sci. 1996;42:405–15.

23. Tibary A, Vaughan J. Reproductive physiology and infertility in male South American camelids: a review and clinical observations. Small Ruminant Res. 2006;61:283–98.

24. Stelleta C, Vencato J, Oztutar F, Milani C, Daskin A, Romagnoli S. Seasonal variation of testicular functionality in alpaca (Vicugna pacos) raised in Italy (abstract). Proceedings of the 31st Meeting of the European Embryo Transfer Association (AETE); Belgium, 2015. A029E. http://www.cbra.org.br/portal/publicacoes/ar/2015/arjs2015.html.

25. Winblad von Walter, Amanda, 2015. Inter-species embryo transfer in South American camelids. Epsilon, SLU, Uppsala. http://stud.epsilon.slu.se/7975/.

26. Fowler ME. Medicine and Surgery of Camelids. 3rd ed. Ames: Wiley-Blackwell; 2010.

27. Miragaya MH, Chaves MG, Agüero A. Reproductive biotechnology in South American camelids. Small Ruminant Res. 2006;61:299–310.

28. Nolan CJ, Neuendorff DA, Godfrey RW, Harms PG, Welsh TH, McArthur NH, Dandel RD. Influence of energy intake on prepubertal development of Brahman bulls. J Anim Sci. 1990;68:1087–96.

29. Brito LFC, Barth AD, Wilde RE, Kastelic JP. Effect of growth rate from 6 to 16 months of age on sexual development and reproductive function in beef bulls. Theriogenology. 2012;77:1398–405.

30. Juyena NS, Vencato J, Pasini G, Vazzana I, Stelleta C. Alpaca semen quality in relation to different diets. Reprod Fertil Dev. 2013;25:683–90.

31. Vaughan J. Selection of fertile alpacas, Size really does matter! Alpaca World Magazine. 2005. Available on: http://www.alpacaseller.com/DisplayArticleList.php?PHPSESSID=lr1n6h7k0gbgbk106i8ikk3dt5. Accessed June 2015.

15

Long-term follow-up on recovery, return to use and sporting activity: a retrospective study of 236 operated colic horses in Finland (2006–2012)

Isa Anna Maria Immonen[1]*[iD], Ninja Karikoski[1], Anna Mykkänen[1], Tytti Niemelä[1], Jouni Junnila[2] and Riitta-Mari Tulamo[1]

Abstract

Background: Surgical treatment of colic is expensive and complications may occur. Information on the prognosis and the use of the horse after surgery for colic is important for surgeons and owners. Current literature on return to athletic function after celiotomy is limited. The present study reviewed surgical cases of the Veterinary Teaching Hospital, Helsinki, Finland for 2006–2012. The aim was to follow the population of horses of different breeds for surgical findings, postsurgical complications, long-term recovery and prognosis. The findings and their influence on survival, return to previous or intended use and performance were assessed.

Results: Most of the operated horses (82.6%; 195/236) recovered from anesthesia and 74.9% (146/195) were discharged. The total follow-up time was 8 years and 10 months and the median survival time 79.2 months. Age of the horse, location of the abdominal lesion (small vs. large intestine), incidence of postoperative colic, surgical site infection, incisional hernia or convalescence time after surgery, did not significantly affect the probability of performing in the previous or intended discipline after the surgery. A majority of the discharged horses (83.7%) was able to perform in the previous or intended discipline and 78.5% regained their former or higher level of performance. Operated horses had 0.18 colic episodes per horse-year during the long-term follow-up. The incidence of colic was 20.0% within the first year after surgery. Horses operated for large intestinal colic were 3.3-fold more prone to suffer postoperative colic than horses operated for small intestinal colic. The majority of the owners (96.3%) were satisfied with the veterinary care and nearly all (98.5%) evaluated the recovery after the colic surgery to be satisfactory or above.

Conclusions: If the horse survives to discharge, prognosis for long-term survival and return to previous level of sporting activity and performance was good after colic surgery in a population of horses of different breeds. None of the factors studied were found to decrease the probability of performing in the same or intended discipline after surgery. The majority of horses were able to return to their previous activity and perform satisfactorily for several years after surgery.

Keywords: Colic, Surgery, Complication, Hernia, Survival, Long-term, Return to use, Performance, Retrospective, Owner satisfaction

*Correspondence: isa.immonen@fimnet.fi
[1] Department of Equine and Small Animal Medicine, Faculty of Veterinary Medicine, University of Helsinki, 00014 Helsinki, Finland
Full list of author information is available at the end of the article

Background

It is important to assess long-term survival for horses that have been operated on for colic. Location and severity of the lesion, surgical procedures performed, age of the horse, complications and incidence of postoperative colic episodes affect the convalescence time and subsequent performance capacity of the horse. Therefore, obtaining more information and clarifying these factors is helpful to clinicians attempting to prognosticate the long-term outcome for individual horses and for their owners to take the most feasible decision.

Several studies that evaluated the recovery of horses after a colic surgery showed that 66–91% of horses were alive for at least 1 year after the celiotomy [1–8]. Comprehensive studies on long-term survival and return to use and performance are challenging as substantial numbers of the horses and information is often lost to follow-up [7]. The most common long-term complications that affect the return to use and performance are incisional hernia and postoperative colic [2–4]. Horses that developed an incisional hernia, were 7–14 times less likely to return to athletic use [6, 7]. According to previous reports postoperative colic is more common in horses with strangulating small intestinal lesions or right dorsal displacement of the colon and it occurs within 100 days after surgery [1, 9, 10]. The incidence of postoperative colic in long-term follow-up for longer than 1.7 years and the effect on performance has not been documented to our knowledge. Postoperative racing performance and use have been studied mainly in Thoroughbred horses, and 63–76% of the operated horses returned to racing [11–13]. Two recent studies have evaluated the return to previous sporting activity and also to the previous performance level in a population of horses of different breeds. In addition, the horse-owners' levels of satisfaction were assessed. According to these two reports, owners expressed that 76–86% of the horses to have regained their previous or intended uses [6, 7].

The objectives of this retrospective study were to evaluate the long-term effect of celiotomy in a heterogeneous (for sex and breed) population of horses in Finland and specifically to determine: First, the short-term and long-term survival of horses over 8 years after colic surgery. Second, evaluate the effect that the age of the horse, location of the surgical lesion (small intestine vs. large intestine), postoperative complications (surgical site infection SSI, incisional hernia, colic), has upon postoperative convalescence time and return to athletic function. Third, determine the incidence rate of colic episodes long-term after the colic surgery (small vs. large intestine lesion). Fourth, evaluate owner satisfaction regarding the outcome after colic surgery and incorporate it into this study.

The hypotheses were that a majority of horses discharged from the hospital after colic surgery would return to their intended use and regain their previous level of performance and that the owners would be satisfied with the end results. It was also hypothesised that horses with small intestinal lesions would have longer postoperative convalescence time and shorter long-term survival time compared with the horses with large intestinal lesions. Horses with small intestinal lesions were therefore hypothesised to be more prone to postoperative colic episodes than horses with large intestinal lesions. The final hypothesis was that postoperative colic episodes and incisional complications or incisional hernia would have a negative effect on the return to use and performance.

Methods

This retrospective study included 236 horses that had undergone ventral midline celiotomy in the Helsinki University Equine Teaching Hospital, Finland during the 2006 to 2012 period. Patients were followed either until their death or until the end of the study (30th November 2014).

Patient records were reviewed for patient data including: age (0–14 years/$\geq$15 years [7]); breed (Standardbred/Warmblood/Finnhorse/other horse breed/pony); gender (mare/stallion/gelding); insurance status (yes/no); location of the lesion (small intestine/large intestine); diagnosis category, surgical findings and treatment procedures (intestinal gas removal yes/no; enterotomy yes/no; resection yes/no); postoperative complications during hospitalization (SSI/incisional dehiscence defined as partial or complete rupture of one or more layers of stitches/incisional hernia/reflux/ileus/continuous pain or colic/peritonitis/laminitis); re-laparotomy (time/cause/surgical findings and treatment); death postoperatively during hospitalization and the date of the discharge were recorded. National competition records were searched for both pre- and postoperative entries in national and international show jumping, dressage, eventing and harness racing to evaluate postoperative performance (Heppa® database of the Finnish Trotting Association Hippos, Helsinki, Finland; Kipa® database of The Equestrian Federation of Finland, Valo, Finland). The short-term survival period was defined as the time from the recovery after anesthesia to the time of discharge. The long-term survival was defined as time from the discharge till the end of the study/death of the horse.

A telephone interview was held with the owners of 125 discharged horses. Ten owners preferred to answer the same questions in a questionnaire sent by e-mail, and 11 were not reached at all. The first follow-up was conducted during 2010 and the second during 2014. The following information about the horse was recorded: alive/dead; date and reason for death; general owner estimated status (poor/satisfactory/good); estimated convalescence time in months (defined as the time it took to return to athletic function after discharge); SSI (defined as purulent or serous discharge from the laparotomy incision for over a 24 h period); incisional hernia and possible repair (yes/no); estimated size of hernia (in cm); number of postoperative colic episodes (during the first/second/third/fourth/fifth postoperative year or later); re-laparotomy (date/cause/outcome); pre- and postoperative use of the horse (ridden sport horse/hobby horse/harness racing/young or in training/breeding/pasture or company horse/retired or geriatric/did not recover); recovery to the previous or intended use (yes/no); return to or start of sporting activity (yes/no); performance capacity compared with the pre-surgical level (worse/same/better); owner satisfaction, cost of treatment and the total cost (euros) of surgery. For young horses, return to use was considered if the horse achieved the preoperatively expected or intended performance capacity and discipline. Horses aged 15 years or older were defined as geriatric [7]. When the horse had more than one surgery, follow-up data were collected following the last surgery, horses with more than one surgery were included in the analysis once. SSI was defined as a long-term complication and thus it was also included in the owner interview. In all SSI cases, horses were discharged before the infection had resolved. In some patients, SSI developed after the horse had been discharged.

Data analysis

Median survival time after colic surgery was calculated and survival curves were constructed using the Kaplan–Meier method to estimate the survival function in the whole study population (236 horses). Kaplan–Meier lifetable-method with un-stratified log-rank tests combined with un-stratified Cox proportional hazard models were used to compare and investigate postsurgical long-term survival between the following groups: age group of the horse (0–14 years/$\geq$15 years), location of the lesion (small intestine/large intestine), breed (Standardbred/Warmblood/Finnhorse/other horse breed/pony) and enterotomy (yes/no) during the surgery.

The effects of pre-selected explanatory variables on owner estimated "Return to the previous/intended use", "Incidence of postoperative colic episodes", and "Death during operation (yes/no)" were analyzed with univariable logistic regression. The explanatory variables were age group; location of the lesion; post-operative colic incidences: yes/no; post-operative hernia: yes/no) for "Return to the previous/intended use", lesion location

and enterotomy during surgery for "Incidence of postoperative colic episodes" and enterotomy for "Death during operation (yes/no)". Each explanatory variable was analyzed separately. Upon finding few statistically significant results with the univariate analyses, it was decided that multivariate models or other advanced statistics were not indicated.

Mann–Whitney U-tests were used to clarify the association between convalescence time (in months) and selected explanatory variables (age group, location of the lesion, SSI: yes/no and incidence of post-operative colic). Convalescence time was used as the response and explanatory variable as the grouping variable. As the distribution of convalescence time clearly differed from the normal distribution, a non-parametric approach was selected. Owner satisfaction was assessed during the interview and the median owner satisfaction was derived from these subgroups and rounded to the nearest integer. The relationship between the median owner satisfaction and the explanatory variables (hospitalization time in days, convalescence time in months, end sum of the discharge bill, owner estimated return to the same/intended use, postoperative SSI, incidence of post-operative colic) were investigated using cumulative logistic regression separately for each explanatory variable. The analyses were constructed to estimate the probability for higher owner satisfaction values.

In the survival analyses, the results were quantified with Hazard ratios (HR) and their 95% confidence intervals (CI). In the logistic regression and cumulative logit-models the results were quantified with odds ratios (OR) and their 95% confidence intervals. P value <0.05 was considered statistically significant. All statistical analyses were performed using SAS® System for Windows, version 9.3 (SAS Institute, Cary, NC, USA).

Results

Signalment

Gender, age, breed and preoperative use of the operated horses are presented in Table 1. The mean age of the horses at the time of the surgery was 8.9 years (median 8.5, range 4 days–22.2 years). Warmblood horses were the most prominent breed with 38.6% of the study population. The group 'Other horse breed' (n = 28) comprised 9 Icelandic horses, 6 horses of mixed breeds, 3 Irish cobs, 2 Toric horses, 2 Friesians, 2 Shire horses, 1 Estonian native horse, 1 Arabian horse, 1 North Swedish horse and 1 Haflinger. The group 'Pony' (n = 12) comprised 5 ponies of mixed breeds, 4 Shetland ponies, 1 Gotland Russ, 1 New Forest and 1 Connemara pony. Approximately two-thirds of the horses (67.4%; 159/236) were insured at the time of the first laparotomy, and 85.8% (12/14) at the time of the re-laparotomy.

Table 1   The signalment, short- and long-term outcome and pre- and postoperative use of the operated horses

Signalment	Small intestine (%[a])	Large intestine (%[a])	Total (n = 236)
Operated patients in total	72 (30.5%)	164 (69.5%)	236
Gender			
Mare	30 (25.9%)	86 (74.1%)	116 (49.2%)
Gelding	23 (29.1%)	56 (70.9%)	79 (33.5%)
Stallion	19 (46.3%)	22 (53.7%)	41 (17.4%)
Age group (years)			
0–14	58 (29.1%)	141 (70.9%)	199 (84.3%)
Over 15	14 (37.8%)	23 (62.2%)	37 (15.7%)
Breed			
Warm blood	24 (26.4%)	67 (73.6%)	91 (38.6%)
Finnhorse	19 (25.0%)	57 (75.0%)	76 (32.2%)
Standardbred	17 (58.6%)	12 (41.4%)	29 (12.3%)
Other horse breed	7 (25.0%)	21 (75.0%)	28 (11.9%)
Pony	5 (41.7%)	7 (58.3%)	12 (5.1%)
Use of the horse	**Preoperative (n = 135)**	**Postoperative (n = 135)**	
Ridden sport horse	48 (35.6%)	39 (28.9%)	
Hobby horse	46 (34.1%)	54 (40.0%)	
Harness racing	19 (14.1%)	20 (14.8%)	
Young/in training	13 (9.6%)	1 (0.7%)	
Breeding	8 (5.9%)	11 (8.1%)	
Pasture/company horse	1 (0.7%)	4 (3.0%)	
Retired/geriatric	0 (0.0%)	1 (0.7%)	
Did not recover back to use	–	5 (3.7%)	
Outcome	**Small intestine (n = 72)**	**Large intestine (n = 164)**	**Total (n = 236)**
Recovered from anesthesia	53 (73.6%)	142 (86.6%)	195 (82.6%)
Euthanasia during operation	19 (26.4%)	22 (13.4%)	41 (17.4%)
Death during hospitalization postop	15 (20.8%)	34 (20.7%)	49 (20.8%)
Discharged from hospital	38 (52.8%)	108 (65.9%)	146 (61.9%)
No information, long-term follow-up[b]	2 (2.8%)	6 (3.7%)	8 (3.4%)
No information after discharge[c]	1 (1.4%)	2 (1.2%)	3 (1.3%)

Horses (n = 236) operated for colic between 2006 and 2012 in University of Helsinki, Equine Teaching Hospital, Finland

[a] Percentages calculated out of the values in the Total-column

[b] Horses whose owners could not be reached and therefore specific data on postsurgical convalescence could not be acquired. These horses were included in the survival analysis as the date and reason of death were available from the hospital records and national databases (Heppa® database of the Finnish Trotting Association Hippos, Helsinki, Finland)

[c] Horses of which no records and information were available after discharge. These horses were excluded from all the statistical analyses

Surgery and short-term survival

Survival from surgery and outcome of the operated horses is presented in Table 1. In total 17.4% (41/236) of the operated horses were euthanized during surgery, 82.6% (195/236) recovered from anesthesia, and subsequently 20.8% (49/236) were euthanized during hospitalization after the surgery and 74.9% (146/195) of the horses that survived the surgery were discharged. Diagnosis categories, surgical findings, procedures and postsurgical complications are presented in Table 2. Most common diagnosis during the surgery were non-strangulating displacement of the large intestine (37.3%; 88/236), strangulation of small intestine (22.0%; 52/236) and strangulating displacement of large intestine (20.3%; 48/236). Five of the operated patients had a gastric rupture or bowel perforation with no other findings. Enterotomy was performed in 50.4% of the operated patients. Postsurgical reflux (defined as reflux of more than 2 l) was the most common complication immediately after surgery and it affected 27.2% of the operated patients. The effect of enterotomy during surgery and lesion location on discharge rate, incidence of postoperative colic and

Table 2 Categorised diagnosis, surgical findings, procedures and complications of the operated horses

Diagnosis category (n = 236)			Total		%
Small intestine					
Strangulating displacement			52		22.0
Simple obstruction			8		3.4
Large intestine					
Non-strangulating displacement and obstruction			55		23.3
Non-strangulating displacement			33		14.0
Strangulating displacement and obstruction			27		11.4
Simple obstruction			26		11.0
Strangulating displacement			21		8.9
Other					
Anterior enteritis			5		2.1
Gastric/bowel perforation with no other findings			5		2.1
Primary gas accumulation			4		1.7

Surgical findings[a] (n = 236)	Small intestine	Caecum	Colon	Small colon	Total
Displacement of large intestine	–	–	136	–	136 (57.6%)
Right dorsal displacement	–	–	49	–	49
Other displacement			36		36
Flexion, large intestine	–	–	27	–	27
Left dorsal displacement	–	–	24	–	24
Intestinal herniation	32	–	–	–	32 (13.6%)
Foramen epiploicum	13	–	–	–	13
Inguinal	10	–	–	–	10
Other	9	–	–	–	9
Sand accumulations	–	–	28	–	28 (11.9%)
Mesenterial anomaly	17	–	1	–	18 (7.6%)
Ruptured bowel	–	–	11	–	11 (4.7%)
Lipoma	10	–	–	–	10 (4.2%)
Foreign objects	–	–	–	3	3 (1.3%)
Adhesions	1	–	1	–	2 (0.8%)
Roundworm	1	–	–	–	1 (0.4%)

Surgical procedures[a] (n = 236)	Small intestine	Caecum	Colon	Small colon	Total
Enterotomy	2	–	117	–	119 (50.4%)
Gas removal[b]	NI	NI	NI	NI	95 (40.3%)
Resection	17	–	1	–	18 (7.6%)

Postsurgical complications			Total		%
Short-term (n = 195)					
Reflux/ileus			53		27.2
Peritonitis			14		7.2
Re-laparotomy[c]			11		5.6
Incisional dehiscence			4		2.1
Laminitis			3		1.5
Cardiac failure			2		1.0
Liver failure and coagulopathy			1		0.5
Long-term: (n – 135)					
Colic episodes in 8y10mo			52		38.5
Colic in the first year postop			27		20.0
Only one colic episode			21		15.6

Table 2 continued

Postsurgical complications	Total	%
Re-laparotomy due to colic	3	2.2
Colic episodes/horse year	0.18	
Surgical site infection SSI	39	28.9
Incisional hernia	15	11.1

Horses (n = 236) operated for colic between 2006 and 2012 in University of Helsinki, Equine Teaching Hospital, Finland

[a] One horse may have had more than one finding or procedure, therefore the listed findings and procedures do not exclude each other

[b] Segment of intestine: *NI* no information

[c] Re-laparotomy during hospitalization due to continuous pain, colic, reflux, or incisional dehiscence

the probability of returning to the same use are presented in Table 3. A second laparotomy was performed in 5.9% (14/195) of the operated patients, 11 of which occurred during the immediate postoperative period and 3 were performed later after discharge due to postoperative colic. Two horses had to be euthanized during the second surgery. The mean hospitalization time after surgery was 7.2 days (median 6.5 days, range 0–31 days); for horses with small intestinal lesion 6.0 d (median 5.0, range 0–21 days) and large intestinal lesion 7.7 days (median 7.0, range 0–31 days), respectively.

Patterns of survival

Figures 1, 2, 3 and 4 illustrate the patterns of survival for the operated colic horses. A marked mortality can be seen immediately following surgery in Fig. 1. Figure 2 illustrates the overall survival of the discharged horses. After 5 years, the cumulative survival was approximately 0.6 and 0.4 after 8 years and 10 months when the follow-up study was ended. Figure 3 illustrates the survival between small and large intestinal lesion groups. Mortality was higher in horses with small intestinal lesions up till approximately 40 months after surgery when cumulative survival was 0.4. The survival was similar between the two groups from 3 to 7 years. Figure 4 illustrates the pattern of overall survival of the different age groups of horses. Geriatric horses (≥15 years) had a less steep

curve initially but from 30 to 70 months the curves of both age groups had the same gradient. The cumulative survival of the geriatric horses from 6 to 9 years after surgery was 0.1.

Long-term convalescence

Survival information (date and reason of death) was obtained from 97.9% (143/146) of the discharged horses. We did not obtain follow-up information after discharge for eight of the discharged horses. These eight horses were, therefore, excluded from the rest of the study except for the survival analysis. Full follow-up data (information including convalescence after discharge) were acquired in 92.5% (135/146) horses and completed at 8 years and 10 months. The median survival time for the discharged 143 horses was 79.2 months (Fig. 2). The survival rates at 6, 12, 24, 36, 48 and 60+ months were as follows: 90.2% (129/143), 83.9% (120/143), 73.4% (105/143), 52.4% (75/143), 37.1% (53/143) and 28.7% (41/143). Age group (0–14 years/≥15 years) or location of the lesion (small intestinal/large intestinal) had no significant effect on the overall probability for survival of the patient after colic surgery long-term.

The mean owner-reported convalescence time of the horse was 6.0 months (median 6.0, range 0–20 months). A majority of the owners (87.4%; 118/135) reported the horse to be in good or satisfactory condition after this

Table 3 The effect and significance of different variables on outcome parameters

Response	Explanatory variable	P value	Odds ratio	95% CI[a]
Discharge from the hospital	Enterotomy (no vs. yes)	0.09	0.63	0.37; 1.07
Postoperative colic	Enterotomy (no vs. yes)	0.31	0.69	0.34; 1.40
	Lesion location (LI vs. SI[b])	0.01	3.27	1.31; 8.19
Return to the same/intended use	Age group (0–14 vs. ≥15)	0.88	1.10	0.33; 3.62
	Postoperative colic (no vs. yes)	0.47	1.41	0.56; 3.54
	Hernia (no vs. yes)	0.74	0.77	0.16; 3.68
	Lesion location (LI vs. SI[b])	0.49	1.42	0.53; 3.83

[a] 95% CI 95% confidence interval

[b] Large intestinal vs. small intestinal lesion

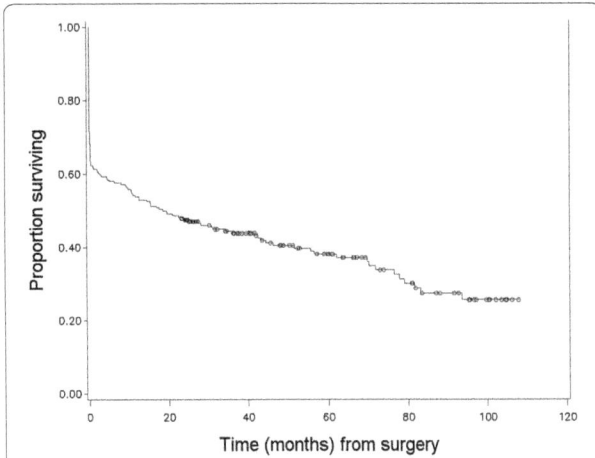

Fig. 1 Kaplan–Meier-plot of the overall survival rate following colic surgery. Number of operated horses 236, time 0 = time of surgery

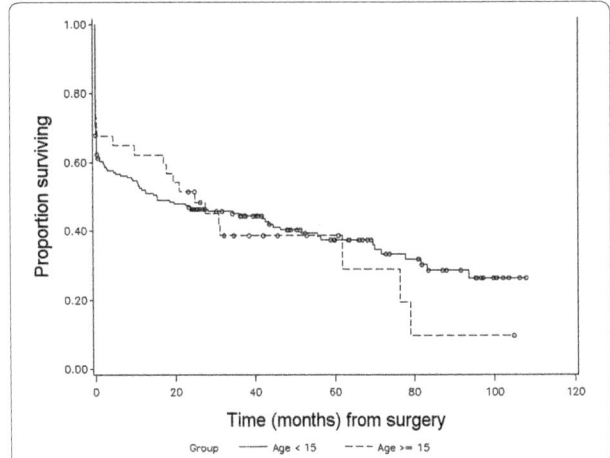

Fig. 2 Kaplan–Meier-plot of the overall survival rate following colic surgery. Number of discharged horses 143, time 0 = discharge from hospital

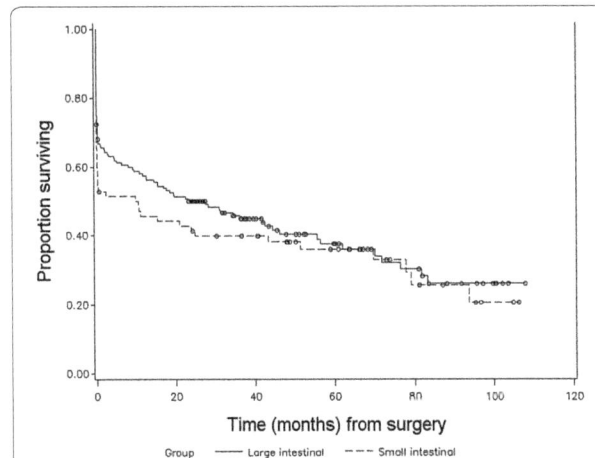

Fig. 3 Kaplan–Meier-plot of overall survival between small and large intestinal lesions. Number of operated horses 236, time 0 = date of surgery

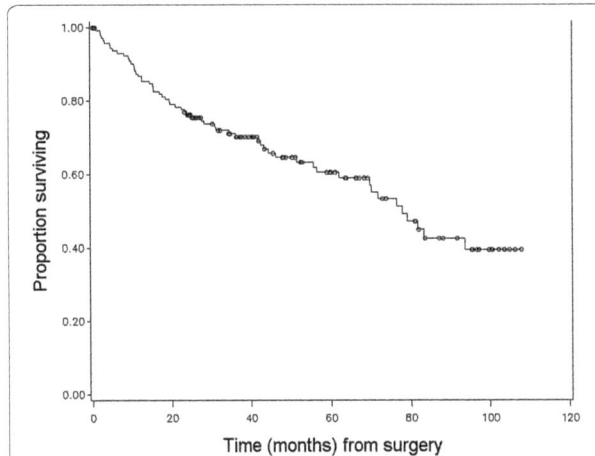

Fig. 4 Kaplan–Meier-plot of overall survival rate between age groups. Number of operated horses 236, time 0 = date of surgery. Horses between 0 and 14 years and horses ≥15 years

period. The effects of age group, lesion location, postoperative colic and SSI variables on the convalescence time are presented in Table 4. Horses with a small intestinal lesion tended to have a slightly longer time postoperatively to return to expected athletic function compared to the horses with large intestinal lesion (Table 4, $P = 0.06$). SSI seemed to lengthen the convalescence time but this increase was not statistically different (Table 4).

Long-term complications

Long-term complications and different variables that affect them are presented in Tables 2 and 3. During the first postoperative year 20.0% (27/135) of the horses suffered from one or more colic episodes. Postoperative colic was documented in 38.5% (52/135) of the discharged horses during the long-term surveillance. The incidence of colic in the operated horses was 0.18 per horse year. The horses with a large intestinal lesion were 3.3-fold more prone to have postoperative colic episodes (CI 1.3; 8.2, $P = 0.01$) compared with the horses with small intestinal lesion. Three horses (2.2%; 3/135) had to be operated after discharge because of colic. Surgical

Table 4 The association and significance of explanatory variables on the convalescence time

Effect of the parameter on the convalescence time (months)	Z value	P value
Age group (0–14 vs. ≥15)	−0.59	0.55
Lesion location (LI vs. SI[a])	1.90	0.057
Postoperative colic (no vs. yes)	−1.42	0.15
Wound infection/SSI (no vs. yes)	0.99	0.32

[a] Large intestinal vs. small intestinal lesion

site infection, defined as incisional drainage, was evident in 28.9% (39/135) cases and 11.0% (15/135) of the discharged horses developed an incisional hernia at some point postoperatively.

Postoperative performance

Pre- and postoperative use of the horses is presented in Table 1. The majority of the operated horses (83.7%; 113/135) were estimated to have reached previous or intended use after the colic surgery, 78.5% (106/135) reached their preoperative or better level of performance. Owners estimated that 72.8% (59/81) of the horses which had been used in previous competitions had also competed at least once postoperatively during the study period and that 89.8% (53/59) performed on the same or at an better level than preoperatively. When the official national database records were searched, 48.9% (66/135) preoperatively and 35.6% (48/135) postoperatively of the discharged horses had competed in one or more discipline. The effects of different variables on the probability of returning to the same/intended use are presented in Table 3. None of the variables were found to have had a significant effect on the patient's probability of regaining previous or intended level of performance.

Owner satisfaction

Nearly all, 96.3% of the owners graded the veterinary care and 98.5% rated their satisfaction toward colic surgery to range from satisfactory to good. Different variables (the length of hospitalization time; number of postoperative colic episodes; SSI; the length of the convalescence time in months; whether or not the horse returned to the same use; the sum of the total cost of veterinary care) did not have a significant negative effect on the median owner satisfaction level.

Discussion

This study is a retrospective follow-up on the long-term survival up to 8 years and 10 months after colic surgery. Long-term retrospective studies are challenging as from 14 to 44% of the horses are lost to follow-up [2, 7, 14–16]. Missing data and small study population sizes may cause bias in statistical analysis and interpretation of results. Information on survival in this study was obtained for nearly all of the discharged horses (97.9%; 143/146) and full follow-up data with complications and their effect on the use and postoperative performance were obtained for 92.5% (135/146) of the discharged horses.

Short-term survival rate after colic surgery was somewhat lower (82.6%; 195/236) compared with previous studies (85.7–87.0%) [11, 17, 18]. Two-thirds (67.4%; 159/236) of the horses were insured at the time of the first surgery, and (85.7%; 12/14) at the time of the second

surgery. Most insurance companies in Finland will not pay out the life insurance compensation sum unless the indicated and possible abdominal surgery has actually been attempted. Therefore, the insurance status may have necessitated horses with poor prognosis to be operated on and then euthanized during surgery or shortly afterwards. Additionally, there are only two 24-h equine emergency hospitals in the southern part of Finland. This might cause delays in the initiation of the treatment, which worsens short- and long-term prognosis for colic patients [14, 16, 17, 19].

The incidence of postoperative colic during the first year after the surgery was 20.0% (27/135) and for the whole study period the incidence was 0.18 colic cases per horse year. Postoperative colic is reported by several other studies to be the most common long-term complication after colic surgery, documented in between 11 and 35% of the patients, which is a negative factor for postoperative survival [1–4, 14, 17, 19, 20]. A study by Tinker and colleagues [21] reported the incidence of colic in a large population of horses that had not had colic surgery, to vary between 0 and 30%. The crude incidence density rate of colic cases has been estimated as 0.106 colic cases per horse year [21]. Horses in this study had postoperatively 1.7 times higher incidence of colic than the naive horse population with no history of colic surgery that was reported by Tinker and colleagues [21]. Previous reports found that operated horses have had 2.8–7.6 times higher incidences of colic compared to non-operated horses [1].

The number of postoperative colic episodes in this study was estimated subjectively by the owner. Not all episodes required veterinary treatment. Therefore, the capability of owners to recognize colic can be questioned and this circumstance may introduce some bias in the results. However, postoperative colic in this study was found to be 3.3-fold more common in horses that had been operated because of a large intestinal lesion compared with the small intestinal lesion. A total of 28 horses in the present study had large sand accumulations in the large colon. Previous reports of sand accumulations in the large intestine were found to be a common cause of colic and abdominal discomfort with the Finnish horse population [22]. If the management of the horse is not changed or the risk factors are not removed, then the horse can be more prone to suffer repeated colic episodes later in life. Enterotomy due to secondary impaction, was performed in the majority of the operated cases in the pelvic flexure in the present study. However, it did not statistically increase the incidence of postoperative colic. Therefore, the increased risk of postoperative colic cannot solely be explained with the existence of possible peritonitis and adhesion formation subsequent to enterotomy. During the immediate postoperative period, 5.6%

(11/195) of the patients underwent a second laparotomy due to recurrent colic, ileus or incisional dehiscence.

Re-laparotomies were performed in 7.2% (14/195) of the horses; 11 during the immediate post-operative period and 3 later on after discharge. The number of re-laparotomies has been higher in other studies (9.6–20.0%) [1, 11, 22–25]. The financial situation of the owners and the use of horses most likely played a role in deciding on re-operating, as most of the horses in this study were hobby horses. It should be noted, however, that a majority of re-operated patients in this study were insured and it is assumed that the insurance status played an important role when deciding whether to re-operate. Owners with no insurance who had instead decided to have their horses euthanatized than to be subjected to a second colic surgery most likely did so due to financial limitations.

Surgical site infection was recorded both during hospitalization and also in the owner questionnaire in this study. SSI was categorized as a long-term complication, as in all cases the horses were discharged before the infection had resolved. In some cases, infection became evident only after discharge. The occurrence of SSI often leads to incisional hernia [2] and incisional hernia in this study developed in 11.1% (15/135) of the cases. A total of 3 hernias had to be corrected surgically, the size of the deficit being approximately 10, 30 and 35 cm, respectively. Hernias are usually identified 2–12 weeks postoperatively [14]. The extended follow-up enabled us to document incisional complications that had also developed later after discharge. Interestingly, the development of hernia did not have a negative effect on the owner-reported return to use and performance level attained for these horses. In other studies, SSI has been reported in 11–42% [1, 14, 19] and incisional hernia in 6–17% of horses following laparotomy [6, 7, 14]. Horses that develop an incisional hernia have been reported to have a poorer outcome and be 7–14 times less likely to return to sporting activity or athletic use [6, 7]. However, in previous studies, the number of horses with incisional hernia is limited: 12/195 horses in one study [7]. The number of horses with incisional hernia was not actually reported in the other study of 79 horses and the ORs those authors calculated were also associated with wide confidence intervals [6]. Limited owner finances, which prevented hernia repair, may have also encouraged the owners to attempt to train and use the horses for the intended activity and performance. In our experience, a small abdominal wall defect does not incapacitate the horse from athletic activity.

If the horse survived to discharge, the overall estimated median survival time was 79.2 months (Fig. 2). Survival at 12 months (83.9%; 120/143) is comparable with an earlier report from Denmark by Christophersen and colleagues (86.6%) [6]. The overall survival between their study and our present data are very similar up to 36 months after surgery. The horses in our study were older (mean 9.2 years vs. 6 years), the population was also larger (143 vs. 79 horses) and the follow-up time was longer (8 years 10 months vs. 5 years) [6]. The decline in survival rate from 5 years onwards probably follows the life expectancy of horses. As expected, survival of horses operated for small intestinal (Fig. 3) lesion was somewhat poorer compared to horses operated for large intestinal lesion in long-term follow-up till about 36–40 months after surgery. Interestingly, after 40 months, the survival graphs were similar between the large and small intestinal groups, till about 90 | months. Complications are common during and after small intestinal surgery, and according to other reports these horses tend to have slightly poorer postoperative prognosis [1, 2, 11, 14, 22, 26]. However, this study supports the finding that a number of horses operated for small intestinal colic are able to live and perform surprisingly long, even up to 10 years after surgery [14]. The age of the horse (0–14 years/≥15 years) did not have a significant effect on overall survival (Fig. 4). Similar findings have been reported in the short-term follow-up in two previous studies [4, 27] but long-term follow-up studies are missing. The number of aged horses was small in this study, 16% of the population.

A high prevalence of discharged horses in the present study returned to the intended use (83.7%; 113/135) and the horses were also able to perform on the same or even at a better level (78.5%; 106/135) after the colic surgery. At the time of surgery, 13 horses were young or were in training and by the time of the postoperative interview 12 of these horses had already moved into a particular discipline and were performing in their intended use. Athletic performance was subjectively determined by the horses' owners, they can be considered to be reliable in assessing performance levels and/or changes within a certain time frame. Nevertheless, a subjective opinion cannot be compared to numerical objective data, such as racing earnings or the number of starts, which reflect the measurable results and changes in performance. It should be noted that most of our horses were, however, hobby horses and therefore could not be categorized or analyzed using only information on competition records. Nevertheless, the information on prognosis, use and capacity to perform is also important to the owners.

We also studied the official competition record databases, which support this as 72.8% (59/81) of horses with a competition history had officially competed postoperatively. The difference between the owner estimation and actual national database records can be explained by the fact that smaller competitions are not included in the national databases. Only a few studies about the long-term performance ability and competing after colic surgery in a population of horses of different breeds exist [6, 7]. Moreover, differences in the study populations and use of the horses between the few studies that do exist may affect the results. A recently published paper studied the operated horses surviving past 6 months after discharge. As much as 86.1% (68/79) of the horses with sporting activity before surgery had resumed by 6 months post-operation and 83.5% (66/79) reached their pre-surgical level of performance [6]. Another report documented that at 12 months after discharge, 76% (145/190) of the horses were performing in their intended use, and 66% (101/153) were doing so at the previous or better level of performance activity [7]. Thoroughbreds have been studied as racing or competitive horses but they are often retired early from their career [11–13]. Two studies on racing Thoroughbreds, respectively reported majorities of 69.0% (59/85) and 76.0% (45/59) that had returned to racing at least once after colic surgery with no marked changes in performance levels [12, 13]. Differences in study populations and the use of the horses most likely affects the results to some extent and therefore the results in their present form are not entirely comparable.

Conclusions

The findings of the present study suggest that horses with small intestinal lesions tended to have a longer convalescence time than horses with large intestinal lesions and that the incidence of postoperative colic was relatively low compared with earlier reports. However, horses operated because of large intestinal lesion were 3.3 times more prone to have postoperative colic compared with horses with small intestinal lesions. Additionally incisional hernia and incidence of postoperative colic—in contrast to previous studies—as well as the age of the horse, location of the surgical lesion and convalescence time, did not decrease the probability of performance after the surgery. Most importantly, the majority of discharged horses had a good prognosis for long-term survival, were able to return to their intended use, compete postoperatively on a satisfactory level and also perform for several years after the operation. A majority of owners estimated that the veterinary care and general satisfaction to be satisfactory or above and also expressed their general satisfaction.

Authors' contributions

II and TR-M participated in the design of the study and drafted the manuscript. JJ performed the statistical analyses in this study. KN, MA and NT participated in drafting the manuscript. All authors read and approved the final manuscript.

Author details

[1] Department of Equine and Small Animal Medicine, Faculty of Veterinary Medicine, University of Helsinki, 00014 Helsinki, Finland. [2] 4 Pharma, 20520 Turku, Finland.

Acknowledgements

The authors acknowledge and thank the surgeons that took part in operating and treating the colic horses during the study period. The authors also thank all the horse owners for their special interest, excellent collaboration and dedication and for their compliance towards this study.

Competing interests

The authors declare that they have no competing interests.

Funding

The first part of this study (2010) was supported by a student grant from the Morris Animal Foundation. The results were presented in *Morris Animal Foundation Research Congress 2011*; Portland, USA as a poster and short oral presentation by Isa Immonen.

References

1. Proudman CJ, Smith E, Edwards GB, French NP. Long-term survival of equine surgical colic cases. Part 1: patterns of mortality and morbidity. Equine Vet J. 2002;34:435–7.
2. Mair TS, Smith LJ. Survival and complication rates in 300 horses undergoing surgical treatment of colic. Part 3: long-term complications and survival. Equine Vet J. 2005;37:310–4.
3. Mezerova J, Zert Z. Long-term survival and complications of colic surgery in horses: analysis of 331 cases. Vet Med Czech. 2008;53:43–52.
4. Krista KM, Kuebelbeck KL. Comparison of survival rates for geriatric horses versus nongeriatric horses following exploratory celiotomy for colic. J Am Vet Med Assoc. 2009;235:1069–72.
5. Müller JMV, Wehli-Eser M, Waldmeier P, Rohn K, Feige K. Short- and long-term survival of surgical colic patients. Small intestinal resection does not influence the prognosis of horses with small intestinal colic following their first laparotomy. Tierarztl Prax. 2009;4:247–54.
6. Christophersen MT, Tnibar A, Pihl H, Andersen PH, Ekstrom CT. Sporting activity following colic surgery in horses: a retrospective study. Equine Vet J. 2011;43(Suppl 40):3–6.
7. Davis W, Fogle CA, Gerard MP, Levine JF, Blikslager AT. Return to use and performance following exploratory celiotomy for colic in horses: 195 cases (2003–2010). Equine Vet J. 2013;45:224–8.
8. Freeman DE, Hammock P, Baker GJ, Goetz T, Foreman JH, Schaeffer DJ, Richter RA, Inoue O, Magid JH. Short- and long-term survival and prevalence of the postoperative ileus after small intestinal surgery in the horse. Equine Vet J. 2000;32(Suppl 32):42–51.
9. Smith LJ, Mair TS. Are horses that undergo an exploratory laparotomy for correction of a right dorsal displacement of the large colon predisposed to post operative colic, compared to other forms of large colon displacement? Equine Vet J. 2010;42:44–6.
10. Proudman CJ, Edwards GB, Barnes J, French NP. Factors affecting long-term survival of horses recovering from surgery of the small intestine. Equine Vet J. 2005;37:360–5.
11. Santschi EM, Slone DE, Embertson RM, Clayton MK, Markel MD. Colic surgery in 206 juvenile thoroughbreds: survival and racing results. Equine Vet J. 2000;32(Suppl 32):32–6.
12. Tomlinson JE, Boston RC, Brauer T. Evaluation of racing performance after colic surgery in thoroughbreds: 85 cases (1996–2010). J Am Vet Med Assoc. 2013;243:532–7.
13. Hart S, Southwood LL, Aceto HW. Impact of colic surgery on return to function in racing thoroughbreds: 59 cases (1996–2009). J Am Vet Med Assoc. 2014;244:205–11.
14. Freeman DE, Schaefer DJ, Cleary OB. Long-term survival in horses with strangulating obstruction of the small intestine managed without resection. Equine Vet J. 2014;46:711–7.

15. Stewart S, Southwood LL, Aceto HW. Comparison of short- and long-term complications and survival following jejunojejunostomy, jejunoileostomy and jejunocaecostomy in 112 horses: 2005–2010. Equine Vet J. 2014;46:333–8.

16. Freeman KP, Southwood LL, Lane J, Lindborg S, Aceto HW. Post operative infection, pyrexia and perioperative drug use in surgical colic patients. Equine Vet J. 2012;44:476–81.

17. Mair TS, Smith LJ. Survival and complication rates in 300 horses undergoing surgical treatment of colic. Part 1: short-term survival following a single laparotomy. Equine Vet J. 2005;37:296–302.

18. Muños E, Argüelles D, Areste L, San Miguel L, Prades M. Retrospective analysis of exploratory laparotomies in 192 Andalusian horses and 276 horses of other breeds. Vet Rec. 2008;162:303–6.

19. Mair TS, Smith LJ. Survival and complication rates in 300 horses undergoing surgical treatment of colic. Part 2: short-term complications. Equine Vet J. 2005;37:303–9.

20. Granot N, Milgram J, Bdolah-Abram T, Shemesh I, Steinman A. Surgical management of sand colic impactions in horses: a retrospective study of 41 cases. Aust Vet J. 2008;86:404–7.

21. Tinker MK, White NA, Lessard P, Thatcher CD, Pelzer KD, Davis B, Carmel DK. Prospective study of equine colic incidence and mortality. Equine Vet J. 1997;29:448–53.

22. Niinistö K, Hewetson M, Kaikkonen R, Sykes BW, Raekallio M. Comparison of the effect of enteral psyllium, magnesium sulphate and their combination for removal of sand from the large colon of horses. Vet J. 2014;202:608–11.

23. Gorvy DA, Edwards GB, Proudman CJ. Intra-abdominal adhesions in horses: a retrospective evaluation of repeat laparotomy in 99 horses with acute gastrointestinal disease. Vet J. 2008;175:194–201.

24. Smith LJ, Mellor DJ, Marr CM, Reid SWJ, Mair TS. Incisional complications following exploratomy celiotomy: does an abdominal bandage reduce the risk? Equine Vet J. 2007;39:277–83.

25. Mair TS, Smith LJ. Survival and complication rates in 300 horses undergoing surgical treatment of colic. Part 4: early (acute) re-laparotomy. Equine Vet J. 2005;37:315–8.

26. Archer DC, Pinchbeck GL, Proudman CJ. Factors associated with survival of epiploic foramen entrapment colic: a multicentre, international study. Equine Vet J. 2011;43(Suppl 39):56–62.

27. Gazzerro DM, Southwood LL, Lindborg S. Short-term complications after colic surgery in geriatric versus mature non-geriatric horses. Vet Surg. 2014;44:256–64.

16

Campylobacter jejuni and *Campylobacter coli* in wild birds on Danish livestock farms

Birthe Hald[1,6*], Marianne Nielsine Skov[2,7], Eva Møller Nielsen[2,8], Carsten Rahbek[3,5,9], Jesper Johannes Madsen[3], Michael Wainø[1,10], Mariann Chriél[4,11], Steen Nordentoft[1,12], Dorte Lau Baggesen[2,6] and Mogens Madsen[1,13]

Abstract

Background: Reducing the occurrence of campylobacteriosis is a food safety issue of high priority, as in recent years it has been the most commonly reported zoonosis in the EU. Livestock farms are of particular interest, since cattle, swine and poultry are common reservoirs of *Campylobacter* spp. The farm environment provides attractive foraging and breeding habitats for some bird species reported to carry thermophilic *Campylobacter* spp. We investigated the *Campylobacter* spp. carriage rates in 52 wild bird species present on 12 Danish farms, sampled during a winter and a summer season, in order to study the factors influencing the prevalence in wild birds according to their ecological guild. In total, 1607 individual wild bird cloacal swab samples and 386 livestock manure samples were cultured for *Campylobacter* spp. according to the Nordic Committee on Food Analysis method NMKL 119.

Results: The highest *Campylobacter* spp. prevalence was seen in 110 out of 178 thrushes (61.8 %), of which the majority were Common Blackbird (*Turdus merula*), and in 131 out of 616 sparrows (21.3 %), a guild made up of House Sparrow (*Passer domesticus*) and Eurasian Tree Sparrow (*Passer montanus*). In general, birds feeding on a diet of animal or mixed animal and vegetable origin, foraging on the ground and vegetation in close proximity to livestock stables were more likely to carry *Campylobacter* spp. in both summer ($P < 0.001$) and winter ($P < 0.001$) than birds foraging further away from the farm or in the air. Age, fat score, gender, and migration range were not found to be associated with *Campylobacter* spp. carriage. A correlation was found between the prevalence (%) of *C. jejuni* in wild birds and the proportions (%) of *C. jejuni* in both manure on cattle farms ($R^2 = 0.92$) and poultry farms ($R^2 = 0.54$), and between the prevalence (%) of *C. coli* in wild birds and the proportions (%) of *C. coli* in manure on pig farms ($R^2 = 0.62$).

Conclusions: The ecological guild of wild birds influences the prevalence of *Campylobacter* spp. through the behavioural patterns of the birds. More specifically, wild birds eating food of animal or mixed animal and vegetable origin and foraging on the ground close to livestock were more likely to carry *Campylobacter* spp. than those foraging further away or hunting in the air. These findings suggest that wild birds may play a role in sustaining the epidemiology of *Campylobacter* spp. on farms.

Keywords: *Campylobacter* spp. epidemiology, *C. jejuni*, *C. coli*, Wild birds, Livestock farms, Ecological guild, Cattle, Pig, Poultry

Background

Human campylobacteriosis has been the most commonly reported zoonosis in the European Union (EU) since 2005, with 214,779 confirmed cases in 2013 according to the European Food Safety Authority (EFSA) [1]. The disease burden was calculated at 35,000 disability-adjusted life years (DALYs) per year and the annual cost in the EU at around €2.4 billion [2]. The global number of DALYs was calculated to be 7,541,000 per year [3]. The cause of campylobacteriosis is *Campylobacter* spp. (primarily *C. jejuni* and *C. coli*)—a Gram-negative, spiral, microaerophilic bacterium and a common commensal inhabitant of the intestinal microflora of food production animals such as cattle, pigs and poultry [4]. It is estimated that 50–80 %

*Correspondence: bhal@food.dtu.dk
[6] Present Address: National Food Institute, Technical University of Denmark, 2860 Søborg, Denmark
Full list of author information is available at the end of the article

of *Campylobacter* spp. strains infecting humans originate from the chicken reservoir, 20–30 % from the cattle reservoir and a small proportion from other reservoirs including wild animals [5]. As a consequence, the entire meat production chain and end products may be contaminated with *C. jejuni* or *C. coli*. In the EU, the pathways to humans are mainly through food, though environmental transmission and direct animal contact are also possible [6]. Therefore, reducing the occurrence of campylobacteriosis in the EU is a food safety issue of high priority, yet one which presents challenges [7].

According to a recent and extensive systematic review of 95 published studies of *Campylobacter* spp. sources around broiler farms [8], several wild animals (including wild birds) are known to be carriers. However, only a small number of the reviewed studies had a primary focus on wild birds living in close proximity to the farms. On a broiler farm in Athens GA, USA, 10 % (of 124) wild birds—mainly House Sparrow (*Passer domesticus*) and Common Starling (*Sturnus vulgaris*)—carried *C. jejuni* [9]. Colles et al. [10] found *C. jejuni* in 50.2 % of droppings from 331 Canada Goose (*Branta canadensis*) and Greylag Goose (*Anser anser*), and in 29.9 % of 954 Common Starling on a free-range broiler farm. Concerning cattle farms, a study in central Iowa, USA sampled 188 wild birds on dairy cattle, sheep and goat farms and found *Campylobacter* spp. in 4.8 % [11].

During the past decade, source attribution studies including multilocus sequence typing (MLST) have been conducted to compare the similarity of *C. jejuni* strains from wild birds with those from chicken and cattle [10–15] and with isolates from human disease [10, 12, 13, 15–17]. The overall conclusion is that the vast majority of *C. jejuni* strains are highly host specific. However, the studies also all identified a small proportion of strains with genotypes overlapping wild birds, farm animals [10–15] and human disease isolates [10, 13, 15–17].

Several studies on *Campylobacter* spp. carriage rates in wild birds in urban areas report a prevalence from 0–90 % [18–24]. Although it would appear that wild birds living in cities (mainly sparrows, pigeons, doves and starlings) have low carriage rates [19, 20, 22], French et al. [16] suggested that wild birds in city parks could contribute to campylobacteriosis in preschool children. The overall highest reported carriage rates have been found in gulls and crows foraging on refuse dumps in urban areas of Norway, Sweden, England, Japan, Spain and USA [18–21, 23–25].

Some of the large discrepancies in wild bird *Campylobacter* spp. prevalence between different studies may be attributed to host taxonomy or differences in the ecological guilds present. Bird ecological guilds are groupings of birds that exploit environmental resources in a

similar way [26, 27]. The significance of different ecological guilds on the carriage rates of *Campylobacter* spp. was shown in a study of 1794 birds (the majority of which were migratory), sampled at Ottenby Bird Observatory on the island Oeland, Sweden [28]. The highest prevalence of *Campylobacter* spp. was found among ground-foraging guilds of short-distance migratory birds wintering in Europe.

The aim of our study was to estimate the prevalence of *Campylobacter* spp. in farm related wild bird species. Additionally, to investigate an association between *Campylobacter* spp. contaminated farm environments and wild birds around cattle, pig and poultry farms by performing an analysis of factors associated with *Campylobacter* spp. carriage of the wild birds.

Methods

Study design and selection of farms

The study covered four cattle farms, four slaughter pig farms, and four free-range poultry farms in Denmark, together with the wild bird populations living inside production buildings or within a 100 m radius from the farms. The study was conducted during January and February (winter) and during August and September (summer) in 2001. Two farms were sampled per week, and visited every weekday in order to get as many wild bird samples as possible. The cattle and pig farms were initially selected for a project investigating the occurrence of *Salmonella* in wildlife near Danish cattle and pig farms during 2001 and 2002 [29], while the poultry farms were included in this study only. The sampling schemes for *Campylobacter* spp. and *Salmonella* were conducted simultaneously in 2001.

Sampling

Wild birds

Birds were caught and ringed following the EURING system (http://www.euring.org/) by licensed ringers with mist-nets, traps, or by hand, thus ensuring that each bird was only sampled once per sampling event. The birds were released again after sampling. To ensure that a sufficient number of birds were caught during the winter months, several feeding places were established at each herd, using sterilised birdseed. We sampled as many birds as possible, and data on the estimated age, fat score, gender and exact place of capture were noted. Cloacal swab samples were obtained from the wild birds, using slim aluminum cotton swabs (DANSU, Ganløse, Denmark) and placed in Brain Heart Infusion (BHI) transport medium (DIFCO, Sparks, MD, USA) containing 5 % (v/v) calf blood (National Veterinary Institute, Copenhagen, Denmark) and 0.5 % agar (Oxoid Ltd., Basingstoke, Hampshire, UK).

Production animals

To detect *Campylobacter* spp. in cattle and pig herds, manure was collected at numerous places in the livestock facilities or among herds in pasture, and mixed into approximately twenty 200 ml containers (Dispatch Container Nunc, Life Technologies, Nærum, Denmark) per herd in each sampling round (i.e. 5–10 manure samples per container equalling 150–180 ml of manure) in order to obtain a representative measure of the within-herd *Campylobacter* spp. status. In order to sample poultry flocks, material from the litter surface was collected on a pair of boot socks whilst walking through the flock's resting house [30].

Bacteriological examination and species characterisation

All samples were transported to the laboratory on the sampling day at ambient temperature, refrigerated overnight between 2 and 4 °C, and *Campylobacter* spp. cultivation was initiated the following day. For the number of samples tested, see Table 1.

Cloacal swabs

Campylobacter spp. were isolated by streaking a swab with the faecal material directly on to modified Charcoal Cefoperazone Deoxycholate Agar (mCCDA) (CM0739, SR0155) (Oxoid) [31], and the plates were incubated under microaerobic conditions (6 % O_2, 6 % CO_2, in 88 % N_2) at 42 °C for 48 h. *Campylobacter* spp.-like colonies were purified on blood agar and identified to species level using standard procedures including tests for hippurate and indoxyl acetate hydrolysis, catalase production and susceptibility to cephalotin and nalidixic acid according to NMKL 119 [32]. *Campylobacter* spp. isolates were identified as *C. jejuni*, *C. coli*, *C. lari*, *C. upsaliensis*, *C. hyointestinalis* or *Campylobacter* spp.

Manure

The manure was diluted to 1 g per 9 ml of buffered peptone water (CM1049, Oxoid), and 10 μl of the suspended material was streaked on mCCDA and incubated as described above.

Boot socks

Each pair of boot socks was placed in a stomacher bag, and after being diluted in 1:10 w/w in buffered peptone water (CM1049, Oxoid), faeces were released by gentle manipulation and 10 μl of the suspension was spread on mCCDA and incubated as described above.

Data analysis

The dependent variable was defined as a positive isolation of *Campylobacter* spp. from a wild bird. Descriptive

Table 1 *Campylobacter* spp. prevalence and species distribution

Origin of sample	Number of samples	Total number (%) positive	Number of *C. jejuni* (%)	Number of *C. coli* (%)	Number of other *C.* spp. (%)
Winter					
Cattle farms					
Wild birds	268	36 (13.4)	22 (8.2)	13 (4.9)	1 (0.4)
Cattle manure	81	36 (44.4)	32 (39.5)	2 (2.5)	2 (2.5)
Pig farms					
Wild birds	288	64 (22.2)	33 (11.5)	27 (9.4)	4 (1.4)
Pig manure	81	72 (88.9)	0 (0.0)	69 (85.2)	3 (3.7)
Poultry farms					
Wild birds	150	16 (10.7)	10 (6.7)	6 (4.0)	0 (0.0)
Poultry manure	8	1 (12.5)	1 (12.5)	0 (0.0)	0 (0.0)
Summer					
Cattle farms					
Wild birds	253	38 (15.0)	36 (14.2)	0 (0.0)	2 (0.8)
Cattle manure	83	55 (66.3)	54 (65.1)	0 (0.0)	1 (1.2)
Pig farms					
Wild birds	330	69 (20.9)	68 (20.6)	1 (0.3)	0 (0.0)
Pig manure	83	54 (65.1)	4 (4.8)	50 (60.2)	0 (0.0)
Poultry farms					
Wild birds	318	73 (23.0)	70 (22.0)	1 (0.3)	2 (0.6)
Poultry manure	50	45 (90.0)	41 (82.0)	4 (8.0)	0 (0.0)

The number of samples tested for *Campylobacter* spp., the total number and percentage of positive samples, and the numbers of *C. jejuni*, *C. coli* and other *Campylobacter* spp. positive samples isolated in wild birds and in livestock manure on each farm type in winter and summer

statistics were performed using bivariate analysis [33] on *Campylobacter* spp. positive samples from wild birds. The association between independent variables was assessed using the Chi square test with a statistical significance threshold of $P < 0.05$. The evaluation of a possible association between *Campylobacter* spp. positive samples in the wild birds and in the herd was carried out separately for the two seasons (winter and summer).

Six potential factors associated with *Campylobacter* spp. carriage were included: (1) age (old, young); (2) herd type (cattle, pig, poultry); (3) proximity (in stable, around stable); (4) ecological guild with ≥ 10 samples (i.e. aerial insectivorous, foliage-gleaners, insectivorous seedeaters, open-land insectivorous, tit-like birds, sparrows, passerine seedeaters, terrestrial and low fly-catching feeders and thrushes); (5) fat score (0–8) [34], and (6) gender (male, female, not determined).

Based on the characteristic behaviour patterns of each ecological guild, the following five factors were selected: (1) feed (animal, mix, vegetable); (2) forage area (aerial, ground, vegetation); (3) proximity to stables (in stable, around stable); (4) contact with slurry (no, yes), and (5) migration range (long, medium, short, partial, none). This analysis included only the summer sampling, as more guilds were present, and the birds exhibited a wider range of behavioural patterns during the summer season than in winter.

Multivariate analyses [33] were carried out in all sampled wild birds organised in an ecological guild structure based on Gotellia et al. [27], using SAS Enterprise guide ver. 3.0.2. The logistic regression analyses were carried out using SAS PROC GENMOD. The modelling procedure assumed a binomial distribution and used logit as the link function. Goodness of fit was assessed by likelihood ratio statistics. The model was adjusted for overdispersion using the PSCALE option. In the analysis, non-significant variables were removed using stepwise backwards elimination. Statistical significance of the covariates was assessed using the likelihood ratio test based on $P \leq 0.05$. The odds ratio (OR) and the 95 % confidence interval were reported for statistically significant variables.

In order to evaluate the impact of different herd types and season on the *C. jejuni* and *C. coli* carriage rates, sparrows (n = 616) were selected for the analysis, since this guild of non-migratory wild birds was the only one to be caught in a sufficient number on all farms during both winter and summer sampling. Correlation coefficients (R^2) were calculated between the prevalence (%) of *C. jejuni* and *C. coli* in sparrows and the proportions (%) *C. jejuni* and *C. coli* in manure from each of the three herd types.

Results

Campylobacter spp. prevalence in sampled wild birds

In total, 1607 wild birds were sampled. The overall *Campylobacter* spp. carriage rate was significantly lower in winter (15.9 %, 112 positive samples out of a total of 706) than in summer (20.0 %, 180 positive samples out of a total of 901; OR = 1.32, 1.02–1.71, $P = 0.03$). For the species of *Campylobacter* spp. detected in each farm type, and the carriage rate among wild birds in winter and summer, see Table 1. For the prevalence of *Campylobacter* spp. in each bird species, see Table 2 and grouped in ecological guilds, see Table 3.

The *Campylobacter* spp. carriage rates varied considerably between ecological guilds. The highest prevalence was found within two guilds: thrushes with 61.8 % (110/178) positive samples and sparrows with 21.3 % (131/616) positive samples (Table 2). Combined, these guilds were responsible for 82.5 % (241 out of 292) of the positive wild bird samples. The main bird species of these two guilds were the Common Blackbird (*Turdus merula*; n = 174), House Sparrow (n = 366) and Eurasian Tree Sparrow (*Passer montanus*; n = 250). They were also the most frequently sampled wild birds on the farms. Other birds that were frequently present were the Barn Swallow (*Hirundu rustica*; n = 128), Great Tit (*Parus major*; n = 129), European Greenfinch (*Carduelis chloris*; n = 90) and Common House Martin (*Delichon urbica*; n = 83), all of which had a low *Campylobacter* spp. prevalence (Table 2).

Factors associated with Campylobacter spp. carriage in wild birds

Analysis of the six selected risk factors for *Campylobacter* spp. carriage in wild birds (age, herd type, proximity, ecological guild, fat score and gender) revealed that the ecological guild was significantly associated with *Campylobacter* spp. carriage during both winter and summer (Table 3). Thrushes and open-land insectivorous birds were more likely to carry *Campylobacter* spp. than sparrows (used as a reference guild), whereas all other guilds had lower odds than sparrows. In general, herd type, fat score, gender and age were not significantly associated with *Campylobacter* spp. prevalence in wild birds (all sampled birds). Proximity was significant in summer (see proximity to stables in Table 4) but not in winter (data not shown).

Patterns of behaviour in summer

Concerning the impact of particular patterns of behaviour in summer (i.e. feed, forage area, proximity to stables, contact with slurry and migration range), there was significantly increased odds for *Campylobacter* spp. carriage in

Table 2 The prevalence of *Campylobacter* spp. in wild birds and the allocation of bird species to ecological guild

Ecological guilds	Species	Common name	Number tested W/S	Number positive W/S	% *Campylobacter* positive W/S
Aerial insectivorous	*Delichon urbicum*	Common house martin	0/83	0/0	0.0/0.0
	Delichon urbicum (brood)	Common house martin, brood	0/2	0/0	0.0/0.0
	Hirundu rustica	Barn swallow	0/128	0/10	0.0/7.8
	Hirundu rustica (brood)	Barn swallow, brood	0/21	0/4	0.0/19.0
Bud-browser and seedeaters	*Pyrrhula pyrrhula*	Eurasian bullfinch	1/5	0/0	0.0/0.0
Columbids	*Columba livia domesticus*	Feral pigeon	3/3	1/0	33.3/0.0
	Columba palumbus	Common wood pigeon	0/1	0/0	0.0/0.0
	Streptopelia decaocto	Eurasian collared dove	2/3	0/0	0.0/0.0
Flycatcher	*Muscicapa striata*	Spotted flycatcher	0/2	0/1	0.0/50.0
Foliage-gleaners	*Fringilla coelebs*	Common chaffinch	26/2	0/0	0.0/0.0
	Hippolais icterina	Icterine warbler	0/1	0/0	0.0/0.0
	Phylloscopus collybita	Common chiffchaff	0/12	0/0	0.0/0.0
	Phylloscopus trochilus	Willow warbler	0/18	0/3	0.0/16.7
	Sylvia atricapilla	Eurasian blackcap	0/9	0/2	0.0/22.2
	Sylvia borin	Garden warbler	0/9	0/0	0.0/0.0
	Sylvia communis	Common whitethroat	0/44	0/5	0.0/11.4
	Sylvia curruca	Lesser whitethroat	0/9	0/3	0.0/33.3
Gallinaceous birds	*Phasianus colchicus*	Common pheasant	1/0	0/0	0.0/0.0
Gulls	*Larus canus*	Mew gull	2/0	0/0	0.0/0.0
Insectivorous seedeaters	*Emberiza citrinella*	Yellowhammer	2/19	0/3	0.0/15.8
	Emberiza calandra	Corn bunting	0/3	0/1	0.0/33.3
Marshwarblers	*Acrocephalus palustris*	Marsh warbler	0/5	0/0	0.0/0.0
	Acrocephalus scirpaceus	Eurasian reed warbler	0/1	0/0	0.0/0.0
Omnivorous corvidae	*Corvus frugilegus*	Rook	2/0	0/0	0.0/0.0
Open-land insectivorous	*Alauda arvensis*	Eurasian skylark	0/1	0/0	0.0/0.0
	Anthus trivialis	Tree pipit	0/1	0/0	0.0/0.0
	Motacilla alba	White wagtail	0/7	0/4	0.0/57.1
	Motacilla alba (brood)	White wagtail, brood	0/1	0/1	0.0/100.0
Passerine seedeaters	*Carduelis cannabina*	Common linnet	0/5	0/0	0.0/0.0
	Carduelis carduelis	European goldfinch	0/3	0/0	0.0/0.0
	Carduelis chloris	European greenfinch	70/20	0/1	0.0/5.0
	Carduelis flammea	Common redpoll	3/0	0/0	0.0/0.0
Scolopacids	*Tringa ochropus*	Green sandpiper	0/1	0/0	0.0/0.0
Sparrows	*Passer domesticus*	House sparrow	214/152	38/51	17.8/33.6
	Passer montanus	Eurasian tree sparrow	81/169	1/41	1.2/24.3
Stream specialist	*Motacilla cinerea*	Grey wagtail	0/1	0/0	0.0/0.0
Terrestrial and low fly-catching feeders	*Erithacus rubecula*	European robin	25/4	0/0	0.0/0.0
	Luscinia luscinia	Thrush nightingale	0/1	0/0	0.0/0.0
	Oenanthe oenanthe	Northern wheatear	0/1	0/0	0.0/0.0
	Phoenicurus phoenicurus	Common redstart	0/3	0/0	0.0/0.0
	Prunella modularis	Dunnock	9/9	4/2	44.4/22.2
	Saxicola rubetra	Whinchat	0/3	0/0	0.0/0.0
	Troglodytes troglodytes	Eurasian wren	16/18	0/0	0.0/0.0
Thrushes	*Turdus merula*	Common blackbird	119/55	63/44	52.9/80.0
	Turdus pilaris	Fieldfare	3/0	3/0	100.0/0.0
	Turdus viscivorus	Mistle thrush	1/0	0/0	0.0/0.0

Table 2 continued

Ecological guilds	Species	Common name	Number tested W/S	Number positive W/S	% *Campylobacter* positive W/S
Tit-like birds	*Certhia brachydactyla*	Short-toed treecreeper	1/0	0/0	0.0/0.0
	Certhia familiaris	Eurasian treecreeper	0/1	0/0	0.0/0.0
	Cyanistes caeruleus	Eurasian blue tit	30/15	0/0	0.0/0.0
	Lophophanes cristatus	European crested tit	1/0	0/0	0.0/0.0
	Parus major	Great tit	86/43	2/1	2.3/2.3
	Poecile palustris	Marsh tit	5/3	0/0	0.0/0.0
	Regulus regulus	Goldcrest	1/0	0/0	0.0/0.0
	Sitta europaea	Eurasian nuthatch	1/0	0/0	0.0/0.0
No guild	*Bombycilla garrulus*	Bohemian waxwing	1/0	0/0	0.0/0.0
	Sturnus vulgaris	Common starling	0/4	0/3	0.0/75.0

The species and number of birds tested for *Campylobacter* spp., and the prevalence in each bird species in winter (W) and summer (S)

Table 3 *Campylobacter* spp. prevalence in ecological guilds

Guild	Winter			Summer		
	Number of samples	Prevalence (%)	OR (95 % CI)	Number of samples	Prevalence (%)	OR (95 % CI)
Aerial insectivorous	–	–	–	234	6.0	0.2 (0.1–0.3)
Foliage-gleaners	26	0.0	NA[a]	104	12.5	0.4 (0.2–0.7)
Insectivorous seedeaters	–	–	–	22	18.2	0.6 (0.2–1,7)
Open-land insectivorous	–	–	–	10	50.0	2.5 (0.7–8.8)
Passerine seedeaters	73	0.0	NA	28	3.6	0.1 (0.01–0.7)
Sparrows	295	13.2	1.0 (reference)	321	28.7	1.0 (reference)
Terrestrial and low fly catching feeders	50	8.0	0.6 (0.2–1.7)	39	5.1	0.1 (0.03–0.6)
Thrushes	123	53.7	7.6 (4.6–12.4)	55	80.0	9.9 (4.9–20.1)
Tit-like birds	125	1.6	0.1 (0.03–0.5)	62	1.6	0.04 (0.01–0.3)
Total	692			875		

The odds-ratios (OR) and 95 % confidence interval (95 % CI) from the multivariate analysis of *Campylobacter* spp. prevalence in ecological guilds with ≥10 birds sampled in winter and summer, with sparrows used as a reference

[a] Not applicable due to zero positive samples

birds eating food of animal or mixed animal and vegetable origin foraging on the ground and in vegetation close to the production buildings (Table 4). No association was found between *Campylobacter* spp. carriage and contact with slurry or migration range (data not shown).

Herd type and *Campylobacter* species distribution

C. jejuni was the most commonly isolated *Campylobacter* species in wild birds on all farm types, comprising 78.3 % (58 out of 74) of wild bird isolates on cattle farms, 75.9 % (101 out of 133) on pig farms and 89.9 % (80 out of 89) on poultry farms (Table 1). The remaining isolates were almost entirely *C. coli*, of which 46 out of 48 isolates were found at the winter sampling.

Looking at the proportions of *Campylobacter* species in herd manure and the prevalence in wild birds at each of the 12 individual farms revealed a strong correlation between the prevalence of *C. jejuni* in both wild birds and the proportions in manure on cattle farms ($R^2 = 0.92$), and a moderate correlation on poultry farms ($R^2 = 0.54$). Likewise, a moderate correlation was found between *C. coli* in both wild birds and in pig manure ($R^2 = 0.62$; Fig. 1). In contrast, no correlation was seen between *C. coli* in wild birds and in manure on cattle and poultry farms, or between *C. jejuni* in wild birds and in manure in pig herds (Fig. 1).

Discussion

A seasonal peak in the prevalence of *Campylobacter* spp. in wild birds was observed in summer. This was also found in a study of farm related Common Starling in the UK [12], and a study of Black-headed Gull (*Larus ridibundus*) in Sweden [23]. The underlying causes of

Table 4 Factors associated with *Campylobacter* spp. carriage and specific bird behaviour during summer

Factor	Odds Ratio (95 % CI)
Feed	
Animal origin	8.0 (4.3–15.0)
Mixed animal and vegetable origin	22.6 (7.4–68.6)
Vegetable origin	1.0 (reference)
Forage area	
In the air	0.03 (0.0–0.1)
On the ground	1.03 (0.4–2.8)
In the vegetation	1.0 (reference)
Proximity to stables	
In or at stables	42.72 (14.2–128.5)
Around stables	1.0 (reference)

seasonality in the epidemiology of *Campylobacter* spp. are not fully understood. However, seasonality is also a recognised factor in the pattern of *Campylobacter* spp. infections in poultry [2], and in the occurrence of human campylobacteriosis [1]. The vast majority (82.5 %) of *Campylobacter* spp. in wild birds in our study was

isolated from thrushes and sparrows (Tables 2, 3), representing some of the most common wild bird species in Denmark (i.e. Common Blackbird, House Sparrow and Eurasian Tree Sparrow).

The *Campylobacter* spp. carriage rates of the farm-related wild birds were found to be closely associated with the ecological guild (Table 3). Studies from Sweden [28] and Italy [35] have reported results for ecological guilds sampled at bird stations. The Swedish study found the highest *Campylobacter* spp. prevalence in wagtails, Common Starling and thrushes [28], in agreement with the results presented here. Common bird species such as the European Greenfinch, European Robin (*Erithacus rubecula*), Great Tit and Common Chaffinch (*Fringilla coelebs*) showed low *Campylobacter* spp. prevalence in both the Swedish study and the present study (Table 2). Our analysis identified feeding habit, forage area and proximity to stables as factors significantly associated with the carriage of *Campylobacter* spp. in wild birds (Table 4). This is in line with the results of the Italian study [35], where feeding habit was considered an important factor, and carnivorous birds foraging on the ground showed the highest prevalence of *Campylobacter* spp. A

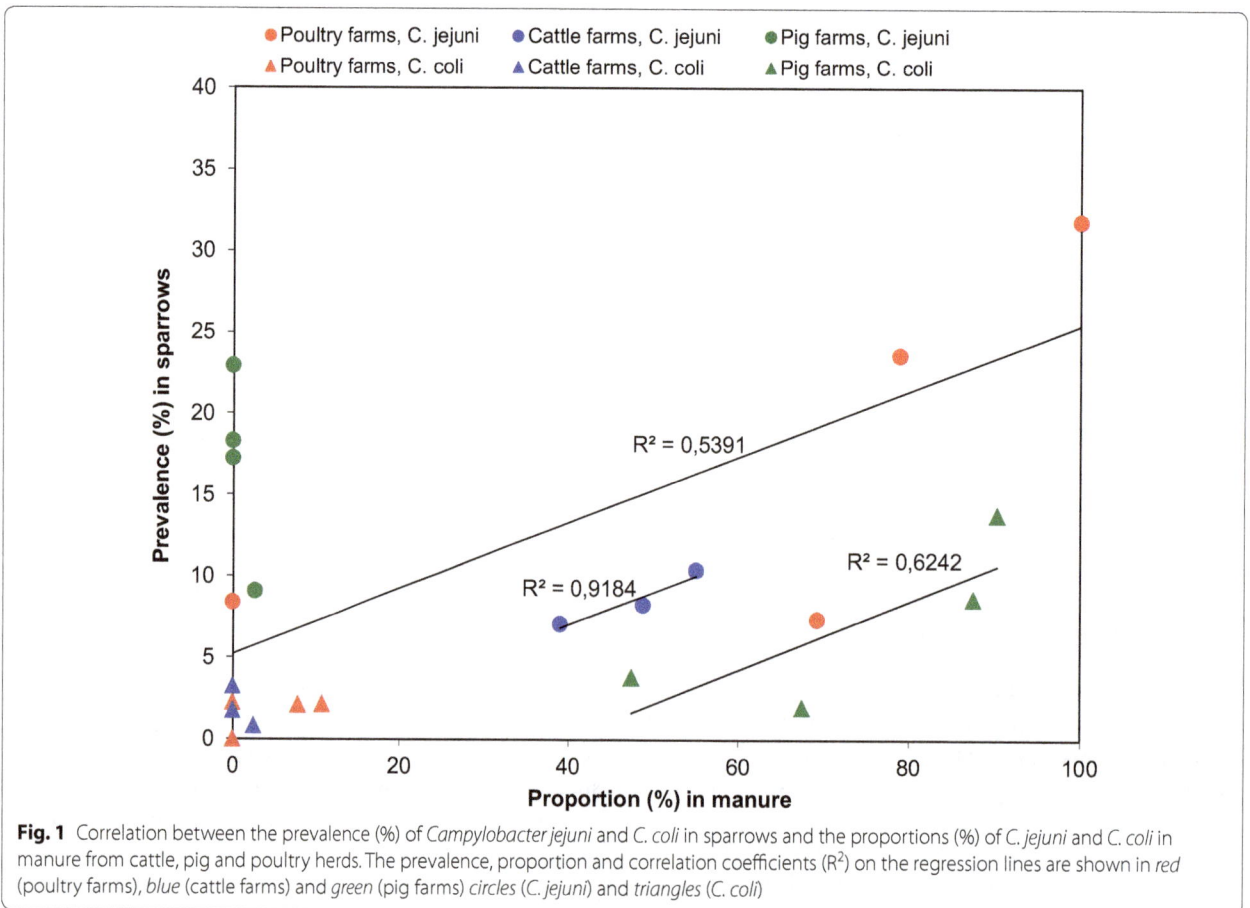

Fig. 1 Correlation between the prevalence (%) of *Campylobacter jejuni* and *C. coli* in sparrows and the proportions (%) of *C. jejuni* and *C. coli* in manure from cattle, pig and poultry herds. The prevalence, proportion and correlation coefficients (R²) on the regression lines are shown in *red* (poultry farms), *blue* (cattle farms) and *green* (pig farms) *circles* (*C. jejuni*) and *triangles* (*C. coli*)

Japanese study [20] examined the correlation between the crop and actual stomach content and the prevalence of *C. jejuni*, and found a negative correlation between vegetable stomach content and *C. jejuni* colonisation. Several other studies have reported that omnivorous birds such as crows and gulls foraging close to areas with human garbage and sewage have a particular risk of high carriage rates [19, 20, 24, 25].

We found a correlation between the prevalence of *C. jejuni* in wild birds and proportions in both manure on cattle and poultry farms, and between *C. coli* in wild birds and pig manure (Fig. 1). However, this correlation can only account for part of the *Campylobacter* spp. epidemiology on the farms, since some of the *C. jejuni* and *C. coli* detected in the wild birds (i.e. the *C. jejuni* in birds on pig farms and the *C. coli* in birds on the cattle farms) could not be explained by the correlation to farm manure (Fig. 1, Table 1). It is likely that bird-to-bird transmission, or sources not included in this study were responsible for the observed *Campylobacter* spp. It is also possible that the farm animals and the wild birds both acquired *Campylobacter* spp. from the same sources, but became colonised by different species adapted to their specific gut environments. An interesting aspect for further research would be to investigate why the isolation rate of *C. coli* in the wild birds during the summer sampling was so low on all farms, and why the proportion of *C. coli* in the pig manure was also lower in summer (60.2 %) than in winter (85.2 %; Table 1).

Our study showed that in summer, sparrows caught at poultry or pig farms were more likely to carry *Campylobacter* spp. than sparrows caught at cattle farms. The reason for this remains speculative, though the majority of cows were at pasture during the summer months, thus potentially resulting in minimal contact with the sparrows close to the farm buildings. Further investigation should be performed in order to evaluate this.

We anticipated that wild birds and livestock occupying very close living space might share strains locally and that this might be a key point to understand the epidemiology of *Campylobacter* spp. in wild birds on livestock farms. We realise however, that our study suffers from an inferior resolution depth, as we summarised our results at the *Campylobacter* species level and not the genotype level. We may therefore have emphasised farm factors over strain factors, which were not measured. More recent studies using MLST have shown a large degree of host specificity [12, 17, 36, 37] and minimal overlap in MLST profiles of *Campylobacter* spp. from wild birds and from poultry, cattle and humans. There was a greater similarity between the level of *C. jejuni* found in Common Starling in Sweden and Common Starling in the UK, than there was between *C. jejuni* from Swedish Common Starling

and their Swedish environment [37]. This segregation between the *Campylobacter* spp. strains in wild birds and the livestock reservoir is supported by a host attribution study [38] investigating the host association in seven housekeeping loci in 2732 published *C. jejuni* isolates from a number of sources including chicken, farm ruminants, and wild birds (passerine birds, ducks and geese). The main finding was that phylogenetically distinct *C. jejuni* lineages were associated with distinct wild birds, whereas in the farm environment, phylogenetically distant farm animals shared several *C. jejuni* lineages. Likewise, a possible adaptation of certain clonal complexes to flocks of barnacle geese in Finland has been found in a recent study [39]. Some studies note that wild birds may have a minor role in transmitting pathogenic *C. jejuni* strains to cattle [11, 13, 15] and to humans [10, 13, 15, 16, 39], whereas others found no evidence of transmission [12]. A recent study [40] found wild bird *C. jejuni* strains to be a consistent source of human disease in the UK, suggesting the existence of some more obscure epidemiological pathways between the wild bird reservoir and humans. From 2003 to 2013, the burden of campylobacteriosis cases attributed to wild birds was estimated at 10,000 per year in the UK. Therefore, it appears that the development of methods to control the transmission of *Campylobacter* spp. between livestock, humans, and wild birds requires better elucidation and understanding of the dynamics of transmission.

Conclusions

Based on the findings in this study, we conclude that the carriage of *C. jejuni* and *C. coli* in wild birds on livestock farms is correlated to the proximity to stables, feeding habits and forage areas on the ground and in vegetation. Birds with forage areas further away from livestock buildings or in the air, carried less *Campylobacter* spp. These findings suggest that wild birds may play a role in sustaining the epidemiology of *Campylobacter* spp. on farms, although this study is not able to elucidate the direction of the transmission, and further studies including genotyping are required.

Authors' contributions
MM, DLB, CR planned the study. BH coordinated the study and the laboratory work. MNS, JJM organised all sampling. JJM sampled the birds and MNS, SN sampled the livestock. EMN, MW, SN performed the *Campylobacter* spp. analyses. MC performed the data management and statistics. All authors read and approved the final manuscript.

Author details
[1] Danish Veterinary Laboratory, Department of Poultry, Fish and Fur Animals, 8200 Aarhus N, Denmark. [2] Department of Microbiology, Danish Veterinary Laboratory, 1870 Frederiksberg C, Denmark. [3] Natural History Museum of Denmark, University of Copenhagen, 1350 Copenhagen K, Denmark. [4] The Danish Meatboard, 1609 Copenhagen V, Denmark. [5] Center for Macroecology, Evolution, and Climate, Natural History Museum of Denmark, University of Copenhagen, 2100 Copenhagen Ø, Denmark. [6] Present Address: National

Food Institute, Technical University of Denmark, 2860 Søborg, Denmark. [7] Present Address: Research Unit for Clinical Microbiology, University of Southern Denmark, 5000 Odense C, Denmark. [8] Present Address: Department of Microbiology and Infection Control, Statens Serum Institut, 2300 Copenhagen S, Denmark. [9] Present Address: Imperial College London, Silwood Park Campus, Ascot, Berkshire SL5 7PY, UK. [10] Present Address: Chr. Hansen, 2970 Hørsholm, Denmark. [11] Present Address: National Veterinary Institute, Technical University of Denmark, 1870 Frederiksberg C, Denmark. [12] Present Address: Novo Nordisk, 4400 Kalundborg, Denmark. [13] Present Address: Dianova Ltd., 8200 Aarhus N, Denmark.

Acknowledgements
We would like to thank the farmers and their families for their kindness and collaboration, and Klaus B. Fries, Henning Heldbjerg, Per A. Kjær, Jan B. Kristensen, Søren H. Nielsen and Lars U. Rasmussen for their assistance with the collection of bird samples. We would also like to thank the laboratory technicians at the National Food Institute and the National Veterinary Institute for their technical support, and Monica Takamiya Wik for help with the manuscript. This project was supported by the Danish Ministry of Food, Fisheries and Agriculture under the programme for *Campylobacter* surveillance of livestock and mapping of environmental *Campylobacter* sources (1998–2001), grant No. FØSI00–6.

Competing interests
The authors declare that they have no competing interests.

References
1. European Food Safety Authority. The European Union summary report on trends and sources of zoonoses, zoonotic agents and food-borne outbreaks in 2013. EFSA J. 2015. doi:10.2903/j.efsa.2015.3991.
2. EFSA Panel on Biological Hazards (BIOHAZ). Scientific Opinion on *Campylobacter* in broiler meat production: control options and performance objectives and/or targets at different stages of the food chain. EFSA J. 2011. doi:10.2903/j.efsa.2011.2105.
3. Murray CJL, Vos T, Lozano R, Naghavi M, Flaxman AD, Michaud C, et al. Disability-adjusted life years (DALYs) for 291 diseases and injuries in 21 regions, 1990–2010: a systematic analysis for the Global Burden of Disease Study 2010. Lancet. 2012;380:2197–223. doi:10.1016/S0140-6736(12)61689-4.
4. Ray JCG, Ryan K. Sherris Medical Microbiology. 4th ed. New York: McGraw-Hill Medical; 2003. p. 378–80. doi: http://dx.doi.org/10.1036/0838585299.
5. EFSA Panel on Biological Hazards (BIOHAZ). Scientific Opinion on Quantification of the risk posed by broiler meat to human campylobacteriosis in the EU. EFSA J. 2010. doi:10.2903/j.efsa.2010.1437.
6. Friesema IHM, Havelaar AH, Westra PP, Wagenaar JA, van Pelt W. Poultry culling and campylobacteriosis reduction among humans, the Netherlands. Emerg Infect Dis. 2012;18:466–8. doi:10.3201/eid1803.111024.
7. Wagenaar JA, French NP, Havelaar AH. Preventing *Campylobacter* at the source: why is it so difficult? Clin Infect Dis. 2013;57:1600–6. doi:10.1093/cid/cit555.
8. Agunos A, Waddell L, Léger D, Taboada E. A systematic review characterizing on-farm sources of *Campylobacter* spp. for broiler chickens. PLoS ONE. 2014;9:e104905. doi:10.1371/journal.pone.0104905.
9. Craven SE, Stern NJ, Line E, Bailey JS, Cox NA, Fedorka-Cray P. Determination of the Incidence of *Salmonella* spp., *Campylobacter jejuni*, and *Clostridium perfringens* in Wild Birds near Broiler Chicken Houses by Sampling Intestinal Droppings. Avian Dis. 2000;44:715–20. doi:10.2307/1593118.
10. Colles FM, Dingle KE, Cody AJ, Maiden MCJ. Comparison of *Campylobacter* populations in wild geese with those in starlings and free-range poultry on the same farm. Appl Environ Microbiol. 2008;74:3583–90. doi:10.1128/AEM.02491-07.
11. Sippy R, Sandoval-Green CMJ, Sahin O, Plummer P, Fairbanks WS, Zhang Q, et al. Occurrence and molecular analysis of *Campylobacter* in wildlife on livestock farms. Vet Microbiol. 2012;157:369–75. doi:10.1016/j.vetmic.2011.12.026.
12. Colles FM, McCarthy ND, Howe JC, Devereux CL, Gosler AG, Maiden MCJ. Dynamics of *Campylobacter* colonization of a natural host, *Sturnus vulgaris* (European starling). Environ Microbiol. 2009;11:258–67. doi:10.1111/j.1462-2920.2008.01773.x.
13. Kwan PSL, Barrigas M, Bolton FJ, French NP, Gowland P, Kemp R, et al. Molecular epidemiology of *Campylobacter jejuni* populations in dairy cattle, wildlife, and the environment in a farmland area. Appl Environ Microbiol. 2008;74:5130–8. doi:10.1128/AEM.02198-07.
14. Hughes LA, Bennett M, Coffey P, Elliott J, Jones TR, Jones RC, et al. Molecular epidemiology and characterization of *Campylobacter* spp. isolated from wild bird populations in northern England. Appl Environ Microbiol. 2009;75:3007–15. doi:10.1128/AEM.02458-08.
15. French N, Barrigas M, Brown P, Ribiero P, Williams N, Leatherbarrow H, et al. Spatial epidemiology and natural population structure of *Campylobacter jejuni* colonizing a farmland ecosystem. Environ Microbiol. 2005;7:1116–26. doi:10.1111/j.1462-2920.2005.00782.x.
16. French NP, Midwinter A, Holland B, Collins-Emerson J, Pattison R, Colles F, et al. Molecular epidemiology of *Campylobacter jejuni* isolates from wild-bird fecal material in children's playgrounds. Appl Environ Microbiol. 2009;75:779–83. doi:10.1128/AEM.01979 08.
17. Broman T, Waldenstrom J, Dahlgren D, Carlsson I, Eliasson I, Olsen B. Diversities and similarities in PFGE profiles of *Campylobacter jejuni* isolated from migrating birds and humans. J Appl Microbiol. 2004;96:834–43. doi:10.1111/j.1365-2672.2004.02232.x.
18. Rosef O. The occurrence of *Campylobacter fetus* subsp. *jejuni* and *Salmonella* bacteria in some wild birds. Nord Vet Med. 1981;33:539–43.
19. Kapperud G, Rosef O. Avian wildlife reservoir of *Campylobacter fetus* subsp. *jejuni, Yersinia* spp., and *Salmonella* spp. in Norway. Appl Environ Microbiol. 1983;45:375–80.
20. Ito K, Kubokura Y, Kaneko K, Totake Y, Ogawa M. Occurrence of *Campylobacter jejuni* in free-living wild birds from Japan. J Wildl Dis. 1988;24:467–70. doi:10.7589/0090-3558-24.3.467.
21. Whelan CD, Monaghan P, Girdwood RWA, Fricker CR. The significance of wild birds (*Larus* sp.) in the epidemiology of *Campylobacter* infections in humans. Epidemiol Infect. 1988;101:259–67. doi:10.1017/S0950026800054170.
22. Chuma T, Hashimoto S, Okamoto K. Detection of Thermophilic *Campylobacter* from Sparrows by Multiplex PCR: the role of sparrows as a source of contamination of broilers with *Campylobacter*. J Vet Med Sci. 2000;62:1291–5. doi:10.1292/jvms.62.1291.
23. Broman T, Palmgren H, Bergstrom S, Sellin M, Waldenstrom J, Danielsson-Tham M-L, et al. *Campylobacter jejuni* in Black-Headed Gulls (*Larus ridibundus*): prevalence, genotypes, and influence on C. *jejuni* epidemiology. J Clin Microbiol. 2002;40:4594–602. doi:10.1128/JCM.40.12.4594-4602.2002.
24. Ramos R, Cerdà-Cuéllar M, Ramírez F, Jover L, Ruiz X. Influence of refuse sites on the prevalence of *Campylobacter* spp. and *Salmonella* serovars in seagulls. Appl Environ Microbiol. 2010;76:3052–6. doi:10.1128/AEM.02524-09.
25. Keller J, Shriver IWG, Waldenström J, Griekspoor P, Olsen B. Prevalence of *Campylobacter* in wild birds of the mid-atlantic region, USA. J Wildl Dis. 2011;47:750–4. doi:10.7589/0090-3558-47.3.750.
26. Simberloff D, Dayan T. The guild concept and the structure of ecological communities. Annu Rev Ecol Syst. 1991;22:115–43. doi:10.1146/annurev.es.22.110191.000555.
27. Gotelli NJ, Graves GR, Rahbek C. Macroecological signals of species interactions in the Danish avifauna. Proc Natl Acad Sci USA. 2010;107:5030–5. doi:10.1073/pnas.0914089107.
28. Waldenstrom J, Broman T, Carlsson I, Hasselquist D, Achterberg RP, Wagenaar JA, et al. Prevalence of *Campylobacter jejuni, Campylobacter lari,* and *Campylobacter coli* in different ecological guilds and taxa of migrating birds. Appl Environ Microbiol. 2002;68:5911–7. doi:10.1128/AEM.68.12.5911-5917.2002.
29. Skov MN, Madsen JJ, Rahbek C, Lodal J, Jespersen JB, Jørgensen JC, et al. Transmission of *Salmonella* between wildlife and meat-production animals in Denmark. J Appl Microbiol. 2008;105:1558–68. doi:10.1111/j.1365-2672.2008.03914.x.
30. Skov MN, Carstensen B, Tornoe N, Madsen M. Evaluation of sampling methods for the detection of *Salmonella* in broiler flocks. J Appl Microbiol. 1999;86:695–700. doi:10.1046/j.1365-2672.1999.00715.x.

31. Wedderkopp A, Rattenborg E, Madsen M. National surveillance of *Campylobacter* in broilers at slaughter in Denmark in 1998. Avian Dis. 2000;44:993. doi:10.2307/1593078.
32. Anonymous. Nordic Committé on Food Analysis, 2nd ed. Methodic no. 119: *Campylobacter jejuni/coli* detection in foods. Esbo, Finland: Statens Tekniska Forskningscentral; 1990.
33. Dohoo IR, Martin W, Stryhn HE. Veterinary Epidemiologic Research. Charlottetown: P.E.I: University of Prince Edward Island; 2003. p. 335–69.
34. Kaiser A. A new multi-category classification of subcutaneous fat deposits of songbirds. J F Ornithol. 1993;64:246–55.
35. Sensale M, Cuomo A, Dipineto L, Santaniello A, Calabria M, Menna LF, et al. Survey of *Campylobacter jejuni* and *Campylobacter coli* in different taxa and ecological guilds of migratory birds. Ital J Anim Sci. 2006;5:291–4. doi:10.4081/ijas.2006.291.
36. de Haan CPA, Lampén K, Corander J, Hänninen M-L. Multilocus sequence types of environmental *Campylobacter jejuni* isolates and their similarities to those of human, poultry and bovine *C. jejuni* isolates. Zoonoses Public Health. 2013;60:125–33. doi:10.1111/j.1863-2378.2012.01525.x.
37. Griekspoor P, Colles FM, McCarthy ND, Hansbro PM, Ashhurst-Smith C, Olsen B, et al. Marked host specificity and lack of phylogeographic population structure of *Campylobacter jejuni* in wild birds. Mol Ecol. 2013;22:1463–72. doi:10.1111/mec.12144.
38. Sheppard SK, Colles FM, McCarthy ND, Strachan NJC, Ogden ID, Forbes KJ, et al. Niche segregation and genetic structure of *Campylobacter jejuni* populations from wild and agricultural host species. Mol Ecol. 2011;20:3484–90. doi:10.1111/j.1365-294X.2011.05179.x.
39. Llarena A-K. Skarp-de Haan CPA, Rossi M, Hänninen M-L. Characterization of the *Campylobacter jejuni* population in the barnacle geese reservoir. Zoonoses Public Health. 2015;62:209–21. doi:10.1111/zph.12141.
40. Cody AJ, McCarthy ND, Bray JE, Wimalarathna HML, Colles FM, van Rensburg MJ, et al. Wild bird associated *Campylobacter jejuni* isolates are a consistent source of human disease, in Oxfordshire, United Kingdom. Environ Microbiol Rep. 2015. doi:10.1111/1758-2229.12314.

17

Prevalence of helminth and coccidian parasites in Swedish outdoor cats and the first report of *Aelurostrongylus abstrusus* in Sweden: a coprological investigation

Giulio Grandi[1]* ⓘ, Arianna Comin[2], Osama Ibrahim[1], Roland Schaper[3], Ulrika Forshell[4] and Eva Osterman Lind[1]

Abstract

Background: This study was performed in order to gather recent epidemiological data on feline endoparasites in Swedish cats. Faecal samples from 205 outdoor cats were collected by their owners and submitted to the National Veterinary Institute for analysis. The study population was comprised of cats with access to an outdoor environment and with no history of anthelmintic treatment within the last 3 months. Intestinal parasites were detected with a centrifugal flotation technique and Baermann larval sedimentation was performed to detect metastrongylid lungworms. Eggs, larvae and oocysts were identified morphologically by microscopic examination. The following information was collected from cat owners: breed, sex, age, anthelminthic medication last used, observation of cestode proglottids and residential address.

Results: Endoparasites were detected in 25% of samples. Eggs of *Toxocara cati* were found in 21% of samples, followed by taeniid eggs (4%), oocysts of *Cystoisospora felis/C. rivolta* and capillarid eggs (both 1%). One cat tested positive for *Toxoplasma gondii*-like oocysts. Larvae of *Aelurostrongylus abstrusus* were detected in one cat, which is the first published observation of this parasite in Sweden.

Conclusions: The occurrence of intestinal parasites is rather high in outdoor cats in Sweden, which could indicate the need for more intensive deworming routines in the population. Clinical practitioners should be aware of the possible occurence of *A. abstrusus* in Swedish cats when considering potential causes of respiratory problems in cats in the future.

Keywords: Feline parasites, *Toxocara cati*, *Aelurostrongylus abstrusus*

Background

A survey carried out in 2012 on the feline population in Sweden reported 1,159,000 cats, which is a slight decrease compared to a previous study performed in 2006 [1]. About 20% of them lived in households with children, that together with other categories, i.e. pregnant women and immunocompromised individuals are at high risk of being infected and develop diseases related to feline parasites [1]. Apart from the anecdotal cosmopolitan distribution of the most common feline endoparasitic helminths, like *Toxocara cati*, *Toxascaris leonina*, *Taenia (Hydatygera) taeniaeformis* and *Aelurostrongylus abstrusus* [2–4], little is known about the status of infection in outdoor cats in Sweden, since they are not routinely tested for parasitic infections. The majority of faecal samples submitted for parasitological examination comes from cats showing clinical signs such as expulsion of helminths and diarrhoea. Moreover, little is known about the deworming frequency, partly because most anthelmintics for cats are purchased without the involvement of a veterinarian, making it difficult to collect figures about common deworming

*Correspondence: giulio.grandi@sva.se
[1] Department of Microbiology, National Veterinary Institute (SVA), Ulls väg 2B, 75189 Uppsala, Sweden
Full list of author information is available at the end of the article

practices. Moreover, it is difficult to quantify the use of fenbendazole for deworming since this drug is also frequently used in cats for (off-label) treatment/control of *Giardia* spp. infection.

Regarding ascarids, the Swedish Medical Products Agency recommends the first treatment to be carried out between the fourth and the sixth week of life and repeated every 2–4 weeks, depending on the substance, until the kittens are delivered to their new owners. The queen should be dewormed at the same time. Further treatments of adult cats against ascarids (and cestodes) are recommended when there is evidence of infection [5]. Since indoor cats are generally less exposed to the risk of helminth infections from the environment [6], the main goal of the present study was to investigate the prevalence of endoparasitic infections in outdoor cats. The other two aims were to carry out for the first time a large scale parasitological survey of metastrongylid lungworms in Sweden and to investigate potential risk factors related to animal management for the presence of parasites. Beyond the lack of any previous information, a deeper epidemiological study regarding *A. abstrusus* was needed due both to the reported presence of this parasite in bordering countries (Denmark and Norway, see [7, 8]) and to the relatively high frequency of findings of *Crenosoma vulpis* in Swedish dogs during the last years. In fact, between 9.4 and 9.7% of canine faecal samples analysed with the Baermann test (more than 500 samples have been tested yearly at the National Veterinary Institute (SVA) during the last 3 years) showed the presence of *C. vulpis* (SVA, unpublished data). This phenomenon addresses at least some geographical areas of Sweden as a favorable environment for the development of carnivore metastrongylid lungworm infection. The collection of information about antiparasitic treatments coupled to the sample collection represented also a chance to gather some information about deworming routines, e.g. used compounds and administration frequency.

Methods

Study population

A total of 205 cats coming from all regions of Sweden were included in the study. Information regarding the study was spread via social media (Facebook) and local Veterinary Clinics across Sweden. Households with one to three cats could participate in the study and faecal samples from a maximum of two individuals per household were submitted for analysis. Further inclusion criteria were that cats should have access to outdoor environment and no anthelmintic treatment should have been undertaken within 3 months prior to sampling. If these criteria were fulfilled, the cat owner received a submission kit with instructions and a referral form including relevant information on cats (i.e. breed, age,

gender, neutering). A questionnaire was added to the referral form to get information on deworming practices. The owners had to reply to three questions: (a) "When was the last time you dewormed your cat and with which drug?" (b) "How often do you deworm your cat?" and (c) "Have you observed white parasitic fragments (i.e. cestode proglottids) around the anus or on the fur of your cat?".

Sample collection and parasitological examination

From each cat three samples from three different occasions within 1 week were collected directly from the ground or from the litter box and placed in individual plastic bags. The total sample volume should be at least 50 ml. Multiple samples were requested in order to increase the probability of finding parasites. Samples were stored at 4–6 °C until shipment to SVA, where they were analysed on the day of arrival. Gastrointestinal parasites were detected with a centrifugal flotation technique employing a flotation solution of saturated salt and 500 g/l sugar (specific gravity 1.28). Briefly, faeces from each of the three samples, totally between 3 and 5 g, were dissolved in the flotation solution, passed through a sieve (150 μm aperture), transferred to a Clayton-Lane centrifuge 15 ml tube. A glass coverslip 18 × 18 mm was placed on the tube that was then centrifuged at $214 \times g$ for 5 min in a Thermo Fisher Scientific—Sorvall ST40 centrifuge (Life Technologies Europe BV, Stockholm, Sweden) equipped with a swing out rotor [15, 16]. After centrifugation, the coverslip was transferred to a microscope slide and examined for parasites at a magnification of 100–400× by one of two experienced biomedical scientists. A minimum of 10 fields were carefully examined at 400×. The reading was done in a blinded fashion, i.e. without any information about the cats. Results were recorded semi-quantitatively as follows: no, few, low number, moderate number, high number and very high number of eggs/oocysts. This technique does not allow the detection of protozoan parasites like *Giardia* and *Cryptosporidium*. Since taeniid cestode eggs are not shed in the intestine but originate from disintegrating proglottids, flotation is not considered the best method for cestode diagnosis; for this reason, the observation of cestode proglottids by the owner was recorded as information to be used in the risk factor analysis.

Presence of metastrongylid lungworms was assessed with a modified Baermann larval sedimentation. Approximately 10 g of faeces were enclosed in cotton-gauze, placed in a glass funnel closed at the bottom extremity with metal clumps and incubated at least 24 h at 20 °C. The first 15 ml were collected then from the bottom of the Baermann apparatus and centrifuged at $214 \times g$ for 5 min. The sediment in the test tube was transferred onto microscope slides, mixed with a drop of Lugol's iodine stain and examined at the magnification of 100×.

Parasitic elements (PE: eggs, oocysts, larvae) were identified morphologically according to [16, 17]. Eggs of *T. cati*, oocysts of *C. felis/C.rivolta* and larvae of *A. abstrusus* could be identified to species level based on their morphology and or size, while capillarid eggs were not identified to species level. Since no molecular analyses were employed, "small" coccidia were defined as *Toxoplasma*-like oocysts, even if this definition can include other parasites as *Hammondia* sp. Molecular identification performed in other cases of Swedish cats have shown that these oocysts belong to *Toxoplasma gondii* (SVA, unpublished results). Regarding taeniid eggs, different species are morphologically indistinguishable and since no polymerase chain reaction (PCR) was performed, species could not be determined and it cannot be excluded that some of them were eggs of *Echinococcus multilocularis*, even if it has been shown that are only rarely infected by this parasite and moreover in Sweden *E. multilocularis* eggs or DNA have only been detected in faeces from foxes [18, 19]. Based on previous data from necropsy studies performed on Swedish cats the likelihood that these eggs belong to *T. taeniaeformis* is very high.

Statistical analysis

The study population was characterized according to (i) animal-level variables: gender (female vs. male), neutering (no vs. yes), age (≤1 year vs. >1 year old), breed (purebred vs. crossbred); (ii) temporal variables: season of testing (first, second, third of fourth quarter of the year); (iii) managerial variables: occurrence of last deworming treatment (never, <1 year before, ≥1 year before), deworming frequency (never, once/year, twice/year or more), and observation of cestode proglottids (no vs. yes).

To investigate the role of the above-mentioned variables as potential risk factors for the presence of feline endoparasites, a multivariate logistic regression analysis was performed. The selection of variables to include in the final model followed the approach proposed by Bursac et al. [20]. Briefly, the selection process began with a univariate analysis of each variable. Any variable having a p value for the Wald test exceeding 0.25 was selected as a candidate for the multivariate analysis. Subsequently, variables were checked for possible confounding and or effect modification, by looking at crude and adjusted odds ratios. At the end of this iterative process of deleting, refitting, and verifying, the model contained significant covariates, interactions and confounders. At this point any variable not selected for the original multivariate model was added back one at a time, to identify those which were not significantly related to the outcome but made an important contribution in the presence of other variables. The final multivariate model included the variables breed, observation of cestodes, deworming frequency and interactions between breed and observation of cestodes and between deworming frequency and observation of cestodes.

Results

The majority (80%; n = 137) of cat owners in the present study (n = 171) sent faecal samples from one cat, while only 20% (n = 34) sampled two cats from the same household. Totally, 25% of the cats tested positive for parasitic faecal stages (Table 1). The most frequent parasites were ascarids, with eggs of *T. cati* being diagnosed in 20% of the samples, followed by 4% of samples positive for taeniid eggs and only 1% other endoparasites, oocysts of coccidia (*C. felis/C. rivolta*) and capillarid eggs. One cat tested positive for *T. gondii*-like oocysts. *A. abstrusus* larvae were observed in one cat from the county of Scania; the same cat shed capillarid eggs. This is the first published observation of *A. abstrusus* in Sweden.

Regarding intensity of infection, a variability was observed only for *T. cati*, those eggs were detected

Table 1 Results of the parasitological examination

Parasite	Samples (n)	% of positive samples	95% exact binomial confidence interval
Toxocara cati	43	20.98	[15.62–27.20]
Taeniid eggs	8	3.90	[1.70–7.54]
Capillarid eggs	3	1.46	[0.30–4.22]
Cystoisospora felis	1	0.49	[0.00–2.69]
Cystoisospora rivolta	1	0.49	[0.00–2.69]
Toxoplasma gondii-like	1	0.49	[0.00–2.69]
Aelurostrongylus abstrusus	1	0.49	[0.00–2.69]
Total positive samples	52	25.36	[19.56–31.90]
Total amount of collected samples	205	–	

between few number and very high number, in most cases between moderate and high number (data not shown).

Regarding the drugs used to deworm cats (Table 2), 44% of the owners did not provide information regarding substances used to deworm the cats. As expected the two most commonly used drugs were the prescription-free ones (milbemycin + praziquantel and fenbendazole), used by 62% of the owners that provided this information. The third most commonly used product (used by 16% of the owners that provided information on deworming products) was a combination of emodepside + praziquantel, that is sold on prescription.

According to the univariate logistic analysis, crossbreed (vs. purebred) and observation of cestodes seemed potential risk factors for having endoparasites (Table 3). However, results of the multivariate logistic analysis—which is more comprehensive since it allows to consider several variables at the same time and to correct for possible confounding and interactions—showed that none of the investigated variables were significant risk factors for the study population.

Discussion

The scope of this study was to investigate the occurrence of parasites in privately owned outdoor cats by faecal analyses. The results confirm that *T. cati* and taeniid cestodes are the most common feline endoparasites in Sweden. The occurrence was higher than previously thought—higher than in samples analysed within the

Table 2 Drugs used by cat owners included in the study at the latest deworming occasion

Drug	% of cats (n = 205)	% of households (n = 171)
Milbemycin + praziquantel	22.4 (n = 46)	20.5 (n = 35)
Fenbendazole	13.7 (n = 28)	14 (n = 24)
Pyrantel embonate + praziquantel	2.9 (n = 6)	2.9 (n = 5)
Praziquantel	3.4 (n = 7)	3.5 (n = 6)
Emodepside + praziquantel	8.3 (n = 17)	8.8 (n = 15)
Selamectin	1 (n = 2)	0.6 (n = 1)
Pyrantel embonate	5.4 (n = 11)	5.3 (n = 9)
Not specified/applicable	42.9 (n = 88)	44.4 (n = 76)

Table 3 Characterization of the study population: number, proportion, 95% exact binomial confidence intervals (CI) and results of univariate logistic analyses of the parasite-positive cats by the main variables (outcome variable = presence of parasites yes/no)

Variable	Trait	Number of positive samples	Number of samples	Proportion of positive samples	Exact binomial 95% CI	Wald test	p value
Gender	Female	21	96	0.22	[0.14–0.31]	1.20	0.28
	Male	31	109	0.28	[0.20–0.38]		
Neutering	No	31	127	0.24	[0.17–0.33]	0.16	0.69
	Yes	21	78	0.27	[0.18–0.38]		
Age	<1 year	7	22	0.32	[0.14–0.55]	0.12	0.73
	≥1 year	45	180	0.25	[0.19–0.32]		
Breed	Purebred	7	50	0.14	[0.06–0.27]	4.60	*0.032*
	Crossbred	44	148	0.30	[0.23–0.38]		
Testing period	Jan–Mar	12	49	0.24	[0.13–0.39]	1.30	0.73
	Apr–Jun	6	20	0.30	[0.12–0.54]		
	Jul–Sep	6	33	0.18	[0.07–0.35]		
	Oct–Dec	28	103	0.27	[0.19–0.37]		
Observation of proglottids on fur	No	21	122	0.17	[0.11–0.25]	11.2	*0.0008*
	Yes	30	77	0.39	[0.28–0.51]		
Last deworming treatment	Never	2	13	0.15	[0.02–0.45]	1.60	0.44
	<1 year before	29	95	0.31	[0.21–0.41]		
	≥1 year before	16	65	0.25	[0.15–0.37]		
Deworming frequency	Never	11	53	0.21	[0.11–0.34]	2.50	0.25
	Once/year	21	83	0.25	[0.16–0.36]		
	Twice/year or more	19	56	0.34	[0.22–0.48]		

Italic values indicate p < 0.05

routine diagnostics, where 5% of the cats shed helminth eggs (SVA, unpublished data, 2015–2016). Furthermore, it was assessed that none of the tested animal- and managerial-level variables was a significant risk factor for the presence of such parasites.

Cats can acquire infection by *T. cati* by different routes, either by ingesting infective eggs from the environment or ingesting larvae contained in rodents and other paratenic hosts or by ingestion of larvae passed in the milk by the queen (transmammary infection). Even if it has not been assessed which one of these routes is the most frequently involved in the transmission of the parasite, based on previous studies [2] it seems that ingestion of larvae present in paratenic hosts linked to hunting behavior of cats is considerably significant.

Regarding the most common cestode parasite of cats (*T. taeniaeformis*), cats become infected exclusively by ingesting the metacestode stage (strobilocercus) that develops in several species of rodents and potentially even in lagomorphs that have acquired infection through the ingestion of taeniid eggs [2].

In the case of coccidia, cats can become infected both by direct ingestion of sporulated oocysts or by ingestion of tissues of paratenic hosts containing coccidian sporozoites and usually infection is more common in kittens [2]. Since the cat population considered in the present study is biased towards adult cats, it is not surprising that these parasites occurred only in few animals.

The only results available from coprological analyses in Swedish cats come from a published summary of the results from 1371 samples submitted to SVA between the years 1958 and 1970 [9]. In comparison to our study, a similar amount of eggs of *T. cati* (19.4%) was detected whereas a higher amount of taeniid eggs (9.1%) and oocysts of *Cystoisospora* spp. (4%) were recorded. Moreover, eggs of several other helminths that were not recorded in the present study (*Toxascaris leonina, Uncinaria stenocephala, Cryptocotyle linguae, Opistorchis felineus, Diphyllobotrium latum, Dipylidium caninum*) were found, indicating that new available anthelmintics as well as improved deworming routines may have reduced the spectrum of parasitic infections in cats during the last decades. However, data collected from diagnostic routine cannot be regarded as representative of a general cat population.

Few other data are available regarding endoparasitic infections in Swedish cats. Two necropsy studies have been previously carried out in Sweden on a random population of cats. In the first one—performed on 83 cats from the area of Stockholm, Sweden [10]—19.3% of the cats were infected by *T. cati* and 9.6% of the cats were infected by *T. taeniaeformis*. One of the cats was infected

by *Mesocestoides lineatus*. In the second study—performed on 100 cats from the county of Halland, Sweden [11]—61 and 31% of outdoor cats (n = 70) were infected with *T. cati* and *T. taeniaeformis*, respectively. Moreover, *Ancylostoma tubaeforme* was found in one cat and *Eucoleus aerophilus* in another. Even though these results come from necropsy studies, where more data on the occurrence of immature stages, species identification and intensity of infections can be recorded, both studies are in agreement with present observations, i.e. that *T. cati* and taeniid cestodes are the most common feline parasites in Sweden.

Analysis by a concentration McMaster technique of faecal samples (n = 95) from a population of necropsied Danish cats showed a much higher prevalence of parasitic infection (77.9%) in comparison to the present study. Eggs of *T. cati* were the most common (69.5%), followed by capillarid type eggs (16.8%), taeniid eggs (9.5%), oocysts of *C. felis* (2.1%) and strongyle type eggs (1.1%) [12]. A possible explanation for such high prevalence values can be the characteristics of the sampled population (92 of 99 cats examined by necropsy were feral). Another survey performed by flotation of faecal samples of 719 Danish shelter cats showed prevalence figures similar to our study (35.6 and 3.5% of cats infected by *T cati* and *T. taeniaeformis*, respectively, followed by lower prevalence of coccidia and *E. aerophilus*), but a slightly higher variety of parasites (*T. leonina* and *U. stenocephala* were found) [13].

Another recent survey carried out in Finland on faecal samples from 411 cats (63.5% with access to outdoor environment), also showed that the most common parasites were *T. cati* and *T. taeniaeformis* (5.4 and 1.7% of cats were infected, respectively). *T. leonina* and *C. felis* were found in few animals; *Giardia* sp. was detected in 3.2% of the cats using an ELISA kit. Outdoor cats showed a higher prevalence of infection for *T. cati* (7.28%) than indoor cats (2.50%), an observation that supports the higher exposure to infection of this class of animals. Also, cats receiving homemade food in the diet, as well as cats from rural areas showed higher risk of being infected by *T. cati*. In agreement with the present study, also cats where the owners had seen proglottids and non-purebred cats had a higher chance of being infected by *T. cati* [14].

Based on the present results clinicians should be aware that cats with access to outdoor environment can harbour feline ascarids as well as taeniid cestodes, and therefore an implementation of deworming routines is needed. Our suggestion is that a regular, monthly deworming of outdoor cats with substances active against nematodes and cestodes should be performed during the "hunting season", i.e. whenever they have access to prey.

Regarding feline metastrongylid lungworms, this is the first published observation of their occurrence in Sweden. The cat that was shedding *A. abstrusus* larvae in the present study was a five-and-a-half-year-old female that was born on a farm and had never travelled abroad. Moreover, she had been dewormed in May 2014 (6 months before the time of sampling) with a product containing milbemycin oxime and praziquantel. Cats can become infected by *A. abstrusus* by ingesting third larval stages of the parasite that develop into several molluscan intermediate hosts; several paratenic hosts have been identified (rodents, birds, reptiles). It is unclear how often infection is due to direct ingestion of intermediate hosts rather than ingestion of paratenic hosts. According to recent studies infective larvae can even be released into the environment by snails, thus increasing the chances of cats to become infected [3]. The present finding is not surprising since the presence of *A. abstrusus* in Norway was documented long ago [8] and since this parasite is relatively common in Denmark [12]. In a recent Danish study, the prevalence of *A. abstrurus* in 147 outdoor cats from Zealand, Møn and Falster regions ranged between 13.6 and 15.6% depending on the method employed; in the Southern regions prevalence peaked to 72.7% [12]. It is difficult to say if *A. abstrusus* has been recently introduced into Sweden but probably this parasite has been unnoticed until now because of its low prevalence in Swedish cats, its uneven geographical distribution and because of the fact that few cats are tested for metastrongylid lungworms and common flotation methods do not allow detection of this parasite.

Even if more data is needed to assess the importance of feline zoonotic endoparasites as a source of human infections it can be assumed that the presence of such parasites (*T. cati* and probably *T. gondii*) can represent a potential source of environmental contamination. This information should be taken in account by all healthcare professionals. Faecal analysis could be useful for diagnosing patent *T. cati* infections. Taeniid cestode eggs are more difficult to detect by flotation since they generally are not liberated from the proglottids.

It is desirable that in the near future figures from necropsies of outdoor feral cats, as well a more widespread testing of cats for metastrongylid lungworms will provide a more detailed picture of the parasitic populations of Swedish cats, both in terms of intensity and of variety.

Conclusions

The results indicated that outdoor cats in Sweden are regularly exposed to endoparasitic infections and the predominant role of *T. cati* was confirmed, followed by taeniid parasites. Current Swedish deworming recommendations assume that the prevalence of feline parasites in adult cats in Sweden is quite low, a statement that according to the present study is not true in the case of cats with outdoor access. Such cats—including adult ones—should receive regular anthelmintic treatments whenever they access to prey or whenever parasites are observed. Demonstrated presence of feline *A. abstrusus* in Sweden should be also taken in account by practitioners as one of the causes of respiratory signs.

Authors' contributions

GG, EOL and UF planned the study, GG and UF managed collection of samples, OI analyzed the samples and interpreted the results. AC performed statistical analysis. GG and EOL wrote the manuscript. UF and RS commented on the manuscript. All the authors read and approved the final manuscript.

Author details

[1] Department of Microbiology, National Veterinary Institute (SVA), Ulls väg 2B, 75189 Uppsala, Sweden. [2] Department of Disease Control and Epidemiology, National Veterinary Institute (SVA), Ulls väg 2B, 75651 Uppsala, Sweden. [3] Bayer Animal Health GmbH, Monheim, Germany. [4] Bayer Animal Health AB, Solna, Sweden.

Acknowledgements

Many veterinary clinics in Sweden helped with sample collection and spreading of information regarding the project. Eva Wattrang, Anna Lundén and Holly Cedervind (SVA) reviewed language of the manuscript. Staff at SVA—Parasitology is thanked for helping in managing samples and recording samples' data.

Competing interests

The authors declare that they have no competing interests. Ulrika Forshell is employee at Bayer AB, Solna, Sweden. Roland Schaper is employee at Bayer Animal Health, Leverkusen, Germany.

Funding

This study was funded by Bayer AB, Solna, Sweden that covered the costs of the analyses.

References

1. Statistiska Centralbyrån (Statistics Sweden). Hundar, katter och andra sällskapsdjur 2012. Statistiska Centralbyrån; 2012. p. 33. http://www.skk.se/Global/Dokument/Om-SKK/SCB-undersokning-Hundar-katter-och-andra-sallskapsdjur-2012.pdf. Accessed 24 Nov 2016.
2. Bowman DD, Hendrix CM, Lindsay DS, Barr SC. Feline clinical parasitology. 1st ed. Ames: Iowa State University Press; 2002.
3. Elsheikha HM, Schnyder M, Traversa D, Di Cesare A, Wright I, Lacher DW. Updates on feline aelurostrongylosis and research priorities for the next decade. Parasit Vectors. 2016. doi:10.1186/s13071-016-1671-6.

4. Di Cesare A, Veronesi F, Grillotti E, Manzocchi S, Perrucci S, Beraldo P, et al. Respiratory nematodes in cat populations of Italy. Parasitol Res. 2015;114:4463–9. doi:10.1007/s00436-015-4687-5.

5. Läkemedelsverket (Swedish Medical Products Agency). Ekto-och endo-parasiter hos hund och katt—ehandlingsrekommendation. In: Information från Läkemedelsverket. 2014; 25 Suppl: 12–3.

6. Fisher M. Toxocara cati: an underestimated zoonotic agent. Trends Parasitol. 2003;19(4):167–70.

7. Olsen CS, Willesen JL, Pipper CB, Mejer H. Occurrence of *Aelurostrongylus abstrusus* (Railliet 1898) in Danish cats: a modified lung digestion method for isolating adult worms. Vet Parasitol. 2015;210:32–9. doi:10.1016/j.vetpar.2015.03.016.

8. Berg C. *Aelurostrongylus abstrusus* in cats—a case report. Norsk VetTidsskr. 1979;91:503–7 **(In Norwegian)**.

9. Persson L. Endoparasites in dogs and cats. Svensk VetTidn. 1971;23:73–8 **(In Swedish)**.

10. Persson L. Roundworms and tapeworms in cats from Stockholm. Svensk VetTidn. 1973;25:214–6 **(In Swedish)**.

11. Persson L. Gastrointestinal parasites in cats from Halland. Svensk VetTidn. 1982;34:569–72 **(In Swedish)**.

12. Takeuchi-Storm N, Mejer H, Al-Sabi MN, Olsen CS, Thamsborg SM, Enemark HL. Gastrointestinal parasites of cats in Denmark assessed by necropsy and concentration McMaster technique. Vet Parasitol. 2015;214:327–32. doi:10.1016/j.vetpar.2015.06.033.

13. Ingstrup A. Parasites in Danish cats—the prevalence in 719 cats. Thesis in companion animal and clinical sciences. University of Copenhagen; 2008. https://www.ddd.dk/sektioner/fagdyrl%C3%A6geforeninger/hundkatsmaedyr/opgaver/Documents/2009-01%20Astrid%20Ingstrup.pdf. Accessed 20 Mar 2017 **(In Danish)**.

14. Nareaho A, Puomio J, Saarinen K, Jokelainen P, Juselius T, Sukura A. Feline intestinal parasites in Finland: prevalence, risk factors and anthelmintic treatment practices. J Feline Med Surg. 2012;14:378–83. doi:10.1177/1098612x12439257.

15. Anon. Manual of veterinary parasitological laboratory techniques. 3rd ed. London: Ministry of Agriculture, Fisheries and Food. London: Her Majesty's Stationary Office; 1986.

16. Soulsby EJL. Helminths, Arthtopods and protozoa of domesticated animals. 7th ed. London: Bailliere Tindall; 1982.

17. Thienpont D, Rochette F, Vanparjs OFJ. Diagnosing helminthiasis through coprological examination. Beerse: Janssen Research Foundation; 1979.

18. Miller AL, Olsson GE, Sollenberg S, Skarin M, Wahlstrom H, Hoglund J. Support for targeted sampling of red fox (*Vulpes vulpes*) feces in Sweden: a method to improve the probability of finding *Echinococcus multilocularis*. Parasit Vectors. 2016. doi:10.1186/s13071-016-1897-3.

19. Oksanen A, Siles-Lucas M, Karamon J, Possenti A, Conraths FJ, Romig T, et al. The geographical distribution and prevalence of *Echinococcus multilocularis* in animals in the European Union and adjacent countries: a systematic review and meta-analysis. Parasit Vectors. 2016. doi:10.1186/s13071-016-1746-4.

20. Bursać Z, Gauss CH, Williams DK, Hosmer DW. Purposeful selection of variables in logistic regression. Sour Code Biol Med. 2008. doi:10.1186/1751-0473-3-17.

18

Systemic inflammation in dogs with advanced-stage heart failure

Aleksandra Domanjko Petrič* ⓘ, Tajda Lukman, Barbara Verk and Alenka Nemec Svete

Abstract

Background: Although human studies have shown that inflammation plays a role in the development of congestive heart failure, scarce information exists on white blood cell count (WBC) and differential cell counts in various stages of heart failure in man and dogs. A few studies demonstrated increased concentrations of C-reactive protein (CRP), a major acute-phase protein, in cardiac diseases In dogs. Our research aimed to investigate whether CRP concentration, WBC and neutrophil count (NEUT), as markers of systemic inflammation, are elevated in canine cardiovascular patients. We also aimed to find out whether there is an association between CRP concentration and WBC and NEUT, as well as associations between these inflammatory markers and selected echocardiographic parameters. Sixty-two client-owned canine cardiac patients and 12 healthy dogs were included in the study. The patients were classified into International Small Animal Cardiac Health Council classes (ISACHC I–III). The serum CRP concentration was determined using a canine CRP test kit. WBC and NEUT were determined using an automated hematology analyzer.

Results: Significantly higher serum CRP concentration, WBC and NEUT were found in the decompensated stage of heart failure (ISACHC III) compared with healthy dogs and with patients in ISACHC group II and ISACHC group I. Serum CRP concentration significantly positively correlated with WBC ($r = 0.65$, $P < 0.001$) and NEUT ($r = 0.58$, $P = 0.002$) in the ISACHC III group, while no significant correlations were found in the ISACHC I and II groups. A significant negative correlation between serum CRP concentration and the left ventricular ejection fraction ($r = -0.49$, $P = 0.046$) and a significant positive correlation between CRP and the E wave velocity of the mitral valve inflow ($r = 0.52$, $P = 0.046$) were found in the ISACHC III group.

Conclusions: The CRP concentration, WBC and NEUT were significantly increased in advanced-stage heart failure patients in comparison with compensated patients and healthy dogs, which indicate the presence of systemic inflammation. However, normal CRP concentration and normal WBC and NEUT can also be present in heart failure.

Keywords: Congestive heart failure, C-reactive protein, Dogs, Leukocytes, Neutrophils

Background

Inflammation plays a role in the pathogenesis and progression of many forms of heart failure, and biomarkers of inflammation have become the subject of intensive investigations in human and veterinary medicine [1, 2]. In humans, C-reactive protein (CRP), measured using a high sensitivity CRP assay (hsCRP assay), as marker of inflammation has received the most attention [3–5]. Concentrations of CRP previously considered to be normal have been shown to predict future cardiovascular events independently in initially healthy individuals, as well as in human cardiovascular patients [4–8]. CRP is a major acute-phase protein in dogs that is characterized by a marked change in serum concentration consistent with systemic inflammatory activity [9–12]. It is produced primarily by the liver in response to proinflammatory cytokines, such as interleukin-1, interleukin-6 and tumor necrosis factor alpha [9, 12].

Several clinical studies have demonstrated significant alterations in some of the inflammatory markers in canine cardiovascular patients [13–18]. Increased concentrations of CRP have been demonstrated in acquired [14, 16–18] and congenital [19] cardiac diseases in dogs.

*Correspondence: aleksandra.domanjko@vf.uni-lj.si
Small Animal Clinic, Veterinary Faculty, University of Ljubljana, Gerbičeva 60, 1000 Ljubljana, Slovenia

In these studies, the CRP Enzyme-Linked ImmunoSorbent Assay [14, 18], automated canine-specific hsCRP assay [17] or human turbidimetric CRP assay, validated for use in dogs [16], were used for determination of CRP concentrations in serum or plasma. Moreover, in dogs with myxomatous mitral valve disease (MMVD) and dilated cardiomyopathy, plasma CRP concentration was associated with disease severity [17, 18]. However, no associations were found between serum CRP concentration, measured using a hsCRP assay, and severity of asymptomatic MMVD [17].

White blood cell count (WBC) is a marker of systemic inflammation, but data on its association with heart failure risk are limited in humans [20–22] and dogs [13, 23]. Moreover, WBC and the percentages of neutrophils, lymphocytes and eosinophils upon admission were found to be significant predictors of the development of congestive heart failure (CHF) in patients with acute myocardial infarction [24]. During years of clinical work, we observed that dogs in CHF had elevated WBC and neutrophil count (NEUT), which leads many practitioners to unjustified use of antibiotics (personal observations). Higher WBC and NEUT and markedly lower total lymphocyte count, as well as percentages of lymphocyte subpopulations in dogs in severe CHF in comparison to the control group were observed also by Farabaugh et al. [13] and Deepti and Yathiraj [23] recently found leukocytosis in CHF dogs.

We hypothesize that canine heart failure patients have elevated markers of systemic inflammation (CRP, WBC and NEUT). Components of the inflammatory process contribute to the worsening and progression of heart failure and imbalance of regulatory mechanisms that maintain cardiac homeostasis [25, 26]. Our research aimed 1) to investigate whether CRP concentration, WBC and NEUT, as markers of systemic inflammation, are elevated in canine cardiovascular patients; 2) to find out whether there is an association between CRP concentration and WBC and NEUT, as well as associations between these inflammatory markers and selected echocardiographic parameters.

Methods
Animals
Eighty-one client-owned dogs of various breeds, sex, age and weight were recruited. Sixty-nine dogs were cardiovascular patients prospectively recruited, and 12 healthy dogs served as controls. The 12 control dogs were from the active rescue dog team and were judged to be healthy based upon normal history, normal clinical examination and the results of hematological and biochemical analyses. All dogs included in the study were regularly dewormed and vaccinated and none of the dogs showed eosinophilia indicative of a parasitic or allergic condition.

Cardiovascular disease was confirmed on the basis of history, clinical examination, radiographic examination of the thorax, standard electrocardiogram and echocardiography using two-dimensional, M-mode, and color and spectral Doppler modes (Vingmed System Five, General Electric Healthcare, Milwaukee, Wisconsin, USA). Nine-lead electrocardiogram was performed in the right lateral recumbence or in standing position, depending of the dog's status. Echocardiography was done according to the recommendations [27]. Left ventricular internal dimensions in diastole and systole were indexed to body weight in kg raised by the exponent according to Cornell et al. [28]. Left ventricular ejection fraction was calculated by the Teichholz method derived from M-mode measurements. Echocardiographic parameters, including left atrium dimension and diameter of the aorta ratio (LAD/Ao), percentage fractional shortening (pctFS), left ventricular dimension at end diastole index (LVDdI), left ventricular ejection fraction (LVEF), left ventricular dimension at end systole index (LVDsI) and E wave velocity of the mitral valve inflow (MVE) were used for correlation analysis to find out whether there is an association between these parameters and inflammatory markers. Dogs with concomitant non-cardiac diseases, including other diseases such as neoplasia, infections or metabolic disorders, were excluded based on the results of hematologic and biochemical analyses, ancillary laboratory tests (urinalysis, *Anaplasma phagocytophilum* (serologic and polymerase chain reaction assay), *Borrelia burgdorferi* serological testing) and abdominal ultrasound. Patients were classified into the International Small Animal Cardiac Health Council (ISACHC) classes [29]. Asymptomatic dogs with documented cardiac disease were included in ISACHC I; however, this class was not further divided. In the ISACHC II group we included dogs with documented cardiac disease and compensated, i.e. well controlled heart failure with cardiac therapy and no overt clinical signs of decompensation. In compensated heart failure, symptoms are stable and many overt features of fluid retention and pulmonary edema are absent. In the ISACHC III group, we included dogs that were in uncontrolled/decompensating heart failure at the time of inclusion. Decompensated heart failure refers to deterioration, which may present either as an acute episode of pulmonary edema or as lethargy and reduction in exercise tolerance and increasing tachypnea/dyspnea on exertion. These later dogs were either first time patients without CHF therapy or worsening of already diagnosed CHF. Criteria for the diagnosis of CHF were based on clinical signs and subjectively assessed thoracic radiography. An interstitial or alveolar pulmonary pattern compatible with pulmonary edema with left atrial enlargement and clinical signs of CHF were used to confirm CHF.

Written consent of the owners was obtained. All procedures were approved by the Ethical Committee of the Ministry of Agriculture, Forestry and Food, Veterinary Administration of the Republic of Slovenia (Animal Protection Act UL RS 43/2007).

Blood sampling and analysis

Blood was taken from the jugular or cephalic vein from fasted dogs. Blood samples for determining complete blood count (CBC) and white cell differential count (WCDC) were collected into tubes containing the anticoagulant ethylenediaminetetraacetic acid (BD Microtainer; Becton–Dickinson, Franklin Lakes, New Jersey, USA). Blood samples for determining the biochemical profile (urea, creatinine, electrolytes (sodium, potassium and chloride), alkaline phosphatase, and alanine aminotransferase; data not shown) and CRP concentrations were collected in serum separator tubes (Vacuette; Greiner Bio-One, Kremsmünster, Austria). Blood samples were centrifuged for 10 min at $1300 \times g$. CBC and WCDC were determined within 1 h after collection of the blood samples using an automated laser-based hematology analyzer (ADVIA 120, Siemens, Munich, Germany) and multispecies software, developed by the manufacturer. All settings in the software were used as provided, without adjustment or modification.

The biochemical profiles, with the exception of electrolytes, were determined with an automated biochemical analyzer (RX Daytona, Randox, Crumlin, United Kingdom) on the day of blood sample collection. The concentrations of electrolytes were determined with an electrolyte analyzer (ILyte, Instrumentation Laboratory, Lexington, MA, USA) on the day of sample collection. Serum samples for CRP measurements were frozen at − 80 °C and analyzed within 2 months. Serum CRP concentrations were determined with the canine CRP test kit (LifeAssays® Canine CRP test kit, LifeAssays®, Lund, Sweden), which is a one-step 11-min magnetic permeability based canine-specific two-site immunoassay [30, 31]. The linear range of the test kit is 10–210 mg/L. All samples were analyzed in duplicate and the mean CRP concentration was used for statistical analyses. The canine CRP control, included in the canine CRP test kit, was used to confirm the efficacy of the reagents and correct performance of the test. The control samples were analyzed according to the same procedure as for a canine sample. The detection limit (DL) of the assay was 10 mg/L. Therefore, the samples with CRP concentration of less than the DL of the assay were assigned a concentration of 10 mg/L and for statistical analysis used as such or treated with special methods.

Statistical analysis

The data were analyzed with commercial software (SPSS version 22.0, SPSS Inc, Chicago, Illinois, USA and R statistical program [32]. A value of $P < 0.05$ was considered significant. Descriptive statistics was used to describe the basic features of the data. The Shapiro–Wilk test was performed to test whether the data were normally distributed. A one-way ANOVA with Tukey Honest Significant Difference post hoc test was used to test for statistically significant differences in age between healthy dogs and individual groups of cardiac patients (ISACHC I–III). Kruskal–Wallis analysis followed by multiple comparisons was performed to compare the measured parameters (WBC, NEUT), as well as weight, between healthy dogs and individual groups of cardiac patients (ISACHC I–III). For the comparison of CRP (ISACHC I–III) a two-part model combining χ^2 and Kruskal–Wallis test [33] was used to account for the values below DL (see supplement). To control for the confounding variables (age, sex and disease etiology) two multiple linear regression models for $(\log_{10})$WBC and $(\log_{10})$NEUT each were performed (disease etiology could be controlled for only in the subset of diseased patients). A two-part model combining logistic and linear regression on diseased patients was used to account for the values below DL in CRP.

Spearman's rank correlation coefficient analysis was performed to determine the correlation between the CRP concentration and WBC and NEUT, as well as selected echocardiographic parameters (LAD/Ao, pctFS, LVDdI, LVEF, LVDsI, and MVE). The same method was used to determine correlations between CRP concentrations and the intensity of cardiac murmur grades 1–6.

Results

Seven cardiovascular patients were excluded from the group of 69 patients, due to various reasons: antibiotic therapy and dental disease (2 dogs), allergy, hypothyroidism, antibiotic therapy with suspected endocrine disorder, cachexia and lost blood sample. Sixty-two dogs of 25 different breeds with confirmed cardiovascular diseases were divided in three groups according to the ISACHC classification, based on a complete cardiovascular examination. Medication regimens included diuretics (furosemide and spironolactone), beta-blockers (atenolol), calcium-channel blockers (diltiazem), ACE (angiotensin-converting enzyme) inhibitors, an inodilator (pimobendan), and digoxin (Table 1). Cardiovascular patients were of the following breeds: Mixed breed dogs (n = 16), Doberman Pinschers (n = 5), Cavalier King Charles (n = 5), 4 Chihuahuas (n = 4), Great Danes (n = 3), German Boxers (n = 3), Italian Greyhounds (n = 3), Airedale Terriers (n = 2), Rottweilers (n = 2), Saint Bernard dogs (n = 2), German Shepherds (n = 2),

Table 1 Treatment used in groups of canine cardiac patients (ISACHC I–III)

Therapeutics	ISACHC I (N = 10) (n)	ISACHC II (N = 26) (n)	ISACHC III (N = 26) (n)
Salbutemol	1		
Furosemide		26	21
ACE inhibitor		26	13
Pimobendan	1	15	14
Atenolol (beta-blocker)		2	4
Digoxin		5	9
Diltiazem (calcium-channel blocker)		4	4
Spironolactone		4	1
Potassium chloride		5	
Total number of dogs with therapy	2	26	21

ISACHC International Small Animal Cardiac Health Council; *N* number of dogs included in ISACHC group; *n* number of dogs per ISACHC group receiving specific cardiac drug; *ACE* angiotensin-converting enzyme

Table 2 Baseline characteristics in healthy dogs and groups of canine cardiac patients (ISACHC I–III)

Group	Healthy	ISACHC I	ISACHC II	ISACHC III
Number	12	10	26	26
Sex (female/male)	9/3	3/7	8/18	7/19
Age (years) mean ± SD	6.7 ± 3.4	7.3 ± 3.7	10.8 ± 3.9*	10.3 ± 4.1*
Weight (kg)				
Median	28.7	14.0	9.9	26.4
Interquartile range	22.5–33.0	6.2–45.7	6.9–36.0	10.5–32.8

ISACHC International Small Animal Cardiac Health Council; *SD* standard deviation

* $P < 0.05$ in comparison with healthy dogs

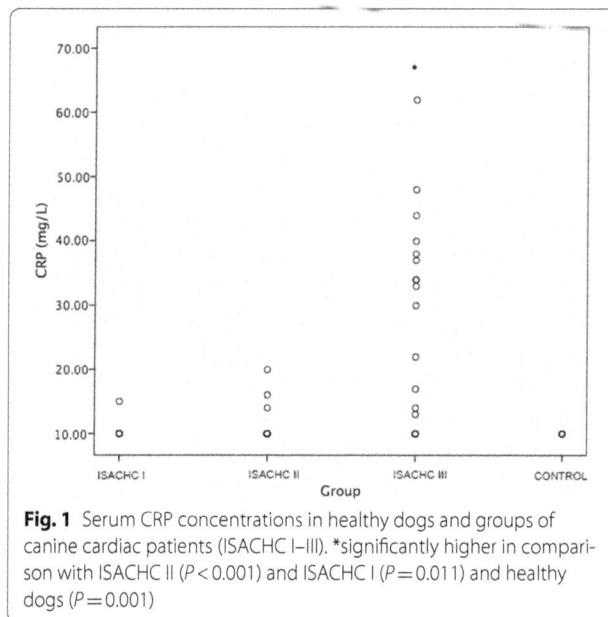

Fig. 1 Serum CRP concentrations in healthy dogs and groups of canine cardiac patients (ISACHC I–III). *significantly higher in comparison with ISACHC II ($P < 0.001$) and ISACHC I ($P = 0.011$) and healthy dogs ($P = 0.001$)

Labrador Retrievers (n = 2) and one dog of each breed: Pekingese, Japanese Chin, Shih-Tzu, Newfoundland Dog, Boston Terrier, Miniature Poodle, Tibetan Terrier, Rhodesian Ridgeback, Beagle, Dogue de Bordeaux, Dachshund, American Staffordshire Terrier and Schipperke. Twelve healthy dogs were enrolled as controls in the study. The following breeds were included in the control group: Labrador Retrievers (n = 6), Golden Retrievers (n = 3), Mixed breed dogs (n = 2), and Border Collie (n = 1). Dog characteristics other than breed are summarized in Table 2.

Cardiovascular patients had the following diseases: myxomatous mitral valve disease (MMVD; ISACHC I, n = 6; ISACHC II, n = 19; ISACHC III, n = 14), dilated cardiomyopathy (ISACHC I, n = 2; ISACHC II, n = 5; ISACHC III, n = 9), subaortic stenosis (ISACHC I, n = 2) and patent ductus arteriosus (ISACHC II, n = 2; ISACHC III, n = 3).

A significantly higher serum CRP concentration (Fig. 1) was found in the decompensated stage of heart failure (ISACHC III; median 15.5 mg/L, interquartile range 10.0–34.8 mg/L) compared with healthy dogs ($P = 0.001$; median 10.0 mg/L, interquartile range 10.0–10.0 mg/L)

and with patients in ISACHC group II ($P < 0.001$; median 10.0 mg/L, interquartile range 10.0–10.0 mg/L) and ISACHC group I ($P = 0.011$; median 10.0 mg/L, interquartile range 10.0–10.0 mg/L). We found a significantly higher WBC (Fig. 2) in ISACHC III dogs (median 14.0×10^9/L, interquartile range 10.4–18.0×10^9/L) compared with healthy dogs ($P = 0.005$; median 9.0×10^9/L, interquartile range 7.8–10.2×10^9/L), ISACHC I dogs ($P = 0.004$; median 8.4×10^9/L, interquartile range 6.3–11.2×10^9/L) and ISACHC II dogs ($P < 0.001$; median 9.1×10^9/L, interquartile range 7.6–10.8×10^9/L). In addition, a significantly higher NEUT (Fig. 3) was observed in ISACHC III dogs (median 10.4×10^9/L, interquartile range 7.2–12.2×10^9/L) compared with

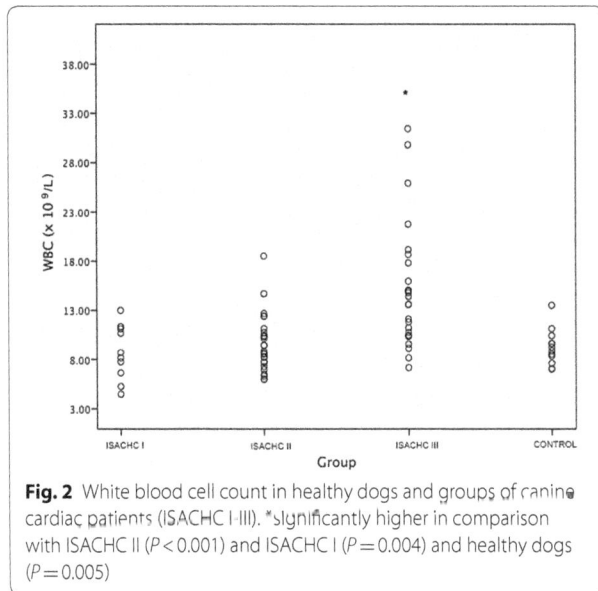

Fig. 2 White blood cell count in healthy dogs and groups of canine cardiac patients (ISACHC I-III). *significantly higher in comparison with ISACHC II (P < 0.001) and ISACHC I (P = 0.004) and healthy dogs (P = 0.005)

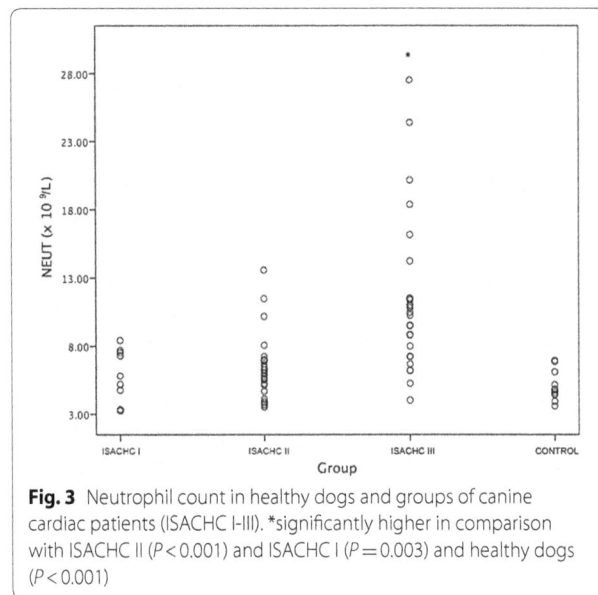

Fig. 3 Neutrophil count in healthy dogs and groups of canine cardiac patients (ISACHC I-III). *significantly higher in comparison with ISACHC II (P < 0.001) and ISACHC I (P = 0.003) and healthy dogs (P < 0.001)

healthy dogs (P < 0.001; median 4.8×10^9/L, interquartile range $4.4–5.9 \times 10^9$/L), ISACHC I dogs (P = 0.003; median 5.5×10^9/L, interquartile range $3.3–7.6 \times 10^9$/L) and ISACHC II dogs (P < 0.001; median 6.0×10^9/L, interquartile range $4.5–7.0 \times 10^9$/L).

In the multivariate analyses, where we controlled for age, sex (and disease), ISACHC group III still had significantly larger expected values of all the three inflammatory parameters ($\log_{10}$WBC, $\log_{10}$NEUT or CRP) compared to ISACHC group II (P < 0.001). Expected values of inflammatory parameters for ISACHC group I in

the multivariate model were never significantly different from the expected values for inflammatory parameters in group II (see Additional file 1).

Serum CRP concentration significantly positively correlated with WBC (r = 0.65, P < 0.001) and NEUT (r = 0.58, P = 0.002) in the ISACHC III group, while no significant correlations were found in ISACHC I and II groups. There were no statistically significant correlations between the serum CRP concentration and heart murmur intensity (grades 1 to 6) in any of the ISACHC groups. A significant negative correlation between serum CRP concentration and LVEF (r = −0.49, P = 0.046) and a significant positive correlation with MVE (r = 0.52, P = 0.046) were found in the ISACHC III group. There were no significant correlations between the CRP concentration and other selected echocardiographic parameters in any of the ISACHC groups.

Discussion

The present study is the first to report on serum CRP concentration in association with WBC and neutrophil count in patients with severe heart failure. Our results demonstrate that systemic inflammation may be present in patients with severe heart failure, irrespective of the etiology. The role of inflammation in the development and progression of heart failure has been described [15, 34–37]. Inflammation can contribute not only to myocardial dysfunction but also to detrimental consequences such as endothelial dysfunction and cardiac cachexia. Inflammatory mediators may be released from the failing myocardium itself, and also from circulating leukocytes, blood platelets, endothelial cells, and from the liver and lungs [36]. Acute phase proteins as markers of inflammation, including CRP, have been found to be increased in acute and chronic inflammatory diseases and heart failure [10, 17, 38–42].

Our study showed a significantly higher serum CRP concentration in ISACHC III heart failure patients in comparison with ISACHC II, ISACHC I and healthy dogs, although the median value of CRP concentration in ISACHC III group did not exceed the upper value of reference range [31] and more than a half of the patients in this group had CRP concentrations within the reference range. Regardless the method for measurement of circulating CRP concentration used, recent studies have reported significantly higher serum CRP concentration in dogs with CHF due to MMVD or dilated cardiomyopathy compared to clinically healthy dogs [17, 18] or in comparison to asymptomatic dogs [16, 17], which is in accordance with our results. Similarly, in the study of Reimann et al. [17], CRP was not increased in dogs with different stages of MMVD without CHF in comparison with control dogs; however, the presence of CHF significantly increased serum CRP concentration. Contrary to our results, Rush et al. [14] found no significant difference in CRP concentration between MMVD dogs with CHF and without CHF; however, CRP concentration was significantly higher in dogs with MMVD (with and without CHF) in comparison with healthy dogs. The differences between the results of our study and that of Rush et al. [14] might be attributed to differences in dogs included in studies and different CRP assays used. Ljungvall et al. [43] found no significant differences in CRP concentration between healthy dogs and dogs at different stages of MMVD that were not in CHF. It has been suggested that renin–angiotensin–aldosterone system with sympathetic system contribute to constant inflammation in CHF. Studies have shown that angiotensin II activates leukocytes in circulation and plays a role in their adhesion to the endothelium. Additionally, lymphocytes and monocytes express beta-adrenergic receptors and beta-adrenergic stimulation may modulate cytokine production in these cells [37]. Our results may indicate that the progression of CHF is the major cause of increased levels of systemic markers of inflammation. Studies with human CHF patients have revealed that WBC and CRP may be implicated in the development of heart failure by the immune system acting as a modulator of myocyte injury and inflammatory reactions contributing to the structural and functional deterioration observed in failing human hearts [44]. Additionally, CRP may be an independent marker of improvement and readmission in heart failure [45]. Higher levels of plasma CRP concentration, measured using a hsCRP assay, have been associated with more severe heart failure and independently associated with morbidity and mortality [6, 39]. Our study revealed a significant positive correlation between CRP and MVE in ISACHC III, which indicates that higher serum CRP concentrations are associated with higher left atrial pressure and thus more severe CHF. Moreover, CRP concentration significantly negatively correlated with LVEF, which additionally supports our results that higher CRP concentrations are associated with more severe CHF and myocardial dysfunction. On the other hand, we did not find a significant correlation between murmur grade and CRP concentration in any of the ISACHC groups. Similarly, Rush et al. [14] found no significant correlation between murmur grade and CRP concentrations in dogs with chronic valvular disease.

In our study, CRP concentration significantly positively correlated with WBC and NEUT in the ISACHC III group. In this group of patients, WBC and NEUT were significantly higher compared with that in ISACHC II and ISACHC I and healthy dogs. In the ISACHC III group, the median values of WBC and NEUT exceeded the upper value of reference ranges in dogs

[46], indicating leukocytosis and neutrophilia in CHF dogs, which suggests that systemic inflammation may be present in advanced stage of heart failure. In addition, authors believe that WBC needs to be judged on an individual basis and not blindly compared to the reference values. Farabaugh et al. [13] found significantly higher WBC and NEUT in CHF dogs (ISACHC III) compared with ISACHC II and the control group, which is in accordance with our results. Deepti and Yahtiraj [23] also found higher mean WBC in CHF dogs compared to the reference values from the literature; however, they did not have their own control group. Few human studies have demonstrated a correlation between WBC and CHF. In human patients with acute myocardial infarction, increased levels of WBC and NEUT and decreased levels of lymphocytes and eosinophils were found to be associated with early development of CHF [24]. Higher incidence of in-hospital deaths of human patients due to decompensated heart failure were found to be associated with higher CRP concentration, higher leukocyte and neutrophil counts and lower lymphocyte count, which supports our findings [47]. A high number of leukocytes may affect the electrical stability of the heart. It has been shown that high WBC is a significant predictor of ventricular fibrillation in patients with acute myocardial infarction [20]. Additionally, high WBC have been associated with the development of new CHF or shock [20]. Mechanisms by which leukocytes may affect the progression of CHF include proteolytic damage, leukocyte aggregation, microvascular obstruction, electrical instability and impaired revascularization [20, 24, 48]. Neutrophils may not directly contribute to contractile dysfunction but may be an indicator of other inflammatory mediators that may be directly involved in the pathogenesis of cardiac dysfunction. Moreover, neutrophils as phagocytes undergo a cellular respiratory burst and release free oxygen radicals, which are toxic to cells. Interaction between neutrophils and inflammatory cells within the myocardium can occur, which results in the release of lysosomal enzymes and arachidonic acid metabolites, thus causing myocardial dysfunction [49–51].

Our study has some limitations. These include quite high DL (10 mg/L) of the canine CRP test used, which disables more sensitive determination of CRP concentration. However, hsCRP assays with much lower detection limits were unable to discriminate between degrees of MMVD without CHF but were able to detect the significant difference in CRP concentration between patients with and without CHF [17], as well as between CHF patients and healthy dogs [17, 18]. The same results were obtained by the CRP test used in our study. In a clinical setting, it is important to recognize that systemic inflammation may be present in acute decompensated heart failure of already treated or new heart failure patients in order not to interpret the results as infection. We would like to point out that practitioners should consider CHF as a differential diagnosis in case of elevated CRP, WBC and NEUT. In this case irrational use of antibiotics can be avoided. The CRP assay used in our study is widely available and may be used by a practitioner because it is easy to use, rapid (it takes only 11 min to get the result) and does not require trained laboratory personnel. In cases of CRP concentrations below the detection limit, CHF needs to be considered in patients with typical clinical signs that may include tachypnea/dyspnea, cough, tachycardia, a heart murmur, a weak femoral pulse and/or arrhythmias. For confirmation of CHF, additional, more specific methods should be used (N-terminal pro-B-type natriuretic peptide, thoracic radiography and echocardiography). Another limitation could be relatively low number of dogs included in the study and the inclusion of more than one heart disease into CHF classes; however, the multiple regression analysis showed that etiology had no effect on the results presented. Another limitation might be that the control dogs had no echocardiographic examination done; however, these were all active rescue dogs without any clinical signs and blood-work abnormalities. In addition, the control group was not breed matched with patient groups; majority of control dogs consisted mostly of large breeds. Control dogs were also significantly younger compared to ISACHC II and III groups; however, no significant age-related differences in CRP concentrations were observed in healthy beagle dogs [52]. Moreover, no associations between CRP and age, body weight or breed were found in canine cardiac patients [18]. In humans, CRP concentration increased with age; however, it remained within the normal range [53]. We cannot totally exclude possible effect of age and breed on hematological variables [54]. Another limitation might be the fact that elderly dogs may have a higher prevalence of comorbidities (periodontal disease, osteoarthritis) that may result in increased values of inflammatory markers [55, 56]; however, dogs with advanced periodontal disease and symptomatic osteoarthritis were not included in this study. The majority of our patients had therapy, which may influence the inflammatory markers [57–59]. In humans, neutrophilia and lymphopenia were more pronounced in CHF patients that were not taking beta-blockers versus those taking this treatment [57]. Another human study showed that administration of specific beta-blockers could be associated with attenuation of inflammation [58]. Short-term inotropic support reduced indices of inflammation in patients with decompensated CHF [59].

This study demonstrated that irrespective of etiology, CHF may be associated with inflammatory process, as evident from significantly increased levels of inflammatory markers (CRP concentration, WBC and NEUT) in decompensating or severe heart failure in comparison with compensated patients and healthy dogs; however, normal CRP concentration and normal WBC/NEUT can also be present in heart failure. It is worth noting that all three measured parameters show an increasing trend with the stage of cardiac disease. Our results give an additional evidence of the inflammatory nature of severe heart failure in dogs as it was already documented with the use of CRP and cytokines in humans [34–36, 42] and dogs [15, 17, 18]. Practitioners should be aware of the presence of inflammation when interpreting complete blood count, white cell differential count or CRP concentration in canine cardiovascular patients.

Conclusions

The study reported here demonstrated significantly increased levels of CRP and WBC and NEUT in dogs with severe, i.e. decompensated CHF in comparison with compensated patients and healthy dogs. However, normal CRP concentration and normal WBC and NEUT can also be present in heart failure. Furthermore, in the group of patients with severe CHF, a significant association between CRP concentration and WBC and NEUT was found. Our results support the hypothesis that systemic inflammation may be present in patients with severe heart failure. This information may help also the practitioners to be aware that systemic inflammation may be present in heart failure in order not to interpret the results of WBC, NEUT and CRP as infection; however, it should be kept in mind that these markers are unspecific and should be interpreted with the history and clinical signs as well as other more specific diagnostic modalities.

Abbreviations

ACE: angiotensin-converting enzyme; ANOVA: analysis of variance; CBC: complete blood count; CHF: congestive heart failure; CRP: C-reactive protein; DL: detection limit; hsCRP: high sensitivity C-reactive protein; ISACHC: International Small Animal Cardiac Health Council; LAD/Ao: left atrium dimension and diameter of the aorta ratio; LVDdI: left ventricular dimension at end diastole index; LVDsI: left ventricular dimension at end systole index; LVEF: left ventricular ejection fraction; MMVD: myxomatous mitral valve disease; MVE: E wave velocity of the mitral valve inflow; NEUT: neutrophil count; pctFS: percentage fractional shortening; SD: standard deviation.

Authors' contributions

ADP and ANS participated in the design of the study and revised the manuscript. ADP carried out the clinical, electrocardiographic and echocardiographic examinations and interpretation of X-rays. ANS and TL performed the analyses for CRP. TL drafted the manuscript. BV helped with the clinical assessment of patients. TL and BV performed hematology and documented the medical record data. ADP and ANS performed the statistical analyses and interpretation of data. All authors read and approved the final manuscript.

Acknowledgements
The authors would like to extend their sincerest thanks and appreciation to the laboratory technician Aleksander Jenko for his help with blood samples processing.

The authors are grateful to Assist. Prof. Dr. Nataša Kejžar for performing the multivariate analysis.

Competing interests
The authors declare that they have no competing interests.

Funding
The authors acknowledge the financial support of the Slovenian Research Agency (research program P4-0053).

References
1. Boswood A. Biomarkers in cardiovascular disease: beyond natriuretic peptides. J Vet Cardiol. 2009;11:S23–32.
2. Braunwald E. Biomarkers in heart failure. N Engl J Med. 2008;358:2148–59.
3. Hirschfield GM, Pepys MB. C-reactive protein and cardiovascular disease: new insights from an old molecule. QJM. 2003;96:793–807.
4. Ridker PM. Clinical application of C-reactive protein for cardiovascular disease detection and prevention. Circulation. 2003;107:363–9.
5. Yousuf O, Mohanty BD, Martin SS, Joshi PH, Blaha MJ, Nasir K, et al. High-sensitivity C-reactive protein and cardiovascular disease: a resolute belief or an elusive link? J Am Coll Cardiol. 2013;62:397–408.
6. Kaneko K, Kanda T, Yamauchi Y, Hasegawa A, Iwasaki T, Arai M, et al. C-reactive protein in dilated cardiomyopathy. Cardiology. 1999;91:215–9.
7. Lagrand WK, Visser CA, Hermens WT, Niessen HW, Verheugt FW, Wolbink GJ, et al. C-reactive protein as a cardiovascular risk factor: more than an epiphenomenon? Circulation. 1999;100:96–102.
8. Yin WH, Chen JW, Jen HL, Chiang MC, Huang WP, Feng AN, et al. Independent prognostic value of elevated high-sensitivity C-reactive protein in chronic heart failure. Am Heart J. 2004;147:931–8.
9. Ceron JJ, Eckersall PD, Martýnez-Subiela S. Acute phase proteins in dogs and cats: current knowledge and future perspectives. Vet Clin Pathol. 2005;34:85–99.
10. Nakamura M, Takahashi M, Ohno K, Koshino A, Nakashima K, Setoguchi A, et al. C-reactive protein concentration in dogs with various diseases. J Vet Med Sci. 2008;70:127–31.
11. Cray C, Zaias J, Altman NH. Acute phase response in animals: a review. Comp Med. 2009;59:517–26.
12. Kjelgaard-Hansen M, Jacobsen S. Assay validation and diagnostic applications of major acute-phase protein testing in companion animals. Clin Lab Med. 2011;31:51–70.
13. Farabaugh AE, Freeman LM, Rush JE, George KL. Lymphocyte subpopulations and hematologic variables in dogs with congestive heart failure. J Vet Intern Med. 2004;18:505–9.
14. Rush JE, Lee ND, Freeman LM, Brewer B. C-reactive protein concentration in dogs with chronic valvular disease. J Vet Int Med. 2006;20:635–9.
15. Zois NE, Moesgaard SG, Kjelgaard-Hansen M, Rasmussen CE, Falk T, Fossing C, et al. Circulating cytokine concentrations in dogs with different degrees of myxomatous mitral valve disease. Vet J. 2012;192:106–11.
16. Polizopoulou ZS, Koutinas CK, Cerón JJ, Tvarijonaviciute A, Martínez-Subiela S, Dasopoulou A, et al. Correlation of serum cardiac troponin I and acute phase protein concentrations with clinical staging in dogs with degenerative mitral valve disease. Vet Clin Pathol. 2015;44:397–404.
17. Reimann MJ, Ljungvall I, Hillström A, Møller JE, Hagman R, Falk T, et al. Increased serum C-reactive protein concentrations in dogs with congestive heart failure due to myxomatous mitral valve disease. Vet J. 2016;209:113–8.
18. Cunningham SM, Rush JE, Freeman LM. Systemic inflammation and endothelial dysfunction in dogs with congestive heart failure. J Vet Intern Med. 2012;26:547–57.
19. Saunders AB, Smith BE, Fosgate GT, Suchodolski JS, Steiner JM. Cardiac troponin I and C-reactive protein concentrations in dogs with severe pulmonic stenosis before and after balloon valvuloplasty. J Vet Cardiol. 2009;11:9–16.
20. Madjid M, Awan I, Willerson JT, Casscells WS. Leukocyte count and coronary heart disease: implications for risk assessment. J Am Coll Cardiol. 2004;44:1945–56.
21. Engström G, Melander O, Hedblad B. Leukocyte count and incidence of hospitalizations due to heart failure. Circ Heart Fail. 2009;2:217–22.
22. Pfister R, Sharp SJ, Luben R, Wareham NJ, Khaw KT. Differential white blood cell count and incident heart failure in men and women in the EPIC-Norfolk study. Eur Heart J. 2012;33:523–30.
23. Deepti BR, Yathiraj S. Hematological and biochemical variables in congestive heart failure in dogs. Int J Sci Environ Technol. 2015;4:836–40.
24. Cruz-Torres L, Griño R, Relos J. Correlation of total white blood cell and differential count in the development of congestive heart failure in patients with acute myocardial infarction. Philipp J Intern Med. 2011;49:185–90.
25. Oikonomou E, Tousoulis D, Siasos G, Zaromitidou M, Papavassilioi AG, Stefanadis C. The role of inflammation in heart failure: new therapeutic approaches. Hellenic J Cardiol. 2011;52:30–40.
26. Chen O, Patel J, Mohamed E, Greene M, Moskovits N, Shani J. The immunoregulatory role of cytokines in congestive heart failure. Interdiscip J Microinflammation. 2014;1:1–6.
27. Thomas WP, Gaber CE, Jacobs GJ, Kaplan PM, Lombard CW, Moise NS, et al. Recommendations for standards in transthoracic two-dimensional echocardiography in the dog and cat. Echocardiography Committee of the Specialty of Cardiology, American College of Veterinary Internal Medicine. J Vet Intern Med. 1993;7:247–52.
28. Cornell CC, Kittleson MD, Della Torre P, Häggström J, Lombard CW, Pedersen HD, et al. Allometric scaling of M-mode cardiac measurements in normal adult dog. J Vet Intern Med. 2004;18:311–21.
29. Fox PR, Moïse NS, International Small Animal Cardiac Health Council. Recommendations for diagnosis of heart disease and treatment of heart failure in small animals. In: Fox PR, Sisson D, Moïse NS, editors. Textbook of canine and feline cardiology. 2nd ed. Philadelphia: WB Saunders Co.; 1999. p. 883–96.
30. Ibraimi F, Kriz K, Merin H, Kriz D. Magnetic permeability based diagnostic test for the determination of the canine C-reactive protein concentration in undiluted whole blood. J Magn Magn Mater. 2009;321:1632–4.
31. Paul C, Hansson LO, Sejerstad SL, Kriz K. Canine C-reactive protein—a clinical guide. Lund: LifeAssays AB; 2011. p. 1–13.
32. R Core Team. R: a language and environment for statistical computing. R Foundation for Statistical Computing, Vienna, Austria. 2016. https://www.R-project.org/. Accessed 2 Feb 2018.
33. Lachenbruch PA. Comparisons of two-part models with competitors. Stat Med. 2001;20:1215–34.
34. Seta Y, Shan K, Bozkurt B, Oral H, Mann DL. Basic mechanisms in heart failure: the cytokine hypothesis. J Card Fail. 1996;2:243–9.
35. Bozkurt B. Activation of cytokines as a mechanism of disease progression in heart failure. Ann Rheum Dis. 2000;59(Suppl 1):i90–3.
36. Yndestad A, Damås JK, Oie E, Ueland T, Gullestad L, Aukrust P. Systemic inflammation in heart failure—the whys and wherefores. Heart Fail Rev. 2006;11:83–92.
37. Yndestad A, Damås JK, Øie E, Ueland T, Gullestad L, Aukrust P. Role of inflammation in the progression of heart failure. Curr Cardiol Rep. 2007;9:236–41.
38. Huang WP, Yin WH, Jen HL, Chiang MC, Feng AN, Young MS. C-reactive protein levels in chronic congestive heart failure. Acta Cardiol Sin. 2004;20:7–14.
39. Anand IS, Latini R, Florea VG, Kuskowski MA, Rector T, Masson S, et al. C-reactive protein in heart failure: prognostic value and the effect of valsartan. Circulation. 2005;112:1428–34.
40. Mueller C, Laule-Kilian K, Christ A, Brunner-La Rocca, Perruchoud AP. Inflammation and long-term mortality in acute congestive heart failure. Am Heart J. 2006;151:845–50.
41. Pye M, Rae AP, Cobbe SM. Study of serum C-reactive protein concentration in cardiac failure. Br Heart J. 1990;63:228–30.
42. Wojciechowska C, Romuk E, Tomasik A, Skrzep-Poloczek B, Nowalany-Kozielska E, Birkner E, et al. Oxidative stress markers and C-reactive protein

are related to severity of heart failure in patients with dilated cardiomyopathy. Mediators Inflamm. 2014. https://doi.org/10.1155/2014/147040.

43. Ljungvall I, Höglund K, Tidholm A, Olsen LH, Borgerelli M, Venge P, et al. Cardiac troponin I is associated with severity of myxomatous mitral valve disease, age, and C-reactive protein in dogs. J Vet Intern Med. 2010;24:153–9.

44. Devaux B, Scholz D, Hirche A, Klövekorn WP, Schaper J. Upregulation of cell adhesion molecules and the presence of low grade inflammation in human chronic heart failure. Eur Heart J. 1997;18:470–9.

45. Alonso-Martínez JL, Llorente-Diez B, Echegaray-Agara M, Olaz-Preciado F, Urbieta-Echezarreta M, et al. C-reactive protein as a predictor of improvement and readmission in heart failure. Eur J Heart Fail. 2002;4:331–6.

46. Harvey JD. Veterinary haematology: a diagnostic guide and color atlas. St. Louis: Elsevier Saunders; 2012. p. 328–35.

47. Ostrowska M, Ostrowski A, Łuczak M, Jaguszewski M, Adamski P, Bellwon J, et al. Basic laboratory parameters as predictors of in-hospital death in patients with acute decompensated heart failure: data from a large single-centre cohort. Kardiol Pol. 2017;75:157–63.

48. Madjid M, Fatemi O. Components of the complete blood count as risk predictors for coronary heart disease: in-depth review and update. Tex Heart Inst J. 2013;40:17–29.

49. Yusuf S, Wittes J, Friedman L. Overview of results of randomized clinical trials in heart disease: I treatments following myocardial infarction. JAMA. 1988;260:2088–93.

50. Kyne L, Hausdorff JM, Knight E, Dukas L, Azhar G, Wei JY. Neutrophilia and congestive heart failure after acute myocardial infarction. Am Heart J. 2000;139:94–100.

51. Ypil WM, Tria R, Abad SJG. Absolute neutrophilia as predictor for the development of early-onset congestive heart failure in patients admitted for acute myocardial infarction. Philipp Heart Center J. 2002;9:2–7.

52. Kuribayashi T, Shimada T, Matsumoto M, Kawato K, Honjyo T, Fukuyama M, et al. Determination of serum C-reactive protein (CRP) in healthy Beagle dogs of various ages and pregnant beagle dogs. Exp Anim. 2003;52:387–90.

53. Wyczalkowska-Tomasik A, Czarkowska-Paczek B, Zielenkiewicz M, Paczek L. Inflammatory markers change with age, but do not fall beyond reported normal ranges. Arch Immunol Ther Exp (Warsz). 2016;64:249–54.

54. Brenten T, Morris PJ, Salt C, Raila J, Kohn B, Schweigert FJ, et al. Age associated and breed-associated variations in haematological and biochemical variables in young Labrador Retriever and miniature schnauzer dogs. Vet Rec Open. 2016. https://doi.org/10.1136/vetreco-2015-000166.

55. Hurter K, Spreng D, Rytz U, Schawalder P, Ott-Knusel F, Schmokel H. Measurements of C-reactive protein in serum and lactate dehydrogenase in serum and synovial fluid of patients with osteoarthritis. Vet J. 2005;169:281–5.

56. Yu G, Yu Y, Li YN, Shu R. Effect of periodontitis on susceptibility to atrial fibrillation in an animal model. J Electrocardiol. 2010;43:359–66.

57. von Haehling S, Schefold JC, Jankowska E, Doehner W, Springer J, Strohschein K, et al. Leukocyte redistribution: effects of beta blockers in patients with chronic heart failure. PLoS ONE. 2009. https://doi.org/10.1371/journal.pone.0006411.

58. Nagatomo Y, Yoshikawa T, Kohno T, Yoshizawa A, Anzai T, Meguro T, et al. Effects of beta-blocker therapy on high sensitivity C-reactive protein, oxidative stress, and cardiac function in patients with congestive heart failure. J Card Fail. 2007;13:365–71.

59. White M, Ducharme A, Ibrahim R, Whittom L, Lavoie J, Guertin MC, et al. Increased systemic inflammation and oxidative stress in patients with worsening congestive heart failure: improvement after short-term inotropic support. Clin Sci (Lond). 2006;110:483–9.

19

Questionnaire survey of detrimental fur animal epidemic necrotic pyoderma in Finland

Heli Nordgren[1*], Katariina Vapalahti[1], Olli Vapalahti[1,2,3], Antti Sukura[1] and Anna-Maija Virtala[1]

Abstract

Background: In 2007, a previously unrecorded disease, fur animal epidemic necrotic pyoderma (FENP), was detected in farmed mink (*Neovision vision*), foxes (*Vulpes lagopus*) and Finnraccoons (*Nyctereutes procyonoides*) in Finland. Symptoms included severe pyoderma with increased mortality, causing both animal welfare problems and economic losses. In 2011, an epidemiologic questionnaire was mailed to all members of the Finnish Fur Breeders' Association to assess the occurrence of FENP from 2009 through the first 6 months of 2011. The aim was to describe the geographical distribution and detailed clinical signs of FENP, as well as sources of infection and potential risk factors for the disease.

Results: A total of 239 farmers (25%) returned the questionnaire. Clinical signs of FENP were observed in 40% (95% CI 34–46%) of the study farms. In addition, the survey clarified the specific clinical signs for different animal species. The presence of disease was associated with the importation of mink, especially from Denmark (OR 9.3, 95% CI 2.6–33.0). The transmission route between Finnish farms was associated with fur animal purchases. Some risk factors such as the farm type were also indicated. As such, FENP was detected more commonly on farms with more than one species of fur animal in comparison to farms with, for example, only foxes (OR 4.6, 95% CI 2.4–8.6), and the incidence was higher on farms with over 750 breeder mink compared to smaller farms (OR 3.8, 95% CI 1.6–9.0). Contact between fur animals and birds and other wildlife increased the risk of FENP on farms. Responses also indicated that blocking the entry of wildlife to the animal premises protected against FENP.

Conclusions: FENP was most likely introduced to Finland by imported mink and spread further within the country via domestically purchased fur animals. Some potential risk factors, such as the type and size of the farm and contact with wildlife, contributed to the spread of FENP. Escape-proof shelter buildings block the entry of wildlife, thus protecting fur animals against FENP.

Keywords: *Arcanobacterium phocae*, Fur animals, Fur animal epidemic necrotic pyoderma FENP, *Neovison vison*, *Nyctereutes procyonoides*, *Vulpes lagopus*

Background

In 2007, Finnish fur farmers noticed clinical signs of a novel disease in their animals. Mink (*Neovison vison*) developed necrotic pyoderma on their feet and head, foxes (*Vulpes lagopus*) had severe conjunctivitis that spread aggressively to pyoderma of the eyelids or the facial skin and Finnraccoons (*Nyctereutes procyonoides*, a raccoon dog bred for the fur industry) developed painful abscesses between their toes. The disease continued to spread between and within farms, typical of a contagious infectious disease. It caused severe and even fatal clinical signs that dramatically affected animal welfare and caused considerable financial loss to fur farmers and to the entire fur industry.

Similar lesions in mink were first documented in the USA in 1970s and in Canada in 1996 [1]. Other pelt-producing countries have also reported the disease [2]. In 2010, the Finnish Fur Breeders' Association (FFBA), Finnish Food Safety Authority (Evira) and the University of Helsinki (UH) initiated a joint project to investigate

*Correspondence: heli.nordgren@helsinki.fi
[1] Department of Veterinary Biosciences, Faculty of Veterinary Medicine, University of Helsinki, Helsinki, Finland
Full list of author information is available at the end of the article

the macroscopic and histological lesions and to identify the causative agents of the disease. The disease was named fur animal epidemic necrotic pyoderma (FENP) due to the lesions seen in all fur animal species. *Arcanobacterium phocae* in addition to a possible role of a novel *Streptococcus* spp. has been identified as potential causative agents [2]. *A. phocae* has its origin in marine mammals [3], which is compatible with observations by North American farmers who linked similar clinical signs in mink to feeding on seal byproducts [1]. Furthermore, Canadian researchers recently found an association between *A. phocae* and pododermatitis in mink [4]. FENP is potentially a multifactorial disease, where the environment, the host's immunology and specific infectious agents may be involved. We report here the results of a retrospective epidemiologic survey based on a questionnaire carried out in 2011. The purpose of this survey was to investigate the clinical presentation and farm-level prevalence of FENP in Finland in mink, foxes and Finnraccoon. Our objectives were also to identify potential farm-level risk factors for FENP, to determine how the disease was introduced to Finland and to identify and implement control measures against the disease.

Methods
Study design
Data were collected using an epidemiologic questionnaire which was sent to fur animal farms in Finland in either Finnish or Swedish language depending on the language of the farmer. The questionnaire focused on the period 2009–2011 (through the first 6 months of 2011). The questionnaire and a cover letter describing the clinical signs of FENP were sent in the summer 2011 to all fur farms that belonged to FFBA (n = 958). In order to determine the farm-level prevalence of FENP, we aimed for a sample size of 270 farms, assuming 40% disease prevalence at a 5% precision using a 95% confidence interval (CI). This calculation was based on the assumption that farmers held a near-perfect competency in recognizing the clinical signs of FENP [5]. In addition, reminder letters were sent to farmers in August and September 2011. The questionnaire consisted of multiple-choice questions, yes or no questions and questions requiring numerical or written responses. Many of the respondents left portions of the 13-page questionnaire incomplete; eight questionnaires were excluded due to severe incompleteness. To elucidate the response percentage for each variable, the number of missing responses are shown in Additional file 1.

The questionnaire covered the following topics:

1. Clinical signs of FENP (chosen from a list of clinical and visible signs), the year clinical signs were first detected, the species affected, the number of diseased or dead animals due to FENP, color phase of the affected animals, seasonal appearance of the clinical signs, the signs detected and the potential treatment's effect on FENP-diseased animals.
2. Characteristics of the farm and farmer including the location and the size of the farm according to the number of breeding animals, the housing system, the animal species on the farm, the sex and age of each farmer and the employment of the farmer on the farm as full or part-time.
3. Fur animal imports and purchases.
4. Other diseases on the farm, and prophylactic and therapeutic practices.
5. Fur animal management including sources of food and water, feeding procedures, the drinking water system, bedding materials, manure handling and the storage of succumbed and culled animals before rendering.
6. Biosecurity on the farm including the use of fences, entry of wildlife and birds to animal premises, visitors and traffic, cleaning and disinfection routines and quarantine procedures.

Definitions of the variables
Data were analyzed by logistic regression. The farms were divided into cases or controls for which risk factors were retrieved from the questionnaire data. A case farm was a farm with FENP in at least one fur animal species during the period 2009 through 2011, while a control farm was a farm with no FENP in any species during the same period. If information about whether a farm was affected by FENP during the study period was missing, FENP presence was inferred using other questionnaire responses, such as procedures used in the treatment of FENP, the number of animals that had died or recovered from FENP and medication used to treat FENP.

Farms were divided into four types: (1) mink farms (solely mink), (2) fox farms (solely foxes), (3) Finnraccoon farms (solely Finnraccoons) and (4) mixed farms (at least two species). In cases where an insufficient response to the question concerning farm type was provided, farm type was inferred from the information provided regarding the number of mink, foxes and Finnraccoons on the farm, medication and vaccines administered to different species and purchases or shelter buildings specified for species.

We categorized farms as small or large according to the number of breeder animals: mink, >750 vs ≤750; fox, >320 vs ≤320; and Finnraccoon, >125 vs ≤125. In farms with more than one species, size was based on the most numerous species. For example, a farm with 600 mink and 200 Finnraccoons was considered a small farm because there were more mink than Finnraccoons, and fewer than 750 mink.

In some cases, it was necessary to study variables for all farms that had mink, foxes or Finnraccoons regardless of whether there were one or several species on the farm. In these cases, the farms were referred to as "farms with mink", "farms with foxes" and "farms with Finnraccoons" to distinguish them from exclusive mink, fox and Finnraccoon farms.

We collected information at annual level, although for some events it was sufficient to know if an event had occurred at all during any of the years in question. Therefore, for variables regarding diseases other than FENP, medication given, vaccinations administered and purchases and the importation of animals, we created new combined variables that summed annual data appropriately. If necessary, both annual and combined variables were analyzed. All variables are listed in Additional file 1.

Statistical analysis

The included farms and farmers (i.e., respondents) were compared with all Finnish fur farms and farmers to determine the representativeness of the study population. Information on all Finnish fur farms was obtained via a questionnaire distributed by FFBA in 2010. The distributions for different species, the geographical distribution of the farms and the main characteristics of the farmers were compared statistically.

The frequencies of all variables in the study were counted in groups of cases and controls. Crude odds ratios (OR, with only one independent variable in the model at a time) and their 95% confidence intervals (95% CIs) were calculated for all variables. A multivariable logistic regression analysis was performed on four groups based on the animal species composition of the farm: (1) all farms, (2) mixed farms only, (3) farms with mink (also including mixed farms with mink) and (4) farms with foxes (also including mixed farms with foxes). For each group, the variables with a significant crude OR at 95% confidence level were included in the model. We tested the effect of missing values by running models that also included missing values for variables recoded as "no".

Multicollinearity was tested using the phi coefficient for binary variables [6] and by considering wideness of CIs in occasion of more than two category variables. Interactions up to the second order were tested between all variables. The Pearson's goodness-of-fit statistic (Pearson GOF) and the McFadden's and Cox and Snell R^2 statistics [7, 8] were used to identify the most parsimonious model.

All statistical analyses were performed using SAS version 9.3 (SAS Institute, Cary, NC, USA). The Proc Freq statement with the Chisq and Fisher options was used to test differences and associations among categorical data. The Proc Npar1way statement with the Wilcoxon option (producing the Kruskal–Wallis test) was used for data with more than two categories. The Proc Logistic statement was used for the logistic regression analysis to define the most important factors in the transmission of FENP to the farm and its further spread on a farm.

Results

Description of the study farms

Questionnaires were returned by 239 farmers (25%). A comparison of the farms included in the study and all Finnish fur farms showed that study farms and farmers well represented fur farms and farmers in Finland in general based on the farm type (Chi square, P = 0.71), age group (Kruskal–Wallis, P = 0.29) and gender (Chi square, P = 0.96) of the farmers (Figs. 1, 2).

In Finland, 97% of fur farms are located in the western part of the country [9], which was similar to the geographical distribution of the respondents' farms (94%). Most farms in this study had traditional shelter buildings, seven had both shelter buildings and halls and only two had halls alone. Standard cages were used for animal housing. Due to new legislation on fox cage sizes (introduced 1 January 2011), 81% of fox farms had recently changed their cages. The distance between individual farms varied. We found that about half were more than 500 meters apart (Additional file 1).

Most farmers were men, while only a few were women or farmed by a couple. About half of the farmers were under 50 years old, and the age ranged from 22 to 71 years (Fig. 2). On 80% of farms, fur farming was reported as the main occupation (data not shown).

Occurrence of FENP in the study farms

The survey showed that FENP had spread to all areas where fur farming is practiced in Finland during the period from 2009 to 2011 (Fig. 3). Clinical signs of FENP were detected on all fur animal species. FENP was reported by 92 (40%; 95% CI 34–46%) of the responding farms, including 16 (39%; 95% CI 26–54%) mink farms, 25 (24%; 95% CI 17–33%) fox farms and 51 (61%; 95% CI 50–70%) mixed farms. The number of affected farms increased during each study year (Fig. 4).

New animals had been bought either from domestic markets or imported from other countries by 89% of all study farms. More specifically, 93% of the farms that reported clinical signs of FENP and 88% of the farms without clinical signs of FENP bought new animals. Animals were imported by 24% of all study farms, by 35% of farms reporting clinical signs of FENP and by 18% of farms without clinical signs of FENP (Additional file 1).

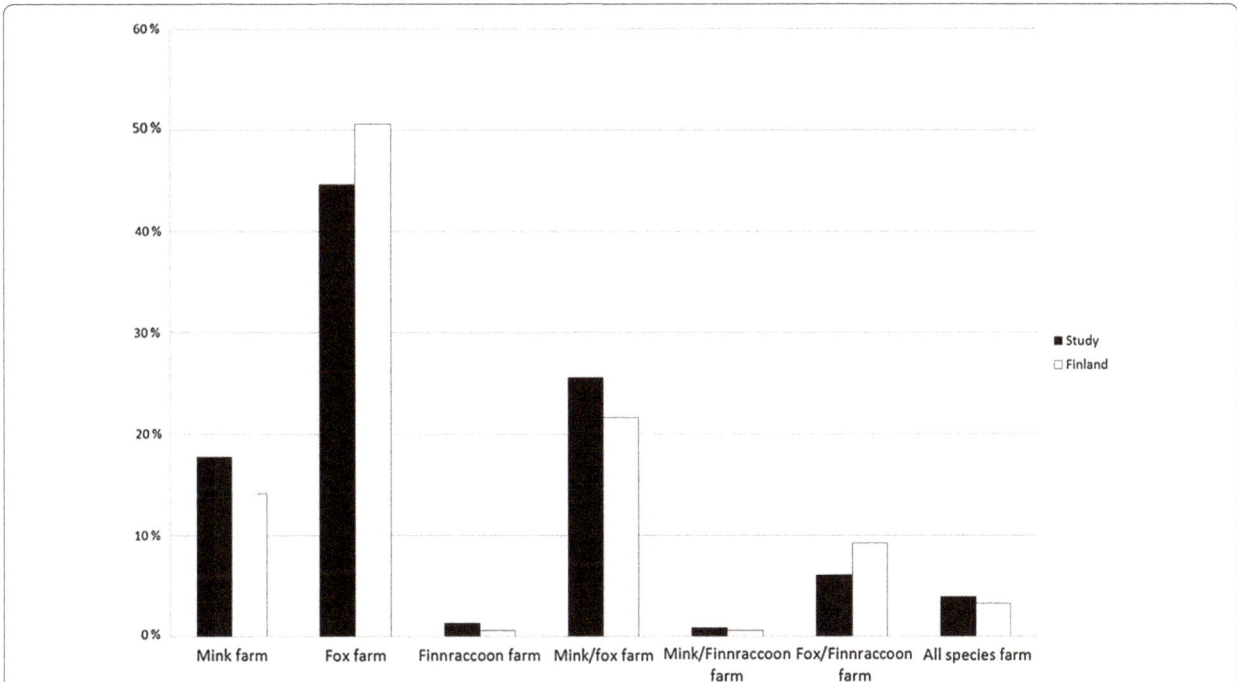

Fig. 1 Characteristics of the fur farms included in the study and all Finnish fur farms (2010). Farms in the study compared with all farms in Finland according to the fur animal species farmed. The information for Finnish fur farms was obtained from the Finnish Fur Breeders' Association (FFBA)

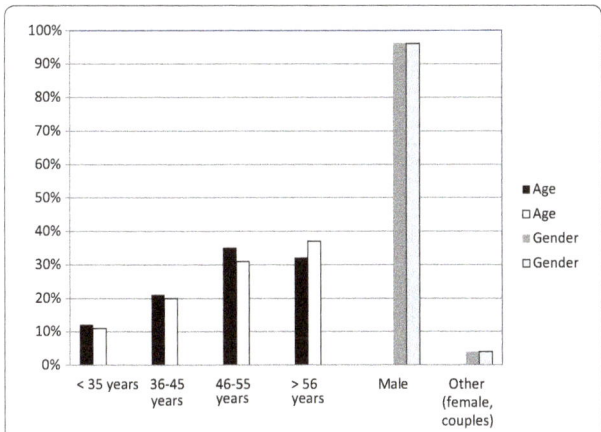

Fig. 2 Characteristics of fur farmers included in the study and all Finnish fur farmers (2010). The age and gender of the fur farmers in the study compared to fur farmers in Finland. The information for Finnish fur farmers was obtained from the Finnish Fur Breeders' Association (FFBA)

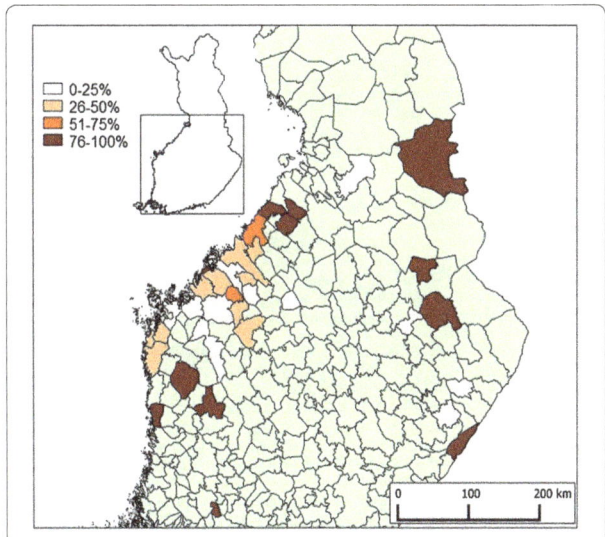

Fig. 3 Fur animal epidemic necrotic pyoderma (FENP) on participating farms. The geographic distribution of the farms and percentage of farms reporting FENP during the period from 2009 through 2011. Areas in *green*: no participants

Farms with clinical signs of FENP imported more mink from Denmark than farms without clinical signs during all study years (Table 1).

In 2009, farms purchasing from domestic sources alone had significantly more FENP than farms without any purchases. However, when the entire period from 2009 to 2011 was included in the analysis, domestic purchases did not significantly increase risk (OR 3.7, 95% CI 0.8–17.1; Table 2).

Farms with clinical signs of FENP sold animals to other farms more than those farms without clinical signs of

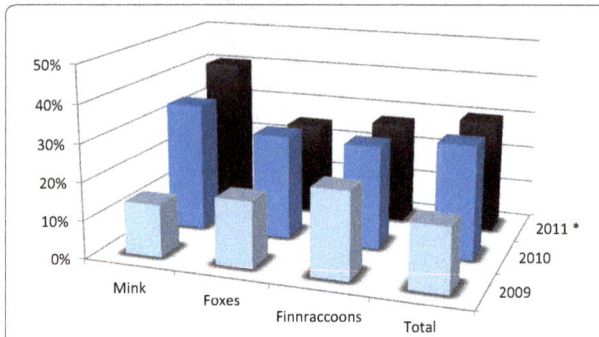

Fig. 4 Occurrence of fur animal epidemic necrotic pyoderma (FENP) on Finnish fur farms. Occurrence of FENP in mink, fox, Finnraccoon and all study farms during the period from 2009 through 2011. *Asterisks* first 6 months of 2011

FENP (FENP + 37% vs FENP −28%); however, the difference was not statistically significant (Chi square, P = 0.14).

Only 25% of all farms that had imported animals used some form of quarantine on their farm. Animals purchased from Finnish farms were kept in quarantine by

14% of farms. In addition, fences were built to enclose the animal premises to avoid fur animals escaping and to keep wildlife from entering the farm on 54% of mink farms, 60% of farms with foxes and 86% of farms with Finnraccoons. According to respondents, wildlife and birds had access to many farms. Both birds and other wildlife were seen inside the farm significantly more often on fenced farms with mink than on unfenced farms with mink (Fisher's exact test, P < 0.0001 and P = 0.001, respectively), while birds were detected inside the farm significantly more often on fenced farms with foxes than on the unfenced farms with foxes (Chi square test, P < 0.0001; Additional file 1).

In addition to FENP, farmers also reported other diseases on their farms. Among these diseases, pre-weaning diarrhea ("sticky kits") (42%), plasmacytosis (32%) and urolithiasis (25%) were most frequently reported on mink farms. Among foxes, the most common diseases consisted of conjunctivitis (55%), fertility disorders (abortion 32%, endometritis 23%) and cystitis (51%). Diarrhea, which is one of the most common diseases, was not included in the options listed on the questionnaire for

Table 1 Fur animal imports by the study farms

Country of origin[a]		Denmark			Poland			Norway		
	FENP	Yes (%)	No (%)	P[b]	Yes (%)	No (%)	P[b]	Yes (%)	No (%)	P[b]
2009	+	9 (24)	29 (76)	0.001	0 (0)	38 (100)	1.000	1 (3)	37 (97)	1.000
	−	7 (5)	141 (95)		1 (1)	147 (99)		7 (5)	141 (95)	
2010	+	12 (18)	56 (82)	0.011	5 (7)	63 (93)	0.536	3 (4)	65 (96)	0.396
	−	8 (6)	130 (94)		7 (5)	131 (95)		11 (8)	127 (92)	
2011	+	5 (7)	62 (93)	0.044	9 (13)	58 (87)	0.001	3 (4)	64 (96)	0.394
	−	2 (2)	130 (98)		2 (2)	130 (98)		12 (9)	120 (91)	

Fur animal imports from Denmark, Poland and Norway during the period from 2009 through 2011 for FENP-positive (+) and FENP-negative (−) farms

[a] In 2010 and 2011 combined imports of the year in question and the previous year because of the unknown incubation time of FENP

[b] Fisher's exact test P value

Table 2 Domestic fur animal purchases by study farms

	FENP	Domestic purchases[a]		
		Yes (%)	No (%)	P[b]
2009	+	26 (100)	0 (0)	0.002
	−	109 (71)	45 (29)	
2010	+	44 (94)	3 (6)	0.052
	−	103 (82)	23 (18)	
2011	+	47 (94)	3 (6)	0.091
	−	110 (85)	20 (15)	

Domestic fur animal purchases for the period from 2009 through 2011 among FENP-positive (+) and FENP-negative farms (−)

[a] In 2010 and 2011, we combined purchases for the year in question and the previous year because of the unknown incubation period for FENP

[b] Chi square test, P value

foxes. In Finnraccoons, the most common diseases included parvovirus enteritis (11%) and abortion (11%). The most commonly used medical treatments on the farms responding were penicillin as an injectable antibiotic and tetracycline, lincomycin and ivermectin (foxes and Finnraccoons) mixed in with feed (data not shown).

Cleaning routines varied between farms. As such, 30% of farms had their own defined schedule of regularly washing cages, 19% washed their cages only after a disease outbreak and 21% of farms did not wash the cages at all. Disinfection was performed regularly (based on the farm's own schedule) on 7% of farms, after a disease outbreak on 30 and 41% did not disinfect the cages at all. Over half of the farms used drinking nipples (80% of mink farms, 44% of fox farms and 68% of mixed farms), while the rest used cups or both nipples and cups. Only mink farms had beddings in nests relying on several different materials (e.g., straw, saw dust, hay, shavings and turf; Additional file 1).

On affected farms, farmers reported signs of pyoderma in the head and on the feet of affected mink. Discharge from the eyes and pyoderma in the head was reported as affecting foxes. Affected Finnraccoons experienced lesions on the paws (Table 3).

Farmers reported having performed the following procedures on FENP diseased animals: medication only, culling all diseased animals without any medication only or both medicating and culling. To treat FENP, farmers primarily used penicillin as an injectable antibiotic in animals with a diminished appetite and oral administration of tetracycline and lincomycin mixed in with the feed in other animals. In addition, when a parasitic skin disease was assumed before the diagnosis of FENP was established, medication with ivermectin was used to treat foxes and Finnraccoons. Farmers reported that animals benefitted from medication with antibiotics, particularly penicillin (data not shown). However, only a few farms (n = 31) having animals with clinical signs of FENP used medication instead of culling.

Risk factors for FENP on the study farms

A clear connection between the incidence of FENP and importing mink from Denmark and Poland emerged compared to farms that did not import from these countries. By contrast, imports from Norway and the USA were not associated with increased risk of FENP (Table 4; Additional file 2).

Larger sized farms (according to the number of breeding animals) had a higher risk of FENP than smaller sized farms across all farm types. However, this risk was not significant on farms with solely mink or solely foxes (Additional file 2). Nearly half of the farms with more than 750 breeder mink had imported animals, whereas the percentage on smaller mink farms having imported animals was 26%. However, the difference in imported animals between different sized farms was not significant (Chi square test, P = 0.079).

Mixed farms had a higher risk for FENP than farms with only mink or only foxes (Table 4). Mixed farms with one FENP affected species also had a higher risk for FENP in other fur animal species on that farm. For instance, in 2010, when mink on a farm were FENP affected, foxes on the same farm had a 22-fold higher risk of developing FENP-positive compared to farms with no diseased mink (data not shown). The occurrence of FENP on farms with mink was associated with wildlife contact. For instance, a significant risk on farms with mink was associated with contact to wild animals and birds compared to farms without such contact. Furthermore, farms using fences around the shelter buildings had a significantly higher risk of FENP than farms with no fences.

Pre-weaning diarrhea [10] exhibited a significant positive association and plasmacytosis in mink exhibited a negative association with development of FENP, whereas feeding with on-farm formulated or commercial feed, feeding procedures or water sources were not associated with FENP. Mink farms that used hay as bedding material had a significantly lower risk for FENP than farms that used other bedding materials. Cleaning and disinfection routines and vaccinations on farms had no effect on the occurrence of FENP (Table 4). Clinical signs of FENP were detected in all color phases, but were least common in the brown color phase in mink. Within foxes, blue foxes were more frequently affected by FENP based on the frequency data from the study (data not shown).

Table 3 Clinical signs of fur animal epidemic necrotic pyoderma (FENP) in mink, foxes and Finnraccoons

Clinical signs	Mink (n = 32)		Fox (n = 47)		Finnraccoon (n = 6)	
	n	(%; 95% CI)	n	(%; 95% CI)	n	(%; 95% CI)
Periocular	1	(3; 0–16)	33	(70; 56–81)	0	(0; 0–39)
Head	14	(44; 28–61)	26	(55; 41–69)	0	(0; 0–39)
Paw	28	(88; 72–95)	2	(4; 0–14)	6	(100; 61–100)
Other parts	6	(19; 9–35)	3	(6; 0–17)	1	(17; 3–56)

Table 4 The crude odds ratios of relevant risk factors for fur animal epidemic necrotic pyoderma (FENP)

Risk factor	Case farms (n = 92)		Control farms (n = 134)		OR (95% CI)
	Exposed (n)	Non-exposed (n)	Exposed (n)	Non-exposed (n)	
All farms					
Farm type					
Mixed farm vs mink farm	51	33	16	24	2.3 (1.1–5.0)
Mixed farm vs fox farm	51	33	25	74	4.6 (2.4–8.6)
Purchases					
Domestic purchases	86	2	118	15	3.7 (0.8–17.1)
All imports combined	32	56	24	96	2.3 (1.2–4.3)
Imports from Denmark	17	71	3	117	9.3 (2.6–33.0)
Imports from Poland	10	78	2	118	7.6 (1.6–35.5)
Drinking system					
Cup	22	68	58	72	0.4 (0.2–0.7)
Nipple	67	23	66	64	2.8 (1.6–5.1)
Farms with mink (including mixed farms)					
Fence around the mink premises	38	19	21	28	2.7 (1.2–5.9)
Access by birds to shelter buildings	25	34	10	38	2.8 (1.2–6.7)
Access by wild animals to shelter buildings	13	42	2	43	6.7 (1.4–31.3)
Size of the farm: >750 vs ≤750 breeder mink	39	13	19	24	3.8 (1.6–9.0)
Hay as bedding material	9	48	18	31	0.3 (0.1–0.8)
Pre-weaning diarrhea	31	30	15	34	2.3 (1.1–5.2)
Plasmacytosis	13	48	23	26	0.3 (0.1–0.7)
Farms with foxes (including mixed farms)					
Access by wild animals to shelter buildings	22	44	18	75	2.1 (1.0–4.3)
Size of the farm: >320 vs ≤320 breeder foxes	44	20	44	54	2.7 (1.4–5.2)
Mixed farms					
Size of the farm large vs small (based on the most numerous species)	26	18	13	19	3.0 (1.2–7.9)
Fence around mink premises	33	9	12	13	4.0 (1.4–11.7)

Number (n) and crude odds ratios (OR, with only one factor in the logistic regression model at a time) for the most prominent risk factors for FENP

The results of the multivariable logistic regression analyses are presented in Table 5. The best model for all farms (model 1) included the variables "farm type", "imports from Denmark" and "imports from Poland". The best model for mixed farms (model 2) included the variables "bird access to mink farm" and "nipple drinking system". The best model for all mink farms (model 3) included the variables "imports to the farm during 2009–2011", "size of the farm" and "wildlife access to mink farm". Finally, the best model for all farms with foxes (model 4) included the variables "farm type", "wildlife access to mink farm" and "nipple drinking system".

All of the variables included in the models were significant risk factors for FENP, except for the variable "farm type" when comparing mink farms to fox farms in model 1. We detected no interaction and only a slight multicollinearity between the variables included in the models. Instead, severe multicollinearity was found between the use of fences around animal shelters and wildlife and bird access to animal shelters, indicating a strong association between these variables.

Discussion

In 2007, Finnish fur animal farms experienced a novel disease designated as FENP. This study revealed that FENP is a detrimental disease in Finnish fur animals and appeared to have spread within and between farms over the study period. The disease also caused severe, sometimes lethal, disease, thereby clearly adversely impacting animal welfare and causing considerable financial loss to farmers.

The clinical signs reported by farmers included pyoderma on the head and feet of mink, conjunctivitis which spread to an inflammation of the eyelids and facial skin areas of foxes and the development of abscesses on the paws of Finnraccoons. These clinical signs are consistent with previous observations in a Finnish study that described the clinical outcome and pathological findings of FENP [2].

Farmers suspected that FENP originally arrived in Finland via imported fur animals. We found an association between the occurrence of FENP and mink importation, particularly from Denmark. Farmers suspected that the further spread of disease in Finland was connected to animal purchases between Finnish fur farms. This putative mechanism agrees with our finding that farms affected by FENP purchased more from domestic sources, particularly in 2009. Our study indicated that quarantine procedures were not a common practice on Finnish fur farms during the outbreak. Thus, in order to avoid the spread of infectious diseases, sufficient quarantine procedures are also crucial on fur farms.

In addition, our study showed that wildlife and birds may act as carriers of FENP, thus spreading the infection on as well as between farms. Unexpectedly, our results showed that FENP was more often detected on farms enclosed by a fence. However, according to the Finnish certification system, farms without a fence are required to construct shelter buildings that entirely prevent fur animals from escaping the premises (escape-proof shelter buildings). Escape-proof shelter buildings much more effectively hinder wildlife access to animal premises and better block contact between wildlife and fur animals than fences. This indicates that high-level biosecurity procedures including the control of wildlife access to farms could limit the spread of FENP.

The FENP risk varied between different types of farms. Farms with a higher number of breeder mink also exhibited a higher risk of FENP. In addition, larger mink farms imported more animals than smaller farms. However, both the size of mink farms and the importation of

animals independently affected the risk for FENP. Mixed farms with more than one fur animal species had a higher risk of FENP than farms with only one species. We found that if one species on a mixed farm was FENP-positive, then other species experienced a higher risk for FENP infection. It may be that FENP susceptibility varies across species and some species may spread disease without showing obvious clinical signs. Furthermore, in mink the different color phases seemed to carry different risks for acquiring FENP. In general, FENP was detected in all color phases, but the brown phase, known as the most vigorous [11], appeared to accompany more resistance to FENP on the farms.

FENP was associated with the occurrence of other diseases. For example, pre-weaning diarrhea in mink occurred more on farms that also had FENP. Pre-weaning diarrhea is a multi-causal disease where viral, bacterial, environmental and dietary factors are all involved [10]. Mink that survive pre-weaning diarrhea may hypothetically be weaker and more prone to other diseases due to a compromised immunity. Alternatively, pathogens causing FENP could already be present at birth, even when no typical lesions are present, thus predisposing minks to pre-weaning diarrhea. It is also possible that similar environmental factors, such as hygiene and management, serve as predisposing factors in the occurrence of both diseases. Surprisingly, farms with plasmacytosis carried a lower risk of FENP. Plasmacytosis (Aleutian disease)

Table 5 Multivariable logistic regression analyses of significant risk factors for fur animal epidemic necrotic pyoderma (FENP)

Model	Cases (n)/ Controls (n)	Risk factors	OR (95% CI)	Goodness-of-fit statistics		
				Test	Value	P
Model 1	88/118	Farm type				
		Mink farm vs fox farm	1.3 (0.5–3.1)	McFadden's R^2	0.147	
		Mixed farm vs fox farm	3.8 (1.9–7.6)	Cox-Snell R^2	0.182	
		Imported from Denmark	6.0 (1.6–22.8)	Pearson	0.721	0.608
		Imported from Poland	7.2 (1.4–37.3)			
Model 2	42/23	Access by birds	4.6 (1.2–16.8)	McFadden's R^2	0.188	
		Nipple	8.4 (2.0–35.0)	Cox-Snell R^2	0.217	
				Pearson	0.411	0.675
Model 3	42/34	Imports	5.3 (1.6–18.0)	McFadden's R^2	0.241	
		Access by wildlife	13.6 (1.5–121.0)	Cox-Snell R^2	0.282	
		Size of the farm > 750 vs ≤ 750 mink	3.1 (1.0–9.0)	Pearson	0.561	0.847
Model 4	65/90	Mink farm vs fox farm	4.5 (2.1–9.4)	McFadden's R^2	0.179	
		Access of wildlife	2.3 (1.0–5.4)	Cox-Snell R^2	0.216	
		Nipple	3.3 (1.6–7.0)	Pearson	0.658	0.621

Model 1 all farms, *Model 2* mixed farms *Model 3* farms with mink *Model 4* farms with foxes

Number (n) of case farms and control farms in the model and odds ratios (OR) of the variables included in the model. In all of the goodness-of-fit tests, a test value of 1 indicates a particular well-fitting model; a Pearson's value <0.05 indicates which model should be rejected. The variable "farm type" has three categories: mink, fox and mixed farms where fox farms serve as the reference group

is a parvoviral mink disease that attenuates the immune system, thereby predisposing animals to other diseases [12, 13]. There is no effective vaccination against plasmacytosis. However, serological screening and control systems conducted on Finnish mink farms [14] divide farms into categories based on the plasmacytosis seroprevalence. It may be that plasmacytosis-positive farms do not check their animals as thoroughly as plasmacytosis-negative farms, whereby they missed some cases of FENP believing that death or clinical signs resulted from plasmacytosis.

Feed might represent one potential source of acquiring FENP. For instance, North American farmers and researchers [1] linked the onset of similar clinical signs to feeding mink with seal byproducts. However, in the current study we found no association between feed sources or feeding systems and the detection of clinical signs of FENP. The original source of the epidemic has probably been seal meat in the mink feed, but due a species shift of the causative agent from marine mammals to mink, FENP is currently transmitted between fur animals [2]. Very little variation occurs in the raw materials utilized in all feed kitchens and no seal byproducts are used in Finland. Clinical signs of FENP were also detected more often on farms that used drinking nipples instead of cups. In general, a nipple water dispensing system is considered more hygienic than a cup system. However, the cups are cleaned regularly whereas the nipples are cleaned less often. Contact between oral mucous membranes and nipple structures might thus act as a predisposing factor for FENP. Furthermore, occasionally cages have sharp wires that can cause wounds, and any sharp protruding structures, such as wires, near the drinking nipple could cause skin trauma, particularly to the head or the feet when an animal is drinking. Experimental infection of mink with *A. phocae* indicated that a skin trauma is needed to transmit the infection [15]. Thus, the role of feed as a possible source of infection and a nipple drinking system as a predisposing factor require further investigation.

We also found that various types of bedding materials were used on mink farms. Hay seemed to protect against FENP. This result is, however, controversial since hay can also cause problems whereby the thick and sharp coarse stalks can traumatize the mucosa in the mouth and cause abscesses, especially when mink are in the sapphire color phase [16]. Differences in the quality of the hay used on the farm exist and softer, less coarsely textured hay may not possess these negative side effects. We did not, however, specifically ask about the hay quality. In addition, hay may also provide solid insulation in the nests and protect against the cold, another external stressor affecting mink.

Limitations

This study carries certain limitations. We cannot completely eliminate the possibility of a nonresponse error [17], since farms that had FENP may have been more motivated to participate in the survey. Alternatively, these same farms might have avoided participating due to the fear of being identified, despite the anonymity of their responses. Responding to this comprehensive questionnaire was time-consuming, thus potentially lowering the response rate and leading to incomplete responses. This may have caused an information bias due to some of the inferences we had to make as well as a measurement error in our results [17]. Despite the low response rate, however, the survey responses adequately represented Finnish fur farms, and included diseased and non-diseased farms (Figs. 1, 4).

Furthermore, it is possible that the descriptions of the clinical signs of FENP provided prompted farmers to report more cases than they actually had. It is, however, also possible that some of the reported cases of FENP in this study were misdiagnosed by farmers since other skin lesions such as biting wounds occur in mink [18]. In foxes, entrophia or ectopic cilia [19] may cause eye inflammations resembling FENP, while the clinical signs in these diseases are much milder. However, we assumed that the farmers were well informed of and competent in recognizing the clinical signs of FENP.

Conclusions

Our study provides further evidence that FENP is a detrimental disease to Finnish fur farms. We found that FENP was likely to have been introduced to Finland via imported mink, particularly those imported from Denmark, and then spread to other farms via domestic purchases and the transfer of infected animals. Other possible causes of the spread of disease between animals and to other farms included fur animal contact with wildlife and birds. FENP occurred more on larger farms and on mixed farms, and one diseased species increased the risk of cross infection to other fur animal species on the same farm. These results provide areas of focus for control measures against FENP.

Additional files

Additional file 1. Frequencies of all variables included in the study in groups of all farms/mink farms (solely mink)/fox farms (solely foxes)/Finnraccoon farms (solely Finnraccoon)/mixed farms, all farms/mink farms (solely mink)/fox farms (solely foxes)/Finnraccoon farms (solely Finnraccoon)/mixed farms with FENP and all farms/mink farms (solely mink)/fox farms (solely foxes)/Finnraccoon farms (solely Finnraccoon)/mixed farms with no FENP.

Additional file 2. Crude odds ratios (OR) with 95% confidence intervals (CI) of all variables included in the epidemiologic study of FENP in Finland: All farms, mixed farms, mink farms, fox farms and adjusted by the farm type.

Authors' contributions
HN participated in the study and questionnaire design and the statistical analyses. KV participated in the study and questionnaire design and the statistical analyses. AS and OV participated in the study and questionnaire design and participated in the analysis. AMV participated in the study and questionnaire design, coordinated the distribution of questionnaires, created the maps in the article and participated in the analysis. All authors contributed to writing the manuscript. All authors read and approved the final manuscript.

Author details
[1] Department of Veterinary Biosciences, Faculty of Veterinary Medicine, University of Helsinki, Helsinki, Finland. [2] Department of Virology and Immunology, HUSLAB, Hospital district of Helsinki and Uusimaa, Helsinki, Finland. [3] Department of Virology, Faculty of Medicine, University of Helsinki, Helsinki, Finland.

Acknowledgements
We thank Maija Mäkinen for her valuable work on preparing the returned questionnaires for statistical analysis, Heidi Rosengren, DVM for participating in the study and questionnaire design, Anna-Maria Moisander-Jylhä, DVM for participating in the questionnaire design and FFBA for funding the study and sending the questionnaires to farmers.

Competing interests
The authors declare that they have no competing interests.

Funding
This work was funded by the Finnish Fur Breeders' Association (FFBA).

References
1. Bröjer C. Pododermatitis in farmed mink in Canada. M.Sc. Thesis, The University of Guelph, Canada. 2000.
2. Nordgren H, Aaltonen K, Sironen T, Kinnunen PM, Kivistö I, Raunio- Saarnisto M, et al. Characterization of a new epidemic necrotic pyoderma in fur animals and its association with *Arcanobacterium phocae* infection. PLoS ONE. 2014;9:10.
3. Johnson SP, Jang S, Gulland FMD, Miller MA, Casper DR, Lawrence J, et al. Characterization and clinical manifestations of *Arcanobacterium phocae* infections in marine mammals stranded along the central California coast. J Wildl Dis. 2003;39:136–44.
4. Chalmers G, Mclean J, Hunter DB, Brash M, Slavic D, Pearl DL, et al. *Staphylococcus* spp., *Streptococcus canis* and *Arcanobacterium phocae* of healthy Canadian farmed mink and mink with pododermatitis. Can J Vet Res. 2015;79:129–35.
5. Sergeant ESG. Epitools epidemiological calculators. AusVet Anim Health Serv Aust Biosecurity Coop Res Cent Emerg Infect Dis. 2011.
6. Ekström J. The phi-coefficient, the tetrachoric correlation coefficient, and the Pearson-Yule Debate. UCLA: Department of Statistics; 2011.
7. McFadden D. Conditional logit analysis of qualitative choice behavior. In: Zarembka P, editor. Frontiers in Econometrics. Cambridge: Academic Press; 1974. p. 105–42.
8. Cox DR, Snell EJ. Analysis of binary data. 2nd ed. London: Chapman & Hall; 1989.
9. Basic information about fur farms in Finland in Turkistieto.fi. http://www.turkistieto.fi/Basic_Information. Accessed 20 Dec 2016.
10. Clausen TN, Dietz HH. Wet kits in mink, a review. Scientifur. 2004;28:87–90.
11. Belliveau AM, Farid A, O'Connell M, Wright JM. Assessment of genetic variability in captive and wild American mink (*Mustela vison*) using microsatellite markers. Can J Anim Sci. 1999;79:7–16.
12. Porter DD, Larsen AE, Porter HG. The pathogenesis of Aleutian disease of mink. 1. In vivo viral replication and the host antibody response to viral antigen. J Exp Med. 1969;130:575–89.
13. Porter DD, Larsen AE, Porter HG. The pathogenesis of Aleutian disease of mink. 3. Immune complex arteritis. Am J Pathol. 1973;71:331–44.
14. Knuuttila A, Aronen P, Saarinen A, Vapalahti O. Development and evaluation of an enzyme-linked immunosorbent assay based on recombinant VP2 capsids for the detection of antibodies to Aleutian mink disease virus. Clin Vaccine Immunol. 2009;16:1360–5.
15. Nordgren H, Aaltonen K, Raunio- Saarnisto M, Sukura A, Vapalahti O, Sironen T. Experimental infection of mink enforces the role of *Arcanobacterium phocae* as causative agent of Fur Animal Epidemic Necrotic Pyoderma (FENP). PLoS ONE. 2016;11:12.
16. Affolter TW, Gorham JR. Bacterial diseases of mink. In: Blue book of farming. 2001;32:20–43.
17. Dillman DA, Smyth JD, Christan LM. Internet, phone, mail, and mixed-mode surveys: the tailored design method. 4th ed. Wiley. 2014;1–18.
18. Jespersen A, Agger JF, Clausen T, Bertelsen S, Jensen HE, Hammer AS. Anatomical distribution and gross pathology of wounds in necropsied farmed mink (*Neovison vison*) from June and October. Acta Vet Scand. 2016;58:1.
19. Kempe R, Strandén I. Breeding for better eye health in Finnish blue fox (*Vulpes lagopus*). J Anim Breed Genet. 2016;133:51–8.

20

Overweight in adult cats: a cross-sectional study

Malin Öhlund[1]* ⓘ, Malin Palmgren[2] and Bodil Ström Holst[1]

Abstract

Background: Overweight in cats is a major risk factor for diabetes mellitus and has also been associated with other disorders. Overweight and obesity are believed to be increasing problems in cats, as is currently seen in people, with important health consequences. The objectives of the present study were to determine the prevalence of overweight in cats from two different cohorts in a cross-sectional study design and to assess associations between overweight and diagnoses, and between overweight and demographic and environmental factors. Data were obtained from medical records for cats (n = 1072) visiting an academic medical center during 2013–2015, and from a questionnaire on insured cats (n = 1665). From the medical records, information on body condition score, breed, age, sex, neutering status, and diagnosis was obtained. The questionnaire included questions relating to the cat's body condition, breed, age, sex, neutering status, outdoor access, activity level, and diet. Data were analyzed by multivariable logistic regression.

Results: The prevalence of overweight was 45% in the medical records cohort and 22% in the questionnaire cohort, where owners judged their pet's body condition. Overweight cats in the medical records cohort were more likely to be diagnosed with lower urinary tract disease, diabetes mellitus, respiratory disease, skin disorders, locomotor disease, and trauma. Eating predominantly dry food, being a greedy eater, and inactivity were factors associated with an increased risk of overweight in the final model in the questionnaire cohort. In both cohorts, the Birman and Persian breeds, and geriatric cats, were less likely to be overweight, and male cats were more likely to be overweight.

Conclusions: The prevalence of overweight cats (45%) as assessed by trained personnel was high and in the same range as previously reported. Birman and Persian cats had a lower risk of overweight. The association with dry food found in adult, neutered cats is potentially important because this type of food is commonly fed to cats worldwide, and warrants further attention. Drawbacks related to the study design need to be acknowledged when interpreting the results, such as a potential for selection bias for cats visiting an animal hospital, and an information bias for questionnaire data. The high occurrence of overweight in cats needs to be addressed because it negatively affects their health.

Keywords: Dry food, Epidemiology, Feline, Logistic regression, Obesity, Type 2 diabetes

Background

Overweight and obesity are considered to be increasing problems in cats [1]. In humans, overweight and obesity are rapidly escalating problems, contributing to the global epidemic of type 2 diabetes mellitus (T2DM) [2, 3]. Overweight and obesity are also important risk factors for diabetes mellitus (DM) in cats [4–7]. The prevalence of overweight and obesity in cats ranges from 7 to 63% in different populations [8–16]. Obesity, together with physical inactivity, are believed to be the main contributors to the insulin resistance associated with T2DM in both cats and people [17–19]. Furthermore, overweight and obesity are associated with an increased risk of other diseases, such as lower urinary tract disease, dermatoses, oral cavity disease, and lameness [4, 6, 20]. Skin problems associated with overweight and obesity are mostly

*Correspondence: malin.ohlund@slu.se
[1] Department of Clinical Sciences, Swedish University of Agricultural Sciences, P.O. Box 7054, 750 07 Uppsala, Sweden
Full list of author information is available at the end of the article

non-allergic, and authors speculate about whether an inability to groom is a contributing factor to this association [4]. An increased load on weight-bearing joints leading to osteoarthritis (OA) is one explanation for the increased risk of lameness in overweight cats, but human studies have also reported an increased risk of OA even in non-weight-bearing joints, suggesting a more general metabolic abnormality affecting the joint cartilage [4, 21]. In people, cats, and dogs, obesity is associated with an increased prevalence of certain types of cancer, and with a shortened life span [6, 22–25]. Obesity is in itself also considered a major animal welfare problem [26].

There are many studies on prevalence and risk factors for overweight and obesity in people, but studies on cats are scarcer. In Sweden, there are currently no studies reporting prevalence of overweight in cats. Better knowledge on predisposing factors for overweight and obesity is important to identify cats at risk at an earlier stage, to enable use of preventive measures to avoid overweight, and subsequently have a better possibility to prevent development of obesity-related diseases such as DM. The aims of this cross-sectional study were to determine the prevalence of overweight in adult cats, to assess associations between overweight and demographic factors and diagnoses in a cohort of cats visiting a University Animal Hospital, and to add the evaluation on associations between overweight and environmental factors derived from questionnaire data obtained from a cohort of adult, insured cats. Overweight in this study is defined as having a body condition score (BCS) above normal, which therefore includes both overweight and obese cats.

Methods

Study populations

Medical records cohort

This cohort consisted of medical records from all cats (n = 5935) visiting the University Animal Hospital, Swedish University of Agricultural Sciences, during 2013–2014, and records from only purebred cats during the first three quarters of 2015, to collect more pure-bred cat data to enable comparisons between breeds. Medical records were reviewed, and information on BCS, breed, age, sex, neutering status, and diagnosis was obtained. Cats were excluded if younger than 1 year of age at time of the visit to avoid cats that were not fully grown. If BCS was not assessed at all by the examining veterinarian or veterinary student, or if not assessed with a nine-grade scale (the BCS scale normally used at the hospital [27]), cats were also excluded from the study. Cats 1–2 years of age were grouped as "junior", 3–6 years as "prime", 7–10 years as "mature", 11–14 years as "senior", and 15 years of age or older as "geriatric". Only one visit per cat was included in the dataset. Purebred cats with less

than 20 individuals within the breed were grouped as "other purebreds". Cats were grouped as "overweight" for BCS 6–9, which included both overweight and obese cats, and to "not overweight" for scores 1–5, which included normal weight and underweight cats [27, 28]. Diagnostic codes were assigned by the attending veterinarian based on a standardized system with about 8000 diagnostic codes available [29]. Diagnostic codes used were grouped into the following 12 categories: the whole animal (including unspecific diagnoses such as anorexia, fever, and depression), circulatory organs, digestive tract, DM, endocrine diseases other than DM, skin disorders, locomotor apparatus, respiratory tract, upper urinary tract, lower urinary tract, neoplasia, and traumatic injuries. The group with a diagnosis referring to the whole animal was used as a reference for comparisons because the group was large and had a normal mean BCS.

Questionnaire cohort

The second cohort comprised cats (n = 5363) insured by Agria Pet Insurance[1] at any time during 2009–2013. The cats were used in a previous study as a non-diabetic control group, supplying data from a large cohort of randomly selected insured cats. Only cats 5 years of age or older were included in the previous study; therefore, data from younger cats were not available in the questionnaire cohort. Besides this no other selection was made for the cats included in this cohort [7]. All cat owners received an invitation to participate in the study by mail, including a web address to the survey. A web-based questionnaire containing 48 questions (in Swedish) was available during a 4-month period during 2015–2016 through an online survey provider.[2] Questions included information about the age and sex of the respondent, number of adults in the household, the presence of children (< 18 years) in the household, the habitat, as well as questions on the cat's birth year, breed, sex, and neutering status. Owners were asked if their cat was still alive, and if it was not, the cause and year of death. All questions on environmental factors referred to the last year of the cat's life if the cat was no longer alive, or to the most recent year for cats alive at the time of the study. Owners were asked about the cat's body condition, type of diet, feeding regimen, eating behavior, number of cats in the household, presence of other animals in the household, vaccinations, activity level, and about indoor confinement or whether the cat had access to the outdoors. Respondents were given several answering options per question, including the alternative "Other/I wish not to answer this question/I do not know", as well as space for free-text

---

[1] Agria Pet Insurance, P.O. Box 70306, SE-107 23, Stockholm, Sweden.

[2] Netigate®, Lästmakargatan 20, SE-111 44, Stockholm. Sweden.

answers. Answers were mandatory to proceed through the survey, and most often with only one answer per question possible. It was possible for respondents to return to previous questions and change their answers. Depending on the answer, some questions led the respondents to a set of extra questions. Questions on type of diet allowed several answers. Owners were asked to give only one answer if the cat's diet consisted mainly of one type of food (≥ 75%), and two answers if the cat ate about 50% of each type of food. It was not possible to give more than two answers to this question. For the question on eating behavior, the respondent could choose between "greedy" (finishes meal immediately), finishes meal within hours, nibbles several times daily (grazer), or "picky" (leaves food). For activity level, the following options were available: very active, normal activity level, and inactive. Alternatives for the question on feeding regimen were ad libitum, once daily, twice daily, or three times daily.

All answers from the questionnaire were thoroughly scrutinized and all incomplete answers were excluded. In case of conflicting answers, e.g. birth year after time of death, contact with the respondent was made if possible, and answers were then corrected or excluded. All free text answers were reviewed and replies were corrected in case of obvious misinterpretation of the question, e.g. a change of breed category to "domestic" if the owner stated that the cat was in fact a mix between two breeds. Purebred cats with less than 20 individuals within the breed were grouped as "other purebreds". Cats 5–6 years of age were grouped as "prime", 7–10 years as "mature", 11–14 years as "senior", and 15 years or older as "geriatric". Answers on type of diet were grouped according to the following categories: "dry" if ≥ 75% dry food, "mixed" if about 50% dry and 50% wet food, and "wet" if ≥ 75% wet food. Wet food included all types of wet or other high moisture food, excluding table scraps.

Respondents estimated their cat's BCS using a five-grade scale with illustrations and accompanying instructions [30]. We chose the five-grade scale in order to facilitate body condition scoring for the owners. Cats were grouped to "overweight", with estimated BCS of 4–5, which included both overweight and obese cats, and to "not overweight" for scores 1–3, which included normal weight and underweight cats.

Data analysis

Data on BCS was dichotomized into the groups overweight and not overweight to be able to use the same type of regression analysis for both cohorts because different scales were used for the body condition scoring. The outcome of interest in the present study was overweight, defining both overweight and obese cats as overweight, which was the second reason for dichotomizing the outcome for analysis. Univariable logistic regression was used to assess associations between overweight and all explanatory variables included in the questionnaire cohort and the medical records cohort separately. Potential 2-way interactions were also assessed between all variables in each cohort. Multicollinearity between explanatory variables was not assessed. The answering option "I wish not to answer this question/I do not know" rendered very few replies per question, and these answers were therefore imputed to the most commonly used answering alternative if used by less than 2% of respondents. A backwards elimination approach with stepwise removal of nonsignificant main effects was then applied to a multivariable logistic regression analysis performed on each dataset, based on a lowered Akaike information criterion (AIC) as a measure of best goodness of fit of the final statistical model. Odds ratios (OR) for risk of overweight for all significant variables from the multivariable regression analysis were calculated in SAS by exponentiation of the parameter estimates, with 95% confidence intervals (CI). Comparisons between cohorts were performed with a *t-test* for mean age, and a Chi square test for the proportions of male, neutered, domestic, and overweight cats. Mean BCS and standard deviation (SD) was calculated for the different diagnostic code groups, and mean age and SD for each cohort. The significance level was set at 5%. Data handling was performed using SAS (version 9.4).[3]

Results

Medical records cohort

A total of 1157 medical records (19%) contained information on BCS and were included, while records from 4778 cats lacked information on BCS and were therefore excluded. An analysis of the medical records lacking information on BCS was not included in this study. Fourteen cats were excluded for using a scale other than the nine-grade. A total of 71 cats were then excluded for being younger than 1 year of age, leaving 1072 individual cats for analysis (18% of all cats visiting the hospital). Cats were predominantly domestic (65%). Fifty-seven percent were male and 43% female. Seventy-eight percent of cats were neutered according to the information available in the medical records. Mean age was 8.3 ± 4.6 years (range 1–21 years).

Questionnaire cohort

The response rate was 32%, with a total of 1716 questionnaires received, of which 1686 were complete. A non-respondent analysis was not performed, due to

---

[3] SAS Institute Inc., Cary, NC 27513, US.

confidentiality, because the respondents most often were anonymous. Twenty-one cats (1.2%) were excluded due to conflicting answers or because birth year was outside the selected range. Questionnaires with data on 1665 cats thus remained for analysis (31% of all cats). Cat owner characteristics did not differ between overweight and non-overweight cats. Respondents comprised 84% females and 16% males. About half of the respondents (47%) lived in towns (200–200,000 inhabitants), 26% lived in larger cities and 27% in the countryside. Seventy-eight percent of the cats lived in a household without children and 25% of the cats lived in a single-person household.

Most cats in the questionnaire cohort were domestic cats (80%), and 20% were purebreds, which was proportionally fewer than in the medical records cohort (P < 0.0001). Fifty-two percent were males and 48% were females, which also differed from the questionnaire cohort (P = 0.04). There were 0.2% intact males, and 1.7% intact females, leaving 98% of cats neutered, which was more than in the medical records cohort (P < 0.0001) Mean age was 13.9 ± 3.1 years (range 5–25 years), higher than for the medical records cohort (P < 0.0001). Fifty-nine percent of the cats were alive at the time their owners took part in the survey.

Prevalence of overweight and results from the regression analyses

There were more overweight cats in the medical records cohort (45%) than in the questionnaire (22%) cohort (P < 0.0001). Descriptive statistics for cats in both cohorts are shown in Table 1, and diagnostic code groups including mean BCS for cats in the medical records cohort in Table 2.

In the univariable analysis on data from the medical records cohort, the following variables were associated with overweight: breed (P = 0.0002), sex (P < 0.0001), age (P < 0.0001), neutering status (P = 0.0026), and diagnostic code group (P < 0.0001). In the questionnaire cohort, the following variables were associated with overweight: breed (P = 0.0038), sex (P = 0.015), age (P = 0.0007), type of food (P = 0.0031), eating behavior (P < 0.0001), and activity level (P < 0.0001). There were no significant interactions present between any of the variables. All variables showing significance in the univariable analyses remained significant in the multivariable logistic regression for both cohorts. Results from the multivariable logistic regression analyses are shown in Figs. 1, 2, 3 and 4. Odds ratios including CIs, and P values, for all significant variables are shown in Additional file 1.

Table 1 Descriptive statistics for both cohorts

	Medical records cohort (n = 1072)		Questionnaire cohort (n = 1665)	
	Total	Number of overweight cats (% within row)	Total	Number of overweight cats (% within row)
Breed (n)				
Birman	43 (4%)	4 (9%)	69 (4%)	2 (3%)
British shorthair	26 (2%)	17 (65%)	n.a.	n.a.
Cornish rex	20 (2%)	8 (40%)	n.a.	n.a.
Domestic cats	701 (65%)*	331 (47%)	1338 (80%)	317 (24%)
Maine Coon	50 (5%)	22 (44%)	20 (1%)	5 (25%)
Norwegian forest cat	51 (5%)	20 (39%)	61 (4%)	7 (11%)
Other purebreds	117 (11%)	58 (50%)	132 (8%)	32 (24%)
Persian	28 (3%)	5 (18%)	45 (3%)	6 (13%)
Ragdoll	36 (3%)	14 (39%)	n.a.	n.a.
Age (years)				
Mean (SD)	8.3 (± 4.6)*	n.a.	13.9 (± 3.1)	n.a.
Sex (n)				
Male	606 (57%)†	307 (51%)	868 (52%)	214 (25%)
Neutering status (n)				
Neutered	841 (78%)*	396 (47%)	1633 (98%)	364 (22%)
Body condition (n)				
Overweight	479 (45%)*	n.a.	369 (22%)	n.a.

General information on cats in the medical records cohort (n = 1072) and questionnaire cohort (n = 1665) with regard to breed, age, sex, neutering status, and body condition, including the number and proportion of overweight cats

n.a. not applicable, *SD* standard deviation

* Difference between cohorts P < 0.0001

† Difference between cohorts P = 0.04

Table 2 Diagnostic code groups and body condition

Diagnostic code group	Number of cats (n = 1072)	Mean body condition score (± SD)
Lower urinary tract	89 (8.3%)	6.2 (± 1.6)
Locomotor apparatus	53 (4.9%)	6.0 (± 1.6)
Respiratory tract	53 (4.9%)	5.9 (± 1.7)
Skin disorders	66 (6.2%)	5.9 (± 1.5)
Diabetes mellitus	23 (2%)	5.8 (± 2.0)
Trauma	160 (14.9%)	5.6 (± 1.3)
Neoplasia	47 (4.4%)	5.2 (± 1.8)
Digestive tract	165 (15.4%)	5.2 (± 1.7)
The whole animal	273 (25.5%)	4.8 (± 1.9)
Circulatory system	40 (3.7%)	4.7 (± 1.7)
Endocrine (other)	32 (3.0%)	4.4 (± 1.5)
Upper urinary system	71 (6.6%)	4.3 (± 1.7)

Number of cats in the medical records cohort (n = 1072) per diagnostic code group, and mean body condition score (scale 1–9) in each group

SD standard deviation

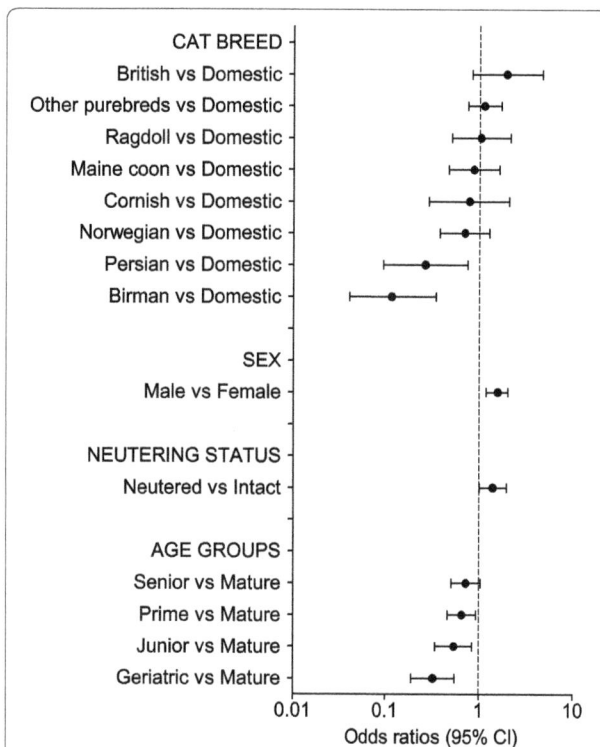

Fig. 1 Multivariable logistic regression on the medical records cohort—demographic factors. Odds ratios for overweight in the medical records cohort (overweight cats n = 479, not overweight n = 593) from the multivariable logistic regression analysis depending on demographic risk factors (breed, sex, neutering status, and age groups). Error bars represent 95% confidence intervals (CI)

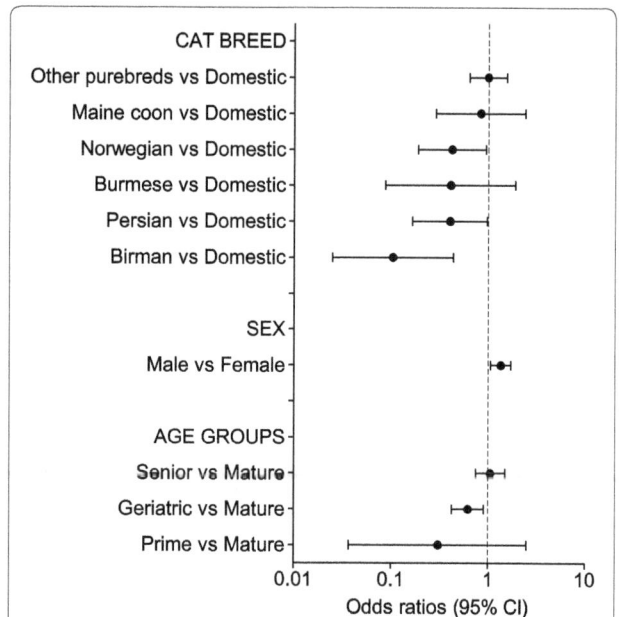

Fig. 2 Multivariable logistic regression on the questionnaire cohort—demographic factors. Odds ratios for overweight in the questionnaire cohort (overweight cats n = 369, not overweight n = 1296) from the multivariable logistic regression analysis depending on demographic risk factors (breed, sex, and age groups). Error bars represent 95% confidence intervals (CI)

In both cohorts, Birman and Persian cats had a lower risk of overweight than domestic cats. In the questionnaire cohort, the Norwegian forest cat breed also showed a decreased risk of overweight. Domestic cats had an increased risk of overweight compared with purebreds in the questionnaire cohort (OR 1.8; 95% CI 1.3–2.5).

Male cats were at increased risk of overweight compared with females in both cohorts (OR 1.6; 95% CI 1.2–2.0 in the medical records cohort, and OR 1.4; 95% CI 1.1–1.7 in the questionnaire cohort). Neutering status was only significant in the medical records cohort, where neutering was associated with an increased risk of being overweight (OR 1.4; 95% CI 1.0–2.0).

In both cohorts, geriatric cats were less likely to be overweight than mature cats (OR 0.3; 95% CI 0.2–0.5 and OR 0.6; 95% CI 0.4–0.9). In the medical records cohort, junior and prime cats were also less likely to be overweight (OR 0.5; 95% CI 0.3–0.8 and OR 0.7; 95% CI 0.5–0.9), compared with mature cats.

In the medical records cohort, several diagnostic code groups were associated with overweight when compared with cats with a diagnosis referring to the whole animal. Cats were more often overweight if they had a diagnosis related to the lower urinary tract (OR 3.4; 95% CI 2.0–5.7), DM (OR 2.7; 95% CI 1.1–6.6), respiratory tract (OR 2.6; 95% CI 1.4–4.8), skin (OR 2.4; 95% CI 1.3–4.2), the locomotor system (OR 1.9; 95% CI 1.1–3.5), or related to trauma (OR 1.6; 95% CI 1.0–2.4).

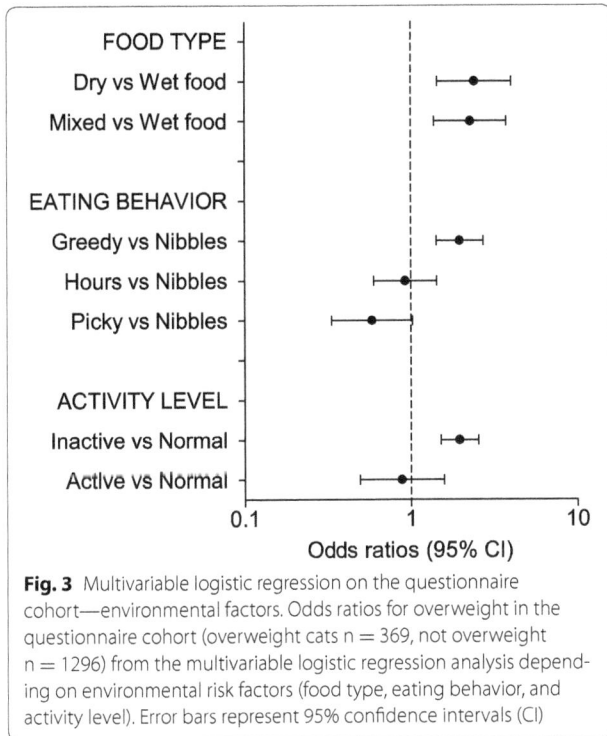

Fig. 3 Multivariable logistic regression on the questionnaire cohort—environmental factors. Odds ratios for overweight in the questionnaire cohort (overweight cats n = 369, not overweight n = 1296) from the multivariable logistic regression analysis depending on environmental risk factors (food type, eating behavior, and activity level). Error bars represent 95% confidence intervals (CI)

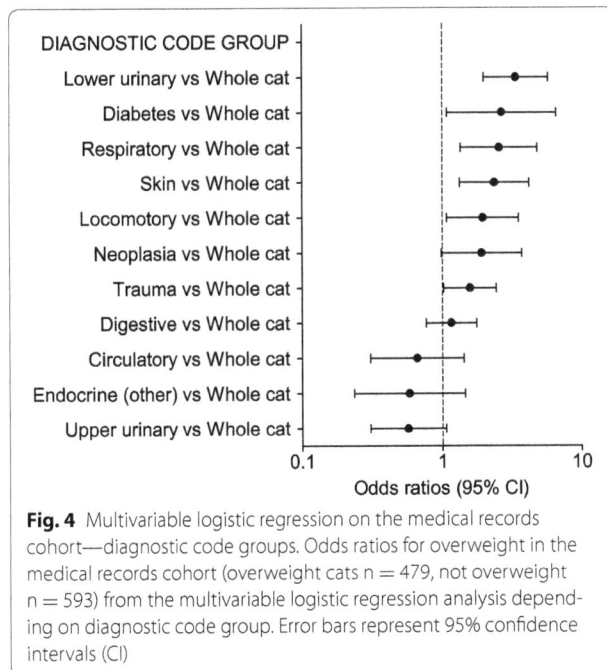

Fig. 4 Multivariable logistic regression on the medical records cohort—diagnostic code groups. Odds ratios for overweight in the medical records cohort (overweight cats n = 479, not overweight n = 593) from the multivariable logistic regression analysis depending on diagnostic code group. Error bars represent 95% confidence intervals (CI)

In the questionnaire cohort, eating predominantly dry food was associated with an increased risk of overweight compared with wet food (OR 2.4; 95% CI 1.4–4.0). Being defined as a greedy eater was also associated with overweight (OR 2.0; 95% CI 1.4–2.7) as compared with cats that preferably nibble several times daily (grazer). Inactive cats were more likely to be overweight compared with cats with a normal activity level (OR 2.0; 95% CI 1.5–2.5).

Variables not associated with overweight in the questionnaire cohort were cat owner characteristics (number of adults in the household, P = 0.79; presence of children in the household, P = 0.93; owner sex, P = 0.21; owner age, P = 0.71), the habitat (P = 0.17), feeding regime (P = 0.22), vaccination status (P = 0.07), number of cats in the household (P = 0.33), presence of other animals in the household (P = 0.67), and outdoor access or indoor confinement (P = 0.43).

Discussion

The prevalence of overweight in adult cats visiting an academic medical center in our study was high, with almost every second cat considered overweight when body condition was assessed by a veterinarian or veterinary student. In the second cohort, where owners estimated their pets' body condition, the prevalence of overweight was lower, with one in five cats considered overweight. The prevalence of overweight found in this study was in the same range as in previous reports [8–11]. Different scales were used for scoring, a nine-grade for the medical records cohort and a five-grade scale for the questionnaire cohort, but because all cats were grouped into only two groups for the analyses, overweight versus not overweight, the influence of using different scales would in our opinion be slight. The divergence between the cohorts can be explained by the actual differences present between the cohorts. There were differences in breed composition, mean age, number of male versus female cats, and neutering status present between cohorts, but the larger proportion of domestic, neutered and older cats in the questionnaire cohort would implicate a higher prevalence of overweight in this group, which was in contrast to what was found. It has previously been described that there is a tendency of owners to underestimate the BCS of their pet, which probably contributes to the lower prevalence seen in the questionnaire cohort [12, 31, 32]. Courcier et al. [31] found that owner misperception was more likely when owners rated cats with BCS 1 (very thin) and 4 (overweight) on a five-grade scale, and in longhaired cats. Moreover, it has been shown that owner underestimation of the cat's BCS is in itself a risk factor for obesity [10, 12, 32]. Because owners tend to underestimate their pet's BCS, we believe that cats judged as overweight in the questionnaire are in fact truly so, strengthening the associations found with overweight in the study. All cats visiting the University Animal Hospital are supposed to have an assessment of their BCS, but in reality only one in five cats was scored, and there is probably also a selection of which cats are actually selected for scoring, which are limitations of the study. It is unknown whether there is a tendency to more often score obese cats, or thin cats. It is possible that healthy cats undergoing routine prophylactic procedures such as vaccinations, and critically ill cats, are not being scored to the same extent as other cats. How this affects our results is unknown. Moreover, cats visiting an animal hospital might not be representative of the general population.

Several diagnostic code groups were associated with overweight. Scarlett and Donoghue reported associations between obesity and lameness, DM, and non-allergic skin disorders [4], similar to the findings in our study, and Lund et al. found associations between obesity and urinary tract disorders [6], also found in our study. Excess weight affects joints mechanically and can lead to OA, but it has also been shown in people that arthrosis is a hormonally mediated disease associated with obesity [21]. The association between DM and overweight in cats is well-known and supported by our findings [1, 4, 7]. Scarlett and Donoghue found a fourfold increased risk of DM in obese cats [4]. Lower urinary tract disease such as urethral obstruction is commonly seen in overweight, neutered, middle-aged male cats [33], similar to our findings. It is not clear from our cross-sectional study design if overweight predisposes cats to certain diseases, or if being overweight is a consequence of disease. It is possible that if overweight predisposes cats to disease, more overweight cats will be encountered at an animal hospital than in the general population.

We found that cats eating predominantly dry food were more often overweight than cats eating predominantly wet food, in a cohort consisting of mature and mainly neutered cats. An association between dry food and overweight in adult cats has to our knowledge not been reported before, although recent studies on younger cats showed feeding a dry diet to be a risk factor for overweight [14, 15]. Rowe et al. [14] showed that cats fed dry food as the only or major part of their diet at about 2 years of age, were twice as likely to be obese compared to those fed a wet or a mixed diet. Because dry food is fed to a vast number of cats worldwide, this finding warrants further investigation. Our group has previously shown an association between dry food and an increased risk of DM in cats assessed as normal weight by their owners [7]. Many studies have investigated associations between food type and risk of overweight, but only associations with therapeutic and premium dry diets have been found, a finding likely to be a confounder because weight loss diets are often prescribed to overweight patients [6, 9, 10, 31, 34–36]. However, the change from a low-carbohydrate diet in feral cats consuming wild prey to a typical high-carbohydrate diet fed to many cats today, has been suggested to be partially responsible for the recent increase in obesity and DM seen in domestic cats [17]. In 1963, Joshua [37] stated that a diet change was not necessary for cats diagnosed with DM because they were already on a very low carbohydrate intake anyway, which reflects the difference in how cats were fed then compared to now, with many cats fed a high-carbohydrate diet such as dry food. High-carbohydrate diets have been shown to lead to higher insulin blood concentrations than high-protein and high-fat diets [38]. The exact macronutrient content in food given to cats in our study is unknown, although a typical commercial dry diet generally contains more carbohydrates than a typical wet diet [39]. Dry food is typically more energy-dense than wet food, which contains more water, which also may contribute to our findings [40]. Cats have been shown to decrease their voluntary energy intake when fed a canned diet *ad lib* compared with a freeze-dried version of the canned diet, indicating that the bulk water might promote weight loss in cats [41]. Because it is not possible to alter one macronutrient without altering another, the difference in BCS between cats fed dry food and cats fed wet food might relate to a protein effect rather than a carbohydrate effect. Studies have shown that increased dietary protein promotes fat loss and reduces loss of lean body mass during weight loss in cats [42]. It has also been shown that high-protein diets can increase energy expenditure, as protein can induce a higher thermic effect than the other macronutrients [43]. Cats are obligate carnivores, whose natural diet consists mainly of protein-rich animal prey [44]. Moreover, cats lack several enzymes involved in carbohydrate metabolism, such as salivary amylase, and have low activities of intestinal amylase and disaccharidases, indicating that they are not adapted to using carbohydrates as a primary energy source, although they can still digest and utilize cooked starch [45, 46].

There was no association between feeding regimen and overweight in our study, in contrast to some previous studies showing conflicting results, with both ad libitum feeding and being fed twice daily as risk factors for obesity [31, 36]. Being defined as a greedy eater, however, was associated with an increased risk of being overweight. Being greedy was an independent risk factor also for DM in a previous study from our group [7]. In people, eating slowly is associated with a lower caloric intake and enhanced satiety [47], but this has to our knowledge not been evaluated in cats.

Activity level was associated with overweight in our study, with inactive cats at higher risk. On the other hand, we could not detect an association between indoor confinement and access to the outdoors and overweight. Some studies have shown indoor confinement to be a risk factor for obesity [9, 15, 34], whereas others have failed to show such an association [12, 31, 36]. Inactivity has been reported as a risk factor for obesity, but others have reported no associations between activity and obesity [9, 10]. According to the present study, it is the activity in itself that is important, not whether it is performed outdoors or indoors. However, in a previous study from our group, investigating risk factors for DM in cats, the opposite was found, with indoor confinement being a more important risk factor for disease than the activity levels [7]. It should be noted that the measurement of activity level is subjectively made, and performed by the owners. Future studies investigating the effect of activity on body weight will benefit from using objective measurements of the cats' activity levels.

Male sex was associated with an increased risk of overweight in both cohorts, similar to what has previously been shown [6, 11, 12, 18, 48]. Male cats have been shown to gain weight more easily than female cats [18]. Neutering was a risk factor found only in the medical records cohort, because almost all cats in the questionnaire cohort were neutered, making comparisons between neutering statuses unfeasible. Neutering can increase daily food intake, decrease the metabolic rate, and cause activity levels to drop, thereby predisposing neutered cats to obesity [48–52]. Caloric restriction is generally required after neutering, and a failure to adjust food supply to meet the lower energy requirements can easily lead to obesity in the neutered cat [50]. Both male sex and neutering have been identified as risk factors also for DM [5, 53]. It is not clear whether the neutering itself causes insulin resistance or whether it indirectly influences the risk of DM by increasing the risk of obesity.

Geriatric cats were less likely to be overweight compared with mature cats in both cohorts, in concordance with previous studies [6, 11, 13, 34, 36]. Sarcopenia is a natural age-related change that likely contributes to this finding, as well as the presence of concurrent diseases causing weight loss more commonly seen in older cats, such as chronic kidney disease, hyperthyroidism, and dental problems [54]. In the medical records cohort, the junior and prime age groups showed less overweight compared with mature cats, but in the questionnaire cohort, the lack of cats younger than 5 years excluded comparisons. It is interesting that the age incidence of DM in cats closely follows the age incidence of overweight, again stressing the importance of obesity as a major risk factor for DM [53].

Birman and Persian cat breeds showed a decreased risk of overweight in our study. We did not identify any particular cat breed at an increased risk of being overweight, but when comparing purebred and domestic cats in the questionnaire cohort, the domestic cats were more often overweight, similar to what has been shown previously [6, 12, 13]. There is also an increased risk for DM in domestic cats compared with purebred cats [53]. The association between breed and overweight likely to some extent reflects the genetic aspect of the condition. Haring et al. have recently shown that a genetic component is responsible for the development of overweight in cats [55]. In the questionnaire cohort, with owners estimating their pet's body condition, the Norwegian cat breed showed a decreased risk of obesity, differing from previous studies [56]. It also differed from our expectations, because the Norwegian forest cat has been shown to have a breed predisposition to DM, and a propensity for obesity was anticipated [53]. The Norwegian forest cat is according to the breed standard a large cat breed, which might lead owners to underestimate their pet's body condition. It should be noted that in the medical record cohort, when BCS was assessed by a veterinarian or veterinarian student, the Norwegian forest cats did not differ in body condition compared with other pedigree cats.

Limitations of our study are mainly related to the study design, particularly the problems with recall bias, because some of the answers in the questionnaire referred to several years back in time, and also the difficulties for owners to accurately assess their cats' BCS which can be a significant confounder. The multiple assessors of the BCS is also a drawback of the study. Moreover, the potential selection bias may also affect the estimated associations of overweight with risk factors and diseases. On the other hand, associations between overweight and demographic factors including age, breed and sex, were similar between cohorts, strengthening the results.

Conclusions
We found a high prevalence of overweight in adult cats, similar to other reports. Having a greedy eating behavior and being inactive were factors associated with overweight, as were diagnoses such as lower urinary tract disease, DM, respiratory disease, skin disorders and locomotor disease. In both cohorts, Birman and Persian cats, and geriatric cats, were less likely to be overweight,

whereas male cats were more likely to be overweight. There was a divergence in the estimated occurrence of overweight between the cohorts, due to differences between groups, but probably also explained by the owners' inability to correctly assess their pets' body condition. Because overweight is a growing problem in both pets and people, there is a risk that our perception of what is actually a normal body condition is being slowly altered. Finally, the association found between dry food and overweight in the group of adult, neutered cats, warrants further investigation because dry food is a common food type fed cats worldwide.

Abbreviations
BCS: body condition score; CI: confidence interval; DM: diabetes mellitus; OA: osteoarthritis; OR: odds ratio; SD: standard deviation; T2DM: type 2 diabetes mellitus.

Authors' contributions
MÖ and MP collected the data. MÖ drafted the manuscript. All authors designed the study, analyzed the data, interpreted the results. All authors read and approved the final manuscript.

Author details
[1] Department of Clinical Sciences, Swedish University of Agricultural Sciences, P.O. Box 7054, 750 07 Uppsala, Sweden. [2] Kumla Animal Hospital, Företagsgatan 7, 692 71 Kumla, Sweden.

Acknowledgements
The authors thank Agria Pet Insurance for access to the database, and the University Animal Hospital, Swedish University of Agricultural Sciences, for access to the medical records.

Competing interests
The authors declare that they have no competing interests.

Funding
The research project was funded by the Future Animal Health and Welfare research platform, Swedish University of Agricultural Sciences.

References
1. German AJ. The growing problem of obesity in dogs and cats. J Nutr. 2006;136:1940–6.
2. Newton W, Jorgensen M, Heymsfield SB. Canaries in the coal mine: a cross-species analysis of the plurality of obesity epidemics. Proc R Soc B. 2011;278:1626–32.
3. Chen L, Magliano DJ, Zimmet PZ. The worldwide epidemiology of type 2 diabetes mellitus-present and future perspectives. Nat Rev Endocrinol. 2012;8:228–36.
4. Scarlett JM, Donoghue S. Associations between body condition and disease in cats. J Am Vet Med Assoc. 1998;212:1725–31.
5. Panciera DL, Thomas CB, Eicker SW, Atkins CE. Epizootiologic patterns of diabetes mellitus in cats: 333 cases (1980–1986). J Am Vet Med Assoc. 1990;197:1504–8.
6. Lund EM, Armstrong PJ, Kirk CA, Klausner JS. Prevalence and risk factors for obesity in adult cats from private US veterinary practices. Int J Appl Res Vet Med. 2005;3:88–96.
7. Ohlund M, Egenvall A, Fall T, Hansson-Hamlin H, Röcklinsberg H, Holst BS. Environmental risk factors for diabetes mellitus in cats. J Vet Intern Med. 2017;31:29–35.
8. Sloth C. Practical management of obesity in dogs and cats. J Small Anim Pract. 1992;33:178–82.
9. Scarlett JM, Donoghue S, Saidla J, Wills J. Overweight cats: prevalence and risk factors. Int J Obes Relat Metab Disord. 1994;18(Suppl 1):22–8.
10. Cave NJ, Allan FJ, Schokkenbroek SL, Metekohy CAM, Pfeiffer DU. A cross-sectional study to compare changes in the prevalence and risk factors for feline obesity between 1993 and 2007 in New Zealand. Prev Vet Med. 2012;107:121–33.
11. Courcier E, Mellor D, Pendlebury E, Evans C, Yam P. An investigation into the epidemiology of feline obesity in Great Britain: results of a cross-sectional study of 47 companion animal practises. Vet Rec. 2012;171:560.
12. Colliard L, Paragon B-M, Lemuet B, Benet J-J, Blanchard G. Prevalence and risk factors of obesity in an urban population of healthy cats. J Feline Med Surg. 2009;11:135–40.
13. Teng KT, McGreevy PD, Toribio J, Raubenheimer D, Kendall K, Dhand NK. Risk factors for underweight and overweight in cats in metropolitan Sydney, Australia. Prev Vet Med. 2017;144:102–11.
14. Rowe EC, Browne WJ, Casey RA, Gruffydd-Jones TJ, Murray JK. Early-life risk factors identified for owner-reported feline overweight and obesity at around 2 years of age. Prev Vet Med. 2017;143:39–48.
15. Rowe E, Browne W, Casey R, Gruffydd-Jones T, Murray J. Risk factors identified for owner-reported feline obesity at around 1 year of age: dry diet and indoor lifestyle. Prev Vet Med. 2015;121:273–81.
16. Vandendriessche VL, Picavet P, Hesta M. First detailed nutritional survey in a referral companion animal population. J Anim Physiol Anim Nutr (Berl). 2017;101(Suppl 1):4–14.
17. Rand JS, Fleeman LM, Farrow HA, Appleton DJ, Lederer R. Canine and feline diabetes mellitus: nature or nurture? J Nutr. 2004;134(8 Suppl):2072–80.
18. Appleton DJ, Rand JS, Sunvold GD. Insulin sensitivity decreases with obesity, and lean cats with low insulin sensitivity are at greatest risk of glucose intolerance with weight gain. J Feline Med Surg. 2001;3:211–28.
19. Porte D. β-cells in type II diabetes mellitus. Diabetes. 1991;40:166–80.
20. Jones B, Sanson R, Morris R. Elucidating the risk factors of feline lower urinary tract disease. NZ Vet J. 1997;45:100–8.
21. Spector T, Campion G. Generalised osteoarthritis: a hormonally mediated disease. Ann Rheum Dis. 1989;48:523.
22. Ogden CL, Carroll MD, Flegal KM. Epidemiologic trends in overweight and obesity. Endocrinol Metab Clin North Am. 2003;32:741–60.
23. Glickman LT, Schofer FS, McKee LJ, Reif JS, Goldschmidt MH. Epidemiologic study of insecticide exposures, obesity, and risk of bladder cancer in household dogs. J Toxicol Environ Health A. 1989;28:407–14.
24. Kitahara CM, Flint AJ, de Gonzalez AB, Bernstein L, Brotzman M, MacInnis RJ, et al. Association between class III obesity (BMI of 40–59 kg/m^2) and mortality: a pooled analysis of 20 prospective studies. PLoS Med. 2014;11:e1001673.
25. Kealy RD, Lawler DF, Ballam JM, Mantz SL, Biery DN, Greeley EH, et al. Effects of diet restriction on life span and age-related changes in dogs. J Am Vet Med Assoc. 2002;220:1315–20.
26. Sandøe P, Palmer C, Corr S, Astrup A, Bjørnvad CR. Canine and feline obesity: a one health perspective. Vet Rec. 2014;175:610–6.
27. Laflamme D. Development and validation of a body condition score system for cats: a clinical tool. Feline Pract. 1997;25:13–8.
28. Bjornvad CR, Nielsen DH, Armstrong PJ, McEvoy F, Hoelmkjaer KM, Jensen KS, et al. Evaluation of a nine-point body condition scoring system in physically inactive pet cats. Am J Vet Res. 2011;72:433–7.
29. Olson P, Kängström LE. Svenska djursjukhusföreningens diagnosregister för häst, hund och katt. Taberg: Svenska djursjukhusföreningen; 1993.
30. Baldwin K, Bartges J, Buffington T, Freeman LM, Grabow M, Legred J, et al. AAHA nutritional assessment guidelines for dogs and cats. J Am Vet Med Assoc. 2010;46:285–96.
31. Courcier EA, O'Higgins R, Mellor DJ, Yam PS. Prevalence and risk factors for feline obesity in a first opinion practice in Glasgow, Scotland. J Feline Med Surg. 2010;12:746–53.
32. Allan FJ, Pfeiffer DU, Jones BR, Esslemont DHB, Wiseman MS. A cross-sectional study of risk factors for obesity in cats in New Zealand. Prev Vet Med. 2000;46:183–96.
33. Gerber B, Boretti F, Kley S, Laluha P, Müller C, Sieber N, et al. Evaluation of clinical signs and causes of lower urinary tract disease in European cats. J Small Anim Pract. 2005;46:571–7.

34. Robertson ID. The influence of diet and other factors on owner-perceived obesity in privately owned cats from metropolitan Perth, Western Australia. Prev Vet Med. 1999;40:75–85.

35. Kienzle E, Bergler R. Human-animal relationship of owners of normal and overweight cats. J Nutr. 2006;136:1947–50.

36. Russell K, Sabin R, Holt S, Bradley R, Harper E. Influence of feeding regimen on body condition in the cat. J Small Anim Pract. 2000;41:12–8.

37. Joshua JO. Some clinical aspects of diabetes mellitus in the dog and cat. J Small Anim Pract. 1963;4:275–80.

38. Keller C, Liesegang A, Frey D, Wichert B. Metabolic response to three different diets in lean cats and cats predisposed to overweight. BMC Vet Res. 2017;13:184.

39. Villaverde C, Fascetti AJ. Macronutrients in feline health. Vet Clin North Am Small Anim Pract. 2014;44:699–717.

40. Zoran DL. The carnivore connection to nutrition in cats. J Am Vet Med Assoc. 2002;221:1559–67.

41. Wei A, Fascetti AJ, Villaverde C, Wong RK, Ramsey JJ. Effect of water content in a canned food on voluntary food intake and body weight in cats. Am J Vet Res. 2011;72:918–23.

42. Laflamme DP, Hannah SS. Increased dietary protein promotes fat loss and reduces loss of lean body mass during weight loss in cats. Int J Appl Res Vet Med. 2005;3:62–8.

43. Wei A, Fascetti A, Liu K, Villaverde C, Green A, Manzanilla E, et al. Influence of a high-protein diet on energy balance in obese cats allowed ad libitum access to food. J Anim Physiol Anim Nutr. 2011;95:359–67.

44. Macdonald ML, Rogers QR, Morris JG. Nutrition of the domestic cat, a mammalian carnivore. Annu Rev Nutr. 1984;4:521–62.

45. Morris JG, Trudell J, Pencovic T. Carbohydrate digestion by the domestic cat (Felis catus). Br J Nutr. 1977;37:365–73.

46. Kienzle E. Carbohydrate metabolism of the cat 2. Digestion of starch. J Anim Physiol Nutr. 1993;69:102–14.

47. Andrade AM, Greene GW, Melanson KJ. Eating slowly led to decreases in energy intake within meals in healthy women. J Am Diet Assoc. 2008;108:1186–91.

48. Donoghue S, Scarlett JM. Diet and feline obesity. J Nutr. 1998;128:2776–8.

49. Hoenig M, Ferguson DC. Effects of neutering on hormonal concentrations and energy requirements in male and female cats. Am J Vet Res. 2002;63:634–9.

50. Harper EJ, Stack DM, Watson TDG, Moxham G. Effects of feeding regimens on bodyweight, composition and condition score in cats following ovariohysterectomy. J Small Anim Pract. 2001;42:433–8.

51. Fettman M, Stanton C, Banks L, Hamar D, Johnson D, Hegstad R, et al. Effects of neutering on bodyweight, metabolic rate and glucose tolerance of domestic cats. Res Vet Sci. 1997;62:131–6.

52. Kanchuk ML, Backus RC, Calvert CC, Morris JG, Rogers QR. Weight gain in gonadectomized normal and lipoprotein lipase—deficient male domestic cats results from increased food intake and not decreased energy expenditure. J Nutr. 2003;133:1866–74.

53. Ohlund M, Fall T, Ström Holst B, Hansson-Hamlin H, Bonnett B, Egenvall A. Incidence of diabetes mellitus in insured Swedish cats in relation to age, breed and sex. J Vet Intern Med. 2015;29:1342–7.

54. Laflamme DP. Nutrition for aging cats and dogs and the importance of body condition. Vet Clin Small Anim Pract. 2005;35:713–42.

55. Haring T, Wichert B, Dolf G, Haase B. Segregation analysis of overweight body condition in an experimental cat population. J Hered. 2011;102(Suppl 1):S28–31.

56. Kienzle E, Moik K. A pilot study of the body weight of pure-bred client-owned adult cats. Br J Nutr. 2011;106:113–5.

21

Prevalence and phylogenetic analysis of hepatitis E virus in pigs, wild boars, roe deer, red deer and moose in Lithuania

Ugne Spancerniene[1]*, Juozas Grigas[1], Jurate Buitkuviene[2], Judita Zymantiene[1], Vida Juozaitiene[3], Milda Stankeviciute[4], Dainius Razukevicius[4], Dainius Zienius[5] and Arunas Stankevicius[1]

Abstract

Background: Hepatitis E virus (HEV) is one of the major causes of acute viral hepatitis worldwide. In Europe, food-borne zoonotic transmission of HEV genotype 3 has been associated with domestic pigs and wild boar. Controversial data are available on the circulation of the virus in animals that are used for human consumption, and to date, no gold standard has yet been defined for the diagnosis of HEV-associated hepatitis. To investigate the current HEV infection status in Lithuanian pigs and wild ungulates, the presence of viral RNA was analyzed by nested reverse transcription polymerase chain reaction (RT-nPCR) in randomly selected samples, and the viral RNA was subsequently genotyped.

Results: In total, 32.98 and 22.55% of the domestic pig samples were HEV-positive using RT-nPCR targeting the ORF1 and ORF2 fragments, respectively. Among ungulates, 25.94% of the wild boar samples, 22.58% of the roe deer samples, 6.67% of the red deer samples and 7.69% of the moose samples were positive for HEV RNA using primers targeting the ORF1 fragment. Using primers targeting the ORF2 fragment of the HEV genome, viral RNA was only detected in 17.03% of the wild boar samples and 12.90% of the roe deer samples. Phylogenetic analysis based on a 348-nucleotide-long region of the HEV ORF2 showed that all obtained sequences detected in Lithuanian domestic pigs and wildlife belonged to genotype 3. In this study, the sequences identified from pigs, wild boars and roe deer clustered within the 3i subtype reference sequences from the GenBank database. The sequences obtained from pig farms located in two different counties of Lithuania were of the HEV 3f subtype. The wild boar sequences clustered within subtypes 3i and 3h, clearly indicating that wild boars can harbor additional subtypes of HEV. For the first time, the ORF2 nucleotide sequences obtained from roe deer proved that HEV subtype 3i can be found in a novel host.

Conclusion: The results of the viral prevalence and phylogenetic analyses clearly demonstrated viral infection in Lithuanian pigs and wild ungulates, thus highlighting a significant concern for zoonotic virus transmission through both the food chain and direct contact with animals. Unexpected HEV genotype 3 subtype diversity in Lithuania and neighboring countries revealed that further studies are necessary to understand the mode of HEV transmission between animals and humans in the Baltic States region.

Keywords: Moose, ORF2, Phylogenetic analysis, Pig, Red deer, Roe deer, Wild boar

Background

Hepatitis E virus (HEV) which causes a food and water borne disease in humans [1], has emerged during the past decade as a causative agent of autochthonous hepatitis in developed countries [2]. Meat and meat-derived products from HEV-infected reservoir animals can transmit the virus to humans and represent a public health concern [3]. The first evidence of the zoonotic transmission of HEV genotype 3 was found in Japan in 2003, when several cases of hepatitis E infection were linked to the consumption of pig and deer meat or organs [4, 5]. More case reports (grilled wild boar meat in Japan, pig meat in

*Correspondence: ugne.spancerniene@lsmuni.lt
[1] Department of Anatomy and Physiology, Faculty of Veterinary Medicine, Lithuanian University of Health Sciences, Tilzes str. 18, Kaunas, Lithuania
Full list of author information is available at the end of the article

Spain, *figatelli* sausage from Corsica) have provided additional evidence that HEV is a zoonosis that can be transmitted via the consumption of contaminated food [6–8]. Admittedly, known viral RNA is an important marker of acute HEV infection, especially during early stages before the antibody response becomes evident [9]. However, until now, viral RNA has not been detected (in the representative sample) in Lithuanian pigs and wild ungulates such as wild boar, roe deer, red deer and moose. Thus, we aimed to gain insight through molecular investigation into HEV in these species as they are frequently used for human consumption. Furthermore, the availability of the generated HEV sequences may serve as a basis for interdisciplinary studies comparing human isolates to identify transmission interactions between animal and human hosts [10].

Methods

The sample set for the study comprised 470 pig serum samples that had been collected randomly from farms by veterinarians within the framework of an official infectious disease surveillance program and 626 (n = 320 liver and n = 306 serum) samples from wild boar *(Sus scrofa)* (n = 505), roe deer *(Capreolus capreolus)* (n = 93), red deer *(Cervus elaphus)* (n = 15) and moose *(Alces alces)* (n = 13) that were hunted in 212 locations of Lithuania during the hunting seasons from 2014 to 2016.

Blood samples obtained from the wildlife were gathered from the heart or thoracic cavity into sterile plastic tubes. The serum was separated from the cellular elements by centrifuging the coagulated blood for 10 min at $2000 \times g$. The extracted serum was stored at -20 °C until further analysis. During the dressing of the carcasses, small pieces of hepatic tissues were also taken and stored at -20 °C prior to further analysis.

HEV RNA extraction and RT-PCR

Viral RNA was isolated from serum or liver samples with the Gene JET RNA Purification Kit (Thermo Fisher Scientific) according to the manufacturer's recommendations. The extracted RNA was analyzed by nested reverse transcription polymerase chain reaction (RT-nPCR) using two HEV-specific sets of primers targeting the ORF1 and ORF2 fragments of the HEV genome (Table 1). The first amplification round was run in 25 µL of reaction mix containing 2.5 µL of extracted RNA, 12.5 µL of Dream Taq Green PCR Master mix (Thermo Fisher Scientific), 1 µL of the forward primer HEV-s (or 3156F), 1 µL of the reverse primer HEV-as (or 3157R), 0.3 µL of RevertAid Reverse Transcriptase (Thermo Fisher Scientific), 0.13 µL of RiboLock RNase Inhibitor (Thermo Fisher Scientific) and 7.12 µL of nuclease-free water (Thermo Fisher Scientific). The cycling conditions were: 42 °C for 30 min, initial denaturation at 95 °C for 5 min followed by 40 cycles of denaturation at 94 °C for 30 s (or 1 min if ORF2 primers were used), annealing at 50 °C for 30 s (or 60 °C for 1 min if ORF2 primers were used) and elongation at 72 °C for 45 s (or 1 min if ORF2 primers were used), followed by a final elongation at 72 °C for 10 min.

Next, 2.5 µL of the product of the first amplification round was transferred to a new PCR mix containing 12.5 µL of Dream Taq Green PCR Master mix (Thermo Fisher Scientific), 1 µL of the forward primer HEV-fn (or 3158Fn), 1 µL of the reverse primer HEV-rn (or 3159Rn) and 8 µL of nuclease-free water (Thermo Fisher Scientific). The second-round cycling conditions were identical to those of the first except that the cycle at 42 °C for 30 min was not required and the annealing temperature of 50 °C was maintained for 30 s (or 55 °C for 1 min if ORF2 primers were used). All reactions were performed in a Mastercycler personal thermocycler (Eppendorf, Hamburg, Germany). The RT-nPCR products were separated on ethidium bromide-stained 1.8% agarose gels and visualized by UV light.

To minimize carryover, different parts of the process were physically separated from one another (in entirely separate working areas). A PCR hood and aerosol-barrier

Table 1 Primer sets used in this study

Primer designation	Sequence (5′ → 3′)	Step	Product length (bp)	Target region
HEV-s	TCGCGCATCACMTTYTTCCARAA	RT-PCR	469	ORF1
HEV-as	GCCATGTTCCAGACDGTRTTCCA			
HEV-fn	TGTTGCCCTGTTTGGCCCLIGGITTAG	Nested RT-PCR	254	
HEV-rn	CCAGGCTCACCRGARTGYTTCTTCCA			
3156F	AATTATGCYCAGTAYCGRGTTG	RT-PCR	731	ORF2
3157R	CCCTTRTCYTGCTGMGCATTCTC			
3158Fn	GTWATGCTYTGCATWCATGGCT	Nested RT-PCR	348	
3159Rn	AGCCGACGAAATCAATTCTGTC			

tips were used for the assembly of all reactions to avoid contamination. In every step, control reactions with no template were performed to check for contamination.

Statistical analyses

Statistical analysis was conducted using the SPSS for Windows 15 statistics package (SPSS Inc., Chicago, IL, USA). The results were significant when $P < 0.05$. The descriptive data are presented as percentages. Fisher's exact test was used to test for differences in prevalence of HEV and different target regions. HEV prevalence was calculated in pigs and wild animal species for the ORF1 and ORF2 sequences with 95% confidence intervals.

Sequencing and phylogenetic analysis

The HEV-positive ORF2 RT-nPCR products were excised from the agarose gel, purified with a GeneJET PCR Purification kit (Thermo Fisher Scientific) and sequenced in both directions using the BigDye Terminator Cycle Sequencing kit v3.1 (Applied Biosystems) and the 3130 × Genetic Analyzer (Applied Biosystems). The sequences of both strands of the ORF2 PCR products were determined using the same primer set and identical cycling conditions as the nested PCR amplification. The sequences were submitted to GenBank.

The obtained ORF2 sequences (Accession Numbers MG739304–MG739318) were compared with the reference set of the selected sequences from GenBank, representing a full range of genetic diversity and geographic locations of the HEV genotype-3. The sequences were aligned using Clustal W software from MegAlign (Lasergene software package, DNASTAR Inc, Madison, USA). Bootstrap values were calculated using CLC Gene Free Workbench software, with bootstrap values based on 100 replicates (v4.0.01, CLC bio A/S, Aarhus, Denmark). Bootstrap values greater than 70% were considered to provide significant evidence for phylogenetic grouping.

Results

The detailed HEV RNA results targeting different parts of the HEV genome are summarized in Table 2.

In total, 155 of 470 (32.98%, 95% CI 28.88–37.35) and 106 of 470 (22.55%, 95% CI 19.01–26.55) domestic pig samples were positive for HEV RNA using RT-nPCR based on ORF1 and ORF2, respectively. The difference in positive detection rates between ORF1 and ORF2 was highly significant ($P = 0.0004$).

In wild animal species, 25.94% (95% CI 22.31–29.93) of wild boar samples, 22.58% of roe deer (95% CI 15.27–32.07) samples, 6.67% (95% CI 1.19–29.82) of red deer samples and 7.69% (95% CI 1.37–33.31) of moose samples were positive for HEV RNA using primers targeting ORF1. Viral RNA was detected in 17.03% (95% CI

14.00–20.55) of wild boar samples and 12.90% (95% CI 7.54–21.21) of roe deer samples targeting ORF2, while no HEV RNA was found in red deer or moose samples. Statistically significant differences in the proportion of the prevalence (%) detected by targeting the ORF1 and ORF2 fragments were observed for all investigated wild animal species except for roe deer.

Samples from different hunting sites and pig farms were sequenced and analyzed to determine the HEV subtypes within different Lithuanian regions and hosts. Phylogenetic analyses based on a 348-nucleotide-long HEV ORF2 region showed that all obtained sequences detected in Lithuanian domestic pigs and wildlife belonged to genotype 3 (Fig. 1). Further subtyping was performed by comparing the obtained sequences with reference sequences representing the 3a, 3b, 3c, 3h, 3i, 3j subtypes of one major clade and the 3e, 3f, 3g subtypes of another major clade. The sequences identified in this study from pigs, wild boars and roe deer clustered within the 3i subtype reference sequences from the GenBank database, showing a homology of 88% (ranging from 86.8 to 88.9%). The 13 sequences from pigs, wild boars and roe deer clustered separately within subtype 3i, showing a mean homology of 96.3% (ranging from 96.3 to 100%). Two sequences from different pig farms clustered within subtype 3f sequences and revealed 85.3% (ranging from 71.6 to 99%) identity to reference strains of this HEV subtype. One HEV wild boar sequence clustered between subtypes 3i and 3h ORF2 reference sequences and exhibited 85.6–92.1% identity to subtype 3i and 87.6–86.4% to subtype 3h sequences.

Discussion

The presence of HEV in food products derived from natural reservoirs of zoonotic HEV or food (fruits, vegetables, shellfish) that is contaminated by surface and irrigation water raises concerns for public health and food safety worldwide [11]. Autochthonous human HEV infections in industrialized countries (due to genotypes 3 and 4) are increasingly reported and are linked to zoonotic transmission, mainly through the consumption of contaminated meat and offal from pigs, Eurasian wild boar and deer that have been deemed to be plausible reservoirs for HEV [12]. Moreover, there is a category of meat from non-domesticated animals (game meat) that are hunted and slaughtered mostly for private consumption, but which can also be found in markets or restaurants. Although game meat represents only a small portion of the European market, its popularity as a luxury food source is growing worldwide. Wild boar and roe deer are the most common sources of game meat in Europe, including Lithuania, and have the largest harvest numbers [12, 13]. In addition, hunting, which is another

Table 2 Prevalence of HEV in domestic pigs and wild animal species using RT-nPCR assay

Investigated host	ORF1 targeting primers			ORF2 targeting primers		
	Sample type (number of HEV positive/tested samples (%))		All types of samples (number of HEV positive/tested (%, 95% CI))	Sample type (number of HEV positive/tested samples (%))		All types of samples (number of HEV positive/tested (%, 95% CI))
	Serum	Liver		Serum	Liver	
Domestic pigs (*Sus scrofa domesticus*)	155/470 (32.98)	–	155/470 (32.98%, 28.88–37.35)	106/470 (22.55)	–	106/470 (22.55%, 19.01–26.55)
Wild boars (*Sus scrofa*)	62/235 (26.38)	69/270 (25.56)	131/505 (25.94%, 22.31–29.93)	41/235 (17.44)	45/270 (16.67)	86/505 (17.03%, 14.00–20.55)
Roe deer (*Capreolus capreolus*)	10/45 (22.22)	11/48 (22.92)	21/93 (22.58%, 15.27–32.07)	7/45 (15.56)	5/48 (10.42)	12/93 (12.90%, 7.54–21.21)
Red deer (*Cervus elaphus*)	1/13 (7.69)	0/2 (0)	1/15 (6.67%, 1.19–29.82)	0/13 (0)	0/2 (0)	0/15 (0%, 0.00–20.39)
Moose (*Alces alces*)	1/13 (7.69)	–	1/13 (7.69%, 1.37–33.31)	0/13	–	0/13 (0%, 0.00–22.81)

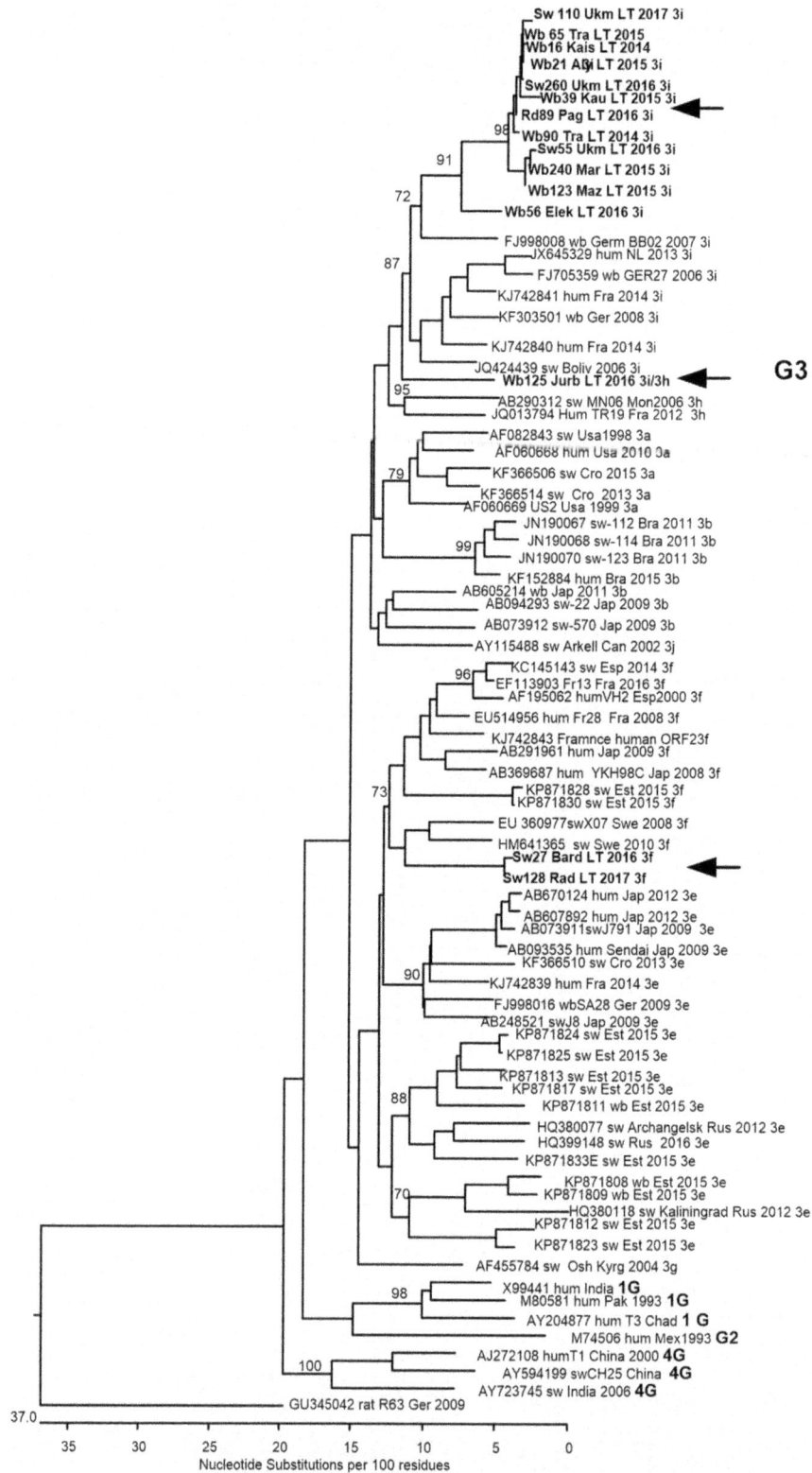

Fig. 1 Phylogenetic analysis of Lithuanian HEV ORF2 sequences. Clustal W algorithm was used for sequence alignment. Numbers adjacent to main branches indicate bootstrap values for different genetic subtypes within HEV genotype3. The reference sequences are marked as follows: GenBank Accession Number, host and name of sequence, country (up to three letter abbreviations), year, subtype. The analysis involved 80-nucleotide partial HEV ORF2 sequences. Only bootstrap values > 70% are indicated. The sequences determined in this study (Accession Numbers MG739304– MG739318) are indicated in bold and with arrows

recognized risk factor for zoonotic HEV transmission, is very common in Lithuania, with approximately 32 624 wild boars and 23 828 roe deer killed during the 2016–2017 hunting season [14]. Thus, the consumption of game meats and offal that may harbor HEV is as risky as eating pork [15].

To date, the detection of HEV is mainly carried out through qualitative or quantitative PCR. Extraction methods and detection protocols can vary significantly, and no gold standard approach has yet been defined for HEV diagnosis. The choice of primers used in RT-PCR assays varies from laboratory to laboratory. The differences in the sensitivity and specificity of various primers often lead to difficulties in comparing results from various studies. Therefore, caution must be taken when interpreting the results. It is known that standard RT-PCR is a sensitive technique, but its sensitivity can be markedly increased by performing nested RT-PCR. The nested strategy increases the specificity of RNA amplification by reducing the background due to non-specific amplification of RNA. Thus, for the direct screening of viral nucleic acids in samples and the ability to use the subsequent positive samples for genotyping, two different PCR assays were applied in this study. For the subtyping of HEV, we needed sequences in the ORF2 region that were 348 bp long. Many real-time RT-PCR products of ORF1, ORF2, and ORF3 are only 76–100 bp in length, which is not long enough for the molecular characterization of prevalent HEV strains.

Domestic pigs had a higher prevalence of HEV (22.55–32.97%) than wild ungulates. A possible reason is that the frequent direct contact among infected pigs reared in confined spaces may enhance the spread of HEV. Pigs housed in the same pen are exposed to the saliva, nasal secretions, urine, and feces of multiple pen mates repeatedly each day. Thus, the pig-farming environment may foster the spread of HEV among pigs compared to the environment of free ranging wild ungulates. The HEV RNA prevalence estimated in domestic pigs in the present study remains within the range found in other countries, such as Croatia (24.5%, [16]) and the USA (35%, [17]). Crossan et al. [18] reported HEV RNA in 44.4% of pig serum samples in Scotland, and Di Bartolo et al. [19] detected a viral prevalence of 64.6% in pigs in Italy, whereas Jori et al. [20] detected HEV RNA in only 8.3% of tested pig samples. The conducted studies have revealed that different viral prevalence exists among countries. This may reflect different infection dynamics related to farm-specific risk factors, such as farming scale, farming practices, biosecurity measures, and seasonal influence. [21].

The viral RNA prevalence in wild boars, roe deer, red deer and moose was 17.03–25.94%, 12.90–22.58%, 0–6.67%, and 0–7.69%, respectively. Despite the high densities of both wild boar and deer in Lithuania, a slightly lower HEV prevalence was observed in cervids (roe deer, red deer, moose) compared to that in wild boars, hinting towards interspecies transmission. Evidence suggests that deer may contract HEV from wild boars in cases where both species share the same habitat [12].

Other studies have identified HEV in 4.2% (24/566), 7.5% (8/106) and 12.3% of tested wild boars in Japan [22], the Netherlands [23] and Croatia [16], respectively. Our results agree with those reported by Mesquita et al. [24], where HEV RNA was detected in 25% (20/80) of the liver samples obtained from wild boars in Portugal. In contrast, the results from most studies of viral RNA prevalence varied widely even within the same country; HEV detection rates of 14.9% (22/148, [10]) and 68.2% (90/132, [25]) were found in wild boars in Germany, and 25% (22/88, [26]) and 0% (0/77, [27]) in Italy. Hence, the RNA detection method is crucial [19]. In fact, our results confirm different sensitivity with different targeted open reading frames, suggesting that the use of several RT-nPCR protocols may increase the sensitivity of HEV RNA detection [28]. The proportion of HEV RNA-positive samples for both open reading frames in this study did not significantly differ except between roe deer (22.58% vs. 12.90%, P = 0.084). However, the sensitivity of RT-PCR assays can vary widely, depending on target regions and HEV genotypes. Furthermore, sensitivity results might be affected by the quality of the RNA extraction procedure [29].

The prevalence of HEV infection among wild cervids has not yet been thoroughly investigated, and data are still inconsistent [3]. In Germany [30], 6.4% (5/78) of roe deer were positive for viral RNA, while an absence of HEV RNA was reported in the Netherlands (0/8) [23] and Sweden (0/29, 0/27) [31]. Our study results (ranging from 12.90 to 22.58% depending on the ORF fragment) are partially consistent with those of Forgach et al. [32], who found that 22% of roe deer (*Capreolus capreolus*) were positive for HEV RNA in Hungary.

In this study, 6.67 and 7.69% of red deer and moose samples were positive for HEV ORF1. The positive result could be caused by specific or unspecific amplification of ORF1 fragment and it is noted these animals HEV strains were not successful sequenced. Moreover, none of the 15 red deer or 13 moose samples were positive for the HEV ORF2 fragment. These results might be affected by a relatively small sample size. The reason for the absence of positive cases might be divergent HEV types that could not be detected by the assay used in this study [31]. Similar findings have been recently reported in Germany, where HEV was detected in 2.0–6.6% of red deer samples [33]. A higher HEV prevalence was noticed in red deer populations in Hungary (10%, [32]), Italy (11%, [34]) and the Netherlands (15%, [23]). There is a lack of surveillance data regarding the prevalence of HEV RNA in moose, which makes it difficult to compare prevalence trends. In another study, 15% of moose samples collected in 2012–2013 in Sweden were positive for viral RNA [35]. Similar results were reported by Roth et al. [31], who detected HEV in 11% (10/66) and 15% (7/11) of Swedish moose samples from 2012 to 2015.

Phylogenetic analyses of partial ORF2 HEV sequences have shown that several genetic subtypes of the HEV genotype 3 are present in Lithuanian pigs and wildlife [36]. The comparison of sequences obtained from wild boar, pig and roe deer samples showed a high degree of homology and clustered within subtype 3i reference sequences. This suggests that only the subtype 3i of HEV genotype 3 is circulating in Lithuanian pigs and wildlife. However, the clustering of the wild boar sequence (Wb125 Jurb LT 2016 3i/3h) between the 3i and 3h subtype sequences show that the wild boar population in Lithuania can also harbor additional subtypes of the HEV 3 genotype. This sequence showed 13.5–14% nucleotide variation compared to 3i subtype reference strains and 15–16% variation compared to subtype 3 h.

The HEV 3i subtype has been detected in Austria, Germany, France, Argentina, Bolivia, and Uruguay in various hosts, including humans [25, 36, 37], wild boars [10, 25] and domestic pigs [37, 38]. The ORF2 nucleotide sequence obtained in this study from roe deer (Rd89 Pag LT 2016 3i) shows that the HEV 3i subtype can be found in this species as well. Until recently, the 3i subtype had only been detected in wild boars in Germany, while in Austria and Argentina it has also been detected in humans [39]. The German wild boar strains of HEV sequences wbGER27 and BB02 were fully sequenced and used as reference HEV 3i subtype sequences [10, 25] in this study.

The sequences obtained from pig farms located in two different counties of Lithuania clustered with HEV strains from Estonia [40], Sweden [41], France [42], Croatia [16], and Hungary [32], and all of them were of the HEV 3f subtype. Interestingly, only one HEV 3f strain was isolated from wild boars, while all other 3f strains were isolated from humans to pigs. The presence of the HEV 3f subtype in Lithuanian pig farms may be due to import of animals from other parts of the EU as HEV strains isolated from wild boars and pigs in the neighboring regions of Estonia and the Kaliningrad district of the Russian Federation, have belonged to the 3e subtype [40].

Conclusions

This study shows that pigs, wild boars, roe deer, red deer and moose in Lithuania may be infected with HEV. This calls for an increased public awareness of the zoonotic risk of HEV infection through food consumption or contact with infected animal populations.

Authors' contributions

AS designed and coordinated the study. JB, US, DZ, DR, MS and JG collected and analysed the samples. AS, US and JG drafted the manuscript. US, JZ and JB performed the literature review. VJ and JG conducted the statistical analyses. All authors read and approved the final manuscript.

Author details

[1] Department of Anatomy and Physiology, Faculty of Veterinary Medicine, Lithuanian University of Health Sciences, Tilzes str. 18, Kaunas, Lithuania. [2] National Food and Veterinary Risk Assessment Institute, J. Kairiukscio str. 10, Vilnius, Lithuania. [3] Department of Animal Breeding and Nutrition, Faculty of Animal Husbandry Technology, Lithuanian University of Health Sciences, Tilzes str. 18, Kaunas, Lithuania. [4] Faculty of Medicine, Lithuanian University of Health Sciences, A. Mickevicius str. 9, Kaunas, Lithuania. [5] Faculty of Veterinary Medicine, Institute of Microbiology and Virology, Lithuanian University of Health Sciences, Tilzes str. 18, Kaunas, Lithuania.

Acknowledgements

The authors are profoundly grateful to the Lithuanian farmers and veterinarians who kindly agreed to help us in this study and also to the hunters who provided wild animal samples.

Competing interests

The authors declare that they have no competing interests.

Funding

This study was supported by the Science Foundation of the Lithuanian University of Health Sciences.

References

1. Hara Y, Terada Y, Yonemitsu K, Shimoda H, Noguchi K, Maeda K. High prevalence of hepatitis E virus in wild boar (*Sus scrofa*) in Yamaguchi Prefecture, Japan. J Wildl Dis. 2014;50:378–83.
2. Dalton HR. Hepatitis E: the "new kid on the block" or an old friend? Transfus Med Hemother. 2014;41:6–9.
3. Serracca L, Battistini R, Rossini I, Mignone W, Peletto S, Boin C, et al. Molecular investigation on the presence of hepatitis E virus (HEV) in wild game in North-Western Italy. Food Environ Virol. 2015;7:206–12.
4. Tei S, Kitajimam N, Takahashim K, Mishirom S. Zoonotic transmission of hepatitis E virus from deer to human beings. Lancet. 2003;362:371–3.
5. Yazaki Y, Mizuo H, Takahasi M, Nishizawa T, Sasaki N, Goatnada Y, et al. Sporadic acute hepatitis E in Hokkaido, Japan, may be food-borne, as suggested by the presence of hepatitis E virus in pig liver as food. J Gen Virol. 2003;84:2351–7.

6.   Li TC, Chijiwa K, Sera N, Ishibashi T, Etoh Y, Shinohara Y, et al. Hepatitis E virus transmission from wild boar meat. Emerg Infect Dis. 2005;11:1958–60.

7.   Riveiro-Barciela M, Rodríguez-Frías F, Buti M. Hepatitis E virus: new faces of an old infection. Ann Hepatol. 2012;12:861–70.

8.   Renou C, Roque Afonso A, Pavio N. Foodborne transmission of hepatitis E virus from raw pork liver sausage, France. Emerg Infect Dis. 2014;20:1945–7.

9.   La Rosa G, Fratini M, Muscillo M, Iaconelli M, Taffon S, Equestre M, et al. Molecular characterisation of human hepatitis E virus from Italy: comparative analysis of five reverse transcription-PCR assays. Virol J. 2014. https://doi.org/10.1186/1743-422x-11-72.

10. Schielke A, Sachs K, Lierz M, Appel B, Jansen A, Johne R. Detection of hepatitis E virus in wild boars of rural and urban regions in Germany and whole genome characterization of an endemic strain. Virol J. 2009. https://doi.org/10.1186/1743-422x-6-58.

11. Doceul V, Bagdassarian E, Demange A, Pavio N. Zoonotic hepatitis E virus: classification, animal reservoirs and transmission routes. Viruses. 2016. https://doi.org/10.3390/v8100270.

12. Boadella M. Hepatitis E in wild ungulates: a review. Small Rumin Res. 2015;128:64–71.

13. Schulp CJE, Thuiller W, Verburg PH. Wild food in Europe: a synthesis of knowledge and data of terrestrial wild food as an ecosystem service. Ecol Econ. 2014;105:292–305.

14. Ministry of environment of the Republic of Lithuania official reports (ME), 2016–2017. http://www.am.lt/VI/index.php#a/18446. Accessed July 15 2017.

15. Lhomme S, Top S, Bertagnoli S, Dubois M, Guerin J, Izopet J. Wildlife reservoir for hepatitis E virus, Southwestern France. Emerg Infect Dis. 2015;21:1224–6.

16. Prpić J, Černi S, Škorić D, Keros T, Brnić D, Cvetnić Z, et al. Distribution and molecular characterization of hepatitis E virus in domestic animals and wildlife in Croatia. Food Environ Virol. 2015;7:195–205.

17. Huang FF, Haqshenas G, Guenette DK, Halbur PG, Schommer SK, Pierson FW, et al. Detection by reverse transcription-PCR and genetic characterization of field isolates of swine hepatitis E virus from pigs in different geographic regions of the United States. J Clin Microbiol. 2002;40:1326–32.

18. Crossan C, Grierson S, Thomson J, Ward A, Nunez-Garcia J, Banks M, et al. Prevalence of hepatitis E virus in slaughter-age pigs in Scotland. Epidemiol Infect. 2015;143:2237–40.

19. Di Bartolo I, Ponterio E, Castellini L, Ostanello F, Ruggeri FM. Viral and antibody HEV prevalence in swine at slaughterhouse in Italy. Vet Microbiol. 2011;149:330–8.

20. Jori F, Laval M, Maestrini O, Casabianca F, Charrier F, Pavio N. Assessment of domestic pigs, wild boars and feral hybrid pigs as reservoirs of hepatitis E virus in Corsica, France. Viruses. 2016. https://doi.org/10.3390/v8080236.

21. Salines M, Andraud M, Rose N. From the epidemiology of hepatitis E virus (HEV) within the swine reservoir to public health risk mitigation strategies: a comprehensive review. Vet Res. 2017. https://doi.org/10.1186/s13567-017-0436-3.

22. Takahashi M, Nishizawa T, Nagashima S, Jirintai S, Kawakami M, Sonoda Y, et al. Molecular characterization of a novel hepatitis E virus (HEV) strain obtained from a wild boar in Japan that is highly divergent from the previously recognized HEV strains. Virus Res. 2014;180:59–69.

23. Rutjes SA, Lodder-Verschoor F, Lodder WJ, Giessen J, Reesink H, Bouwknegt M, et al. Seroprevalence and molecular detection of hepatitis E virus in wild boar and red deer in the Netherlands. J Virol Methods. 2010;168:197–206.

24. Mesquita JR, Oliveira RM, Coelho C, Vieira-Pinto M, Nascimento MS. Hepatitis E virus in sylvatic and captive wild boar from Portugal. Transbound Emerg Dis. 2016;63:574–8.

25. Adlhoch C, Wolf A, Meisel H, Kaiser M, Ellerbrok H, Pauli G. High HEV presence in four different wild boar populations in East and West Germany. Vet Microbiol. 2009;139:270–8.

26. Martelli F, Caprioli A, Zengarini M, Marata A, Fiegna C, Di Bartolo I, et al. Detection of hepatitis E virus (HEV) in a demographic managed wild boar (Sus scrofa scrofa) population in Italy. Vet Microbiol. 2008;126:74–81.

27. Martinelli N, Pavoni E, Filogari D, Ferrari N, Chiari M, Canelli E, et al. Hepatitis E virus in wild boar in the Central Northern part of Italy. Transbound Emerg Dis. 2015;62:217–22.

28. Vasickova P, Psikal I, Widen F, Smitalova R, Bendova J, Pavlik I, et al. Detection and genetic characterisation of hepatitis E virus in Czech pig production herds. Res Vet Sci. 2009;87:143–8.

29. Mokhtari C, Marchadier E, Haïm-Boukobza S, Jeblaoui A, Tessé S, Savary J, et al. Comparison of real-time RT-PCR assays for hepatitis E virus RNA detection. J Clin Virol. 2013;58:36–40.

30. Anheyer-Behmenburg HE, Szabo K, Schotte U, Binder A, Klein G, Johne R. Hepatitis E virus in wild boars and spillover infection in red and roe deer, Germany, 2013–2015. Emerg Infect Dis. 2017;23:130–3.

31. Roth A, Lin J, Magnius L, Karlsson M, Belák S, Widén F, et al. Markers for ongoing or previous hepatitis E virus infection are as common in wild ungulates as in humans in Sweden. Viruses. 2016. https://doi.org/10.3390/v8090259.

32. Forgách P, Nowotny N, Erdélyi K, Boncz A, Zentai J, Szucs G, et al. Detection of hepatitis E virus in samples of animal origin collected in Hungary. Vet Microbiol. 2010;143:106–16.

33. Neumann S, Hackl SS, Piepenschneider M, Vina-Rodriguez A, Dremsek P, Ulrich RG, et al. Serologic and molecular survey of hepatitis E virus in German deer populations. J Wildl Dis. 2015;52:106–13.

34. Di Bartolo I, Ponterio E, Angeloni G, Morandi F, Ostanello F, Nicoloso S, et al. Presence of hepatitis E virus in a red deer (Cervus elaphus) population in Central Italy. Transbound Emerg Dis. 2017;64:137–43.

35. Lin J, Karlsson M, Olofson AS, Belák S, Malmsten J, Dalin AM, et al. High prevalence of hepatitis E virus in Swedish moose—a phylogenetic characterization and comparison of the virus from different regions. PLoS ONE. 2015. https://doi.org/10.1371/journal.pone.0122102.

36. Lu L, Li C, Hagedorn CH. Phylogenetic analysis of global hepatitis E virus sequences: genetic diversity, subtypes and zoonosis. Rev Med Virol. 2006;16:5–36.

37. Mirazo S, Mainardi V, Ramos N, Gerona S, Rocca A, Arbiza J. Indigenous hepatitis E virus genotype 1 infection, Uruguay. Emerg Infect Dis. 2014;20:171–3.

38. Purdy MA. Evolution of the hepatitis E virus polyproline region: order from disorder. J Virol. 2012;86:10186–93.

39. Vina-Rodriguez A, Schlosser J, Becher D, Kaden V, Groschup MH, Eiden M. Hepatitis E virus genotype 3 diversity: phylogenetic analysis and presence of subtype 3b in wild boar in Europe. Viruses. 2015;7:2704–26.

40. Ivanova A, Tefanova V, Reshetnjak I, Kuznetsova T, Geller J, Lundkvist Å, et al. Hepatitis E virus in domestic pigs, wild boars, pig farm workers, and hunters in Estonia. Food Environ Virol. 2015;7:403–12.

41. Widén F, Sundqvist L, Matyi-Toth A, Metreveli G, Belák S, Hallgren G, et al. Molecular epidemiology of hepatitis E virus in humans, pigs and wild boars in Sweden. Epidemiol Infect. 2011;139:361–71.

42. Colson P, Borentain P, Queyriaux B, Kaba M, Moal V, Gallian P, et al. Pig liver sausage as a source of hepatitis E virus transmission to humans. J Infect Dis. 2010;202:825–34.

22

Experimentally induced subclinical mastitis: are lipopolysaccharide and lipoteichoic acid eliciting similar pain responses?

Annalisa Elena Jolanda Giovannini[1], Bart Henricus Philippus van den Borne[2], Samantha Kay Wall[3], Olga Wellnitz[3], Rupert Max Bruckmaier[3] and Claudia Spadavecchia[1*] (iD)

Abstract

Background: Pain accompanying mastitis has gained attention recently as a relevant welfare compromising aspect of disease. Adequate pain recognition and therapy are necessary in the context of a modern and ethically acceptable dairy care. For research purposes mastitis is often induced by intramammary infusion of immunogenic bacterial cell wall components. Lipopolysaccharide (LPS) from *Escherichia coli* and lipoteichoic acid (LTA) from *Staphylococcus aureus* are commonly administered to this end. While the immune response to specific immunogenic components has been well characterized, not much is known about their role on the expression of pain indicators. The aim of this study was to trial the effects of an intramammary challenge of LTA or LPS on the degree of pain and discomfort as indicated by both physiological and behavioral variables in cows. The hypothesis was that a similar degree of pain can be identified in LTA as well as in LPS induced mastitis.

Results: On the challenge day, compared to pre-challenge, total pain index increased for all treatment groups (LPS; LTA and control), the LPS group having significantly higher values than the control group (P = 0.01). Similarly, pain visual analogue scale (VAS) increased significantly in all cows following treatment on the challenge day. Furthermore, compared to baseline, higher VAS were found 3, 4 and 5 h after the challenge in cows of the LPS group ($P_{3h, 4h} < 0.001$ and $P_{5h} = 0.001$) and 7 h after the challenge in cows of the LTA group ($P_{7h} = 0.002$). In the control group, VAS was higher 5 h after the challenge ($P_{5h} = 0.001$). On the challenge day, udder edema was higher in the LPS than in the control group (P = 0.007). Furthermore, 4 h after the challenge, milk cortisol was significantly higher than at baseline in the LPS group (P < 0.001).

Conclusions: When administered at equipotent doses targeting a standard somatic cell count increase, intramammary LPS seems to be accompanied by a higher degree of pain and discomfort than LTA, as suggested by the modifications of the outcome variables total pain index, VAS, udder edema and milk cortisol.

Keywords: Mastitis, Lipoteichoic acid, Lipopolysaccharide, Dairy cow, Pain

Background

Bovine bacterial mastitis has been increasingly recognized as a detrimental disease in dairy herds, leading to major economic losses and premature culling [1]. Mastitis-related pain and discomfort can severely compromise animal welfare and deserve to be specifically addressed [2]. In the last decade several indicators have been proposed to recognize and quantify pain in bovine mastitis. Physiological parameters such as heart rate, respiratory rate and temperature [2], modifications of postural and ingestive behaviors [3, 4], expression of active behavior like stepping, kicking and limb lifting [5, 6] and alteration in nociceptive thresholds [7, 8] have been all applied to this end.

*Correspondence: claudia.spadavecchia@vetsuisse.unibe.ch
[1] Department of Clinical Veterinary Medicine, Anesthesiology and Pain Therapy Section, Vetsuisse Faculty, University of Berne, Laenggassstrasse 124, 3012 Berne, Switzerland
Full list of author information is available at the end of the article

Most of the recent research aiming at characterizing the physiological, immunological and behavioral response to pathogenic invasion of the mammary gland has been conducted on experimentally induced mastitis [6, 7, 9, 10]. Two major immunogenic cell wall components, lipoteichoic acid (LTA) and lipopolysaccharide (LPS), deriving from *Staphylococcus aureus* and *Escherichia coli* respectively, are commonly infused in the bovine mammary gland to elicit experimental disease [10–13]. In spontaneous mastitis, *S. aureus* tend to induce a rather chronic subclinical disease, while *E. coli* is typically isolated in acute clinical cases. Whereas a pathogen-specific immune response of the mammary gland in LPS and LTA-induced mastitis has been confirmed by several studies [10, 13, 14], not much is known about the role of these specific immunogenic components on the expression of clinical pain indicators. Indeed, pain-related physiological and behavioral alterations have been widely investigated in LPS [3, 4, 7] but not in LTA induced mastitis. As *S. aureus* mammary infections lead to breast pain in humans [15], we hypothesized that a similar degree of pain can be identified in LTA as well as in LPS induced mastitis in lactating dairy cows.

The main aim of this study was to trial the effects of an intramammary challenge of LTA or LPS on the degree of pain and discomfort as indicated by both physiological and behavioral variables in cows.

Methods
The study was approved by the Cantonal Committee for Animal Experimentation, Fribourg, Switzerland (FR16/13) and all experimental procedures followed the Swiss law of animal protection.

Animals
Sixteen lactating dairy cows (12 Holstein and 4 Swiss Fleckvieh) in mid lactation (mean DIM = 202 ± 88), involved in a larger immunological study [13], were enrolled in this experiment. Parities of experimental cows ranged from 1 to 4 (average parity = 2.6) and cows were producing >15 l of milk/day (mean milk yield = 18.4 ± 3.9 l/day). They were housed in a stanchion barn and were kept in single rowed tie-stalls (width 250 cm, length 200 cm) on rubber mats bedded with wood shavings and straw. Hay was available ad libitum, as well as water (through individual water bowls); concentrate was fed according to individual production levels. Cows were machine milked at 0530 and 1600 h. Before the trial, animals were allowed to acclimatize to the new environment for at least 1 week.

Inclusion criteria for the experiment were: body condition score (BCS) of 2.5–3, healthy based on clinical examination, negative glutaraldehyde test, normal hematology and blood chemistry, milk somatic cell count (SCC) of each quarter $<150 \times 10^3$ cells/ml and negative milk bacteriology.

Experimental design
The study was designed as a prospective, blinded, controlled experimental trial. Cows were randomly allocated to one of 3 treatment groups: LPS group (n = 6), LTA group (n = 6) and control group (C group, n = 4). For each animal, the trial started 24 h before the intramammary challenge and ended 26 h later. A maximum of two cows were studied at once. On the day preceding the challenge (control day), baseline outcome parameters were measured over 8 h and intramammary infusion, milk and blood sampling were simulated at the same time points as during the challenge day. Once terminated the 8 h data collection, a catheter (length 105 mm −Ø 1.9 × 2.4 mm −13 G, Vygon, Ecouten, France) was introduced in the jugular vein and a liver biopsy was performed. On the challenge day, immediately after morning milking and following aseptic preparation of the teat, animals received an intramammary infusion containing the assigned treatment through a sterile teat cannula (length 100 mm, −Ø 22 mm, Delvo, Switzerland; time 0). The treatments consisted of 0.2 µg LPS (from *E. coli* serotype O26:B6, Sigma-Aldrich, St. Louis, MO, USA) diluted in 10 ml of 0.9% sterile saline for group LPS, 20 µg LTA (from *S. aureus*, Sigma-Aldrich, St. Louis, MO, USA) diluted in 10 ml of 0.9% sterile saline for group LTA, and 10 ml of sterile saline 0.9% alone for group C. Dosages of LPS and LTA were chosen to induce a similar SCC increase. For each animal 2 randomly allocated quarters (one front and one hind) were infused according to the treatment, while the other 2 received an equivalent volume of sterile 0.9% saline. On the challenge day, outcome parameters were collected over 8 h starting from time 0. Once terminated the data collection, a liver and two udder biopsies on the hind quarters were performed. All biopsies, performed for the purpose of the immunological study [13] in all groups, were taken in unsedated but physically restrained cows after skin desensitization with 10 ml of lidocaine (Lidocaine 2%, Streuli Pharma AG, Switzerland). A last clinical examination and recording of outcome parameters was performed 26 h after the challenge. At this time point, rescue analgesia (3 mg/kg ketoprofen IV; Rifen 10%, Streuli Pharma AG, Switzerland) was provided if pain visual analogue scale (VAS) score >3 (for VAS description see below). The investigator performing clinical pain assessment (AEJG) was blinded to the treatment.

Outcome parameters

Physiological parameters

The following physiological parameters were recorded at hourly intervals: heart rate, respiratory rate and rectal temperature. Heart rate was continuously monitored using a portable heart rate monitoring system (Polar RS800CX, Polar Electro Europe BV, Switzerland) inserted in a girth positioned around the cow's chest before the trial started. Respiratory rate was evaluated through visual detection of costoabdominal distension, while rectal temperature was measured with a digital thermometer.

Ingestive and postural behavior

Time spent eating, ruminating, and lying were automatically recorded for 8 h during both the control and the challenge day using a recently validated monitoring system (Rumiwatch, Itin+Hoch GmbH, Switzerland) [16]. On cows standing with parallel hind limbs, hock-to-hock distance was measured every hour with a centimeter-scaled rolling tape as the distance between the middle points of each calcaneal tuberosity [17].

Pain scoring

For pain assessment, a mastitis-specific multidimensional pain scoring system was designed. The scoring system was organized in two main categories of symptoms, general and local, which were further divided in a total of eight sub-categories. Each sub-category was scored using simple numerical rating scales except for the sub-category postural behavior, for which a score of 1 was assigned to each of the observed manifestations. At each specific time point, assigned scores were summed to obtain the total pain index, with a maximum possible value of 42 (Table 1). Furthermore, pain severity was scored using a dynamic-interactive VAS on a 100 mm line (0 meaning no pain, 100 mm meaning the worst possible pain) [18].

Udder parameters

Udder edema and reaction to udder palpation were scored as part of the total pain index (local subcategory items, Table 1) but were also analyzed as separate variables.

Udder temperature was measured using an auto-calibrating thermic camera (InfraVet OptiRes D, VarioCAM, Infra Tech GmbH, Dresden, Germany). Two lateral views of the udder were recorded from a 50 cm distance and on animals left undisturbed for at least 10 min. Median udder surface temperature on predefined area was detected with a dedicated software (Exam Professional 5.8, InfraMedic GmbH, Germany), as previously described [19, 20].

A purpose-built digital hand-held pressure algometer with a contact surface of 0.5 cm^2 was used to test the mechanical nociceptive thresholds (MNT) at the front quarters at 2 h intervals. Force was applied in caudal direction at a constant rate of 5 N/s perpendicularly to the udder surface, dorsally to the teat basis until an avoidance behavioral reaction was observed. Maximal peak force applicable was set at 24.6 N. Two measurements per quarter, taken at 60 s intervals, were averaged for analysis.

Laboratory analysis

During the challenge day, cortisol concentrations in milk and plasma aliquots, collected as described by Wall et al. [14] and stored at −20 °C, were measured at 2 h intervals with methods described elsewhere [21]. Somatic cell count (SCC) in fresh milk samples was measured hourly with a DeLaval cell counter (DCC, DeLaval International AB, Tumba, Sweden) according to the manufacturer's protocol.

Statistical analysis

Statistical analysis of outcome parameters (see Additional file 1) was performed using hierarchical regression models built with PROC GLIMMIX within SAS 9.4 (SAS Institute, Inc., Cary, NC). Cows' activities eating, ruminating and laying were expressed as a percentage over the total recording time and aggregated at day level. The quarter outcome variable "reaction to udder palpation" was also aggregated at day level and represented whether any of the measurements on that day had a value ≥ 1. Presence of udder edema was classified as yes or no applying a binomial distribution. The decimal logarithm of milk and plasma cortisol was taken for the data to follow a normal distribution. Cow level models included the covariates day, time, and treatment as fixed effects and all their 2- and 3-way interactions evaluated. The correlation structure with the best model fit was selected to correct for correlation among repeated measurements based on the Akaike Information Criterion. For quarter-level variables, the same modeling procedure was applied but "quarter" (infusion yes or no) was additionally evaluated as a fixed effect in the above-mentioned model. Moreover, a random intercept was added to correct for clustering of quarters within cows. After Bonferroni correction, significance was defined at P value <0.0045 for cow level outcome variables and at P < 0.01 for quarter level outcome variables to correct for multiple comparisons. Model fit of linear regression models was checked by evaluating normality and homoscedasticity of residuals. Reference categories of significant variables were changed to perform a post hoc analysis to determine significant differences in 2-way or 3-way interaction terms.

Descriptive analysis of cow demographics and spearman rank correlation coefficients between total pain

Table 1 Multidimensional pain scoring system, including general and local items, divided in 8 sub-categories

Category	Sub-category	Manifestation	Assigned value
General	General subjective assessment	No signs of pain	0
			1
			2
			3
		Signs of severe pain	4
	Postural behavior	Low, asymmetric ears	1
		Corrugated upper eyelids	1
		Open nostrils	1
		Restless	1
		Apathy	1
		Wide hind limbs	1
		Other (specify)	1
	Interactive behavior	Interest	0
			1
		No interest	2
	Response to food	Appetite	0
			1
		No appetite at all	2
	Sacrum position	Normal	0
		Downward with arched back	1
	Reaction to back palpation	No reaction	0
			1
		Strong reaction	2
Local	Udder edema	FL	0-1-2-3-4
		FR	0-1-2-3-4
		HL	0-1-2-3-4
		HR	0-1-2-3-4
		0 = no swelling, 4 = very severe swelling	
	Udder palpation	FL	0-1-2
		FR	0-1-2
		HL	0-1-2
		HR	0-1-2
		0 = no reaction, 1 = mild reaction (tail flicking, limb lifting), 2 = strong reaction (kick, moving away)	
	Total pain index	Summation of scores	Max 42

Assigned scores are added to obtain the total pain index

FL front left quarter, *FR* front right quarter, *HL* hind left quarter, *HR* hind right quarter

index and VAS and between total pain index and SCC were calculated using SigmaPlot 12.0 (Systat Software GmbH, Germany).

Results

A total of 16 challenges were performed. One cow of the LTA group was excluded from statistical analysis because it had not responded to the challenge with the expected SCC increase. Thus, variables of 15 cases were evaluated. No significant differences were found among the groups concerning parity and DIM. Similar increases in SCC in infused quarters confirmed the equivalence of the LPS and LTA doses (Fig. 1).

All cows except one recovered well from the trial, as confirmed by the clinical examination 26 h after the challenge. A single cow in the LPS group received rescue analgesia at this time point.

Physiological parameters

No statistical significant difference was detected among groups for the variables heart rate, respiratory rate and rectal temperature (Table 2).

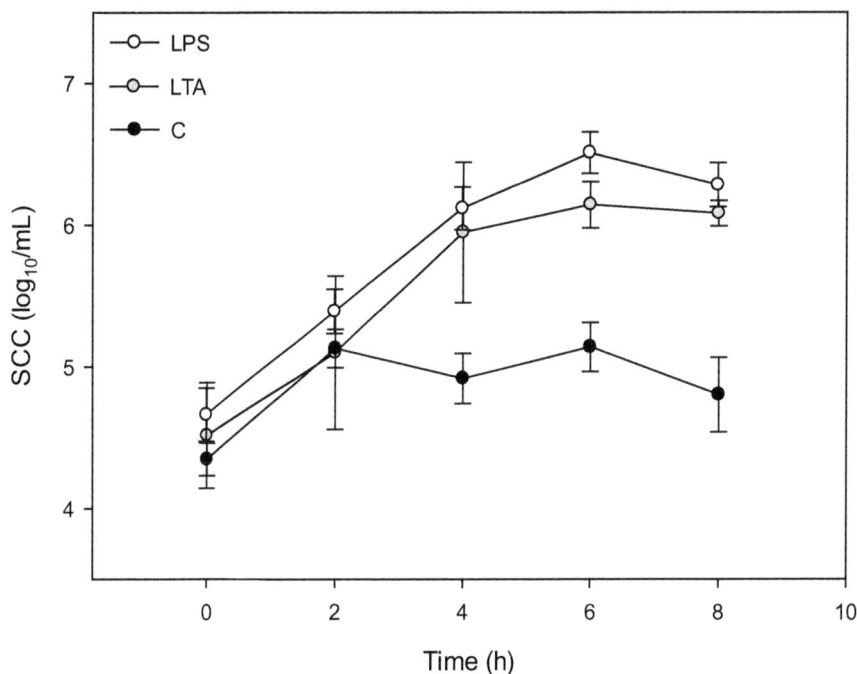

Fig. 1 Somatic cell count of infused quarters. Changes in somatic cell count of infused quarters in the LPS (lipopolysaccharide) (*white circles*), LTA (lipoteichoic acid) (*grey circles*) and control groups (*black circles*) on the challenge day. Data are expressed as mean ± SEM

Ingestive and postural behavior

Independently from the group, all cows spent significantly less time lying on the challenge day compared to the control day ($P < 0.001$). No significant difference among groups could be found for time spent eating and ruminating, although on the challenge day animals of the LPS group tended to eat less than those of the C group ($P = 0.05$) (Table 3). No differences in hock-to-hock distance were found among groups (Table 2).

Pain scoring

The variable total pain index (Fig. 2a, b) had a significant day × time interaction ($P = 0.002$). On the challenge day it increased for all 3 treatment groups, the LPS group having higher values than the control group ($P = 0.01$). Within the multidimensional pain scoring system, the mostly affected sub-categories were appetite, reaction to udder palpation and udder edema score. Results for udder variables are presented in the following paragraph.

Visual analogue scale data (Fig. 2c, d) showed a significant day × time × treatment interaction ($P < 0.001$). On the challenge day, higher VAS were found 3, 4 and 5 h after the challenge compared to t0 in cows of the LPS group ($P_{3h, 4h} < 0.001$ and $P_{5h} = 0.001$) and 7 h after the challenge in cows of the LTA group ($P_{7h} = 0.002$). In the control group, VAS was higher 5 h after the challenge

($P_{5h} = 0.001$). High correlation between total pain index and VAS ($r = 0.817$; $P < 0.001$), as well as between total pain index and SCC of infused quarters ($r = 0.707$; $P < 0.001$) were found (Fig. 3).

Udder parameters

A treatment-independent significant day effect ($P = 0.008$) resulted for reaction to udder palpation, with higher presence of at least mild responses on the challenge day compared to the control day. Udder edema score had a significant day × time interaction ($P < 0.001$): it was increasingly detected over time during the challenge day whereas no such increase was observed on the control day. On the challenge day, udder edema was higher in the LPS than in the C group ($P = 0.007$) and tended to be higher in the LTA group ($P = 0.016$) than in the C group. Moreover, udder edema tended to be higher in infused than in control quarters ($P = 0.013$). For udder temperature, no day nor quarter effect was found but, compared to t0, significantly higher values were found 2 and 8 h after the challenge in the LPS group ($P = 0.002$ and $P = 0.004$, respectively), and 6 and 8 h after the challenge in the LTA group ($P = 0.006$ and $P = 0.001$, respectively). No changes over time were detected for the C group. No statistical significant difference was detected among groups for mechanical nociceptive thresholds (Table 4).

Table 2 Heart rate (HR), respiratory rates (RR), rectal temperature (Rectal T) and hock-to-hock distance (H–H) measured in cows challenged with intramammary LPS (lipopolysaccharide), LTA (lipoteichoic acid) or saline (control group)

Parameter	Control day				Challenge day			
	2 h	4 h	6 h	8 h	2 h	4 h	6 h	8 h
HR (beats/min)								
LPS	76 (69–80)	71.5 (64–73)	71 (64–72)	74.5 (62–78)	69.5 (60–78)	71 (60–75)	71.5 (60–74)	70 (60–78)
LTA	69 (64–79)	71 (66–82)	71 (66–81)	71 (69–79)	67 (65–71)	67 (64–77)	76 (72–77)	70 (64–81)
Control	68 (62–73.5)	66.5 (59.5–72)	61.5 (57–71)	66 (61–70)	62.5 (57.5–67.5)	69 (62–70.5)	63.5 (58.5–66)	61.5 (57–67.5)
RR (breaths/min)								
LPS	30 (28–32)	32 (28–32)	32 (24–40)	32 (28–36)	28 (28–36)	32 (28–36)	30 (24–32)	30 (28–32)
LTA	32 (28–36)	32 (28–40)	36 (32–40)	32 (32–48)	32 (32–44)	32 (28–44)	44 (32–44)	36 (32–40)
Control	32 (28–34)	28 (22–38)	28 (26–42)	32 (30–36)	30 (24–36)	32 (28–38)	28 (24–40)	30 (28–40)
Rectal T (°C)								
LPS	38.1 (37.9–38.4)	38 (37.9–38.4)	38.2 (38.1–38.4)	38.1 (37.9–38.5)	38.2 (37.9–38.5)	38.3 (38.1–39.0)	38.4 (38.3–39.4)	38.8 (38.1–39.2)
LTA	38.3 (38.2–38.5)	38.2 (38–38.3)	38.3 (38.3–38.4)	38.5 (38–38.5)	38.3 (38.2–38.4)	38.4 (38.3–38.4)	38.5 (38.2–38.6)	38.7 (38.4–39.0)
Control	38.1 (37.9–38.3)	38.1 (37.9–38.3)	38.1 (37.9–38.3)	38.2 (38.1–38.3)	38.1 (38–38.1)	38.3 (38.1–38.3)	38.1 (38–38.2)	38.1 (38.1–38.3)
H–H (cm)								
LPS	22.5 (18–25)	21 (17–28)	20 (16–30)	26 (15–28)	22 (20–23)	23.5 (15–26)	20.5 (14–25)	23.5 (17–27)
LTA	23 (20–24)	22 (22–22)	22 (20–24)	22 (20–23)	18 (15–20)	20 (16–25)	23 (22–25)	23 (20–24)
Control	23 (17.5–24.5)	23.5 (17–26)	25 (19.5–28)	25 (20–27.5)	22.5 (17.5–25)	24 (23–26.5)	24.5 (24–27.5)	22 (19–26)

On the control day, the intramammary challenge, milk and blood sampling were simulated. Medians and interquartile ranges (IQR) at 2, 4, 6 and 8 h after the simulated challenge (control day)/challenge (challenge day) are reported

Table 3 Total time spent lying, eating and ruminating by cows challenged with intramammary LPS (lipopolysaccharide), LTA (lipoteichoic acid) or saline (control group)

Parameter	Control day	Challenge day
Lying time (min)		
LPS	88.4 (48.8–118.5)	26.4 (18.2–31.6)
LTA	73.6 (51.4–92.9)	15.4 (0–41.7)
Control	110.6 (80.2–130.3)	39.1 (11.8–71.4)
Eating time (min)		
LPS	104.3 (82.2–110.7)	73.4 (58.9–89.9)
LTA	160 (103–183.3)	124 (68.3–178.9)
Control	146.2 (92.4–215)	167.9 (131.4–208)
Ruminating time (min)		
LPS	186.7 (83.5–201.1)	148.9 (12–146.9)
LTA	161.2 (140.5–221)	127 (85.1–146.9)
Control	142.1 (93.7–174.1)	109.1 (95.2–119.3)

On the control day, the intramammary challenge, milk and blood sampling were simulated. Medians and interquartile ranges are reported. Recordings were performed over 8 h on both the control and the challenge day

Laboratory analysis

For plasma cortisol, no significant difference among groups was found (Fig. 4a) but a significant time × treatment effect (P = 0.003) was identified for milk cortisol. In the LPS group, 4 h after the challenge, milk cortisol was significantly higher than at t0 (P < 0.001); no quarter effect was detected. In the LTA group, 2 h after the challenge, milk cortisol was significantly lower than at t0 (P < 0.001). No changes over time for milk cortisol were observed in the C group (Fig. 4b).

Discussion

Aim of this study was to evaluate and compare the effects of an intramammary challenge of LTA or LPS on the degree of pain and discomfort as indicated by physiological and behavioral variables in cows. Our findings indicate that significant alterations of selected outcome variables occurred mostly in LPS treated cows, thus leading to a rejection of the hypothesis that similar degree of pain occurs in both LTA and LPS experimentally induced mastitis.

In the present study, the physiological outcome variables heart rate, respiratory rate and rectal temperature were evaluated. While these parameters have been shown to be good indicators of disease severity in spontaneously occurring mastitis [17, 22], they were not significantly altered by the LPS and LTA treatments, most probably due to the fact that sub-clinical disease levels were targeted.

On the challenge day, all cows spent less time lying than on the control day. Despite the effort to simulate all manipulations foreseen for the challenge day on the

control day, the presence of more people and equipment in the barn might have provoked a higher degree of disturbance to the cows, independently from the treatment group. Moreover, as udder and liver biopsies were taken at the end of the control day, it cannot be excluded that residual discomfort in the affected area might have prevented the cows from lying down [23]. For time spent lying contrasting results have been previously reported in cows affected by LPS-induced mastitis: while in some studies a clear reduction of the time spent lying was detected after the intramammary challenge [4, 6], in others no differences were found [24]. This discrepancy might confirm that direct comparison of experimental results from studies evaluating endotoxins-induced mastitis should be performed with caution, as targeted levels of severity, and thus clinical and behavioral consequences, might be different.

Several studies on LPS induced mastitis have reported reduced food intake and reduced time spent ruminating following the intramammary challenge [3, 24]. The peak effect seems to occur 3–9 h after the LPS challenge [24], indicating that the evaluation time of 8 h used in the present study should be adequate to detect challenge-induced alterations if present. While a trend for reduced time spent eating was detected in the LPS group, no differences among groups were found for time spent ruminating. Similar results have been previously reported [7] and, as hypothesized above, they might be linked to the severity degree of the disease. The lack of differences among groups for the postural variable hock-to-hock distance corroborates this hypothesis. Wider hind limb stance is expected to occur in cows affected by mastitis due to udder inflammation: increased hock-to-hock distance was found in mild to moderate clinical mastitis cases [17] in one study while it was unchanged in another [5].

For pain evaluation, a condition-specific multidimensional pain scale was designed. The structure of the scoring system was similar to the one used previously in other species [25] but the included items were meant to be specific for bovine mastitis and whenever possible evidence-based. The first item was a simple numerical rating scale allowing the observer to attribute a general subjective pain score. The second item was a list of possible expected manifestations, the first three being related to facial expression. While facial pain scales have not been validated so far for bovines, it is generally accepted that modifications of facial expression accompanying pain are rather conserved among mammal species [26]. Ears, eyelid and nostrils modifications indicating pain have been described in mice [27], rats [28] and horses [29] and were therefore expected to be potentially modified in cows with experimentally induced mastitis. Restlessness [5], apathy

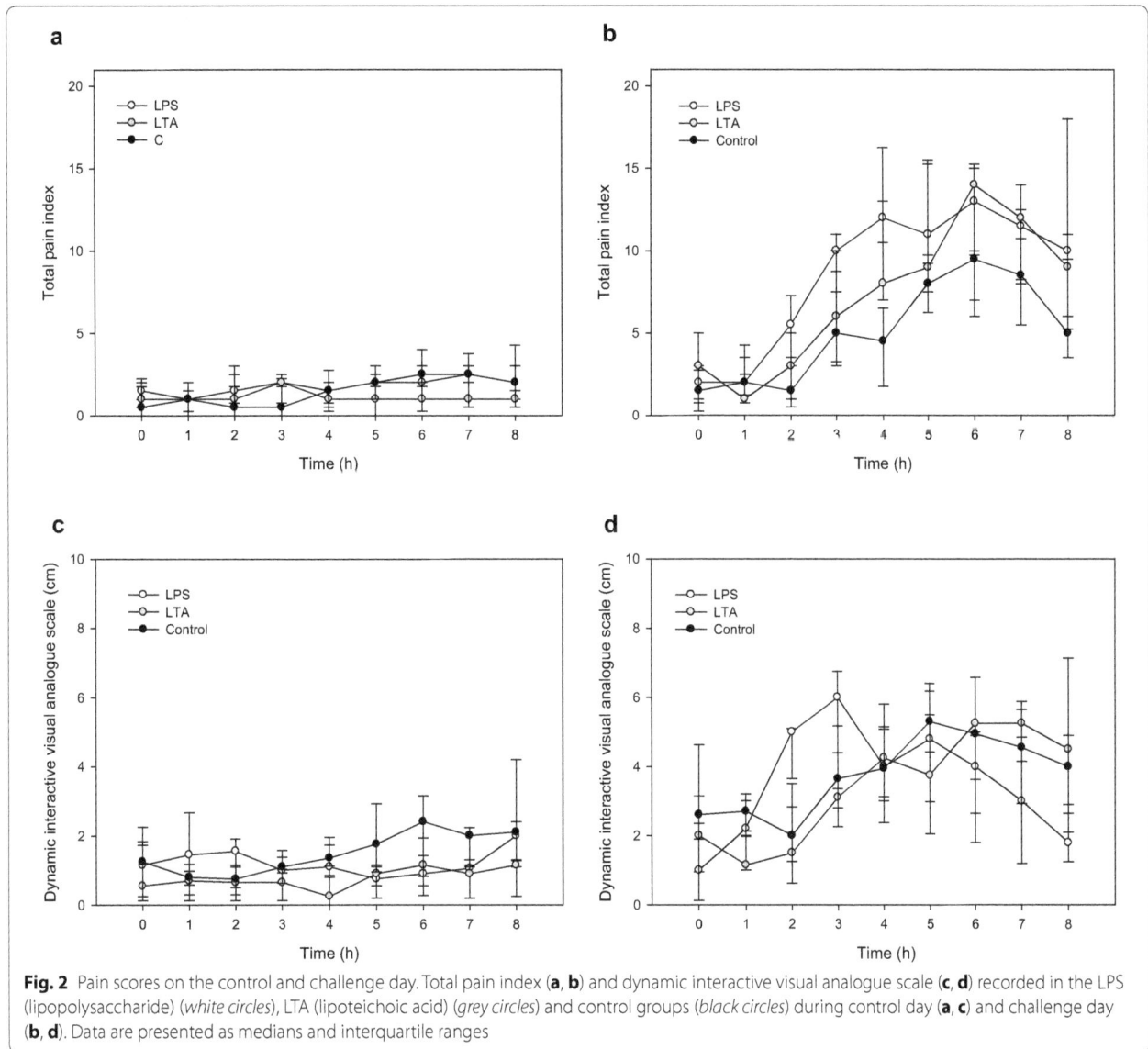

Fig. 2 Pain scores on the control and challenge day. Total pain index (**a**, **b**) and dynamic interactive visual analogue scale (**c**, **d**) recorded in the LPS (lipopolysaccharide) (*white circles*), LTA (lipoteichoic acid) (*grey circles*) and control groups (*black circles*) during control day (**a**, **c**) and challenge day (**b**, **d**). Data are presented as medians and interquartile ranges

[22] and wide hind limb stance [17] have been previously reported in bovine mastitis. Absence of interactive behavior and response to food were included as general sickness indicators [2], while presence of back arch, reported in bovine affected by lameness [30] and metritis [31], had been observed to occur in clinical mastitis cases and was therefore included in the scoring system. Reactivity to back palpation was expected to potentially occur in painful mastitis as a form of secondary hyperalgesia and muscle hypersensitivity due to postural abnormalities. Additionally, the local items udder edema and reaction to udder palpation were meant to provide disease-specific information as previously reported [22]. Total pain index increased in all treatment groups during the challenge day, with significantly higher values for the LPS group

compared to the control group. These findings suggest two considerations. First, a certain treatment-independent day-time effect is detected by the scale, probably representing additional stress provoked by human presence during the challenge day. Second, the total pain index indicates higher degree of pain following the LPS challenge. Similarly, the dynamic-interactive VAS pain scores were mostly affected by the LPS treatment, even if values significantly higher than baseline were found for LTA and control groups at single time points. Visual analogue scales for pain evaluation are daily used in humans [32] and have previously been applied to evaluate pain in ruminants [18, 33]. For veterinary use, dynamic-interactive VAS scales are generally preferred, as the responses to the dynamic interaction with the animal add important

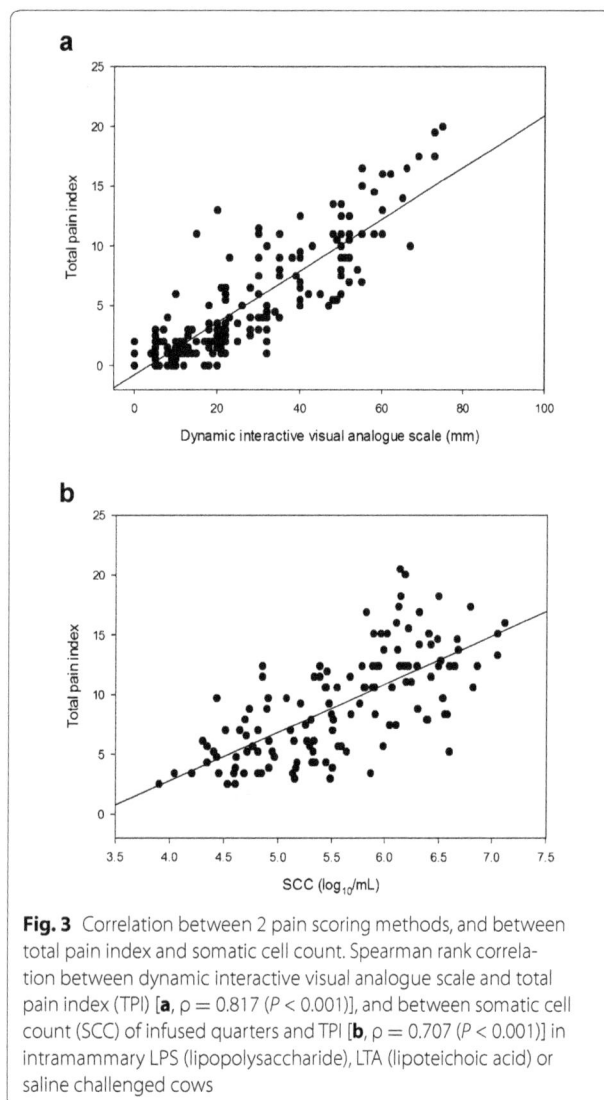

Fig. 3 Correlation between 2 pain scoring methods, and between total pain index and somatic cell count. Spearman rank correlation between dynamic interactive visual analogue scale and total pain index (TPI) [**a**, ρ = 0.817 (P < 0.001)], and between somatic cell count (SCC) of infused quarters and TPI [**b**, ρ = 0.707 (P < 0.001)] in intramammary LPS (lipopolysaccharide), LTA (lipoteichoic acid) or saline challenged cows

induced and naturally occurring coliform mastitis, it does not appear to be a typical sign in staphylococcal mastitis [36]. Indeed, LTA has been demonstrated to induce a weaker effect on vascular permeability [12] than LPS, possibly corroborating our findings.

Udder temperature of cows in the LPS and LTA groups was higher at some time points after the simulated challenge/challenge than at their first early morning measurement. Since no day effect could be detected, the changes were likely due to treatment-unrelated factors. Udder surface temperature has been shown to vary dependently on circadian oscillations, stage of lactation, environmental temperature and physical activity. In the present study the highest values were measured at 2, 6 and 8 h after the simulated challenge/challenge. Similar findings were previously reported for healthy cows, where a rise in udder temperature was observed between 0900 and 1100 and at late afternoon, with minimal values being recorded between 0400 and 0600 [37].

No differences in udder mechanical nociceptive thresholds were detected in the present study. Contrasting results on nociceptive thresholds have been previously reported for mastitic cows. While nociceptive thresholds to hind limb and udder laser stimulations increased during E. coli mastitis indicating hypoalgesia [8], thresholds to thermal hind limb stimulations were lower in cows affected by clinical mastitis compared to healthy controls indicating hyperalgesia [35]. Probably the severity of systemic illness accompanying the inflammation of the mammary gland strongly affects nociceptive thresholds and the reactivity to local stimulation. In presence of severe sickness symptoms like somnolence, lethargy and depression, it is more likely to observe an increase rather a decrease in sensitivity to pain.

While plasma cortisol was not significantly affected by treatment and was within the previously reported range for healthy lactating dairy cows [38], milk cortisol was significantly higher in the LPS group 4 h after the challenge compared to t0. Milk cortisol is considered as a useful indicator of response to acute stressors acting up to 2 h before sampling in lactating dairy cows [39]. As cortisol measured in milk derives from the systemic circulation, higher milk cortisol might reflect a higher permeability of the blood-milk barrier in LPS treated cows. This hypothesis is supported by the finding of higher levels of lactate dehydrogenase in LPS compared to LTA treated cows [14]. In a recent study, significant effects of SCC on milk cortisol were found for SCC above 400 × 10³ cells/ml. This finding suggests that hypothalamic–pituitary–adrenal axis activation following an antigenic stimulation can be detected only in case of a severe inflammatory response [40].

The LPS dose of 0.2 µg used in the present study is lower than what generally described in literature [7], while

information for a correct pain assessment [34]. They are based on subjective assessment of pain following observation and dynamic interaction with the animal. As interobserver variability might be high, it is important to have a single observer throughout the study period when using visual analogue scales. In the present study, total pain index and dynamic-interactive VAS were significantly correlated and led to similar results.

Local signs of disease have been commonly used to evaluate the severity of clinical mastitis [22]. In endotoxins-induced mastitis, rapid influx of neutrophils in the mammary gland occurs [24] accompanied by local signs of inflammation, like edema [7], increased udder temperature [17] and hyperalgesia [35].

In the present study, prevalence of udder edema was higher in the LPS than in the control group. While udder edema has been reported to occur in both experimentally

Table 4 Reaction score to udder palpation (Reaction score), udder edema score (Edema score), udder temperature (Udder T) and mechanical nociceptive threshold (MNT) measured in infused quarters of cows challenged with intramammary LPS (lipopolysaccharide), LTA (lipoteichoic acid) or saline (control group)

Parameter	Control day				Challenge day			
	2 h	4 h	6 h	8 h	2 h	4 h	6 h	8 h
Reaction score								
LPS	0 (0–0)	0 (0–0)	0 (0–0)	0 (0–0)	0 (0–0)	0 (0–0)	0 (0–0)	0 (0–0)
LTA	0 (0–0)	0 (0–0)	0 (0–0)	0 (0–0)	0 (0–0)	0 (0–0)	0 (0–0)	0 (0–0)
Control	0 (0–0)	0 (0–0)	0 (0–0)	0 (0–0)	0 (0–0)	0 (0–0)	0 (0–0)	0 (0–0)
Edema score								
LPS	0 (0–1)	0 (0–0)	0 (0–0)	0 (0–0)	1 (1–1)	2.5 (2–3)	2 (1–3)	1.5 (1–2)
LTA	0 (0–1)	0 (0–1)	0 (0–1)	0 (0–1)	0 (0–0.2)	1 (0.75–2)	1 (0.75–2.25)	1 (0.75–1.5)
Control	0 (0–0)	0 (0–0.5)	0 (0–0)	0 (0–0)	0 (0–0)	0 (0–0)	0 (0–0.5)	1 (0.5–1)
Udder T (°C)								
LPS	36.3 (34.7–36.9)	36.6 (34.7–37.4)	36.2 (35–37)	36.9 (36.6–37.2)	36.1 (36–37.5)	36.4 (35.8–37)	36.8 (36–37.3)	36.4 (36–37.2)
LTA	35.1 (34.1–36.6)	34.7 (34–37.4)	35.9 (34.3–37.1)	35.5 (33.8–37.4)	34.4 (33.6–36.8)	35.2 (34.1–37.0)	36.2 (34.3–37.7)	36.9 (33.9–37.6)
Control	33.9 (32.5–35.1)	34 (32.8–35)	34.3 (32.9–35.7)	34.6 (33–35.8)	33.5 (32.9–34.8)	34.4 (33.3–35.5)	33.9 (33.1–35.2)	34.5 (33.5–36)
MNT (N)								
LPS	22.4 (13.4–24.6)	22 (11–24.6)	22.7 (11.8–24.6)	24.6 (22.6–24.6)	18.3 (13.9–23.4)	23.6 (18.2–24.6)	23.9 (19.1–24.6)	21.8 (15.8–24.6)
LTA	24.6 (24.6–24.6)	23.3 (16.6–24.6)	24.6 (19.7–24.6)	24.6 (17.3–24.6)	24.6 (19.4–24.6)	24.6 (21.7–24.6)	23.9 (17.6–24.6)	18.2 (10.7–24.6)
Control	24.6 (23.8–24.6)	24.6 (24.6–24.6)	20.8 (19.2–24.6)	24.6 (22–24.6)	15.5 (11.5–20.6)	22.1 (20.5–23.9)	18.2 (12–23.6)	20.4 (15.1–24)

On the control day, the intramammary challenge, milk and blood sampling were simulated. Medians and interquartile ranges (IQR) at 2, 4, 6 and 8 h after the simulated challenge (control day)/challenge (challenge day) are reported

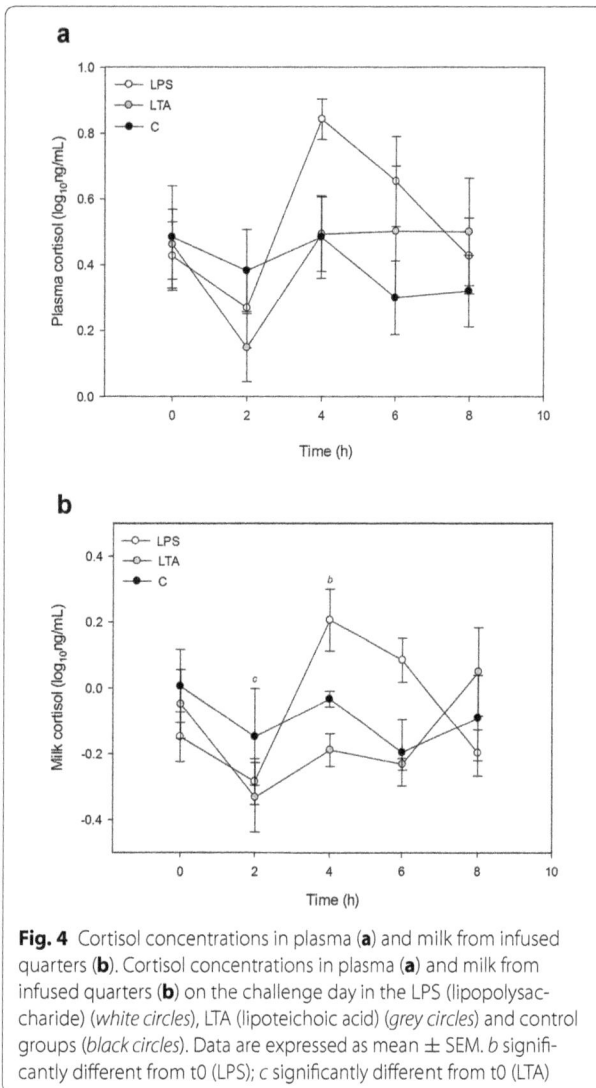

Fig. 4 Cortisol concentrations in plasma (**a**) and milk from infused quarters (**b**). Cortisol concentrations in plasma (**a**) and milk from infused quarters (**b**) on the challenge day in the LPS (lipopolysaccharide) (*white circles*), LTA (lipoteichoic acid) (*grey circles*) and control groups (*black circles*). Data are expressed as mean ± SEM. *b* significantly different from t0 (LPS); *c* significantly different from t0 (LTA)

20 µg LTA has been previously administered to compare LTA and LPS induced immune responses [10]. The highest SCC values, reached approximately 6 h after the challenge, correspond to a subclinical-to-clinical threshold for mastitis. The doses of LPS and LTA were chosen to induce a similar SCC increase as previously reported [41]. Although using other indicators of mastitis severity degree might have led to different results, SCC is a simple quantitative measure used both in clinical and in experimental settings and was considered the most adequate to compare the immune response to this challenge. Interestingly, a high correlation between total pain index and SCC was found, independently from the treatment groups.

Main limitation of the current study is the small size of the treatment groups. As both LPS and LTA experimental models of mastitis are highly standardized and repeatable [41], groups of 6 animals, as determined for the parallel immunological study, were considered to be sufficient for the purpose of this study as well; indeed, statistically significant results could be found even after applying very restrictive Bonferroni corrections. Furthermore, the presence of a small control group in addition to the control day in both LPS and LTA groups, contributed to differentiate between manipulation-induced and treatment-induced changes. Another limitation might be represented by the fact that the cows included were of different breeds and parities. These factors might potentially affect some of the measured outcome variables, like it has been recently described for milk cortisol [40]. Finally, milk and plasma cortisol concentrations, as well as SCC, were not measured on the control day. Therefore, only one pre challenge baseline value was available for these variables.

Conclusions

When administered at equipotent doses targeting a standard SCC increase, intramammary LPS seems to be accompanied by a higher degree of pain and discomfort than LTA, as suggested by the modifications of the outcome variables total pain index, dynamic interactive VAS, udder edema and milk cortisol.

Authors' contributions
AEJG carried out all the measurements and the data collection with exception of the laboratory tests; she also drafted the first manuscript version under supervision of CS. BHPvdB contributed to the development of the statistical models and to the statistical analysis. CS conceived the study design, supervised the development of the pain scoring systems and had major contributions in the drafting of the final manuscript version. SKW was responsible for the intramammary infusion and for the setting of the immunological study, as well as contributed to the final manuscript draft. RMB contributed to the study design, performed the laboratory tests and helped interpreting the results. OW coordinated the study and contributed to the final manuscript draft. All authors read and approved the final manuscript.

Author details
[1] Department of Clinical Veterinary Medicine, Anesthesiology and Pain Therapy Section, Vetsuisse Faculty, University of Berne, Laenggassstrasse 124, 3012 Berne, Switzerland. [2] Veterinary Public Health Institute, Vetsuisse Faculty, University of Berne, Schwarzenburgstrasse 155, 3097 Liebefeld, Switzerland. [3] Veterinary Physiology, Vetsuisse Faculty, University of Berne, Bremgartenstrasse 109a, 3012 Berne, Switzerland.

Acknowledgements
The authors would like to thank the Swiss National Science Foundation for the partial financial support; moreover they are deeply thankful to Claudine Morel and Chantal Philipona (Veterinary Physiology, Vetsuisse Faculty, University of Berne, Switzerland), as well as Dr. Judith Howard (Clinical Laboratory, Vetsuisse Faculty, University of Berne, Switzerland) for their support in the sample analysis.

Experimentally induced subclinical mastitis: are lipopolysaccharide and lipoteichoic acid eliciting...

197

Competing interests

The authors declare that they have no competing interests.

Funding

The project was partially supported by the Swiss National Science Foundation (Bern, Switzerland; Grant No. 149460).

References

1. Hogeveen H, Huijps K, Lam TJ. Economic aspects of mastitis: new developments. NZ Vet J. 2011;59:16–23.
2. Leslie KE, Petersson-Wolfe CS. Assessment and management of pain in dairy cows with clinical mastitis. Vet Clin North Am Food Anim Pract. 2012;28:289–305.
3. Yeiser EE, Leslie KE, McGilliard ML, Petersson-Wolfe CS. The effects of experimentally induced *Escherichia coli* mastitis and flunixin meglumine administration on activity measures, feed intake, and milk parameters. J Dairy Sci. 2012;95:4939–49.
4. Cyples JA, Fitzpatrick CE, Leslie KE, DeVries TJ, Haley DB, Chapinal N. Short communication: the effects of experimentally induced *Escherichia coli* clinical mastitis on lying behavior of dairy cows. J Dairy Sci. 2012;95:2571–5.
5. Medrano-Galarza C, Gibbons J, Wagner S, de Passille AM, Rushen J. Behavioral changes in dairy cows with mastitis. J Dairy Sci. 2012;95:6994–7002.
6. Siivonen J, Taponen S, Hovinen M, Pastell M, Lensink BJ, Pyörälä S, et al. Impact of acute clinical mastitis on cow behaviour. Appl Anim Behav Sci. 2011;132:101–6.
7. Fitzpatrick CE, Chapinal N, Petersson-Wolfe CS, DeVries TJ, Kelton DF, Duffield TF, et al. The effect of meloxicam on pain sensitivity, rumination time, and clinical signs in dairy cows with endotoxin-induced clinical mastitis. J Dairy Sci. 2013;96:2847–56.
8. Rasmussen DB, Fogsgaard K, Rontved CM, Klaas IC, Herskin MS. Changes in thermal nociceptive responses in dairy cows following experimentally induced *Escherichia coli* mastitis. Acta Vet Scand. 2011;53:32.
9. Bannerman DD, Paape MJ, Lee JW, Zhao X, Hope JC, Rainard P. *Escherichia coli* and *Staphylococcus aureus* elicit differential innate immune responses following intramammary infection. Clin Diagn Lab Immunol. 2004;11:463–72.
10. Wellnitz O, Arnold ET, Bruckmaier RM. Lipopolysaccharide and lipoteichoic acid induce different immune responses in the bovine mammary gland. J Dairy Sci. 2011;94:5405–12.
11. Hoeben D, Burvenich C, Trevisi E, Bertoni G, Hamann J, Bruckmaier RM, et al. Role of endotoxin and TNF-alpha in the pathogenesis of experimentally induced coliform mastitis in periparturient cows. J Dairy Res. 2000;67:503–14.
12. Rainard P, Fromageau A, Cunha P, Gilbert FB. *Staphylococcus aureus* lipoteichoic acid triggers inflammation in the lactating bovine mammary gland. Vet Res. 2008;39:52.
13. Wall SK, Wellnitz O, Hernandez-Castellano LE, Ahmadpour A, Bruckmaier RM. Supraphysiological oxytocin increases the transfer of immunoglobulins and other blood components to milk during lipopolysaccharide- and lipoteichoic acid-induced mastitis in dairy cows. J Dairy Sci. 2016;99:9165–73.
14. Wall SK, Hernandez-Castellano LE, Ahmadpour A, Bruckmaier RM, Wellnitz O. Differential glucocorticoid-induced closure of the blood-milk barrier during lipopolysaccharide- and lipoteichoic acid-induced mastitis in dairy cows. J Dairy Sci. 2016;99:7544–53.
15. Witt A, Mason MJ, Burgess K, Flocke S, Zyzanski S. A case control study of bacterial species and colony count in milk of breastfeeding women with chronic pain. Breastfeed Med. 2014;9:29–34.
16. Alsaaod M, Niederhauser JJ, Beer G, Zehner N, Schuepbach-Regula G, Steiner A. Development and validation of a novel pedometer algorithm to quantify extended characteristics of the locomotor behavior of dairy cows. J Dairy Sci. 2015;98:6236–42.
17. Kemp MH, Nolan AM, Cripps PJ, Fitzpatrick JL. Animal-based measurements of the severity of mastitis in dairy cows. Vet Rec. 2008;163:175–9.
18. Flower FC, Weary DM. Effect of hoof pathologies and subjective assessments of dairy cow gait. J Dairy Sci. 2006;89:139–46.
19. Hovinen M, Siivonen J, Taponen S, Hanninen L, Pastell M, Aisla AM, et al. Detection of clinical mastitis with the help of a thermal camera. J Dairy Sci. 2008;91:4592–8.
20. Stewart M, Stafford KJ, Dowling SK, Schaefer AL, Webster JR. Eye temperature and heart rate variability of calves disbudded with or without local anaesthetic. Physiol Behav. 2008;93:789–97.
21. Thun R, Eggenberger E, Zerobin K, Luscher T, Vetter W. Twenty-four-hour secretory pattern of cortisol in the bull: evidence of episodic secretion and circadian rhythm. Endocrinology. 1981;109:2208–12.
22. Wenz JR, Garry FB, Barrington GM. Comparison of disease severity scoring systems for dairy cattle with acute coliform mastitis. JAVMA. 2006;229:259–62.
23. Molgaard L, Damgaard BM, Bjerre-Harpoth V, Herskin MS. Effects of percutaneous needle liver biopsy on dairy cow behaviour. Res Vet Sci. 2012;93:1248–54.
24. Zimov JL, Botheras NA, Weiss WP, Hogan JS. Associations among behavioral and acute physiologic responses to lipopolysaccharide-induced clinical mastitis in lactating dairy cows. Am J Vet Res. 2011;72:620–7.
25. Graubner C, Gerber V, Doherr M, Spadavecchia C. Clinical application and reliability of a post abdominal surgery pain assessment scale (PASPAS) in horses. Vet J. 2011;188:178–83.
26. Guesgen MJ, Beausoleil NJ, Leach M, Minot EO, Stewart M, Stafford KJ. Coding and quantification of a facial expression for pain in lambs. Behav Process. 2016;132:49–56.
27. Langford DJ, Bailey AL, Chanda ML, Clarke SE, Drummond TE, Echols S, et al. Coding of facial expressions of pain in the laboratory mouse. Nat Methods. 2010;7:447–9.
28. Sotocinal SG, Sorge RE, Zaloum A, Tuttle AH, Martin LJ, Wieskopf JS, et al. The rat grimace scale: a partially automated method for quantifying pain in the laboratory rat via facial expressions. Mol Pain. 2011;7:55.
29. Dalla Costa E, Minero M, Lebelt D, Stucke D, Canali E, Leach MC. Development of the horse grimace scale (HGS) as a pain assessment tool in horses undergoing routine castration. PLoS ONE. 2014;9:e92281.
30. Hoffman AC, Moore DA, Vanegas J, Wenz JR. Association of abnormal hind-limb postures and back arch with gait abnormality in dairy cattle. J Dairy Sci. 2014;97:2178–85.
31. Stojkov J, von Keyserlingk MA, Marchant-Forde JN, Weary DM. Assessment of visceral pain associated with metritis in dairy cows. J Dairy Sci. 2015;98:5352–61.
32. Hjermstad MJ, Fayers PM, Haugen DF, Caraceni A, Hanks GW, Loge JH, et al. Studies comparing numerical rating scales, verbal rating scales, and visual analogue scales for assessment of pain intensity in adults: a systematic literature review. J Pain Symptom Manage. 2011;41:1073–93.
33. Welsh EM, Gettinby G, Nolan AM. Comparison of a visual analogue scale and a numerical rating scale for assessment of lameness, using sheep as a model. Am J Vet Res. 1993;54:976–83.
34. Anil SS, Anil L, Deen J. Challenges of pain assessment in domestic animals. J Am Vet Med Assoc. 2002;220:313–9.
35. Peters MD, Silveira ID, Fischer V. Impact of subclinical and clinical mastitis on sensitivity to pain of dairy cows. Animal. 2015;9:2024–8.
36. Petzl W, Zerbe H, Gunther J, Yang W, Seyfert HM, Nurnberg G, et al. *Escherichia coli*, but not *Staphylococcus aureus* triggers an early increased expression of factors contributing to the innate immune defense in the udder of the cow. Vet Res. 2008;39:18.
37. Berry RJ, Kennedy AD, Scott SL, Kyle BL, Schaefer AL. Daily variation in the udder surface temperature of dairy cows measured by infrared thermography: potential for mastitis detection. Can J Anim Sci. 2003;83:687–93.
38. Lefcourt AM, Bitman J, Kahl S, Wood DL. Circadian and ultradian rhythms of peripheral cortisol concentrations in lactating dairy cows. J Dairy Sci. 1993;76:2607–12.
39. Verkerk GA, Phipps AM, Carragher JF, Matthews LR, Stelwagen K. Characterization of milk cortisol concentrations as a measure of short-term stress responses in lactating dairy cows. Anim Welfare. 1998;7:77–86.
40. Sgorlon S, Fanzago M, Guiatti D, Gabai G, Stradaioli G, Stefanon B. Factors affecting milk cortisol in mid lactating dairy cows. Bmc Vet Res. 2015;11:259.

23

Experimental studies on effects of diet on *Lawsonia intracellularis* infections in fattening boars in a natural infection model

Christian Visscher[1]* **ⓘ**, Anne Kruse[1], Saara Sander[1], Christoph Keller[2], Jasmin Mischok[1], Robert Tabeling[3], Hubert Henne[4], Ricarda Deitmer[5] and Josef Kamphues[1]

Abstract

Background: *Lawsonia intracellularis* is one of the most economically important pathogens in swine production. This study tested the hypothesis that the composition of diets for pigs has an impact on the excretion of *L. intracellularis* in a natural infection model.

Results: Fifty boars (~ 90 kg BW) from a SPF-farm with a strict hygiene and management regime for reducing the spread of an *L. intracellularis* infection up to the beginning of the final fattening period were transported, regrouped and randomly allotted to groups of five animals each at the research facility. After a 1-week acclimatisation period groups were fed one of five diets 4 weeks before slaughter. These were either a finely ground pelleted diet (FP) or a coarsely ground meal diet (CM), both consisting of wheat (40.0%), barley (39.3%), soybean meal (16.0%), soybean oil (2.0%) and minor components. In the other meal diets parts of wheat, barley and soybean meal were substituted either with 22% cracked corn (CORN), 16.9% dried whey (WHEY) or 30% raw potato starch (RPS). The animals had a comparable serological status in a blocking-ELISA immediately before the start and at the end of the feeding experiment. Values increased significantly during the trial. In all subgroups (FP/CM/CORN/WHEY/RPS), shedding was detected in week 0 (genome equivalents $=$ GE; $\log_{10}$ GE *L. intracellularis*/g faeces: $2.46 \pm 2.64/3.58 \pm 2.54/3.43 \pm 2.37/2.30 \pm 3.16/2.58 \pm 2.73$). The average number of *L. intracellularis* microbes in faeces during the trial period did not differ between the groups ($\log_{10}$ GE *L. intracellularis*/g faeces: $3.40 \pm 1.53/3.01 \pm 1.41/3.80 \pm 1.71/3.98 \pm 2.20/4.08 \pm 2.13$). In animals fed the WHEY-diet, significantly lower counts of *L. intracellularis* were found in the caecal content. The acetate content in the caecum was negatively correlated with the serological results at the end of the trial ($r = -0.36$; $P = 0.010$). Butyrate concentrations in the caecal content were negatively correlated with the number of *L. intracellularis* in the caecum ($r = -0.32$; $P = 0.023$).

Conclusion: Therefore, this study provides preliminary evidence that there might be specific dietary effects on the course of a *L. intracellularis* infection.

Keywords: Boar, Diet, Infection, *Lawsonia intracellularis*, Whey

Background

The infection with *Lawsonia intracellularis* is a disease present in all pig-producing countries regardless of husbandry systems [1–7]. In a Europe-wide study, a total of 93% of all surveyed fattening units and 97% of all breeding farms were positive for *L. intracellularis*. For Germany, an even higher prevalence was achieved. About 94% of all fattening farms and 99% of the breeding units investigated had been in contact with the pathogen [8].

The degree of severity of the clinical symptoms is reflected by the level of excretion of *L. intracellularis* in faeces [9]. Increasing pathogen concentrations in faeces are significantly associated with significantly reduced daily weight gains [5]. Excretion of only very few

*Correspondence: Christian.Visscher@tiho-hannover.de
[1] Institute for Animal Nutrition, University of Veterinary Medicine Hannover, Foundation, Bischofsholer Damm 15, 30173 Hanover, Germany
Full list of author information is available at the end of the article

numbers of *L. intracellularis* does not seem to have any effects on daily weight gains [5]. However, the extent of this dependency was lower with increasing dry matter (DM) content in faeces [5]. An increase in one log level concerning numbers of *L. intracellularis* in faeces means the probability of that pig having a lower growth rate by a factor of 1.97 [6]. Especially when more than 10^6 pathogens per gramme of faeces were detected, this was also a significant risk factor for a lower body weight gain [6].

So far, only two main dietary factors have been investigated more systematically depending on the course of an *L. intracellularis* infection: on the one hand, the effect of packaging (meal versus pellets or crumbles), on the other hand the possible effects of lactic acid-rich diets. On the basis of a survey conducted on 79 Danish pig farms, a reduced in-herd prevalence of *L. intracellularis* was associated with home-mixed and (or) non-pelleted diets [10]. On farms using commercially prepared pelleted diets the prevalence was higher [10]. Therefore, an indirect influence of diet on *L. intracellularis* colonisation would appear possible. This has already been reported in pigs [11, 12] as well as in hamsters [13]. A relative reduction in the numbers of *L. intracellularis* in the total ileal microbiota of pigs fed a non-pelleted diet could be shown [11]. Overall, an effect of diet on the course of an experimental *L. intracellularis* infection was found [12]. Reproducing the effects with a 'home-mixed diet' (coarsely ground, non-pelleted diet) following experimental infection with *L. intracellularis* failed [12]. Feeding a fermented liquid diet (rich in lactic acid) to pigs following experimental infection with *L. intracellularis* delayed the excretion of the organism [12]. Offering a standard diet in the same study (based on wheat, barley and soybean meal) supplemented with 2.4% lactic acid led to limited pathological lesions in pigs. Examination was done 28 days after inoculation [12].

The present study was based on the hypothesis that both, the packaging and the potential of a diet to foster the concentrations of specific fermentation products (lactic acid, butyrate) specifically minimise the effects of *L. intracellularis* infections in pigs. A natural infection model was used because it simulates the conditions in practice more than an experimental infection approach. Transport and regrouping of subclinically infected individuals from a high health herd was the starting point for the model. This was intended to simulate the phenomenon observed under natural conditions [14]; namely, the spread of infection after transporting animals from a high health herd to other herds. This is the first study testing five diets differing in terms of the nature of the ingredients in a natural *L. intracellularis* infection model in fattening boars in the final finishing phase.

Methods

The study consisted of three stages of sampling, which require an explanation regarding classification in accordance with the German Animal Protection Act or the Council Regulation (EC) No 1099/2009 on the protection of animals at the time of slaughter.

First, serological results from routine examinations of organ samples of boars (*L. intracellularis* serostatus of boars) previously carried out on the supplier farm for boars were provided by the corresponding field veterinarian prior to the trial. The sampling was thus not subject to an approval in accordance with the Animal Protection Act.

Second, before starting the experiments, the feeding trial itself was examined routinely by the Animal Welfare Officer of the University of Veterinary Medicine, Hannover, Foundation, Hanover, Germany. This evaluation categorically stated, that the study was not based on an animal experiment requiring notification or approval in accordance with the Animal Protection Act.

Third, at the end of the trial, the animals were anaesthetised using a new method. This method required notification and approval from the relevant authority (exemption: file 32.22.2, Department of Law and Order, state capital of Hanover). The slaughtering process took place at the abattoir in Hannover. The pigs were subsequently killed by bleeding after finishing the trial.

Natural infection model, animals and housing

Fifty boars from a specific pathogen-free (SPF) pig fattening unit were chosen for the experiments. The animals were selected at a specific date. At ~90 kg body weight (BW) at the farm, already 50% of the animals had been serologically positive for the pathogen in the blocking ELISA (PI value ≥ 30) in the past. This was also the case in the experiment. At this time, it can be assumed that an intensive pathogen exchange can be expected within the following few weeks. In particular, if transport and regrouping additionally take place. Under these circumstances, it can be assumed that the pathogen excretion is high, especially if the herd of origin has a high health status and the infection occurs late [14].

The animals were transported to the Institute for Animal Nutrition, University of Veterinary Medicine Hannover.

The 50 boars from the German Federal Breeding Programme were genetically defined animals of five lines with regard to inheritance factors for androstenone and skatole. Groups of five boars each were newly formed, with one representative of each genetic line per group. The boars were kept in groups of five animals each (Table 1) in 2×3 m boxes with solid floors. Each box

Table 1 Experimental design concerning number of animals, repetitions and group size

Item	Treatment				
	FP	CM	CORN	WHEY	RPS
Group size	5	5	5	5	5
Repetitions/treatment	2	2	2	2	2
Total no. of animals	10	10	10	10	10

FP fine pelleted diet, *CM* coarse meal diet, *CORN* meal diet with 22% cracked corn; *WHEY* meal diet with 16.9% dried whey, *RPS* meal diet with 30% raw potato starch

had two feeding troughs, each 1 m in length. Chains and playing balls were offered as environmental enrichment material. Covered metal pits, each 20 cm wide, were placed at the back of the boxes.

Feeding regime, performance parameters and sampling

The experiments were carried out for a period of about 5 weeks, this being divided into a 1-week acclimatisation phase and a 4-week experimental phase. During the 1-week acclimatisation phase (Time point 1 = TP1), the boars were given a pelleted diet (Vereinigte Saatzuchten Ebstorf-Rosche eG, Ebstorf, Germany). This diet had previously been fed on the farm. The five complete diets used during the 4-week trial period (TP2–5) had been produced at the research institute itself. These differed from one another either in their composition or in their packaging (Table 2). In each case, two boxes received one of the five compound feeds used in the experiment. The grinding of the barley and the wheat was carried out in the hammer mill for all groups. For the control group (fine pelleted = FP), a 1 mm sieve

Table 2 Ingredient and nutrient composition of the experimental diets offered in the experimental period

Item	Diet	FP	CM	CORN	WHEY	RPS
Diet composition (%)						
Wheat		40.0	40.0	27.7	32.4	23.5
Barley		39.3	39.3	30.0	32.2	19.0
Soybean meal		16.0	16.0	16.7	15.0	15.0
Corn		–	–	22.0	–	–
Whey powder		–	–	–	16.9	–
Potato starch		–	–	–	–	30.0
Wheat gluten						6.00
Soybean oil		2.00	2.00	1.00	1.50	3.00
L-Lysine		0.30	0.30	0.20	0.20	0.30
Methionine		0.10	0.10	0.10	0.10	0.10
Salt		0.30	0.30	0.30		0.30
Monocalcium phosphate		–	–	–	–	0.80
Mineral feed[a]		2.00	2.00	2.00	1.70	2.00
Sodium chloride		0.30	0.30	0.30	0.30	0.30
Analysed nutrient composition (g/kg DM)						
ME (MJ/kg DM)		15.6	15.5	15.5	15.2	16.1
Crude ash		46.8	46.7	46.5	50.6	44.8
Crude fat		41.7	42.1	34.8	33.1	50.2
Crude fibre		34.5	40.0	36.2	33.6	28.3
Crude protein		192	187	187	181	189
Starch		482	487	526	405	546
Sugar		44.1	39.5	39.1	125	31.0
Ca		6.90	7.15	6.95	7.45	8.65
P		4.40	4.45	5.10	5.55	5.85
Mg		1.90	2.00	2.05	1.90	1.65
K		6.90	6.70	6.95	10.7	5.60
Na		2.60	3.00	2.65	2.50	2.55
Lysine		13.8	13.5	12.7	12.5	12.9

FP fine pelleted diet, *CM* coarse meal diet, *CORN* meal diet with 22% cracked corn, *WHEY* meal diet with 16.9% dried whey, *RPS* meal diet with 30% raw potato starch

[a] Supplement containing (per kg): Ca 24.50%; P 2.40%; Na 5.10%; Lysine 6.60%; Methionine 1.50%; Threonine 1.00%; 450,000 IU vitamin A; 50,000 IU vitamin D3; 2950 mg vitamin E; 4000 mg Fe; 3500 mg Mn; 3500 mg Zn; 600 mg Cu; 60 I; 13 mg Se; 5 mg Co; 20,000 IU phytases

insert was used, whereas for the other groups either a 6 mm sieve insert (coarse meal = CM) or a 3 mm sieve insert (corn = CORN, whey = WHEY and raw potato starch = RPS) was selected for preparing the diet. Further processing (pelleting) was done for the control group (FP). All other groups received the diet in meal form ad libitum. The amounts of feed consumed were recorded on a daily basis. Quantification was done at group level (n = five animals/group). The animals always had free access to drinking water.

Body weight of finishing boars was measured individually on the day of delivery as well as at the start and at the end of the four-week trial period with a pair of mobile scales (WA 200, Meier-Brackenberg GmbH & Co. KG, Exterlal, Germany). Body weight gain and feed intake on group basis were used to calculate the feed conversion ratio (FCR) per kg gain.

Once a week, samples from all individual animals were collected during defaecation or directly from the rectum. One part of the sample was used for analysis (DM), another part being frozen for further analyses (volatile fatty acids, *L. intracellularis* qPCR).

At the end of the 4-week experimental period (TP6), the animals were killed in a mobile chamber by means of a CO_2:N fumigation (30:70) at the abattoir in Hanover. The slaughtering process was done in small groups. In each group, genetic lineage and feeding variants were equally represented. On the morning before the dissection all the boars were given their respective experimental diets. In order to avoid unnecessary stress for the animals, only those boars were loaded and transported to the abattoir, which were also going to be killed directly afterwards in the chamber.

During the bleeding, blood samples were taken. After the evisceration by the abattoir personnel, the caecum was ligated before at the base of the caecum with a double ligature. Subsequently, the organ was separated with a pair of scissors and removed. The tip of the caecum was opened. The entire contents were collected and cooled until storage for further processing. For the histological examination, a piece tissue from the intestinal wall (about 3×2 cm in size) was taken of each boar in the vicinity of the appendix of the caecum. Care was taken to save the taenia-area. The samples obtained from the caecum wall were clamped on cork plates with needles. Afterwards, tissue was transferred to a cup filled with 10% formalin. After a fixation time of about 24 h, the tissue samples were further processed.

Analytical methods

Diets were analysed by standard procedures in accordance with the official methods of the VDLUFA [15]. The dry matter content (DM) was determined by drying to the weight constancy at 103 °C. The raw ash was analysed by means of incineration in the muffle furnace at 600 °C for 6 h. Determining the crude protein content was done by analysing the total nitrogen content using the catalytic tube combustion method (DUMAS combustion method; Vario Max®, Elementar, Hanau, Germany). The crude fat content was determined after acid digestion in the soxhlet apparatus. The content of crude fibre was determined after washing in dilute acids and alkalis. Starch determination was carried out polarimetrically (Polatronic E, Schmidt und Haensch GmbH & Co., Berlin, Germany). The sugar content was analysed using the Luff-Schoorl method by titration with sodium thiosulphate. The mineral content was determined by atomic absorption spectrometry (Unicam Solaar 116, Thermo, Dreieich, Germany). Amino acids were determined by ion-exchange chromatography (AA analyser LC 3000, Biotronic, Maintal, Germany). The content of volatile fatty acids in the homogenised caecal chyme was measured by means of a gas chromatograph (610 Series, Unicam, Kassel, Germany). After the sample had been mixed with an internal standard (10 mL of formic acid 89% and 0.1 mL of 4-methylvaleric acid), the mixture was centrifuged and then subjected to gas chromatography with a column temperature of 155 °C (injector: 175 °C, detector: 180 °C).

The serological tests were carried out using a sandwich blocking ELISA [16]. This ELISA has a specificity of 98.7% and a sensitivity of 96.5% and works with specific monoclonal antibodies. Cut-off values for the blocking ELISA test are given as percent inhibition (PI) with a cut-off value of PI 30.

The mean *L. intracellularis* content was determined from the aliquot of the homogenised faeces via quantitative PCR using established methods [17]. Results are given in genome equivalents (GE) per gramme faeces.

For histopathological analysis, the fixed tissue specimens were processed by routine methods, embedded into paraffin, and sectioned at 2 μm; three series (with three cuts per series) with a minimum distance of 25 μm were prepared and fixed on microscope slides (Superfrost® plus, Menzel GmbH & Co. KG, Brunswick, Germany) per block.

To measure the crypt depth of the caecal epithelium, a hematoxylin−eosin (HE) staining was performed in accordance with a standard protocol (two tissue sections per animal with a minimum separation of 50 μm). For each boar, these two HE stained sections were examined with regard to the crypt depth of the caecal epithelium. The measurement was carried out with a photomicroscope (Axiophot, Zeiss, Oberkochen, Germany) and the program analysisSIS® 3.0 (Soft Imaging Systems, Münster, Germany). For each slide, ten completely cut crypts were measured from their base to the opening to the intestinal lumen.

Statistical analyses

The statistical analyses were performed using the Statistical Analysis System for Windows SAS®, version 9.3, (SAS Institute Inc., Cary, North Carolina, USA). The group comparison for performance parameters (BW, ADWG), results of serological analyses (PI values), quantitative detection of *L. intracellularis* in faeces and caecal content, DM content in faeces, short chain fatty acids in caecal content and crypt depth of caecal wall were performed by a one-way analysis of variance (ANOVA) for independent samples. The Ryan-Einot-Gabriel-Welsch multiple range test was used for the multiple pairwise means comparisons. The distributions of the residuals from the linear models belonging to the analyses of variance were close to the normal one.

In the case of non-normalised data, overall differences in parameters between groups were assessed by the Kruskal–Wallis equality of populations rank test followed by comparisons with a Wilcoxon signed-rank test. The latter was carried out in pairs to investigate differences in the mean values. The transition from the comparative to the experimental-related error probability was achieved by the so-called "α-adjustment" according to Bonferroni.

Differences in concentration between *L. intracellularis* counts at different time points depending on group as well as differences between DM content in faeces between groups were examined by means of one-way analyses of variance for repeated measures.

For the correlation-analysis of data with normal distribution, the correlation coefficient of Pearson was used. In non-normally distributed residuals the Spearman's rank correlation coefficient was calculated.

All statements of statistical significance were based upon P values smaller than 0.05. This approach controls the comparison-wise error rate.

Results

The experiment ran as planned. There were no animal losses. Changes in faecal consistency, which were associated with the detection of *L. intracellularis*, were not treated with antibiotics due to the short duration of the clinical manifestation.

The experimental diets could be regarded as almost isoenergetic (15.6 ± 0.33 MJ ME/kg DM) and isonitrogenous (187 ± 4.02 g/kg DM). The lysine contents were comparable (13.1 ± 0.55 g/kg DM) as intended when formulating the diets (Table 2).

Performance parameters

Overall, there were no significant differences in the final body weight (Ø at group level: 134 ± 3.42 kg), or in the weight development between the groups (Ø at group level: 1227 ± 82.8 g/day; (Table 3). In numerical terms, the performance in the RPS group was the lowest (1104 ± 336 g/day). If, however, independent of the diet, the mean *L. intracellularis* excretion by category during the experimental period showed numerical differences in terms of performance. Animals with an excretion greater than $5 \times \log_{10}$ GE/g faeces had a numerically lower ADWG ($\log_{10}$ GE/g faeces < 4: 1.246 kg ADWG; $\log_{10}$ GE/g faeces $\geq 4 < 5$: 1.252 kg ADWG; $\log_{10}$ GE/g faeces $\geq 5 < 6$: 1.150 kg ADWG; $\log_{10}$ GE/g faeces ≥ 6: 1.147 kg ADWG).

Blood analysis

The PI values before the start of the experiment (Ø PI values at group level: 29.8 ± 2.77; 50% of animals with PI values ≥ 30) and at the time of slaughter (Ø PI values at group level: 55.5 ± 3.59) did not differ between groups

Table 3 Body weight, average daily weight gain and feed conversion ratio in finishing boars (n = 10/treatment) fed diets with different compositions during the 4-week trial period

Item	Time	Treatment									
		FP		CM		CORN		WHEY		RPS	
		Mean	SD	Mean	SD	Mean	SD	Mean	SD	Mean	SD
Body weight (kg)	TP1 (start)	98.7	6.97	97.0	6.85	99.1	6.77	97.0	7.77	96.1	8.12
	TP6 (final)[a]	138	13.7	135	8.22	136	7.48	133	10.1	129	13.1
ADWG (kg)	Ø TP2–5 (week 1–4)	1.326	0.272	1.273	0.161	1.225	0.164	1.208	0.250	1.104	0.336
ADFI (kg DM)	Ø TP2–5 (week 1–4)	3084		3217		3242		3261		2861	
FCR (kg/kg)	Ø TP2–5 (week 1–4)	2.64		2.87		2.93		2.94		2.94	

FP fine pelleted diet, *CM* coarse meal diet, *CORN* meal diet with 22% cracked corn, *WHEY* meal diet with 16.9% dried whey, *RPS* meal diet with 30% raw potato starch, *ADWG* average daily weight gain, *FCR* feed conversion ratio in kg diet per kg weight gain, Ø abbreviation for mean value, *TP1* time point 1 (start), TP2 (week 1), TP3 (week 2), TP4 (week 3), TP5 (week 4), TP6 (slaughter)

[a] 30 days later; no significant differences between values in a row detectable at P < 0.05

at each time point. There was a significant increase in each single group between PI values from the start of the experiment to slaughter (Table 4). The comparison of delta values in PI values between the start and end-points of the different groups showed no differences.

Faecal analysis

The excretion of *L. intracellularis* with the faeces did not differ between the groups at the different time points, nor did the mean excretion in the experimental period. The difference between the mean excretion in the experimental period (TP2–5) and the initial value (TP1) was positive with the exception of group CM. Group CM, however, showed the highest numbers of *L. intracellularis* in faeces at time TP1 in numerical terms. Within some of the groups (FP, CM, RPS), significant differences were seen as a function of time. In the FP group, the most significant excretion was found for TP3 ($4.32 \pm 3.16 \log_{10}$ GE/g) and TP5 ($4.55 \pm 3.33 \log_{10}$ GE/g). In group CM, on the other hand, the excretion at TP3 was the lowest ($0.59 \pm 1.87 \log_{10}$ GE/g), and the highest at TP4 ($5.83 \pm 2.36 \log_{10}$ GE/g). In group RPS, a significantly higher excretion with faeces was observed at the end of the trial phase (TP4 $7.25 \pm 1.44 \log_{10}$ GE/g; TP5 $5.46 \pm 3.85 \log_{10}$ GE/g).

The DM content in the faeces of the boars did not differ at the beginning of the experiment (Ø DM content at group level: 236 ± 16.8 g/kg). At TP2 in groups WHEY and RPS, at TP3 (numerically), TP4 and TP5, the DM content in group RPS was the lowest, whereas at TP2, TP4 and TP5, the DM content in the control group (FP) was highest. When comparing the average DM content during the experimental period (TP2–5), group FP showed the highest DM content in faeces, group RPS the lowest (P < 0.001). Depending on the time, there were no significant differences within each group.

Caecal content

In the groups CORN and RPS, the *L. intracellularis* genome equivalents were significantly highest (Table 4). In the WHEY group, numbers of *L. intracellularis* in the caecal content were the lowest. The butyrate concentration in the caecal content was the largest in the RPS group, the lowest in the CORN group. In the RPS group the crypt depths were significantly highest.

Correlations

Very strong negative correlations (r – correlation coefficient) occurred between the PI TP1 and the PI Δ TP1 to TP6 (r = − 0.90, P < 0.001) as well as between the $\log_{10}$ GE TP1 and the Δ $\log_{10}$ GE TP2–5 − TP1 (r = − 0.85, P < 0.001; Table 5). A strong positive correlation occurred

between the log GE at TP5 and the log GE in the caecum content (r = 0.66, P < 0.001).

In terms of *L. intracellularis* status in faeces, there were significances between DM at TP1 and crypt depth in the caecum (r = − 0.40, P = 0.006), as well as between the log GE in the caecal content and the butyrate concentration at this location (r = − 0.32, P = 0.023). These correlations were moderate (DM) and weak (butyrate).

At a feeding group level, significant correlations were found between PI TP6 and the mean faecal DM TP2–5 (r = − 0.72, P = 0.020) for group CM as well as positive correlations between butyrate and PI TP6 for the CORN group (r = 0.70, P = 0.024; Table 6). The difference between the PI values correlated significantly negative with the average DM content in faeces of animals in the CM group (r = − 0.74, P = 0.015). The delta PI value correlated positively with the butyrate concentration in the caecal content for the CORN group (r = 0.76, P = 0.010). The counts of *L. intracellularis* (log10 GE) at TP1 correlated negatively with the acetate content in the caecum for the WHEY group (r = − 0.65, P = 0.043). The average $\log_{10}$ numbers of *L. intracellularis* during the experimental period correlated positively with the DM at TP1 (r = 0.78, P = 0.012) and negatively with the average DM content (r = − 0.70, P = 0.025) for the FP group during the experimental phase. For the CORN group, the mean log GE content in ZP2–5 correlated positively with the butyrate content (r = 0.68, P = 0.030). For the CORN group, the difference in the $\log_{10}$ GE *L. intracellularis* between TP2–5 and TP1 correlated negatively with the average DM content during the experimental period (r = − 0.72, P = 0.018). The *L. intracellularis* counts in the caecal content correlated negatively with the DM at TP1 for the WHEY group (r = − 0.71, P = 0.033), there also being a negative correlation for the RPS group to all volatile fatty acids acetate (r = − 0.74, P = 0.015), propionate (r = − 0.74, P = 0.014) and butyrate (r = − 0.70, P = 0.026).

Discussion

In this study, effects of different dietary approaches on the spreading and extent of a natural *L. intracellularis* infection in finishing boars were monitored. The present study is, to our knowledge, the first study on fattening boars, which has analysed the effect of very different diets on the course of a natural *L. intracellularis* infection over several weeks. The experimental conditions were selected in such a way that other factors were minimised. At the same time, different factors were chosen so as to be able to monitor the natural infection. First, boars came from a high health farm with late *L. intracellularis* infections. Second, the chosen animals had a known serological *L. intracellularis* status, 50% of animals being serologically

Table 4 Results of serological investigations, analyses in faeces (qPCR *Lawsonia intracellularis* and DM) as well as counts of *L. intracellularis* and concentrations of short chain fatty acids in caecal content and cecal crypt depth in groups of finishing boars (n = 10/treatment) fed diets with different compositions

Item	Time	Treatment									
		FP Mean	SD	CM Mean	SD	CORN Mean	SD	WHEY Mean	SD	RPS Mean	SD
PI values blocking ELISA	Blood										
	TP1 (start)	31.0[B]	12.9	30.5[B]	16.9	25.5[B]	13.1	29.0[B]	14.7	32.9[B]	14.6
	TP6 (final)	53.7[A]	10.3	50.1[A]	10.3	57.9[A]	4.84	57.3[A]	3.92	58.7[A]	7.15
	Δ TP1 to TP6[†]	22.7	18.9	19.6	23.3	32.4	14.2	28.3	16.2	25.8	17.6
$\log_{10}$ GE *L. intracellularis* (per g)	Faeces										
	TP1 (start)	2.46[AB]	2.64	3.58[AB]	2.54	3.43	2.37	2.30	3.16	2.58[B]	2.73
	TP2 (week 1)	1.08[B]	2.32	1.54[BC]	2.48	2.52	2.68	3.75	3.51	1.90[B]	2.46
	TP3 (week 2)	4.32[A]	3.16	0.59[C]	1.87	3.06	3.32	4.11	2.99	2.45[B]	3.33
	TP4 (week 3)	3.64[AB]	3.23	5.83[A]	2.36	5.06	3.09	5.05	3.28	7.25[A]	1.44
	TP5 (week 4)	4.55[A]	3.33	4.27[A]	3.35	4.98	3.42	3.11	3.37	5.46[A]	3.85
	Ø TP2–5 (weeks 1–4)	3.40	3.23	3.03	3.25	3.78	3.19	3.95	3.23	4.08	3.59
	Δ (ØTP2–5–TP1)	0.93	3.14	−0.57	3.30	0.38	2.65	1.68	3.58	1.51	3.80
DM content (g/kg)	TP1 (start)	237	78.9	247	24.7	254	28.8	248	84.7	240	29.1
	TP2 (week 1)	273[a]	40.9	248[bc]	10.1	266[ab]	24.8	241[c]	19.9	238[c]	32.1
	TP3 (week 2)	259	84.7	238	18.0	257	97.7	245	16.7	214	18.1
	TP4 (week 3)	274[a]	49.2	249[ab]	24.0	246[ab]	17.9	241[ab]	16.8	226[b]	55.4
	TP5 (week 4)	268[a]	27.4	245[ab]	17.7	263[a]	24.6	245[ab]	17.5	222[b]	25.9
	Ø TP2–5 (weeks 1–4)	269[a]	53.0	245[bc]	17.9	258[ab]	51.16	243[bc]	17.2	225[c]	35.4
	Caecal content or rather caecal wall										
$\log_{10}$ GE *L. intracellularis* (per g)	TP6	4.34[ab]	3.83	5.46[a]	3.03	5.16[ab]	3.63	1.57[b]	3.32	5.82[a]	3.51
Starch g/kg DM	TP6	41.4[b]	7.97	164[a]	35.4	136[a]	40.6	85.1[b]	22.4	179[a]	110
Acetate (mmol/kg FM)	TP6	148	6.64	145	8.07	131	14.4	143	6.90	136	27.1
Propionate (mmol/kg FM)	TP6	50.5	3.98	53.8	5.82	51.0	3.03	49.4	2.80	48.6	9.28
Butyrate (mmol/kg FM)	TP6	20.3[b]	3.32	24.8[b]	3.83	21.2[b]	8.38	24.4[b]	6.09	33.7[a]	9.53
Crypt depth caecum (μm)	TP6	482[b]	57.5	473[b]	50.0	499[b]	106	475[b]	66.0	570[b]	189

Upper case letters (A, B) signify differences in columns (vertical) on the level of a specific feeding group between TPs (between TPs (between TP1 and TP6 for "PI values blocking ELISA"; between TP1–5 for "$\log_{10}$ GE *L. intracellularis*", between TP1–5 for "DM content") depending on time point at P < 0.05

Lower case letters (a, b, c) signify differences in a row (horizontal) between feeding groups on parameter and TP-level at P < 0.05

FP fine pelleted diet, *CM* coarse meal diet, *CORN* meal diet with 22% cracked corn, *WHEY* meal diet with 16.9% dried whey, *RPS* meal diet with 30% raw potato starch, Ø abbreviation for mean value, *TP1* time point 1 (start); *TP2* (week 1), *TP3* (week 2), *TP4* (week 3), *TP5* (week 4), *TP6* (slaughter), *PI* percent inhibition, cut-off values for the blocking ELISA test with a cut-off value cf PI 30, *GE* genome equivalents per gramme faeces, [†]30 days later

Table 5 Crosstab regarding intercorrelations between *Lawsonia intracellularis* status, DM content in faeces, volatile fatty acid concentrations in caecal content and ADWG in finishing boars with natural *L. intracellularis* infection

	PI TP1	PI TP6	Δ PI TP1 to TP6	$\log_{10}$ GE L.i. TP1	$\log_{10}$ GE L.i. TP2	$\log_{10}$ GE L.i. TP3	$\log_{10}$ GE L.i. TP4	$\log_{10}$ GE L.i. TP5	Ø $\log_{10}$ GE L.i. TP2–5	Δ $\log_{10}$ GE L.i. (Ø TP2–5–TP1)	DM TP 1	Ø DM TP2–5	$\log_{10}$ GE L.i. caecum (TP6)	Crypt depth caecum (TP6)	Acetate caecum (TP6)	Propionate caecum (TP6)	Butyrate caecum (TP6)	ADWG (TP2–6)
P value																		
PI TP1		− 0.26	− 0.90	0.01	− 0.24	− 0.25	− 0.39	− 0.21	− 0.44	− 0.23	0.20	0.13	− 0.12	− 0.00	0.14	0.04	0.22	0.10
PI TP6	0.070		0.56	− 0.03	0.05	0.26	0.47	0.14	0.37	0.17	− 0.05	− 0.23	− 0.04	0.06	− 0.36	− 0.27	0.08	− 0.26
Δ PI TP1 to TP6	< .001	< .001		− 0.01	0.23	0.34	0.50	0.22	0.51	0.24	− 0.17	− 0.20	0.09	− 0.00	− 0.24	− 0.09	− 0.18	− 0.14
$\log_{10}$ GE L.i. TP1	0.932	0.8109	0.939		0.11	− 0.20	− 0.04	− 0.16	− 0.09	− 0.85	0.29	− 0.03	− 0.01	− 0.22	− 0.04	0.15	− 0.04	− 0.14
$\log_{10}$ GE L.i. TP2	0.099	0.742	0.110	0.450		0.12	0.15	0.19	0.54	0.13	0.14	− 0.12	0.04	0.11	− 0.23	− 0.07	− 0.03	− 0.13
$\log_{10}$ GE L.i. TP3	0.084	0.074	0.015	0.174	0.426		0.33	− 0.18	0.51	0.41	0.10	− 0.09	− 0.24	0.05	0.03	− 0.16	0.11	0.00
$\log_{10}$ GE L.i. TP4	0.007	0.001	< .001	0.770	0.328	0.022		0.39	0.72	0.38	0.07	− 0.34	0.19	0.19	− 0.06	− 0.11	0.11	− 0.05
$\log_{10}$ GE L.i. TP5	0.165	0.362	0.135	0.283	0.203	0.240	0.010		0.57	0.42	− 0.04	− 0.14	0.66	0.30	− 0.02	0.01	− 0.24	− 0.14
Ø $\log_{10}$ GE L.i. TP2–5	0.002	0.008	< .001	0.531	< .001	< .001	< .001	< .001		0.59	0.04	− 0.26	0.14	0.25	− 0.10	− 0.16	0.01	− 0.06
Δ $\log_{10}$ GE L.i. (Ø TP2–5–TP1)	0.104	0.234	0.096	< .001	0.362	0.003	0.009	0.004	< .001		− 0.28	− 0.16	0.06	0.34	0.04	− 0.18	0.08	0.11
DM TP 1	0.182	0.740	0.251	0.048	0.358	0.523	0.671	0.803	0.778	0.058		− 0.08	− 0.06	− 0.40	0.01	0.14	0.14	0.00
Ø DM TP2–5	0.387	0.110	0.155	0.853	0.395	0.552	0.020	0.346	0.073	0.279	0.587		− 0.02	− 0.12	0.19	0.17	− 0.24	− 0.13
$\log_{10}$ GE L.i. caecum (TP6)	0.411	0.777	0.521	0.966	0.782	0.092	0.191	< .001	0.327	0.679	0.707	0.917		0.18	− 0.23	− 0.02	− 0.32	− 0.19
Crypt depth caecum (TP6)	0.991	0.669	0.981	0.118	0.441	0.731	0.200	0.041	0.081	0.015	0.006	0.407	0.214		− 0.05	0.04	0.06	0.16
Acetate caecum (TP6)	0.321	0.010	0.096	0.759	0.101	0.851	0.687	0.891	0.508	0.780	0.941	0.193	0.102	0.734		0.40	0.30	0.25
Propionate caecum (TP6)	0.802	0.057	0.545	0.289	0.647	0.260	0.443	0.926	0.257	0.215	0.353	0.244	0.880	0.787	0.004		− 0.03	0.04
Butyrate caecum (TP6)	0.133	0.589	0.217	0.807	0.859	0.450	0.478	0.115	0.924	0.560	0.353	0.089	0.023	0.681	0.034	0.829		− 0.03
ADWG (TP2–6)	0.499	0.069	0.371	0.318	0.352	0.995	0.724	0.370	0.673	0.437	0.981	0.351	0.194	0.282	0.083	0.790	0.838	

Ø abbreviation for mean value, *TP1* time point 1 (start); TP2 (week 1), TP3 (week 2), TP4 (week 3), TP5 (week 4), TP6 (slaughter), *L.i. L. intracellularis*, *PI* percent inhibition, cut-off values for the blocking ELISA test with a cut-off value of PI 30, *r* Correlation coefficient

P P value, statistical significance is based on P values smaller than 0.05 (italics)

[a] Pearson correlation coefficients—for combination of parameters between grey boxes; Spearman's rank correlation coefficients—combination of unshaded boxes); correlations: 0.00–0.19 "very weak"; 0.20–0.39 "weak"; 0.40–0.59 "moderate"; 0.60–0.79 "strong"; 0.80–1.0 "very strong"

positive in blocking ELISA at the time of transport and regrouping. Third, effects of transport and regrouping were used to provoke the spreading of the pathogen within new groups at the research facility.

Performance parameters

In the present study, no effect of diet on the performance parameters could be seen. If, however, independent of the diet, the mean *L. intracellularis* excretion by category during the experimental period showed numerical differences in terms of performance. In literature, an effect on the ADWG was seen only for an excretion greater than 10^6 GE per gramme faeces [7]. However, these previous experiments were conducted with artificial *L. intracellularis* infection. Also, these animals were only 6 or 9 weeks old at the time of artificial infection. In another study on animals of similar age, an effect of the level of *L. intracellularis* excretion on the ADWG (P < 0.001) was shown [5]. The authors of the study emphasise, however, that this effect was particularly important with low DM content in the faeces. In pigs with higher faecal DM (20%) the association between ADG and *L. intracellularis* was

minimal. In pigs with faecal DM above 25%, no effect on ADWG was reported [5].

In the experimental period of the present study, the group RPS showed the lowest average DM content in faeces (225 ± 35.4 g/kg). The correlation analysis showed only for the group RPS that the average *L. intracellularis* counts in faeces were significantly negatively correlated with ADWG ($r = -0.78$). The present investigations thus confirm that the known relationship applies to RPS. The numerically lowest ADWG in the comparison between the feeding groups was associated with the numerically highest excretion in this group.

In the present study, a negative correlation was observed between the mean values of ADWG of the different feeding groups and excretion levels of *L. intracellularis* between TP2 and TP5 (Spearman's correlation coefficient: $r = -0.90$; $P = 0.038$). At group average level a higher *L. intracellularis* excretion could be the reason for a lower performance. Nonetheless, also factors such as the palatability of the feed can provoke a different feed intake. Thus, this relation could also be a reason for the

Table 6 Crosstab regarding intercorrelations between *Lawsonia intracellularis* status, DM content in faeces, volatile fatty acid concentrations in caecal content and ADWG in finishing boars with natural *L. intracellularis* infection

Item	Item	DM TP1		Ø DM TP2–5		Acetate caecum (TP6)		Propionate caecum (TP6)		Butyrate caecum (TP6)	
		r	P	r	P	r	P	r	P	r	P
PI TP1	FP	−0.28	0.460	0.35	0.322	−0.41	0.241	−0.06	0.803	0.50	0.138
	CM	0.41	0.243	0.58	0.078	0.24	0.513	−0.15	0.679	0.09	0.811
	CORN	0.01	0.977	0.47	0.171	−0.29	0.418	0.08	0.829	−0.57	0.085
	WHEY	0.31	0.410	−0.22	0.541	0.44	0.207	−0.17	0.630	0.60	0.067
	RPS	0.62	0.072	−0.20	0.577	0.27	0.446	0.13	0.716	0.53	0.115
PI TP6	FP	0.11	0.773	−0.32	0.362	−0.17	0.637	−0.32	0.366	−0.36	0.310
	CM	−0.21	0.552	−0.72	0.020	−0.24	0.506	−0.11	0.760	−0.31	0.377
	CORN	0.08	0.832	0.31	0.378	−0.42	0.225	−0.13	0.716	0.70	0.024
	WHEY	−0.22	0.576	0.12	0.751	−0.21	0.556	0.09	0.803	−0.02	0.960
	RPS	−0.07	0.852	−0.06	0.860	−0.26	0.467	0.18	0.627	−0.41	0.235
Δ PI TP1 to TP6	FP	0.25	0.512	−0.41	0.234	0.19	0.607	−0.15	0.676	−0.48	0.162
	CM	−0.39	0.265	−0.74	0.015	−0.28	0.440	0.06	0.869	−0.20	0.577
	CORN	0.02	0.964	−0.33	0.358	0.12	0.736	−0.12	0.746	0.76	0.010
	WHEY	−0.34	0.366	0.14	0.693	−0.46	0.179	0.12	0.737	−0.56	0.089
	RPS	−0.54	0.130	0.15	0.681	−0.44	0.200	0.02	0.960	−0.61	0.063
Log₁₀ GE *L.i.* TP1	FP	−0.02	0.963	0.19	0.604	0.11	0.763	0.12	0.735	−0.05	0.901
	CM	0.19	0.599	−0.52	0.122	0.25	0.483	0.28	0.440	−0.06	0.880
	CORN	0.36	0.304	0.52	0.122	0.42	0.223	0.15	0.672	−0.15	0.672
	WHEY	0.57	0.112	−0.27	0.457	−0.65	0.043	−0.14	0.693	0.17	0.637
	RPS	0.31	0.416	−0.17	0.630	−0.05	0.901	0.01	0.986	−0.06	0.873
Ø log₁₀ GE *L.i.* TP2–5	FP	0.78	0.012	−0.70	0.025	−0.13	0.718	−0.36	0.310	−0.62	0.054
	CM	0.05	0.892	−0.06	0.873	0.15	0.675	−0.12	0.747	0.04	0.916
	CORN	−0.05	0.881	−0.29	0.411	0.02	0.955	−0.08	0.826	0.68	0.030
	WHEY	0.01	0.982	−0.33	0.358	−0.27	0.455	−0.01	0.979	−0.11	0.761
	RPS	−0.32	0.398	0.16	0.654	−0.10	0.777	0.18	0.627	−0.46	0.178
Δ log₁₀ GE *L.i.* (Ø TP2–5−TP1)	FP	0.42	0.251	−0.45	0.188	−0.18	0.618	−0.15	0.676	−0.15	0.676
	CM	−0.17	0.649	0.51	0.136	−0.08	0.820	−0.30	0.396	0.03	0.927
	CORN	−0.40	0.252	−0.72	0.018	−0.16	0.652	−0.38	0.278	0.38	0.277
	WHEY	−0.47	0.202	0.02	0.947	0.53	0.115	0.12	0.751	−0.14	0.706
	RPS	−0.54	0.134	0.22	0.532	0.19	0.603	0.08	0.829	0.01	0.979
log₁₀ GE *L.i. caecum* (TP6)	FP	0.53	0.146	0.09	0.810	−0.22	0.544	−0.11	0.757	−0.31	0.389
	CM	0.01	0.973	0.21	0.555	−0.26	0.477	0.12	0.738	−0.60	0.066
	CORN	0.52	0.122	0.33	0.359	0.15	0.684	0.46	0.186	−0.27	0.445
	WHEY	−0.71	0.033	0.07	0.849	−0.24	0.500	0.03	0.924	−0.59	0.074
	RPS	−0.65	0.057	−0.36	0.309	−0.74	0.015	−0.74	0.014	−0.70	0.026
Crypt depth caecum (TP6)	FP	0.21	0.586	−0.14	0.706	0.52	0.120	0.49	0.150	−0.05	0.881
	CM	−0.19	0.592	0.43	0.210	0.15	0.672	0.37	0.295	0.02	0.964
	CORN	−0.30	0.405	−0.21	0.556	−0.53	0.117	0.22	0.533	0.20	0.580
	WHEY	−0.46	0.208	−0.14	0.702	0.47	0.167	−0.13	0.729	0.16	0.665
	RPS	−0.23	0.546	−0.24	0.511	−0.35	0.328	−0.41	0.244	−0.49	0.150

FP fine pelleted diet, *CM* coarse meal diet, *CORN* meal diet with 22% cracked corn, *WHEY* meal diet with 16.9% dried whey, *RPS* meal diet with 30% raw potato starch; *TP1* time point 1 (start), TP2 (week 1), TP3 (week 2), TP4 (week 3), TP5 (week 4), TP 6 (slaughter); *L.i. L. intracellularis*, *PI* percent inhibition, cut-off values for the blocking ELISA test with a cut-off value of PI 30, *r* Correlation coefficient

P P value, statistical significance is based on P values smaller than 0.05 (italics)

Pearson correlation coefficients—grey boxes; Spearman's rank correlation coefficients—unshaded boxes); correlations: 0.00–0.19 "very weak"; 0.20–0.39 "weak"; 0.40–0.59 "moderate"; 0.60–0.79 "strong"; 0.80–1.0 "very strong"

numerically different weight development between the different feeding groups.

Dynamics of infection and diet

The results of the serological tests are clear in the present study. During the acclimatisation and experimental period, in each group an intense *L. intracellularis* spread within the animal group is to be assumed. In each feeding group, a significant increase in the serological response provided evidence of this confrontation with the pathogen. It is known from the literature that the antibodies can fall off already 2 weeks after the excretion peak [9, 18]. This infers that our investigations took place in an intensive infection phase. Antibody titres were high at the end of the trial. This is the best prerequisite for testing a feeding concept in the field.

The haemorrhagic form of an *L. intracellularis* infection is termed proliferative haemorrhagic enteropathy [14]. This form is commonly observed in replacement gilts and boars from high health herds that are introduced onto a new farm site [14]. In the present experiment, the boars had also been obtained from a high health herd. The farmer raised boars of defined genetics from a German breeding company. The animals were transferred to the research facilities and regrouped. In four animals, the acute form of *L. intracellularis* infection occurred during the experiment (divided into groups: $1\times$FP, $2\times$WHEY, $1\times$RPS). These animals showed numerically significant serological characteristics. The initial PI values were lower (20.2 ± 8.74). The final values tended to be higher (59.1 ± 6.69). The ΔPI values were more pronounced during the experiment (ΔPI: 38.9 ± 7.39). The average excretion was higher in the experimental phase (TP2–5: 5.86 ± 3.45 $\log_{10}$ GE/g) and the ADWG was lower (0.946 ± 0.477). This also indicates the intensive infection in the groups.

Overall, however, during the experimental phase in the present study there was no difference in the quantitative excretion of *L. intracellularis* in faeces as a function of the diet. Feeding of whey powder showed, however, significantly lower *L. intracellularis* levels in the caecum.

In literature, it could be proven that a fermented liquid diet (uncontrolled fermentation for 3–4 days at 24 °C) delayed the excretion of *L. intracellularis* [12]. Furthermore, pigs fed the standard diet supplemented with lactic acid (2.4%) had limited pathological lesions when the intestines were examined 4 weeks after inoculation [12]. High lactate concentrations are also to be expected for the fermented diet. Lactic acid concentration of 5.45% at DM level after an 8 h fermentation process were seen [19]. For a ration with 25% whey on DM basis, an 18–27% share of lactic acid on total organic acids in the caecum was shown [20].

Against this background, for the WHEY group higher concentrations of lactate in the gastrointestinal tract can be presumed. Therefore, it can be assumed that the lactic acid has a certain influence on the level of *L. intracellularis* in the intestine. This could be very promising for future dietetic approaches in swine.

Correlations

Regardless of the diet`s nature, two significant correlations were identified. First, the acetate content in the caecum was negatively correlated with the serological results at the end of the trial. Second, the butyrate contents in the caecum were negatively correlated with the number of *L. intracellularis* in the caecum. This is a first link between parameters describing the extent of an infection and the substrate properties at the site of the main infection (caecum). In both cases, however, the correlation was weak.

A direct effect is not yet known [21]. However, it is known that the concentration and production of volatile fatty acids in the large intestine is a function of substrate availability for fermentation [22]. Therefore, it depends on feed intake. This, in turn, is lower when animals develop *L. intracellularis* infections. In a US study, a reduction in feed intake (1.27 and 7.85, respectively) in animals aged 28 to 49 days could be observed for different inoculation doses (counts per pig: comparison 1: 7.2×10^7 to 3.8×10^5; comparison 2: 7.2×10^7 to 2.2×10^6) [23]. In pigs at 38–58 days of age a reduction in feed intake of about 3.79% after experimental infection (1.26×10^{10} *L. intracellularis* organisms in the inoculum) was demonstrated. As a control animals were treated with 50 ppm tylvalosin for 14 further days after experimental infection [24].

In the present trial, for group FP a positive correlation was found between the DM content in faeces in the acclimatisation phase and the average *L. intracellularis* excretion in the experimental phase. At the same time, however, there was a negative correlation between DM content and *L. intracellularis* excretion during the experimental phase. Animals show more severe clinical symptoms during initial *L. intracellularis* infection [18]. The DM content in the faeces is lower with high excretion of the pathogen [5]. Conversely, this means for our study: The higher dry matter content in the faeces in the acclimatisation phase is indicative of a lower excretion. Therefore, when infected in the experimental phase, these animals will possibly react with a higher level of *L. intracellularis* excretion. During the experimental phase, a negative correlation between the DM content in faeces and the amount of excretion is to be expected. A previous study described that higher excretion is associated with softer faeces [5, 7]. In the present study there was a significant correlation between the ΔPI concerning serological tests and the average excretion in the experimental phase (r = 0.68). The level of excretion is thus also reflected in the extent of the serological response.

For the CM group, the serological response to the infection with *L. intracellularis* was reflected relatively clearly in the faecal consistency. Both, the final PI value and the change in the PI value were negatively correlated with the DM content in the faeces during the experimental phase. An effect of *L. intracellularis* is only relevant to performance when it is also reflected in the DM content [5]. This relationship cannot be confirmed on the basis of the available results for group CM. There was no correlation with the ADWG. Under the conditions of CM feeding the excretion level was too low to lead to performance losses, as described for higher excretion [7].

For the CORN group, there were positive correlations of serological results (PI TP6 and Δ PI) with the butyrate concentration in the caecal content. However, this group was characterised by the numerically lowest butyrate concentrations. At low butyrate concentrations, no positive effect on the excretion of *L. intracellularis* could be observed. Also, in this group there are indications that a clearer response to the pathogen (ΔPI ↑) leads to changes in fecal consistency (softer).

When feeding whey (WHEY), few correlations were detectable. On the one hand, the number of *L. intracellularis* in faeces at TP1 was negatively associated with the acetate content in the caecum. On the other hand, there was a negative correlation between the DM content in faeces in the acclimatisation phase and *L. intracellularis* counts in the caecum. The period between acclimatisation and slaughter is relatively long (more than 30 days). A possible effect can certainly only be achieved if the corresponding feeding regime creates constant conditions in the animal. The measured parameters should also be causally related to the living conditions and characteristics of the pathogen. This is not proven for acetate. For the WHEY group, no correlation between the excretion and DM content in faeces could be determined for TP1 (Spearman: r = 0.57; P = 0.112). It is also known from the literature that high amounts of pathogens in the caecum or adjacent areas need not be found in the colon [25] and therefore could be easily found in faeces.

The RPS group had the highest concentrations of butyrate and the highest *L. intracellularis* counts in the caecum as well as the deepest crypt in the caecum. For this group a negative correlation of all volatile fatty acids with the *L. intracellularis* content in the caecum could be shown. The PI at TP6 as well as the average *L. intracellularis* content in the faeces were negatively correlated with the ADWG (r = −0.66 and r = −0.78), respectively. Thus, the question is whether the disease leads to less substrate

or if less substrate favours the disease. The fact that less *L. intracellularis* was detected at absolutely lower butyrate concentrations in the caecal content of the CORN group rather suggests that the butyrate content within this group is more likely to be an indicator function than it being causally related to *L. intracellularis* counts.

Conclusions

The present investigations indicate that the model of a natural infection in the finishing boars fundamentally works. Therefore, it is a good tool to analyse possible feeding influences on *L. intracellularis* infections. Dietetics can be a starting point for limiting the extent of infection at an early stage. Nevertheless, further tests over longer periods have to be performed first. In this context, feeding concepts with higher original lactic acid contents or provoking lactic acid production, such as from controlled fermentation, could prove promising to limit the effects of an *L. intracellularis* infection on performance and health.

Abbreviations

ADFI: average daily feed intake; ADWG: average daily weight gains; BW: body weight; CM: coarse meal diet; CORN: meal diet with 22% cracked corn; DM: dry matter; FCR: feed conversion ration; FP: fine pelleted diet; GE: genome equivalents *Lawsonia intracellularis*; *L. intracellularis*: *Lawsonia intracellularis*; ME: metabolisable energy; PI: percent inhibition; RPS: meal diet with 30% raw potato starch; SPF: specific pathogen free. The herd was considered free from infection with Porcine reproductive and respiratory syndrome virus and *Actinobacillus pleuropneumoniae* serotype 1/9/11, 5a/b, 2 (serological confirmed); *Pasteurella multocida* (free from—clinical confirmed); TP: time point; VDLUFA: Verband Deutscher Landwirtschaftlicher Untersuchungs- und Forschungsanstalten e. V; WHEY: meal diet with 16.9% dried whey.

Authors' contributions

JK, RT, HH (study itself) and CV (*L. intracellularis* topic) were the initiators of the idea. JK, SS (study itself) and CV (*L. intracellularis* topic) designed the study. AK, SS, CK, JM, RT, CV performed the study and made the analyses. CV did the statistics. CV wrote the paper. All authors read and approved the final manuscript.

Author details

[1] Institute for Animal Nutrition, University of Veterinary Medicine Hannover, Foundation, Bischofsholer Damm 15, 30173 Hanover, Germany. [2] Boehringer Ingelheim Veterinary Research Center GmbH & Co. KG, Bemeroder Str. 31, 30559 Hanover, Germany. [3] Veterinärgesellschaft im BHZP, Veerßer Str. 65, 29525 Uelzen, Germany. [4] BHZP GmbH, An der Wassermühle 8, 21368 Dahlenburg-Ellringen, Germany. [5] Boehringer Ingelheim Vetmedica GmbH, Binger Str. 173, 55218 Ingelheim am Rhein, Germany.

Acknowledgements

We would like to thank Frances Sherwood-Brock for proof reading the manuscript to ensure correct English.

Competing interests

CK is an employee of Boehringer Ingelheim Veterinary Research Center GmbH & Co. KG, Hanover, Germany; RD is an employee of Boehringer Ingelheim Vetmedica GmbH, Ingelheim am Rhein; Germany.

Funding

Parts of the project were supported by funds of the Federal Ministry of Food and Agriculture (BMEL) based on a decision of the Parliament of the Federal Republic of Germany via the Federal Office for Agriculture and Food (BLE) under the innovation support programme. Parts of the study were also financially supported by Boehringer Ingelheim Vetmedica GmbH, D-55216 Ingelheim am Rhein, Germany (qPCR analysis).

References

1. Jacobson M, Fellstrom C, Jensen-Waern M. Porcine proliferative enteropathy: an important disease with questions remaining to be solved. Vet J. 2010;184:264–8.
2. McOrist S, Barcellos D, Wilson R. Global patterns of porcine proliferative enteropathy. Pig J. 2003;51:26–35.
3. Marsteller TA, Armbruster G, Bane DP, Gebhart CJ, Muller R, Weatherford J, et al. Monitoring the prevalence of Lawsonia intracellularis IgG antibodies using serial sampling in growing and breeding swine herds. J Swine Health Prod. 2003;11:127–30.
4. Brandt D, Kaim U, Baumgartner W, Wendt M. Evaluation of Lawsonia intracellularis infection in a group of pigs in a subclinically affected herd from weaning to slaughter. Vet Microbiol. 2010;146:361–5.
5. Pedersen KS, Skrubel R, Stege H, Angen O, Stahl M, Hjulsager C, et al. Association between average daily gain, faecal dry matter content and concentration of Lawsonia intracellularis in faeces. Acta Vet Scand. 2012;54:58.
6. Johansen M, Nielsen M, Dahl J, Svensmark B, Baekbo P, Kristensen CS, et al. Investigation of the association of growth rate in grower-finishing pigs with the quantification of Lawsonia intracellularis and porcine circovirus type 2. Prev Vet Med. 2013;108:63–72.
7. Collins AM, Barchia IM. The critical threshold of Lawsonia intracellularis in pig faeces that causes reduced average daily weight gains in experimentally challenged pigs. Vet Microbiol. 2014;168:455–8.
8. Hardge T, Keller C, Steinheuer R, Tessier P, Salleras J, Rubio P, et al. Serological prevalence of Lawsonia intracellularis across european pig herds. In: Proceedings of the 19th international pig veterinary society congress. Copenhagen: International Pig Veterinary Society; 2006. p. 77.
9. Guedes RMC, Winkelman NL, Gebhart CJ. Relationship between the severity of porcine proliferative enteropathy and the infectious dose of Lawsonia intracellularis. Vet Rec. 2003;153:432–3.
10. Stege H, Jensen TK, Moller K, Baekbo P, Jorsal SE. Risk factors for intestinal pathogens in Danish finishing pig herds. Prev Vet Med. 2001;50:153–64.
11. Molbak L, Johnsen K, Boye M, Jensen TK, Johansen M, Moller K, et al. The microbiota of pigs influenced by diet texture and severity of Lawsonia intracellularis infection. Vet Microbiol. 2008;128:96–107.
12. Boesen HT, Jensen TK, Schmidt AS, Jensen BB, Jensen SM, Moller K. The influence of diet on Lawsonia intracellularis colonization in pigs upon experimental challenge. Vet Microbiol. 2004;103:35–45.
13. Jacoby RO, Johnson EA. Transmissible ileal hyperplasia. In: Streilein JW, editor. Hamster immune responses in infectious and oncologic diseases. New York: Springer; 1981. p. 267–89.
14. Naumann C, Bassler R. Methoden der landwirtschaftlichen Forschungs- und Untersuchungsanstalt, Biochemische Untersuchung von Futtermitteln. Darmstadt: Methodenbuch III (einschließlich der achten Ergänzungen) (VDLUFA); 2012.
15. Keller C, Ohlinger V, Bulay A, Maala C. A blocking ELISA for the detection of antibodies against Lawsonia intracellularis. In: Proceedings of the 18th international pig veterinary society congress. Hamburg: International Pig Veterinary Society; 2004. p. 293.
16. Nathues H, Holthaus K, Beilage EG. Quantification of Lawsonia intracellularis in porcine faeces by real-time PCR. J Appl Microbiol. 2009;107:2009–16.
17. Collins AM, Love RJ. Re-challenge of pigs following recovery from proliferative enteropathy. Vet Microbiol. 2007;120:381–6.
18. Kroll JJ, Roof MB, Hoffman LJ, Dickson JS, Harris DL. Proliferative enteropathy: a global enteric disease of pigs caused by Lawsonia intracellularis. Anim Health Res Rev. 2005;6:173–97.
19. Mikkelsen LL, Jensen BB. Performance and microbial activity in the gastrointestinal tract of piglets fed fermented liquid feed at weaning. J Anim Feed Sci. 1998;7:211–5.
20. Friend D, Cunningham H, Nicholson J. The production of organic acids in the pig. Can J Anim Sci. 1963;43:156–68.
21. Vannucci FA, Gebhart CJ. Recent advances in understanding the pathogenesis of Lawsonia intracellularis infections. Vet Pathol. 2014;51:465–77.
22. Argenzio RA, Southworth M. Sites of organic acid production and absorption in gastrointestinal tract of the pig. Am J Physiol. 1975;228:454–60.
23. Paradis M, McKay R, Wilson J, Vessie G, Winkelman N, Gebhart C, et al. Subclinical ileitis produced by sequential dilutions of Lawsonia intracellularis in a mucosal homogenate challenge model. Am Assoc Swine Vet. 2005;189–91.
24. Guedes RMC, Franca SA, Machado GS, Blumer MA, Cruz ECD. Use of tylvalosin-medicated feed to control porcine proliferative enteropathy. Vet Rec. 2009;165:342–6.
25. Boutrup TS, Boesen HT, Boye M, Agerholm JS, Jensen TK. Early pathogenesis in porcine proliferative enteropathy caused by Lawsonia intracellularis. J Comp Pathol. 2010;143:101–9.

24

Clinical and histopathologic findings in dogs with the ultrasonographic appearance of gastric muscularis unorganized hyperechoic striations

Hock Gan Heng[1], Chee Kin Lim[1]*iD, Sarah Steinbach[1], Meaghan Maureen Broman[2] and Margaret Allan Miller[2]

Abstract

Background: Ultrasonographic appearance of unorganized hyperechoic striations (UHS) has been observed in the canine gastric muscularis layer. The purpose of the study was to determine the prevalence, sonographic and postmortem histologic features, and to determine the clinical significance of canine gastric muscularis UHS. In the prospective study, 72 dogs were included. The presence of gastric muscularis UHS were reviewed to determine its distribution and location. In the retrospective study, 167 dogs that had both abdominal ultrasonography and necropsy were included.

Results: The prevalence of gastric muscularis UHS in dogs was 37.5% in the prospective and 5.4% in the retrospective studies respectively. The higher prevalence in prospective study was due to greater anticipation by the radiologists in search for gastric muscularis UHS. In the ventral gastric wall, the muscularis UHS were better defined when the gastric lumen was empty or non-distended, and were mostly parallel with the serosa when the gastric wall was distended (with gas or fluid). Visualization of the dorsal gastric wall was often obscured by gas shadowing from luminal gas. Histopathology was performed on eight dogs with gastric muscularis UHS, three of which had fibrous tissue observed with Masson's trichrome stain.

Conclusion: Presence of gastric muscularis UHS in dogs may have been attributable to presence of incomplete interfaces between the inner oblique, middle circular and outer longitudinal layers of the gastric tunica muscularis or due to presence of fibrous tissue within the gastric muscularis layer. The clinical significance of canine gastric muscularis UHS is uncertain.

Keywords: Canine, Fibrosis, Gastric muscularis layer, Ultrasonography, Unorganized hyperechoic striations

Background

During routine ultrasonographic examination of the gastrointestinal tract (GIT), the GIT wall thickness and the 5-layered appearance, as well as the function (motility) are often assessed. The 5-layers of the stomach wall (from outermost to innermost) include the serosa, muscularis, submucosa, mucosa and mucosal surface. The alternating echogenicity appearance of these layers has been well-described in veterinary literature. The serosa,

submucosa and mucosal surface are hyperechoic, while the muscularis and mucosa are hypoechoic [1]. The hyperechoic appearance of the mucosal surface is due to trapping of small gas bubbles at the mucosal surface and hence it is not considered as a true histologic layer [1]. Recently, hyperechoic bands paralleling the serosal layers of the muscularis layer of the canine colon wall has been reported and was found to be associated with the presence of fibrous tissue in the myenteric plexus or in the tunica muscularis [2]. Unorganized hyperechoic striations (UHS) have been observed within the canine gastric muscularis layer (Fig. 1) by the authors. This has

*Correspondence: cklim@purdue.edu
[1] Department of Veterinary Clinical Sciences, College of Veterinary Medicine, Purdue University, West Lafayette, IN 47907, USA
Full list of author information is available at the end of the article

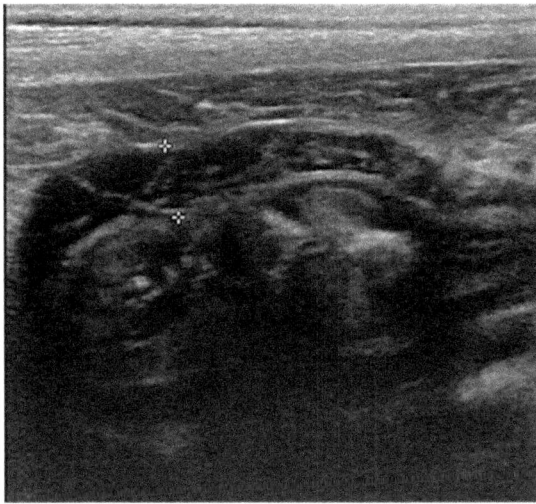

Fig. 1 Sagittal ultrasonographic image of the stomach of a dog from the prospective study. The unorganized hyperechoic striations (UHS) are seen in the gastric muscularis layer (between the asterisks). This dog had no clinical sign related to the gastrointestinal tract

never been reported and the clinical significance of this is unknown.

The aims of this study were to estimate the prevalence of canine gastric muscularis UHS, to characterize the ultrasonographic and histologic features, and to determine the clinical significance of canine gastric muscularis UHS wherever possible.

Methods

This is a single institution, descriptive, cross-sectional study comprising of prospectively and retrospectively recruited sample populations of dogs.

In the prospective part of the study, all dogs that underwent routine abdominal ultrasound examination during a 4-week period (March 2014) were included. There were no exclusion criteria. The standard care of the institute was provided to each animal. All ultrasonographic studies were performed by two board-certified radiologists (HGH & CKL) using the same ultrasound system (Philips iU22 SonoCT system, Philips Ultrasound, Bothell, WA) and machine settings. Both linear (5–12 MHz) and micro-convex (5–8 MHz) transducers were used. The choice of the transducer used depended on the body conformation and size of the dogs. The selection of the location of the focus point varied depending on the type of transducer used. The linear transducer was preferred whenever possible for superior image resolution. This ultrasonographic examination was part of the standard care for the diagnostic evaluation of the patients, thus owner consent was not deemed necessary. The radiologists were not blinded and therefore aware of the clinical

presentation of each dog that was presented for abdominal ultrasound.

The appearance of the gastric muscularis was evaluated to determine the presence of UHS. Still images and video clips were captured and reviewed by two board-certified radiologists (HGH & CKL) to determine the region of the stomach involved: (i) ventral wall, or (ii) dorsal wall, or (iii) both ventral and dorsal walls; and the distribution of UHS: (i) local if only one part of the fundus or body or pylorus in either of the ventral wall or dorsal wall is affected, or (ii) diffuse if more than one part of the fundus or body or pylorus of the ventral wall or dorsal wall is affected. Presence of gas or ingesta that may obscure visualization of the dorsal wall is also noted.

In the retrospective part of the study, all dogs that had both abdominal ultrasound and necropsy from January 2011 to December 2013 were included, without any exclusion criteria. All ultrasonographic studies were performed using the same ultrasound machine and settings used in the prospective part of this study and reviewed by both radiologists to identify dogs with gastric muscularis UHS. Due to the retrospective nature of the study and limited images of the stomach (usually two to three still images in both longitudinal and transverse planes) captured in routine abdominal ultrasound, the presence of gastric muscularis is remarked as present or not present. Once such cases were identified, the original histologic sections of formalin-fixed, paraffin-embedded stomach stained with hematoxylin and eosin (H&E) were reviewed by a board-certified veterinary pathologist (MAM). Additionally, Masson's trichrome stain was used to identify fibrous collagen.

The medical records of dogs with gastric muscularis UHS in both the prospective and retrospective parts of the study including the signalment (gender, age and breed), clinical signs at presentation, previous or current history of GIT problems, current and pertinent laboratory results (including histologic results whenever available) and outcome were reviewed by a board-certified internist (SS) to determine if a dog had any underlying GIT disease.

Results

A total of 72 dogs were evaluated during the prospective part of the study. Gastric muscularis UHS were observed in 27 dogs (37.5%). The entire stomach including the ventral wall and dorsal wall was visible in 10 dogs while only the ventral wall was visible for the remaining 17 dogs due to presence of intraluminal gas within the stomach. All 27 dogs with gastric muscularis UHS had diffuse distribution, involving all regions (fundus, body and pylorus) of the ventral and dorsal stomach wall that were visible. Gastric muscularis UHS were best defined when the gastric lumen was empty or non-distended (Fig. 2). This could be seen on both transverse and sagittal planes, using both micro-convex and linear transducers. The gastric muscularis UHS were subjectively better defined using linear transducer. The gastric muscularis UHS appeared to be parallel to the serosal layer when the gastric wall was distended with fluid or gas (Fig. 2A) but unorganized when the stomach is empty or non-distended. The 27 dogs with gastric muscularis UHS were comprised of 16 neutered female, 10 neutered male and one intact male with a mean age of 10 years 2 months (ranges from 3 years 2 months to 14 years 9 months). There were eight mixed breed dogs, two West Highland White Terriers, two Yorkshire Terriers and one of each of the following breeds: Papillion, English Springer Spaniel, Skye Terrier, Jack Russell Terrier, Greyhound, Rhodesian Ridgeback, Border Collie, Dachshund, Bernese Mountain Dog, English Bulldog, Golden Retriever, Cairn Terrier, Belgian Malinois, Pug and Bichon Frise. Six of 27 dogs with gastric muscularis UHS had some episodes of vomiting as part of their medical history. The vomiting could be attributed to the following underlying medical conditions (one each): acute or chronic renal disease, pyelonephritis, chemotherapy associated, splenic torsion, pyonephrosis, and hemoabdomen. None of the dogs had any evidence of chronic GIT disease. No other ultrasonographic abnormalities of the GIT were noted in these dogs. One other dog showed occasional soft stools likely attributable to receiving piroxicam for treatment of transitional cell carcinoma (TCC).

Still images from a total of 167 abdominal ultrasonographic examinations were reviewed for the retrospective part of the study. Based on the captured still images of the gastric wall available, presence of gastric muscularis UHS was observed only in nine out of the 167 dogs (5.4%), all of which were within the ventral wall only.

The dorsal gastric wall was not visible due to intraluminal gas. The nine dogs were comprised of four neutered females and five neutered males with a mean age of 9 years 9 months (ranges from 5 to 15 years old) and were of the breeds Yorkshire Terrier (n = 2) and English Bulldog, Welsh Corgi, Chow Chow, Beagle, Australian Shepherd, Labrador Retriever (one of each breed) and a mixed breed dog. The nine individual dogs with gastric muscularis UHS and their respective significant findings are shown in Table 1. One dog (Dog 4) had neither clinical nor ultrasonographic signs related to GIT disease. Eight of nine dogs showed either clinical signs and/or ultrasonographic findings related to the GIT. In 4/8 dogs these findings were attributable to their primary disease process: gastric hematoma due to immune-mediated thrombocytopenia (Dog 1) progressive TCC and cholangio-hepatitis (Dog 3), liver failure (Dog 5), and glomerulonephritis and interstitial nephritis (Dog 8). In 2/8 dogs it was difficult to determine the reason for their GIT signs or ultrasonographic changes. Dog 6 was treated for multiple neoplastic diseases and also suffered from primary hyperparathyroidism and had an episode of acute kidney injury at the time of evaluation. This dog was found to have a ruptured hepatic adenoma leading to hemoabdomen. It was unclear what contributed most to his clinical signs, but there was no evidence for primary GIT disease. Dog 9 showed vomiting and lethargy of 12 h duration and multiple liver nodules on abdominal ultrasound. Necropsy was consistent with hepatic adenomas and pulmonary and renal amyloidosis was found concurrently. There was no evidence for primary GIT disease. In 2/8 dogs GIT disease could not be ruled out. Dog 2 suffered from septicemia and showed thickened gastric and duodenal wall on ultrasound. Necropsy confirmed acute pancreatitis with likely secondary enteritis. Dog 7 showed some weight loss on presentation and was diagnosed

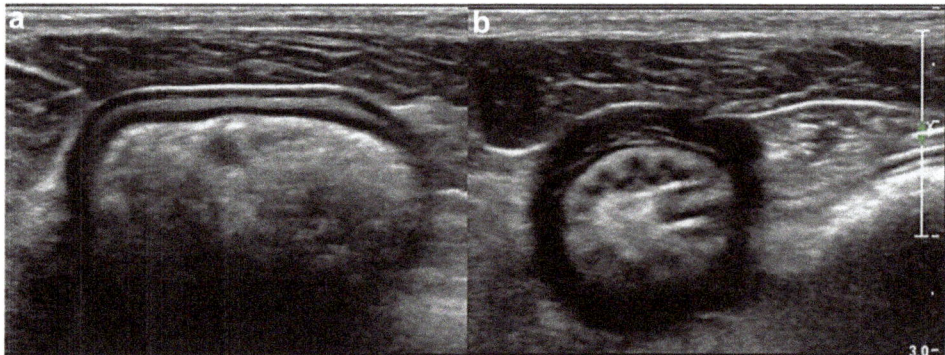

Fig. 2 Transverse ultrasonographic images of one dog with the gastric muscularis UHS from the prospective study. The gastric muscularis UHS were subtle and appeared to be linear and parallel to the serosa when the stomach was relaxed (**a**) but were more prominent when the stomach was contracted (**b**)

Table 1 Dogs with gastric muscularis unorganized hyperechoic striations and their respective clinical and histopathological findings

Animal	Signalment	Clinical signs related to GIT disease	Primary disease process	Histopathology stomach
Dog 1	5 years FS Welsh Corgi	No	Immune-mediated thrombocytopenia	Light patchy (microscopic) mucosal and submucosal hemorrhage; no hemorrhage in muscularis layer
Dog 2	7 years FS Bulldog	Vomiting, hematemesis	Probable immune-mediated thrombocytopenia, DIC, septicemia	Diffuse light submucosal hemorrhage; patchy muscularis hemorrhage (light) and mainly along plexus and extending perivascular into inner and outer layers
Dog 3	15 years MN Yorkshire Terrier	Inappetence, melena	Transitional cell carcinoma, cholangio-hepatitis	Mucosal layer has accentuated deep follicles, but more diffuse lymphoplasmocytic superficial lamina proprial infiltration; parietal cells with swollen hypochromatic nucleus and cytoplasmic pseudoinclusion; cut perpendicular so looks different, but impression is increased mature fibrous tissue through tunica muscularis and serosa
Dog 4	8.5 years MN mixed breed dog	No	Glomerulopathy, cerebral infarcts	Normal mucosal layer; submucosal small arteries, arterioles, and veins have pale amphophilic homogeneous mural deposition (vasculopathy); surrounding fibrous tissue has pale basophilic coarse globular/stippling; inner layer muscularis has areas with drop-out of myofibers
Dog 5	8 years MN Chow Chow	Vomiting (medication related)	Hepatocellular necrosis with liver dysfunction, portal vein thrombosis	Normal mucosa/submucosa layers; increased fibrous tissue in muscularis; perivascular fatty infiltration in muscularis
Dog 6	15 years MN Beagle	Vomiting, diarrhea, anorexia	Acute kidney injury, primary hyperparathyroidism, and multiple neoplastic disease processes (transitional cell carcinoma, hepatocellular adenoma, mantle cell lymphoma, thyroid mass). Ruptured hepatic adenoma with hemoabdomen	No abnormal histopathologic findings
Dog 7	10.5 years FS Australian Shepherd	Weight loss	Spinal meningioma, chronic kidney disease and eosinophilic enteritis	No abnormal histopathologic findings
Dog 8	9 years MN Yorkshire Terrier	Weight loss	Renal tubular dysfunction, membranoproliferative glomerulonephritis with interstitial nephritis	Small portion of the outer layer of tunica muscularis has atrophied bundles); myenteric plexus and ganglia present; space between inner and outer layers expanded by edematous fibrous tissue with dilated lymphatics; submucosa and mucosa layer with mineralization of vessels and basement membrane; fibrin thrombi in mucosal venules (azotemia)
Dog 9	10 years FS Labrador Retriever	Vomiting	Hepatocellular adenoma, pulmonary and renal amyloidosis	No tissue

FS female spayed, MN male neutered

with a spinal meningioma and chronic kidney disease. In addition, mild eosinophilic enteritis was present.

Eight of these nine dogs had postmortem histologic examination of the stomach. Histologically, one dog (Dog 3) had mild lymphoplasmocytic gastritis and one dog (Dog 8) had mucosal mineralization. The muscularis layers of seven dogs were within normal limits in H&E-stained sections (including both dogs with mucosal changes), except for one dog that had increased mature fibrous tissue throughout the muscularis layer. With Masson's trichrome stain, however, fibrous tissue was observed in the gastric muscularis layer in three dogs (Fig. 3). This change was mild to moderate and patchy in the two dogs without obvious fibrosis in H&E-stained sections, and more diffuse and extensive in the dog with apparent muscularis fibrosis in H&E-stained sections.

Discussion

The higher prevalence of canine gastric muscularis UHS in the prospective study (37.5%) than in the retrospective study (5.4%) was expected because the prospective study was designed specifically to assess the presence of UHS in the gastric muscularis layer. In the prospective part of the study, multiple attempts were often made to capture optimal still images and video clips in order to demonstrate the presence of gastric muscularis UHS. In the retrospective part of the study, assessment for UHS in the gastric muscularis layer were only based on few (one or two) captured still images of the gastric wall, and some of these image quality may not have been optimized to illustrate the presence of gastric muscularis UHS. Gastric muscularis UHS were mostly observed in the ventral gastric wall because the evaluation of the dorsal gastric wall were often hampered by presence of artifacts originating from intraluminal gas. The gastric muscularis UHS and the diffuse distribution were best seen in a contracted (non-distended) gastric wall, possibly due to the increased thickness of the fibrous tissue (Fig. 2).

Based on the findings of this study, gastric muscularis UHS may be attributable to the presence of increased fibrous tissue within the muscularis layer. It is difficult to discern fibrous tissue in the gastric muscularis using conventional H&E-stain because smooth muscle and fibrous tissue have similar affinity for the eosin dye. Therefore, Masson's trichrome stain was used in this study to differentiate blue-stained collagen fibers from red smooth muscle. With Masson's trichrome stain, increased fibrous tissue was detected in three of the eight dogs where fibrous tissue was not detected with H&E stain. However, one may argue that fibrous tissue may not be the only possible explanation for presence of gastric muscularis UHS since five of the eight dogs did not have increased fibrous tissue within their tissue sections. The failure to detect an increase in fibrous tissue in the gastric muscularis in these five dogs could reflect sampling differences between the sonographic and the histologic examinations. Difficulties in a histologic search for sonographic lesions may also be due to small focal sample size (versus the entire stomach).

Perhaps a more plausible explanation for the appearance of the gastric muscularis UHS would be the unique nature of three sublayers within the normal canine gastric tunica muscularis: (i) inner oblique layer (ii) middle circular layer (iii) outer longitudinal layer [3, 4]. Presence of connective tissue or interface between these sublayers of the gastric tunica muscularis has been previously reported in humans and has also been corresponded to presence of additional thin hyperechoic layers within the gastric wall on ultrasound [5]. Similarly in veterinary medicine, presence of additional hyperechoic line within the muscularis layer of canine small intestines on ultrasound have also been corresponded to interface between longitudinal and circular layers of the tunica muscularis [6]. The hyperechoic striations appeared 'unorganized' because each of the sublayers of the gastric tunica muscularis were actually incompletely covering the stomach.

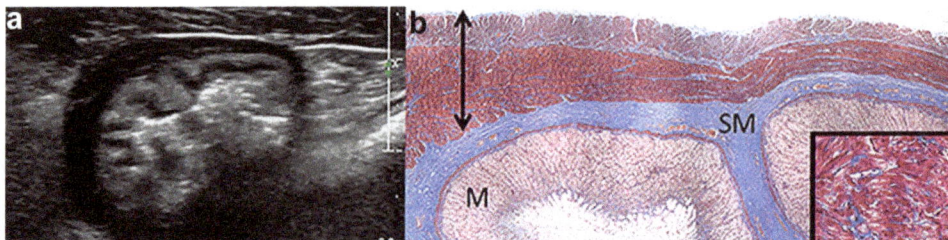

Fig. 3 Transverse ultrasonographic image of a dog's stomach (**a**) and corresponding histologic section with Masson's trichrome stain (**b**) from the retrospective study. The gastric muscularis UHS were more prominent in the contracted portion of the stomach where the muscularis was thicker. In the histologic section, the fibrous tissue (blue) in the thicker part of the muscularis is mostly perivascular (see insertion at the right bottom corner), whereas in the thinner part, the blue-stained fibrous tissue is in the muscularis interstitium parallel to the muscle fibers and to the serosal surface (top). The double-headed arrow spans the muscularis. *M* gastric mucosa, *SM* gastric submucosa

For example, the outer longitudinal layer continues from the outer muscle of the esophagus, spreads widely over the pylorus but is thicker along the curvatures while the middle circular layer is distributed in hoops from the cardia to the pyloric canal [4]. The innermost oblique layer is very incomplete but compensates for the deficiencies in the circular layer as stout fascicles above the cardia and continuing distally to each side of the lesser curvature [4]. The advancement in ultrasonographic technology may have also contributed to increased feasibility of detecting gastric muscularis UHS. The image quality and resolution of the ultrasound equipment has improved tremendously compared to 20 years ago [7, 8]. Measurement of the individual layers of the GIT [9–11], detection of canine colonic muscularis hyperechoic band [2], small nodules in the submucosa layer of colon in dogs and cats [12] and mucosal fibrosis in cats [13] have been published recently due to the improvement of the resolution of ultrasound technology and equipment. In this study, the combination of improved resolution of the ultrasound machine with preferential use of high frequency linear transducer may have increased the likelihood of visualizing gastric muscularis UHS.

In the canine stomach, altered echogenicity of the muscularis layer has not been correlated with any specific disease. However, altered echogenicity of the mucosa layer has been associated with disease. A hyperechoic line at the gastric mucosal-luminal interface is usually secondary to mineralization in dogs with uremic gastropathy [14]. The presence of a gastric mucosal defect with accumulation of hyperechoic specks (microbubbles) is characteristic of gastric ulceration [15]. Presence of submucosal fat in feline stomach may lead to increased thickness and echogenicity of this layer [16, 17]. Fibrosis leading to presence of a linear hyperechoic band in feline mucosal layer has been reported [13]. In the prospective part of our study, 22% (7 of 27) of dogs showed clinical signs such as vomiting, inappetance or anorexia, diarrhea, or weight loss, which can be attributed to GIT disease. However, no dog was identified to have primary GIT disease and the clinical signs could be attributed to the primary disease process in each individual. Seven out of nine dogs in the retrospective part of our study were found to have clinical signs related to the GIT. However, all these animals were severely ill and most of them had multiple medical conditions potentially leading to GIT signs. Only three (Dogs 2, 3, and 7) out of eight dogs were found to have inflammatory changes of their stomach or intestines on histopathology. Dog 2 had mild duodenal and jejunal enteritis on histopathology. This dog was diagnosed with septicemia and pancreatitis, therefore the enteritis was considered more likely to be secondary to acute pancreatitis rather than primary GIT disease. In

Dog 3, no clear association with primary GIT disease could be made. Dog 7 was found to have mild eosinophilic enteritis, which is most commonly seen either due to inflammatory bowel disease or parasitic infestation. The only sign possibly indicating GIT disease was weight loss and the dog was diagnosed with chronic kidney disease and a spinal meningioma. Primary GIT disease cannot be ruled out in this dog.

Canine gastric muscularis UHS were unlikely to be breed or gender specific as they were observed in large variety of canine breeds, ranging from small to large breed dogs, both in male and female. The mean age of the dogs with gastric muscularis UHS was about 10 years old. The lack of younger dog population in this study makes the correlation of age with canine gastric muscularis UHS impossible.

The small number of patients in which histopathology was available was a limitation of this study, though approximately 1/3 of the histopathologic samples evaluated had fibrous tissue present in the muscularis layer.

Conclusions

This study is the first to describe the appearance of gastric muscularis UHS in dogs. Presence of gastric muscularis UHS in dogs may have been attributable to presence of incomplete interfaces between the inner oblique, middle circular and outer longitudinal layers of the gastric tunica muscularis or due to presence of fibrous tissue within gastric muscularis layer. Based on this study, this finding appears to have no significant clinical correlation with primary GIT disease.

Abbreviations

GIT: gastrointestinal tract; H&E: hematoxylin and eosin; TCC: transitional cell carcinoma; UHS: unorganized hyperechoic striations.

Authors' contributions

HGH and CKL carried out the diagnostic imaging procedures, interpretation and wrote the manuscript. SS made intellectual contribution by reviewing medical records of affected dogs. MAM and MMB performed the histopathologic examination and interpretation. All authors read and approved the final manuscript.

Author details

[1] Department of Veterinary Clinical Sciences, College of Veterinary Medicine, Purdue University, West Lafayette, IN 47907, USA. [2] Department of Comparative Pathobiology, College of Veterinary Medicine, Purdue University, West Lafayette, IN 47907, USA.

Competing interests

The authors declared that they have no competing interests.

Funding
None of the authors received any funding for this study.

References

1. Penninck DG, Nyland TG, Fisher PE, Kerr LY. Ultrasonography of the normal canine gastrointestinal tract. Vet Radiol. 1989;30:272–6.

2. Heng HG, Lim CK, Miller MA, Broman MM. Ultrasonographic observation of colonic muscularis hyperechoic band paralleling the serosal layer in dogs. Vet Radiol Ultrasound. 2015;76:666–9.

3. Frappier BL. Chapter 10 digestive system. In: Eurell JA, Frappier BL, editors. dellman's textbook of veterinary histology. Iowa: Blackwell Publishing; 2006. p. 170–211.

4. Dyce KM, Sack WO, Wensing CJG. The digestive apparatus. In textbook of veterinary anatomy, Chapter 3. 3rd ed. Pennsylvania: Elsevier; 2002. p. 100–47.

5. Aibe T, Fuji T, Okita K, Takemoto T. A fundamental study of normal layer structure of gastrointestinal wall visualized by endoscopic ultrasonography. Scand J Gastroenterol Suppl. 1986;123:6–15.

6. Le Roux AB, Granger LA, Wakamatsu N, Kearney MT, Gaschen L. Ex vivo correlation of ultrasonographic small intestinal wall layering with histology in dogs. Vet Radiol Ultrasound. 2016;57:534–45.

7. Taxt T, Jirik R. Superresolution of ultrasound images using the first and second harmonic signal. IEEE Trans Ultrason Ferroelectr Freq Control. 2004;51:163–76.

8. Lin CH, Sun YN, Lin CJ. A motion compounding technique for speckle reduction in ultrasound images. J Digit Imag. 2010;23:246–57.

9. Donato PD, Penninck D, Pietra M, Cipone M, Diana A. Ultrasonographic measurement of the relative thickness of intestinal wall layers in clinically healthy cats. J Fel Med Surg. 2014;16:333–9.

10. Gladwin NE, Penninck DG, Webster CR. Ultrasonographic evaluation of the thickness of the wall layers in the intestinal tracts of dogs. Am J Vet Res. 2014;75:349–53.

11. Winter MD, Londono L, Berry CR, Hernandez JA. Ultrasonographic evaluation of relative gastrointestinal layer thickness in cats without clinical evidence of gastrointestinal tract disease. J Fel Med Surg. 2014;16:118–24.

12. Citi S, Chimenti T, Marchetti V, Millantra F, Mannucci T. Micronodular ultrasound lesions in the colonic submucosa of 42 dogs and 14 cats. Vet Radiol Ultrasound. 2013;54:646–51.

13. Penninck DG, Webster CR, Keating JH. The sonographic appearance of intestinal mucosal fibrosis in cats. Vet Radiol Ultrasound. 2010;51:458–61.

14. Grooters AM, Miyabayashi T, Biller DS, Merryman J. Sonographic appearance of uremic gastropathy in four dogs. Vet Radiol Ultrasound. 1994;35:35–40.

15. Penninck D, Matz M, Tidwell A. Ultrasonography of gastric ulceration in the dog. Vet Radiol Ultrasound. 1997;38:308–12.

16. Heng HG, Teoh WT, Sheikh Omar AR. Gastric submucosal fat in cats. Anat Histol Embryol. 2008;37:362–5.

17. Heng HG, Wrigley RH, Kraft SL, Powers BE. Fat is responsible for an intramural radiolucent band in the feline stomach wall. Vet Radiol Ultrasound. 2005;46:54–6.

25

Changes in energy metabolism, and levels of stress-related hormones and electrolytes in horses after intravenous administration of romifidine and the peripheral α-2 adrenoceptor antagonist vatinoxan

Soile Anja Eliisa Pakkanen[1*], Annemarie de Vries[2], Marja Riitta Raekallio[1], Anna Kristina Mykkänen[1], Mari Johanna Palviainen[1], Satu Marja Sankari[1] and Outi Maritta Vainio[1]

Abstract

Background: Romifidine, an α-2 adrenoceptor agonist, is a widely-used sedative in equine medicine. Besides the desired sedative and analgesic actions, α-2 adrenoceptor agonists have side effects like alterations of plasma concentrations of glucose and certain stress-related hormones and metabolites in various species. Vatinoxan (previously known as MK-467), in turn, is an antagonist of α-2 adrenoceptors. Because vatinoxan does not cross the blood brain barrier in significant amounts, it has only minor effect on sedation induced by α-2 adrenoceptor agonists. Previously, vatinoxan is shown to prevent the hyperglycaemia, increase of plasma lactate concentration and the decrease of insulin and non-esterified free fatty acids (FFAs) caused by α-2 adrenoceptor agonists in different species. The aim of our study was to investigate the effects of intravenous romifidine and vatinoxan, alone and combined, on plasma concentrations of glucose and some stress-related hormones and metabolites in horses.

Results: Plasma glucose concentration differed between all intravenous treatments: romifidine (80 µg/kg; ROM), vatinoxan (200 µg/kg; V) and the combination of these (ROM + V). Glucose concentration was the highest after ROM and the lowest after V. Serum FFA concentration was higher after V than after ROM or ROM + V. The baseline serum concentration of insulin varied widely between the individual horses. No differences were detected in serum insulin, cortisol or plasma adrenocorticotropic hormone (ACTH) concentrations between the treatments. Plasma lactate, serum triglyceride or blood sodium and chloride concentrations did not differ from baseline or between the treatments. Compared with baseline, plasma glucose concentration increased after ROM and ROM + V, serum cortisol, FFA and base excess increased after all treatments and plasma ACTH concentration increased after V. Serum insulin concentration decreased after V and blood potassium decreased after all treatments.

Conclusions: Romifidine induced hyperglycaemia, which vatinoxan partially prevented despite of the variations in baseline levels of serum insulin. The effects of romifidine and vatinoxan on the insulin concentration in horses need further investigation.

Keywords: α-2 adrenoceptor agonist, Glucose, Horse, Hyperglycaemia, Insulin, MK-467, Romifidine, Vatinoxan

*Correspondence: soile.pakkanen@fimnet.fi
[1] Department of Equine and Small Animal Medicine, Faculty of Veterinary Medicine, University of Helsinki, P.O. Box 57, 00014 Helsinki, Finland
Full list of author information is available at the end of the article

Background

Romifidine is an α-2 adrenoceptor agonist which is commonly used to induce sedation and analgesia in horses. In addition to their sedative and analgesic effects, α-2 adrenoceptor agonists have a marked effect on plasma concentrations of glucose and some stress-related hormones and metabolites; romifidine, xylazine and detomidine increase plasma glucose concentrations by inhibiting insulin release from pancreatic β-cells in horses [1, 2], ponies [3] and mice [4]. Detomidine is also reported to increase base excess (BE), indicating metabolic alkalosis [5] and to decrease the plasma concentration of free fatty acids (FFAs, or non-esterified free fatty acids) [3] and cortisol [3, 6] in horses. In contrast, in one study detomidine had no effect on plasma cortisol concentration [7]. Furthermore, plasma cortisol and adrenocorticotropic hormone (ACTH) concentrations decreased in horses after administration of clonidine, another α-2 adrenoceptor agonist [8]. The plasma concentration of potassium (K^+) is reported to be unaffected by α-2 adrenoceptor agonists in horses [9]. In theory, decreased insulin concentration could result in hyperkalemia through diminished cellular K^+ influx, as shown in dogs and humans [10].

The effects of α-2 adrenoceptor agonists on energy metabolism, stress-related hormones and metabolites can be attenuated by α-2 adrenoceptor antagonists. Atipamezole and yohimbine antagonized medetomidine-induced hyperglycaemia, hypoinsulinaemia and decrease in FFA concentration in dogs; the effect of atipamezole was reported to be dose-dependent [11]. Atipamezole also attenuated hyperglycaemia and decrease in FFA concentration in cats [12], and hyperglycaemia in cattle [13] and goats [14]. Contradictory results have also been reported; atipamezole did not affect hyperglycaemia [15] while the α-2 adrenoceptor antagonist tolazoline caused a rapid increase in plasma glucose concentration in horses treated with detomidine [3]. In addition, tolazoline attenuated the detomidine-induced decrease in FFA concentration transiently [3]. All of these α-2 adrenoceptor antagonists reverse, at least partly, both the sedative and analgesic effects induced by α-2 adrenoceptor agonist [3, 16–18], a feature which is often undesired.

Vatinoxan, previously known as MK-467 and L-659,066, is an α-2 adrenoceptor antagonist which poorly penetrates the blood brain barrier. Therefore, it targets mainly peripherally located α-2 adrenoceptors [19]. Vatinoxan prevented the hyperglycaemic effect of clonidine in humans [20] and mice [21]. In dogs, vatinoxan prevented the slight increase of plasma lactate and glucose concentrations and the decrease of insulin and FFA induced by the α-2 adrenoceptor agonist dexmedetomidine [22]. Vatinoxan, in addition, enhanced insulin responses to glucose in mice [21] and to exercise in humans [23]; although, in another study vatinoxan showed no effect on plasma glucose, insulin or insulin response to glucose in humans [24]. The effect of vatinoxan on quality of sedation induced by detomidine or romifidine in horses [25, 26] and dexmedetomidine in dogs [27–29] is only minor because it acts predominantly on peripheral α-2 adrenoceptors.

The aim of this study was to explore whether the intravenous (IV) administration of romifidine or vatinoxan induces changes in plasma concentrations of glucose or some metabolites and stress-related hormones in horses, and whether vatinoxan is able to antagonise the possible effects of romifidine when these agents are administered simultaneously. To the best of our knowledge, there are no previous reports of the effects of romifidine in combination with vatinoxan, on plasma concentrations of glucose or stress-related hormones and metabolites in horses or any other species.

Methods

Seven Finnhorse mares aged 15 ± 5 years (mean $\pm$ SD) and with a body weight (BW) of 586 ± 44 kg were used in this study. The horses were considered healthy based on clinical examination (inspection of mucous membranes, measuring of capillary refill time and body temperature and auscultation of heart, lungs and intestinal sounds). Screening blood samples were not taken before the trials. The routine diet of these horses consisted of hay, silage and concentrates. On the day of the trials, the horses were fed normal hay and silage, but not concentrates, and had free access to water.

Baseline blood samples were drawn in the stables via puncture of jugular vein, after which the horses were taken to examination room and restrained in stocks. Two 14G, 80 mm intravenous catheters (Intraflon 2, Laboratoires Pharmaceutiques Vygon Uk Ltd., UK) were placed in the right jugular vein at least 15 cm apart under local infiltration of the skin with lidocaine (Lidocain 20 mg/mL, Orion Pharma, Espoo, Finland). An 18G, 70 cm central venous catheter (Cavafix Certo, B. Braun Melsungen AG, Melsungen, Germany) was placed in the left jugular vein and a 20G, 45 mm catheter (BD Arterial cannula, Becton–Dickinson India Pvt., India) was placed in the transverse facial artery under local skin infiltration with lidocaine. All catheters were sutured to the adjacent skin, except the caudal jugular catheter, which was used for the administration of medications and was immediately removed after injection. The remaining cranial jugular catheter was used for blood sampling. The arterial catheter was used for sampling for arterial blood gas analysis and for monitoring arterial blood pressure, and the central venous catheter for monitoring central venous blood pressure; these results are a subject of a separate paper

[26]. The horses used in the study were research horses that were accustomed to minor procedures like IV punctures. Some of the horses mildly resisted their placement into the stocks and one horse got agitated by standing in the stocks for a long time without sedation. All the horses tolerated instrumentation without marked resistance. To obtain full immobility during arterial catheter placement, a twitch was used in all of the horses. All the catheters were removed at the end of the trial and replaced at the day of next trial.

Each horse was treated three times by means of a blinded cross-over Latin square design with a minimum washout period of 6 days. Venous blood samples were collected into EDTA, fluoride-oxalate and serum tubes in the stable (baseline) before each horse was taken to the examination room for instrumentation, administration of drugs and monitoring. After instrumentation, the horses were let to settle down for 5 min before administration of the medications. The horses received the following medications intravenously:

1. Romifidine hydrochloride (HCl) (80 µg/kg BW, Sedivet, Boehringer Ingelheim Vetmedica GmbH, Ingelheim, Germany; ROM). 2. Romifidine HCl (80 µg/kg BW) and Vatinoxan HCl (200 µg/kg BW, Vetcare Ltd, Salo, Finland; ROM + V). 3. Vatinoxan HCl (200 µg/kg BW; V).

Vatinoxan HCl was supplied as a powder. For each treatment, the drugs were diluted in saline (Natriumklorid, B. Braun Melsungen AG, Germany) in a single syringe to a total volume of 20 mL, and were administered IV as a bolus injection over 15 s at T0. Venous blood samples were taken 15, 30, 60, 90 and 120 min (T15–T120, respectively) after drug administration. EDTA and fluoride-oxalate tubes were placed in ice water immediately after blood sampling and centrifuged within 10 min to separate the plasma. Fluoride-oxalate plasma for analysis of lactate and glucose was refrigerated until analysis (maximum of 48 h). EDTA plasma was frozen at − 20 °C until ACTH analysis. Tubes for serum samples were kept at room temperature until centrifugation, which was performed on the same day. Serum was frozen at − 20 °C to await cortisol, FFA, triglyceride and insulin analyses. The laboratories analysing the blood samples were unaware of the treatments administered to the horses.

Lactate was analysed with enzymatic lactate oxidase (Konelab™ Lactate PAP, Thermo Fisher Scientific Ltd, Vantaa, Finland), glucose with the photometric glucose hexokinase 2-reagent method (Konelab™ Glucose HK) and triglycerides with the enzymatic colorimetric method (Konelab™ Trigycerides; Konelab 30i Clinical Chemistry Analyzer). The enzymatic colorimetric method was used for the determination of FFAs (NEFA-C, Wako Chemicals GmbH, Neuss, Germany; KONE Pro

Selective Chemistry Analyzer, Thermo Fisher Scientific Ltd). ACTH was analysed with a solid-phase, two-site sequential chemiluminescent immunometric assay and insulin with a solid-phase, enzyme-labelled chemiluminescent immunometric assay (Immulite 2000, Siemens Healthcare Diagnostics Products GmbH, Marburg, Germany). Plasma cortisol concentration was analysed by RIA (Spectria cortisol RIA kit, Orion Diagnostica Ltd, Espoo, Finland), and samples were run as duplicates.

Venous blood gas samples (PICO50 blood gas syringes; Radiometer Medical ApS, Denmark) were taken after instrumentation (baseline) and at T5, T15, T30 and T60 after drug administration for measurement of potassium (K^+), sodium (Na^+), chloride (Cl^-) and base excess (BE) (IDEXX VetSta; ME, USA).

The normality assumptions were evaluated with Shapiro–Wilk tests. Friedman's two-way analysis of variance for related samples was used to compare serum insulin concentrations to baseline within each treatment. Kruskall–Wallis test was used for comparisons of serum insulin concentrations between the treatments. Concentrations of all other variables were compared between the treatments with repeated measures analysis of variance (rmANOVA) and pairwise comparisons within each time point were conducted with Student's t test. All significance values were adjusted by Bonferroni correction for multiple tests. Significance was set at $P < 0.05$.

Results

Romifidine induced sedation in all of the horses and vatinoxan did not significantly affect the quality of sedation. Vatinoxan administered alone caused mild abdominal discomfort and watery faeces in some of the horses, but otherwise it was well tolerated. When romifidine and vatinoxan were administered simultaneously, many of the peripheral cardiovascular and intestinal side-effects of romifidine were alleviated [26].

Plasma glucose concentration showed significant differences between all treatments. The concentration was the highest after ROM and the lowest after V. Compared to baseline, ROM and ROM + V, but not V, significantly increased plasma glucose concentration (Fig. 1).

Serum insulin concentrations of five horses were within the laboratory reference range (0–19 µU/mL, Animal Laboratory Vetlab, Tampere, Finland) at all time-points. The remaining two horses had their values above the reference range at several measuring points; concentrations varied from below detection level (2 µU/mL)–82.9 µU/mL. No significant differences in insulin concentration were detected between treatments, but the inter-individual variation was high. Insulin concentration significantly decreased from baseline after V (Table 1).

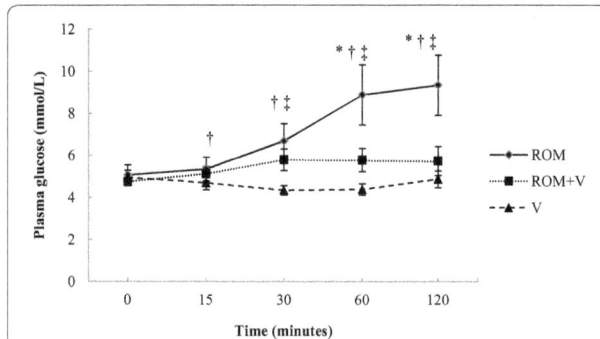

Fig. 1 Mean plasma glucose concentration of seven horses. The horses received romifidine (ROM, 80 µg/kg IV), ROM with vatinoxan (ROM + V, 80 µg/kg + 200 µg/kg IV) and vatinoxan (V, 200 µg/kg IV) at T0. Error bars indicate the standard deviation. Plasma glucose concentrations were significantly different ($P < 0.05$) from baseline at T60 and T120 after ROM and at T30, T60 and T120 after ROM + V. Significant difference ($P < 0.05$) between * ROM and ROM + V, †ROM + V and V and ‡ROM and V

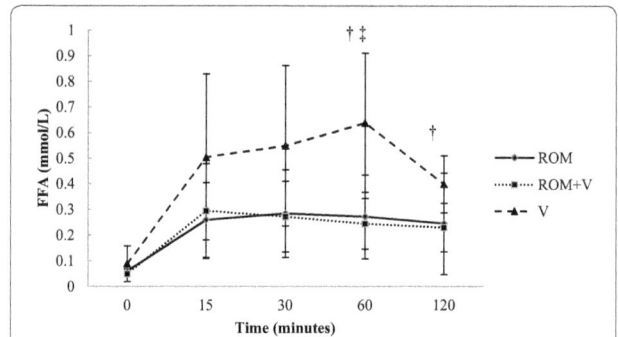

Fig. 2 Mean serum FFA concentration of seven horses. The horses received romifidine (ROM, 80 µg/kg IV), ROM with vatinoxan (ROM + V, 80 µg/kg + 200 µg/kg IV) and vatinoxan (V, 200 µg/kg IV) at T0. Error bars indicate the standard deviation. Serum FFA concentrations were significantly different ($P < 0.05$) from baseline at T30 after ROM, at T15 and T30 after ROM + V and at T30 and T60 after V. Significant difference ($P < 0.05$) between †ROM + V and V and ‡ROM and V

Table 1 Serum insulin concentrations

	Baseline	T15	T30	T60	T120
ROM	6.0 (83)	< 2.0 (49)	< 2.0 (45)	< 2.0 (32)	< 2.0 (42)
ROM + V	4.8 (58)	< 2.0 (45)	< 2.0 (62)	< 2.0 (39)	< 2.0 (59)
V	7.8 (80)	3.2 (74)	< 2.0 (47)*	4.3 (58)	< 2.0 (43)*

Medians (and highest concentrations) of serum insulin concentration of seven horses (µIU/mL). The horses received romifidine (ROM, 80 µg/kg IV), ROM with vatinoxan (ROM + V, 80 µg/kg + 200 µg/kg IV) and MK-467 (V, 200 µg/kg IV) at T0. The lowest concentration after all treatments at all time points was below the detection limit (< 2 µIU/mL)

* Significantly different ($P < 0.05$) from baseline (T0), no significant differences detected between treatments

Serum FFA concentration was higher after V than ROM or ROM + V. Serum FFA concentrations increased from baseline after all treatments (Fig. 2).

Baseline plasma ACTH concentrations were within the reference range (< 35 pg/mL, Animal Laboratory Vetlab) in all but one horse, which had a higher concentration before ROM + V. After the treatments, the values varied from 5.82 to 74.9 pg/mL, except for one measurement in one horse of 185 pg/mL at T120 after ROM. This reading was confirmed by measuring in duplicate. Plasma ACTH concentrations, relative to baseline, increased after MK at T15 and T30, but significant differences were not detected between treatments. Plasma lactate and serum triglyceride concentrations did not differ significantly from baseline or between treatments. Serum cortisol concentrations increased from baseline after all treatments, but no significant differences emerged between treatments (Table 2).

Base excess showed an increasing trend after all treatments and there was a significant difference between baseline and T60 after ROM and V, but no significant differences were detected between the treatments. Potassium, in contrast, decreased after all the treatments and the concentrations were significantly lower than baseline at T15 after ROM and ROM + V, and at T60 after ROM + V and V. There was also a significant difference in K^+ concentrations between ROM + V and V at T15 (Table 2). Sodium and Cl^- concentration were stable trough the monitoring period (data not shown).

Discussion

As far as we are aware, this is the first study reporting the effects of romifidine administered in combination with vatinoxan, on plasma concentrations of glucose or hormones and metabolites in any animal species. In this study, romifidine induced hyperglycaemia in horses and the plasma glucose concentration remained high until the end of the monitoring period of 120 min. This indicates that the effect of romifidine on plasma glucose concentration is long lasting and that plasma glucose concentration may, indeed, have peaked after the last time point of this study. These findings are in agreement with previous studies from horses treated with romifidine [1], detomidine [3, 18] and dogs treated with xylazine, medetomidine and dexmedetomidine [22, 30]. In contrast, Raekallio and co-workers [31] reported a decrease in plasma glucose concentration in dogs after dexmedetomidine administration, but they noted that their monitoring period of 90 min might have been too short to detect possible hyperglycaemia. It is noticeable that the sedative effect of romifidine was already ceased at the point of highest plasma glucose concentration

Table 2 Plasma ACTH and lactate, serum triglyceride, cortisol and blood K⁺, Na⁺ and BE concentrations

Analyte	Treatment	Baseline	T15	T30	T60	T120
ACTH	ROM	16.8 (±3.83)	32.3 (±22.4)	25.0 (±12.5)	18.7 (±7.66)	44.7 (±62.4)
	ROM+V	19.4 (±11.1)	28.5 (±12.4)	21.6 (±8.39)	21.4 (±13.2)	19.1 (±11.1)
	V	17.3 (±6.53)	32.2* (±6.66)	29.0* (±5.71)	23.0 (±5.68)	16.1 (±5.68)
Lactate	ROM	0.60 (±0.30)	0.61 (±0.17)	0.63 (±0.24)	0.49 (±0.11)	0.41 (±0.24)
	ROM+V	0.58 (±0.29)	0.69 (±0.24)	0.70 (±0.27)	0.71 (±0.24)	0.56 (±0.17)
	V	0.50 (±0.59)	0.55 (±0.35)	0.55 (±0.33)	0.61 (±0.30)	0.70 (±0.35)
Triglycerides	ROM	0.30 (±0.10)	0.36 (±0.13)	0.37 (±0.13)	0.36 (±0.13)	0.27 (±0.07)
	ROM+V	0.27 (±0.03)	0.30 (±0.06)	0.30 (±0.09)	0.29 (±0.12)	0.24 (±0.12)
	V	0.28 (±0.08)	0.32 (±0.09)	0.33 (±0.11)	0.30 (±0.10)	0.23 (±0.11)
Cortisol	ROM	59.0 (±13.9)	120* (±34.7)	106 (±37.6)	86.6 (±35.4)	113 (±51.7)
	ROM+V	51.9 (±16.1)	107* (±24.7)	84.1 (±23.1)	76.5 (±29.0)	66.3 (±26.5)
	V	61.2 (±14.7)	131* (±34.2)	120* (±30.4)	102 (±23.5)	79.4 (±32.7)

Analyte	Treatment	Baseline	T5	T15	T30	T60
BE	ROM	4.00 (±0.54)	4.04 (±0.95)	4.47 (±0.47)	4.76 (±0.79)	5.74* (±0.88)
	ROM+V	4.46 (±1.43)	4.19 (±1.32)	4.31 (±1.55)	4.84 (±1.30)	5.41 (±1.06)
	V	3.86 (±0.78)	3.63 (±0.87)	3.96 (±0.96)	4.19 (±0.66)	5.24* (±0.57)
K⁺	ROM	4.30 (±0.26)	4.16 (±0.28)	4.09* (±0.28)	4.16 (±0.30)	4.17 (±0.27)
	ROM+V	4.20 (±0.29)	4.11 (±0.40)	3.87*,$ (±0.28)	3.91 (±0.25)	3.84* (±0.27)
	V	4.44 (±0.36)	4.39 (±0.28)	4.30$ (±0.31)	4.21 (±0.36)	3.94* (±0.31)

Means (±SD) of plasma ACTH (pg/mL), plasma lactate (mmol/L), serum triglyceride (mmol/L), serum cortisol (nmol/mL) and venous blood K⁺ and BE (mmol/L) concentrations of seven horses. The horses received romifidine (ROM, 80 µg/kg IV), ROM with vatinoxan (ROM+V, 80 µg/kg + 200 µg/kg IV) and vatinoxan (V, 200 µg/kg IV) at T0

* Significantly different ($P < 0.05$) from baseline (T0)

$ Significant difference between treatments

[26], which means that its effect on energy metabolism is longer lasting than the sedative action.

Plasma glucose concentration also increased after ROM+V, although to a lesser extent than after ROM. This suggests that V partially prevented romifidine-induced hyperglycaemia. Prevention of the haemodynamic effects of dexmedetomidine by vatinoxan in dogs is reported to be dose-dependent [32]. This could also apply to the effects of vatinoxan on alterations in plasma hormone and metabolite concentrations caused by alpha-2 adrenoceptor agonists. On that basis, we assumed that the dose of 200 µg/kg used in our study might have been inadequate for complete prevention of romifidine-induced hyperglycaemia. In dogs, for example, vatinoxan completely antagonized dexmedetomidine (10 µg/kg) induced hyperglycaemia at the dose of 500 µg/kg [22]. Of the other α-2 adrenoceptor antagonists, antagonism of medetomidine induced hyperglycaemia and hypo-insulinaemia in dogs by atipamezole is also reported to be dose-dependent [11]. In humans, vatinoxan partially inhibited both the clonidine-induced increase of plasma glucose and reduction of plasma insulin concentration. These authors speculated that glucose homeostasis could be only partially regulated by peripheral α-2

adrenoceptors, which would also explain the incompleteness of inhibition [33].

In our study, vatinoxan, when administered alone, did not significantly affect plasma glucose concentration. This finding is in agreement with previous reports in which vatinoxan did not change plasma glucose or insulin concentrations in normoglycaemic fasted mice [21] or humans [33, 34]. In contrast, vatinoxan increased insulin and decreased plasma glucose concentration in hyperglycaemic mice [21]. However, despite no significant difference in plasma glucose concentration, vatinoxan decreased serum insulin concentration in the present study. This might relate to the balance between inhibition of α-2 adrenoceptors in pancreatic β-cells and increased sympathoadrenal output and concentration of catecholamines due to stress caused by restraint of non-sedated horses in stocks. The ability of vatinoxan to decrease serum insulin in horses could be a useful feature in horses suffering from equine metabolic syndrome (EMS), as hyperinsulinaemia is known to predispose these horses to laminitis [35].

Alpha-2 adrenoceptor agonist-related hyperglycaemia is known to result from a reduction of insulin release by a direct action of the α-2 adrenoceptor agonist on pancreatic β-cells [4]. However, in our study this association between hyperglycaemia and hypoinsulinaemia could not be demonstrated, because in the majority of the samples the serum insulin concentration was below the detection limit of the analysing method. In individual horses, romifidine seemed to cause an increase in plasma glucose concentration, while the insulin concentration stayed below the detection limit. This could suggest that even a slight decrease of insulin concentration, which was not detectable in the analysis, may result in hyperglycaemia or there could have been other factors affecting the increase of glucose concentration. Findings in previous studies [11, 30, 36] suggest that the α-2-mediated decrease in plasma insulin concentration might not be the only factor affecting blood glucose concentration in animals treated with α-2 adrenoceptor agonists. We also suggest that some of the effects of romifidine on glucose concentration might have been other than α-2 adrenoceptor activation in pancreas, such as hepatic glycogenolysis induced by α-2-adrenergic agents and gluconeogenesis mediated by α-1 adrenoceptors, as romifidine is stated to be partial α-2 adrenoceptor agonist [37] or to have α-2:α-1 selectivity of 340:1 [38]. Some of the effects might also be mediated by central imidazoline receptors, as romifidine is an imidazoline derivative.

Serum cortisol concentration increased rather quickly after each treatment, after which it slowly decreased again. Plasma ACTH concentrations showed a similar trend, although the increase was significant only after V. These increases are probably due to stress induced by instrumentation and confinement to stocks. Instrumentation procedure was the same before every trial and we assume that the bias caused by stress from instrumentation would be similar throughout the experiment. Short term increases in serum cortisol concentration could be of clinical importance in EMS or pituitary pars intermedia dysfunction (PPID) patients because they are reported to enhance vasoconstriction in laminar veins in vitro, creating a possible risk factor for laminitis [39]. There are conflicting reports on the effects of α-2 adrenoceptor agonists on cortisol concentration in various species. Plasma cortisol concentration is reported to either decrease or to remain constant in horses [3, 6, 7], to remain constant in various other species such as dogs [11, 22, 30] and calves [13] or to increase in dairy cows, sheep and goats [13, 14]. Other factors, such as differences between species, differences in baseline cortisol concentrations and stress related to the environment or sampling procedures, likely affected cortisol concentrations in these studies. Cortisol concentration is known to fluctuate during the day in horses; it is highest from morning until early afternoon (8 a.m.–14 p.m.) and lowest before midnight, around 10–12 p.m. [40–42]. To avoid the effect of diurnal variation in our results, all three treatments were conducted at approximately the same time of the day for each horse.

In the present study, we detected an increase in serum concentrations of FFA after each treatment. The concentration of FFA was significantly higher after V than after ROM or ROM+V, which, in turn, did not differ significantly from each other. This was indicative of stress caused by instrumentation, which most likely increased catecholamine plasma concentrations. This was manifested as increased FFA concentration. Alpha-2 adrenoceptor agonists are previously reported to decrease serum FFA in horses [3] and dogs [22, 30]. In our study, romifidine-induced sedation probably affected serum FFA concentration only partially because the stress increasing the FFA concentrations was induced before the horses received the medications. The stress caused by procedures may also overcome the decreasing actions of α-2 adrenoceptor agonists on serum FFA, which is reported in horses undergoing standing laparoscopy [43]. The greater increase in serum FFA after V could also result partly from a direct effect of vatinoxan on lipolysis as vatinoxan is reported to increase the plasma concentration of FFA [23] and, furthermore, α-2 adrenoceptor antagonists potentiate the lipolytic action of adrenaline in humans [44]. In dogs, plasma FFA concentration showed a biphasic response after the combined administration of vatinoxan with dexmedetomidine. Initially, a similar decrease was noticed after both medications, but later the concentration increased significantly more after the combined administration [22]. The temporal discrepancy was speculated to result from the balance between catecholamine and insulin concentrations since both affect the activity of hormone-sensitive lipase, which is the main regulator of lipolysis [45].

As all lactate concentrations were within the reference range (< 1.5 mmol/L, Laboratory Ellab, Ypäjä, Finland) and the concentrations did not differ significantly from baseline values, which indicates that there was no evidence of tissue hypoxia or lactic acidosis after any of the treatments. In fact, as the BE increased after all treatments, the metabolic state of the horses changed towards metabolic alkalosis during the experiment. This observation is in agreement with previous findings of Raekallio and co-workers [5]. Possible reasons for the change toward alkalosis after romifidine administration in the present study are altered renal function and compensatory response to respiratory acidosis due to decreased respiratory rate and increased arterial carbon dioxide tension [26]. As there was significant increase in BE during this relatively short sampling period, further investigation is needed to examine if the metabolic alkalosis will be clinically relevant for example after long infusions of α-2 adrenoceptor agonists for veterinary standing procedures that have become more common in recent years.

The blood K^+ concentrations of the horses in our study decreased although the change was not clinically relevant. The regulation of blood potassium concentration is complex and involves, for example, aldosterone, insulin, sympathomimetics, and is regulated by the acid–base balance and renal function. Because of the high concentration difference between intracellular and extracellular potassium content, alterations in blood potassium concentrations are often a result of redistribution of potassium between these compartments [46]. Renal excretion of potassium is increased during metabolic alkalosis. Furthermore, both urine production and renal excretion of electrolytes are increased by alpha-2 adrenoceptor agonists [9], and one possible explanation of decreased potassium in the present study is increased loss to urine. Considering the complexity of potassium homeostasis, the effects of romifidine and vatinoxan on blood potassium need further investigation.

Conclusions

Romifidine induced hyperglycaemia in horses is similar to other α-2 adrenoceptor agonists, but its effects on serum insulin warrant further investigations. Vatinoxan was able to alleviate the romifidine induced hyperglycaemia despite of the wide variation in baseline insulin concentrations. Further research is needed to evaluate the metabolic changes under stressful situations, such as veterinary procedures or in compromised patients (e.g. critically ill foals and adult horses with underlying disease processes such as PPID and EMS). In these patients, the metabolic and hormonal changes induced by α-2 adrenoceptor agonists may be of clinical importance, especially because they last longer than the sedative action of romifidine.

Authors' contributions
SP and AdV performed the practical trial, collected samples and prepared major parts of the manuscript. MP contributed to the laboratory work as well as handling samples. AM participated in planning and organizing the study and revision of the manuscript. SS participated in laboratory work, interpretation of results and revision of the manuscript. MR and OV participated in planning and organizing the study, interpretation of the results and critically revised the manuscript. All authors read and approved the final manuscript.

Author details
[1] Department of Equine and Small Animal Medicine, Faculty of Veterinary Medicine, University of Helsinki, P.O. Box 57, 00014 Helsinki, Finland. [2] Davies Veterinary Specialists, Manor Farm Business Park, Higham Gobion, Hertfordshire, UK.

Acknowledgements
We would like to thank Marianna Myllymäki from MTT Agrifood Research Finland for her technical assistance and Ninja Karikoski from University of Helsinki for helping with the interpretation of the results.

Competing interests
The authors declare that they have no competing interests.

Funding
This study was financially supported by the Finnish Veterinary Foundation, Foundation of Kymi Osakeyhtiö 100 years, and Vetcare Ltd. Romifidine was donated by Boegringer Ingelheim. Neither Vetcare Ltd. nor Boehringer Ingelmheim had an impact on study design, collection and analysis of samples or interpretation of data.

References
1. Kullmann A, Sanz M, Fosgate GT, Saulez MN, Page PC, Rioja E. Effects of xylazine, romifidine, or detomidine on hematology, biochemistry, and splenic thickness in healthy horses. Can Vet J. 2014;55:334–40.
2. Thurmon JC, Neff-Davis C, Davis LE, Stoker RA, Benson GJ, Lock TF. Xylazine hydrochloride-induced hyperglycemia and hypoinsulinemia in thoroughbred horses. J Vet Pharmacol Ther. 1982;5:241–5.
3. Carroll GL, Matthews NS, Hartsfield SM, Slater MR, Champney TH, Erickson SW. The effect of detomidine and its antagonism with tolazoline on stress-related hormones, metabolites, physiologic responses, and behavior in awake ponies. Vet Surg. 1997;26:69–77.
4. Angel I, Bidet S, Langer SZ. Pharmacological characterization of the hyperglycemia induced by alpha-2 adrenoceptor agonists. J Pharmacol Exp Ther. 1988;246:1098–103.
5. Raekallio M, Vainio O, Karjalainen J. The influence of atipamezole on the cardiovascular effects of detomidine in horses. J Ass vet Anaesth. 1990;17:50–3.
6. Raekallio M, Leino A, Vainio O, Scheinin M. Sympatho-adrenal activity and the clinical sedative effect of detomidine in horses. Equine Vet J. 1992;24(Suppl):66–8.
7. Raekallio M, Vainio O, Scheinin M. Detomidine reduces the plasma catecholamine, but not cortisol concentrations in horses. Zbl Vet Med A. 1991;38:153–6.
8. Alexander SL, Irvine CH. The effect of the alpha-2-adrenergic agonist, clonidine, on secretion patterns and rates of adrenocorticotropic hormone and its secretagogues in the horse. J Neuroendocrinol. 2000;12:874–80.
9. Nuñez E, Steffey EP, Ocampo L, Rodriguez A, Garcia AA. Effects of alpha 2-adrenergic receptor agonists on urine production in horses deprived of food and water. Am J Vet Res. 2004;65:1342–6.
10. DeFronzo RA, Sherwin RS, Dillingham M, Hendler R, Tamborlane WV, Felig P. Influence of basal insulin and glucagon secretion on potassium and sodium metabolism. Studies with somatostatin in normal dogs and in normal and diabetic human beings. J Clin Invest. 1978;61:472–9.
11. Ambrisko TD, Hikasa Y. The antagonistic effects of atipamezole and yohimbine on stress-related neurohormonal and metabolic responses induced by medetomidine in dogs. Can J Vet Res. 2003;67:64–7.
12. Ueoka N, Hikasa Y. Effects in cats of atipamezole, flumazenil and 4-aminopyridine on stress-related neurohormonal and metabolic responses induced by medetomidine, midazolam and ketamine. J Feline Med Surg. 2015;17:711–8.
13. Ranheim B, Horsberg TE, Søli NE, Ryeng KA, Arnemo JM. The effects of medetomidine and its reversal with atipamezole on plasma glucose, cortisol and noradrenaline in cattle and sheep. J Vet Pharmacol Ther. 2000;23:379–87.
14. Carroll GL, Hartsfield SM, Champney TH, Geller SC, Martinez EA, Haley EL. Effect of medetomidine and its antagonism with atipamezole on stress-related hormones, metabolites, physiologic responses, sedation, and mechanical threshold in goats. Vet Anaesth Analg. 2005;32:147–57.
15. Luna SPL, Taylor PM, Carregaro AB. Atipamezole antagonism of an ACTH stimulation test in ponies sedated with detomidine. J Vet Pharmacol Ther. 2010;34:508–11.
16. Ramseyer B, Schmucker N, Schatzmann U, Busato A, Moens Y. Antagonism of detomidine sedation with atipamezole in horses. Vet Anaesth Analg. 1998;25:47–51.
17. Hubbell JAE, Muir WW. Antagonism of detomidine sedation in the horse using intravenous tolazoline or atipamezole. Equine Vet J. 2006;38:238–41.
18. DiMaio Knych HK, Covarrubias V, Steffey EP. Effect of yohimbine on detomidine induced changes in behavior, cardiac and blood parameters in the horse. Vet Anaesth Analg. 2012;39:574–83.

19. Clineschmidt BV, Pettibone DJ, Lotti VJ, Hucker HB, Sweeney BM, Reiss DR, Lis EV, Huff JR, Vacca J. A peripherally acting alpha-2 adrenoceptor antagonist: L-659,066. J Pharmacol Exp Ther. 1988;245:32–40.

20. Warren JB, Dollery CT, Sciberras D, Goldberg MR. Assessment of MK-467, a peripheral alpha 2-adrenergic receptor antagonist, with intravenous clonidine. Clin Pharmacol Ther. 1991;50:71–7.

21. Goldman ME, Pettibone DJ, Reagan JE, Clineschmidt BV, Baldwin JJ, Huff JR. Blockade of peripheral α2-adrenoceptors by L-659,066 enhances glucose tolerance and insulin release in mice. Drug Develop Res. 1989;17:141–51.

22. Restitutti F, Raekallio M, Vainionpää M, Kuusela E, Vainio O. Plasma glucose, insulin, free fatty acids, lactate and cortisol concentrations in dexmedetomidine-sedated dogs with or without MK-467: a peripheral α-2 adrenoceptor antagonist. Vet J. 2012;193:481–5.

23. Sciberras DG, Reed JW, Elliott C, Blain PG, Goldberg MR. The effects of a peripherally selective alpha 2-adrenoceptor antagonist, MK-467, on the metabolic and cardiovascular response to exercise in healthy man. Br J Clin Pharmacol. 1994;37:39–44.

24. Schafers RF, Elliott HL, Howie CA, Reid JL. A preliminary, clinical pharmacological assessment of L-659,066, a novel alpha 2-adrenoceptor antagonist. Br J Clin Pharmacol. 1992;34:521–6.

25. Vainionpää MH, Raekallio MR, Pakkanen SAE, Ranta-Panula V, Rinne VM, Scheinin M, Vainio OM. Plasma drug concentrations and clinical effects of a peripheral alpha-2-adrenoceptor antagonist, MK-467, in horses sedated with detomidine. Vet Anaesth Analg. 2013;40:257–64.

26. de Vries A, Pakkanen SA, Raekallio MR, Ekiri A, Scheinin M, Taylor PM, Vainio OM. Clinical effects and pharmacokinetic variables of romifidine and the peripheral α2-adrenoceptor antagonist MK-467 in horses. Vet Anaesth Analg. 2016;43:599–610.

27. Honkavaara J, Raekallio MR, Kuusela EK, Hyvärinen EA, Vainio OM. The effects of L-659,066, a peripheral α 2-adrenoceptor antagonist, on dexmedetomidine-induced sedation and bradycardia in dogs. Vet Anaesth Analg. 2008;35:409–13.

28. Restitutti F, Honkavaara JM, Raekallio MR, Kuusela EK, Vainio OM. Effects of different doses of L-659'066 on the bispectral index and clinical sedation in dogs treated with dexmedetomidine. Vet Anaesth Analg. 2011;38:415–22.

29. Rolfe NG, Kerr CL, McDonell WN. Cardiopulmonary and sedative effects of the peripheral α2-adrenoceptor antagonist MK 0467 administered intravenously or intramuscularly concurrently with medetomidine in dogs. Am J Vet Res. 2012;73:587–94.

30. Ambrisko TD, Hikasa Y. Neurohormonal and metabolic effects of medetomidine compared with xylazine in beagle dogs. Can J Vet Res. 2002;66:42–9.

31. Raekallio MR, Kuusela EK, Lehtinen ME, Tykkyläinen MK, Huttunen P, Westerholm FC. Effects of exercise-induced stress and dexamethasone on plasma hormone and glucose concentrations and sedation in dogs treated with dexmedetomidine. Am J Vet Res. 2005;66:260–5.

32. Honkavaara JM, Restitutti F, Raekallio MR, Kuusela EK, Vainio OM. The effects of increasing doses of MK-467, a peripheral alpha2-adrenergic receptor antagonist, on the cardiopulmonary effects of intravenous dexmedetomidine in conscious dogs. J Vet Pharmacol Ther. 2011;34:332–7.

33. Warren JB, Dollery CT, Sciberras D, Goldberg MR. Assessment of MK-467, a peripheral alpha 2-adrenergic receptor antagonist, with intravenous clonidine. Clin Pharmacol Ther. 1991;50:71–7.

34. Schafers RF, Elliott HL, Howie CA, Reid JL. A preliminary, clinical pharmacological assessment of L-659,066, a novel α2-adrenoceptor antagonist. Br J Clin Pharm. 1992;34:521–6.

35. Johnson PJ, Wiedmeyer CE, LaCarrubba A, Ganjam VK, Messer NT 4th. Laminitis and the equine metabolic syndrome. Vet Clin North Am Equine Pract. 2010;26:239–55.

36. Benson GJ, Grubb TL, Neff-Davis C, Olson WA, Thurmon JC, Lindner DL, Tranquilli WJ, Vanio O. Perioperative stress response in the dog: effect of pre-emptive administration of medetomidine. Vet Surg. 2000;29:85–91.

37. Wojtasiak-Wypart M, Soma LR, Rudy JA, Uboh CE, Boston RC, Driessen B. Pharmacokinetic profile and pharmacodynamic effects of romifidine hydrochloride in the horse. J Vet Pharmacol Ther. 2012;35:478–88.

38. Muir WW. Anxiolytics, nonopioid sedative-analgesics, and opioid analgesics. In: Muir WW, Hubbel JAE, editors. Equine anesthesia. St Louis: Saunders Elsevier; 2009. p. 185–209.

39. Keen JA, Mcgorum BC, Hillier C, Nally JE. Short-term incubation of equine laminar veins with cortisol and insulin alterscontractility in vitro: possible implications for the pathogenesis of equine laminitis. J Vet Pharmacol Ther. 2013;36:382–8.

40. Zolovick A, Upson DW, Eleftheriou BE. Diurnal variation in plasma glucocorticosteroid levels in the horse (Equus Caballus). J Endocrinol. 1966;35:249–53.

41. Hemmann K, Raekallio M, Kanerva K, Hänninen L, Pastell M, Palviainen M, Vainio O. Circadian variation in ghrelin and certain stress hormones in crib-biting horses. Vet J. 2012;193:97–102.

42. Bohák Z, Szabó F, Beckers JF, Melo de Sousa N, Kutasi O, Nagy K, Szenci O. Monitoring the circadian rhythm of serum and salivary cortisol concentrations in the horse. Domest Anim Endocrin. 2013;45:38–42.

43. van Dijk P, Lankveld DP, Rijkenhuizen AB, Jonker FH. Hormonal, metabolic and physiological effects of laparoscopic surgery using a detomidine-buprenorphine combination in standing horses. Vet Anaesth Analg. 2003;30:72–80.

44. Wright EE, Simpson ER. Inhibition of the lipolytic action of beta-adrenergic agonists in human adipocytes by alpha-adrenergic agonists. J Lipid Res. 1981;22:1265–70.

45. Langin D, Holm C, Lafontan M. Adipocyte hormone-sensitive lipase: a major regulator of lipid metabolism. P Nutr Soc. 1996;55:93–109.

46. Weiner I, Wingo C. Hypokalemia–consequences, causes, and correction. J Am Soc Nephrol. 1997;8:1179–88.

26

Milk-flow data collected routinely in an automatic milking system: an alternative to milking-time testing in the management of teat-end condition?

Håvard Nørstebø[1,2]* [ID], Amira Rachah[1], Gunnar Dalen[1,2], Odd Rønningen[2], Anne Cathrine Whist[2] and Olav Reksen[1]

Abstract

Background: Having a poor teat-end condition is associated with increased mastitis risk, hence avoiding milking machine settings that have a negative effect on teat-end condition is important for successful dairy production. Milking-time testing (MTT) can be used in the evaluation of vacuum conditions during milking, but the method is less suited for herds using automatic milking systems (AMS) and relationships with teat end condition is poorly described. This study aimed to increase knowledge on interpretation of MTT in AMS and to assess whether milk-flow data obtained routinely by an AMS can be useful for the management of teat-end health. A cross-sectional study, including 251 teats of 79 Norwegian Red cows milked by AMS was performed in the research herd of the Norwegian University of Life Sciences. The following MTT variables were obtained at teat level: Average vacuum level in the short milk tube during main milking (MTVAC), average vacuum in the mouthpiece chamber during main milking and overmilking, teat compression intensity (COMPR) and overmilking time. Average and peak milk flow rates were obtained at quarter level from the AMS software. Teat-end callosity thickness and roughness was registered, and teat dimensions; length, and width at apex and base, were measured. Interrelationships among variables obtained by MTT, quarter milk flow variables, and teat dimensions were described. Associations between these variables and teat-end callosity thickness and roughness, were investigated.

Results: Principal component analysis showed clusters of strongly related variables. There was a strong negative relationship between MTVAC and average milk flow rate. The variables MTVAC, COMPR and average and peak milk flow rate were associated with both thickness and roughness of the callosity ring.

Conclusions: Quarter milk flow rate obtained directly from the AMS software was useful in assessing associations between milking machine function and teat-end condition; low average milk flow rates were associated with a higher likelihood of the teat having a thickened or roughened teat-end callosity ring. Since information on milk flow rate is readily available from the herd management system, this information might be used when evaluating causes for impaired teat-end condition in AMS.

Keywords: Automatic milking, Milk flow, Teat-end callosity

*Correspondence: havard.norstebo@nmbu.no
[1] Department of Production Animal Clinical Sciences, Faculty of Veterinary Medicine, Norwegian University of Life Sciences, PO Box 8146 Dep, 0033 Oslo, Norway
Full list of author information is available at the end of the article

Background

Changes in condition of the teat-end of dairy cattle, as evaluated by thickness and roughness of the callosity ring, have been associated with increased mastitis risk in previous studies from conventional milking systems (CMS) [1, 2]. Factors related to milking machine function, environment such as housing and climate, and general management have been identified as risk factors for alterations of the integrity of teat tissue [3]. One major advantage of automatic milking systems (AMS) over CMS is a reduction of overmilking by individual attachment and detachment of the four teat cups [4, 5]. However, thickening of the skin surrounding the teat orifice, teat-end callosity, is still found also in AMS herds, necessitating further studies on how to manage the problem. AMS was first introduced in Norwegian dairy herds in 2000 [6], and in 2017 more than 30% of Norwegian dairy farms had adopted this technology [7]. AMS continuously records large amounts of data from the milking process. Using such data in decision-support systems enabling the farmer to improve herd health has been subject to extensive research the last decade [8]. This approach has motivated us to explore whether improved utilization of data from the AMS might be useful when investigating causes for impaired teat end condition in AMS herds.

Milking-time tests (MTT) are used under field conditions to assess the potential negative effects of the milking equipment on the teat. MTT is defined as a "test made on a milking machine during milking of live animals" [9]. However, documentation on how MTT variables relate to each other, and to teat-end condition, is limited in AMS herds because most research on the topic has been performed in CMS [10]. Performing MTT in AMS herds is also time demanding because only one cow is milked at a time, making the method less practical.

Several parameters have been established to evaluate the forces applied on the teat by the collapsing liner [11–13]. Spohr and Uhlenbruck [12] described a variable called "drucksumme" (German; "sum of pressure"), estimating the forces acting on the teat-end during the closed phase of the pulsation cycle by using milking-time vacuum recordings from the short milk tube and pulsation tube, and found a strong positive correlation between "drucksumme" and percentage of cows with high degree of teat-end callosity [12]. However, an association between "drucksumme" and teat-end condition on quarter level has not yet been reported.

The vacuum level in the short milk tube, and hence at the teat-end, is one of many parameters used in a standard MTT. This vacuum level is influenced mainly by the system vacuum level and the milk transport through the short and long milk tube [14]. Quarter milk flow rate is related to system vacuum level [15, 16], teat anatomy [17] and pulsation settings [18]. It seems reasonable to assume that for cows milked by the same milking system (i.e. same system vacuum, pulsation settings and liner), individual cow- or teat factors are responsible for variation in vacuum level in the short milk tube, and hence the forces applied on the teat.

The vacuum level in the mouthpiece chamber (MPC) is another parameter often obtained by MTT. MPC vacuum is a proposed measurement for how well the teat fits the liner [19]. A recent study showed that a high MPC vacuum was associated with congestion at the teat-end [20]. However, a possible association between MPC vacuum and long-term changes in teat-end condition, such as teat-end callosity, has not been evaluated so far.

The overall aim of this study was to assess whether data obtained routinely by the AMS can be used as a proxy for MTT variables in the management of teat-end condition in AMS herds. Our first objective was to describe inter-relationships between variables from MTT, the AMS and teat dimension measurements. Secondly, we wanted to assess relationships between these variables and teat-end callosity thickness and roughness, and finally to compare the fit of these models to conclude on the overall aim.

Methods

Herd description and milking machine settings

Our study was performed in the research herd at the Norwegian University of Life Sciences. The herd consisted of 91 Norwegian Red cows divided in two groups, each milked by one AMS (DeLaval VMS, Tumba, Sweden) with identical settings. These 91 cows formed the source population. The two groups were situated in immediate proximity and had identical housing conditions. The teat-cups were equipped with DeLaval 20 M VMS liner (Product No. 92725901). The system vacuum was set to 45 kPa, the pulsator ratio was 65% and the pulsation rate was 60 cycles/min. Quarter take-off limit (switch-level) was set to 0.24 kg/min. The system was set with a low-vacuum period of 6 s and a delay from initiation of detachment to detachment of 4 s. The herd, including housing conditions, management and equipment, is comparable to commercial AMS farms in Norway. Data on parity and days in milk (DIM) in the study herd were obtained from the Norwegian Dairy Herd Recording System [21]. Except from a period of 3–5 days immediately after calving, the included cows had not been milked by CMS in the current lactation. Cows in second or later lactations had been milked by CMS in previous lactations.

Teat-end scoring and teat dimensions

Teats on all 91 lactating cows in the herd were evaluated using a scoring system where the thickness and roughness of the callous ring of the teat orifice was categorized into one of eight classes [22]. Teat length (Length) and width 0.5 cm from apex (Apex) and base (Base) was measured by placing the teat between a white background and a transparent 0.5 cm grid (DeLaval, Tumba, Sweden). In addition, the shape of the teat-end was classified in the following groups; pointed, round, flat or inverted, and the teat position was registered. All registrations were performed once per cow during a 2-day period. The udder and teats were cleaned and stripped prior to the evaluation. The same person performed all scoring and registrations. The time from last milking to teat evaluation was not standardized.

Two outcome variables for logistic regression models were established by transforming the results from the teat-end scoring. The variable THICKNESS was given the value 0 if the thickness of the callosity ring was thin or not visible, and the value 1 if it was classified as medium, thick or extreme according to the scoring system by Neijenhuis et al. [22]. The variable ROUGHNESS was given the value 0 if a smooth callosity ring was registered, and the value 1 if a rough callosity ring was registered. This approach was chosen because previous research has shown that severe degrees of teat-end callosity is significantly related to mastitis risk [2, 23].

Vacuum recordings

VaDia vacuum recorders (BioControl, Rakkestad, Norway) were used to record vacuum at a rate of 200 Hz in the short milk tube, pulsation tube, and MPC in the four individual teatcups during milking in both milking stations. The data were collected during three herd visits, between 1 and 4 weeks after the initial teat-end scoring was performed. We used data from a convenience sample of cows that entered the milking stations voluntarily without interference from the herdsmen. For cases of duplicate vacuum registrations of the same quarter, the recording taken closest to the day of teat-end scoring was used. Cows not entering the milking stations during our visits were excluded from the study. Teats that had been dried-off prior to our observational period and teats where MTT variables could not be calculated due to missing vacuum recordings were also excluded.

Calculation of MTT variables per quarter

In accordance with common procedures for MTT under field conditions, the different periods of the milking were found by evaluating the vacuum recordings [24]. For each milking two main periods were identified, based on the vacuum registrations from the short milk tube and the MPC: (a) the main milking period and (b) the overmilking period. The main milking period was characterized by high milk flow and stable vacuum conditions in the short milk tube. The start of the main milking period was identified by monitoring the average short milk tube vacuum in 10 s periods, until the decline from one period to the next was less than 0.3 kPa. The end of the main milking period, which coincides with the start of the overmilking period, was defined as the point where a marked change in MPC vacuum became apparent as described by Borkhus and Rønningen [19]. Automatic detection of these MPC vacuum changes was set at the point where the MPC vacuum increased at least 30% plus 2 kPa above a weighted running average. The result of the automated procedure was controlled manually and if necessary adjusted taking changes in short milk tube vacuum into account as described previously [19]. The end of the overmilking period was set to the initiation of detachment, i.e. the point where the short milk tube vacuum started to fall markedly ($\geq$ 5 kPa) shortly before the end of milking.

The average vacuum in the short milk tube during the main milking period (MTVAC) was calculated as the mean of all vacuum recordings from the short milk tube within the main milking period. The average vacuum levels in the MPC during the main (MPCVAC) and the overmilking periods (MPCOM) were calculated accordingly.

To estimate the forces applied on the teat-end by the liner during the closed-phase of the pulsation cycle, the variable teat compression intensity (COMPR) was calculated for each teat. This variable is comparable with "drucksumme", as described by Spohr and Uhlenbruck [12]. Vacuum records from the pulsation tube and short milk tube of 10 consecutive pulsation cycles from 60 to 70 s into the main milking period were used for the calculation of COMPR. Differential pressure across the liner wall, i.e. the difference between the short milk tube vacuum and the pulsation tube vacuum, was calculated throughout the 10 pulsation cycles. Touchpoint pressure difference (TPPD) is the pressure difference across the liner wall when two sides of the liner achieves or loses contact during closing and opening respectively [9]. TPPD is traditionally measured without a teat in the teatcup [25]. In this study, however, approximated values for TPPD was derived from the pulsation tube vacuum curves at the points of fastest liner wall movement during opening and closing, respectively [26]. The average of the approximated TPPD at opening and closing was used in further calculations. The closed-phase of the pulsation cycles were defined as the period when the differential pressure across the liner wall was higher than the approximated TPPD. For each of the 10 pulsation cycles, an integral of the differential pressure across the liner wall minus approximated TPPD as a function of time over the liner closed period was calculated. The average of the integrals found in the 10 pulsation cycles represented teat compression intensity, COMPR (kPa s).

Quarter average milk flow rate (AVGFLOW) and quarter peak milk flow rate (PEAKFLOW), for the same milkings in which the vacuum measurements were performed, were obtained from the AMS software (DeLaval, Tumba, Sweden). The milking stations were equipped with ICAR-approved milk meters using near-infrared technology providing in-line data on milk flow and milk yield used in the calculation of these variables.

Statistical analyses

Principal component analysis (PCA) is a multivariate technique that can be used to explore multi-dimensionality of data and to reduce a large set of variables to a small number of latent variables, principal components, which nevertheless retain most of the information in the dataset. PCA is also useful for the analysis of intercorrelation of variables. We applied PCA to study the relationships between the variables obtained from the different registrations, and as suggested by Dohoo et al. [27], we used PCA as a complementary technique in the subsequent model-building process. We used the 2-dimensional scatter plot of loadings for two specified components from PCA, which is most useful for interpreting principal component 1 versus principal component 2, as they contain the most important information in the data. In our application of PCA, we focused on the geometric interpretation of the relationships between variables, plotted as points in the component space using their loadings as coordinates on the "circle of correlations". In addition to PCA, we also used a linear regression model to describe the mathematical relationship between MTVAC and AVGFLOW.

The following variables were evaluated as potential explanatory variables in logistic regression models describing the likelihood of a teat-end having a rough or thickened callosity ring, respectively: DIM, Parity, MTVAC, COMPR, AVGFLOW, PEAKFLOW, MPCVAC, MPCOM, Length, Apex, Base, teat position and overmilking time. Parity was categorized as; first lactation, second lactation, and greater than second lactation.

Linearity between the outcome variables and the explanatory variables was assessed by inspecting lowess smoothing curves obtained with a logit transformation of the outcome variables; THICKNESS and ROUGHNESS (Stata SE/14, Stata Corp., College Station, TX, USA).

To establish logistic regression models for teat-end callosity roughness and thickness, we initially tested each of the explanatory variables in univariable logistic regression models to detect associations with the two outcome variables, THICKNESS and ROUGHNESS. Variables with a P-value less than 0.2 were further evaluated for inclusion in multivariable models. In order to avoid including highly correlated variables in the same model,

variables identified by PCA as belonging either to the same cluster or in clusters aligned on the opposite side of the circle of correlation, were evaluated in separate models. We repeated a backwards selection procedure to build multiple multivariable models for each outcome, and variables with P-value $\geq$ 0.05 were excluded from the final multivariable models. Because teat-end callosity thickness and roughness has been shown to vary between parities and lactation stages, parity and DIM were forced into all multivariable models [1].

We expected registrations between teats within the same cow to be correlated, and to account for this, we included a random intercept at cow level in both the univariable and multivariable models. Because the multivariable models were non-nested, i.e. the predictors in one model could not be considered as subsets of the predictors in other models, Bayesian Information Criterion (BIC) was calculated to compare model fit [27].

Data from different sources were assembled in SAS 9.4 (SAS Institute Inc., Cary, NC, USA) to form a final dataset. We used the STATA meqrlogit procedure for the logistic regression analysis and the regress procedure for the linear regression analysis (Stata SE/14, Stata Corp., College Station, TX, USA). The PCA was conducted using the statistical software JMP Pro version 12 (SAS Institute Inc., Cary, NC, USA).

Results

Out of 91 cows that were assigned teat-end scores, eight cows did not enter the milking stations at any of the visits for MTT. Of the remaining 83 cows, complete vacuum registrations from at least one teat were obtained in 79 cows, while four cows were excluded due to complete or partial loss of vacuum data for all teats. From 79 cows, four teats were excluded because they were dried off, while 61 teats were excluded due to complete or partial loss of vacuum data. This resulted in a study sample including 251 teats in 79 cows.

The parities in the study sample were distributed as follows; 34 cows in first lactation, 13 in second, and 32 in third or higher lactations. Table 1 shows the distribution of teat-end callosity scores in the included teats. The data included 123 front teats and 128 rear teats. Concerning teat-end shape, 145 teat-ends were classified as round, 78 flat, 12 pointed and 16 inverted. The number of roughened teat-ends in the same groups were 54, 15, 9 and 0, respectively. Due to the small number of observations with inverted and pointed teats, the teat-end shape was not included in statistical models. The average DIM at the time of teat-end scoring was 76, ranging from 4 to 167. The average overmilking time was 32 s, and ranged from 16 s to 3 min 17 s. However, 90% of the observations had an overmilking time shorter than 48 s.

Table 1 Frequency of teat-end callosity scores [22] in the study herd

Callosity ring thickness	Callosity ring roughness		Total
	Smooth	Rough	
Not visible	53	–	53
Thin	80	37	117
Intermediate	30	31	61
Thick	10	8	18
Extremely thick	–	2	2
Total	173	78	251

Relationships among milk flow-variables, MTT-variables and teat dimensions

Figure 1 shows the plot of the loadings of the explanatory variables MTVAC, COMPR, MPCVAC, MPCOM, PEAKFLOW AVGFLOW, Length, Apex and Base on the components. Each variable is a point whose coordinates are given by the loadings on the principal components. The first and second principal components described 67.4% of the total variation of these explanatory variables. From this loading plot we distinguished 4 clusters of variables: Cluster 1, consisting of MPCVAC and MPCOM; cluster 2, consisting of Length, Apex, and Base; cluster 3,

including AVGFLOW and PEAKFLOW; cluster 4, consisting of MTVAC and COMPR. Cluster 1 loaded opposite to cluster 2, showing a negative relationship between teat dimensions and vacuum levels in the MPC. MTVAC and COMPR in cluster 4 were negatively correlated with PEAKFLOW and AVGFLOW of cluster 3.

A linear regression model showed a strong linear relationship between MTVAC and AVGFLOW with a coefficient of determination (R^2) of 0.71. The relationship was described mathematically by the following equation:

$$MTVAC = 42.9 - 0.38 \times AVGFLOW$$

The R^2 increased to 0.84 when we omitted the 3 observations with the largest residuals.

Relationships between teat-end callosity and milk flow- and MTT-variables

In the univariable analysis, the outcome variable ROUGHNESS was significantly associated with AVGFLOW, PEAKFLOW, COMPR and MTVAC ($P < 0.05$). No significant association was found between ROUGHNESS and teat position. The results of the univariable analyses are presented as odds ratios in Table 2. Cows with teat-ends classified as normal were the designated comparison group and were assigned the odds ratio (OR) value of 1. OR are multiplicative measures of risk that range from 0 to infinity. OR > 1 is predisposing and implies an increased risk. OR < 1 is preventive and implies an inverse association.

The results from the PCA indicated that the variables AVGFLOW, PEAKFLOW, COMPR and MTVAC were strongly related. To avoid collinearity in the multivariable models, separate model building procedures were performed by including one of these variables in addition to remaining variables from the univariable analyses meeting the inclusion criteria.

The results of the multivariable models showed that MTVAC, COMPR, AVGFLOW and PEAKFLOW were all associated with ROUGHNESS ($P < 0.01$). The model with AVGFLOW as explanatory variable (Table 3) had the lowest BIC (290.59). The models using MTVAC, COMPR and PEAKFLOW had a BIC of 290.70, 297.95 and 291.88, respectively.

For the outcome variable THICKNESS, the univariable analysis showed a significant association with AVGFLOW, PEAKFLOW, COMPR, MTVAC and MPCOM ($P < 0.05$). The results are presented in Table 2. A significant association was not found between THICKNESS and teat position.

MTVAC, COMPR, AVGFLOW and PEAKFLOW were significantly associated with THICKNESS in multivariable models ($P < 0.01$). The model with AVGFLOW as explanatory variable had lowest BIC (281.38) also for this

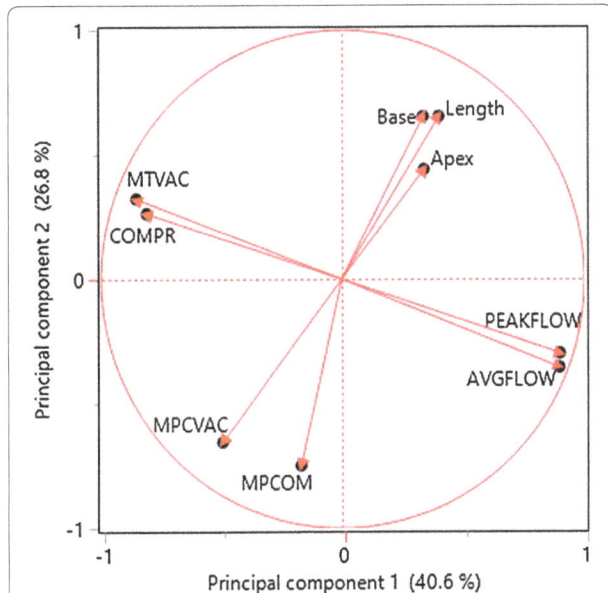

Fig. 1 Principle component loading plot. Loading plot, describing the relationship between milking-time test variables and teat characteristics, derived from principal component analysis. From this loading plot, we distinguished 4 clusters of variables: cluster 1, consisting of MPCVAC and MPCOM; cluster 2, consisting of Length, Apex, and Base; cluster 3, including AVGFLOW and PEAKFLOW; cluster 4, consisting of MTVAC and COMPR

Table 2 Results from univariable analysis for teat-end callosity roughness and thickness

Variable	ROUGHNESS				THICKNESS			
	Odds ratio	P	95% CI		Odds ratio	P	95% CI	
			Lowe	Upper			Lower	Upper
MTVAC, kPa	2.126	0.001	1.357	3.331	1.890	0.008	1.185	3.016
COMPR, kPa s	1.380	0.014	1.069	1.781	1.443	0.016	1.072	1.942
AVGFLOW, kg/min	0.040	0.001	0.006	0.265	0.049	0.005	0.006	0.406
PEAKFLOW, kg/min	0.082	0.001	0.018	0.382	0.146	0.022	0.028	0.761
MPCVAC, kPa	1.008	0.708	0.967	1.050	0.965	0.132	0.921	1.011
MPCOM, kPa	0.979	0.480	0.922	1.039	0.928	0.040	0.865	0.997
Length, cm	1.137	0.665	0.635	2.034	1.054	0.874	0.549	2.024
Apex, cm	0.241	0.099	0.045	1.305	0.843	0.853	0.138	5.136
Base, cm	0.907	0.865	0.295	2.793	1.252	0.714	0.376	4.170
Overmilking time, min	0.916	0.858	0.352	2.384	0.558	0.402	0.143	2.102

MTVAC, average vacuum level in the short milk tube during the main milking period; COMPR, teat compression intensity; AVGFLOW, quarter average milk flow rate; PEAKFLOW, quarter peak milk flow rate; MPCVAC, average vacuum level in the mouthpiece chamber during the main milking period; MPCOM, average vacuum level in the mouthpiece chamber in the overmilking period. Random intercepts at cow level were included in all analyses to account for within cow dependency of the outcome variables

ROUGHNESS, dichotomized outcome variable where smooth teat-end callosity rings form the comparison group and teat-ends with a roughened callosity ring is considered abnormal

THICKNESS, dichotomized outcome variable where teat-ends having a thin or not visible teat-end callosity ring form the comparison group, and medium, thick or extreme are considered abnormal

Table 3 Final multivariable logistic regression models describing the likelihood of a teat having a roughened or thickened teat-end callosity ring, respectively [22]

Outcome and BIC	Variable	Odds ratio	P	95% CI	
				Lower	Upper
ROUGHNESS	DIM	1.016	0.032	1.001	1.030
BIC = 290.59	Parity 1 (reference)	–	–	–	–
	Parity 2	0.291	0.201	0.044	1.928
	Parity ≥ 3	2.943	0.073	0.903	9.593
	AVGFLOW, kg/min	0.020	0.001	0.003	0.160
THICKNESS	DIM	1.024	0.006	1.007	1.041
BIC = 281.38	Parity 1 (reference)	–	–	–	–
	Parity 2	0.386	0.381	0.046	3.249
	Parity ≥ 3	3.969	0.056	0.963	16.362
	AVGFLOW, kg/min	0.019	0.001	0.002	0.181

The models were selected based on having the lowest Bayesian information criterion (BIC) among other models for the same outcome

DIM, days in milk; AVGFLOW, quarter average milk flow rate

ROUGHNESS, dichotomized outcome variable where smooth teat-end callosity rings form the comparison group and teat-ends with a roughened callosity ring is considered abnormal

THICKNESS, dichotomized outcome variable where teat-ends having a thin or not visible teat-end callosity ring form the comparison group, and medium, thick or extreme are considered abnormal

outcome (Table 3). BIC for the models using MTVAC, COMPR and PEAKFLOW were 283.22, 282.86 and 285.33, respectively.

The random intercept term signifying the correlation between teats within the same cow was highly significant (P < 0.001) in all models.

Discussion

Relationships among milk flow-variables, MTT-variables and teat dimensions

The clustering of variables identified by the PCA shows that recording and evaluating a smaller number of variables might be sufficient for MTT in AMS herds. Cluster 1 was based on vacuum recordings from the MPC, cluster 2 represented the measured teat dimensions, cluster 3 displayed milk flow recordings, and cluster 4 was based on vacuum recordings from the short milk tube.

We observed a strong negative relationship between MTVAC and AVGFLOW. This is in agreement with previous studies [16, 28]. The relationship between system vacuum, claw vacuum and milk flow has been described in previous experimental studies [10, 15, 16]. The system vacuum was the same for all observations, and the system has no claw. Based on the strong relationship between MTVAC and AVGFLOW it seems possible to use average milk flow as a proxy for the vacuum level in the short milk tube during milking in an AMS. Increasing the system vacuum will increase the physical forces acting on the teat. Our findings indicates that cows with a low milk flow responded with poor teat-end condition even at a standard system vacuum level. Increasing system vacuum level is likely to increase the number of cows with this problem.

The PCA showed that MTVAC and COMPR were closely related. This indicates that COMPR and MTVAC contain similar information. Because COMPR accounts for both duration of the pulsation cycle, vacuum level in the pulsation tube and liner type, this variable might be better suited for comparisons between herds [12]. Since every milking was performed using the same liner and the same pulsation settings, and there was little variation in vacuum conditions in the pulsation tube between cows, COMPR was mainly influenced by the vacuum level in the short milk tube. The PCA also showed a negative relationship between the milk flow variables (AVGFLOW and PEAKFLOW) and COMPR, which is likely due to the strong association between the milk flow variables and vacuum level in the short milk tube.

In agreement with previous research on teat anatomy and milk flow rate in CMS [17], the PCA showed that there were no apparent association between teat dimensions and the milk-flow variables AVGFLOW and PEAKFLOW. Accordingly, no evident association was found between teat dimensions and the MTT-variables MTVAC and COMPR. The quarter milk flow rate has been shown to be a consequence of the canal anatomy, such as length and diameter, but sophisticated tools such as ultrasonography is required to acquire this kind of information [17].

The PCA also showed that teat dimensions were related to MPC vacuum; larger teat dimensions were associated with lower MPC vacuum. This finding is in agreement with results from a previous study performed in a CMS [19]; a high vacuum level in the MPC can be observed when the teat is too small relative to the diameter of the liner barrel, allowing the vacuum in the short milk tube to propagate to the MPC. A low vacuum level in the MPC is observed when the liner fits the teat, making a tight seal in the liner barrel. Low MPC vacuum levels may also be a result of air leakage due to the mouthpiece opening being too large relative to the base of the teat [19].

Relationships between teat-end callosity and milk flow- and MTT-variables

The multivariable logistic regression models showed that MTVAC, COMPR, AVGFLOW, and PEAKFLOW were all associated with the outcome variables THICKNESS and ROUGHNESS. The negative relationship between the milk flow variables AVGFLOW and PEAKFLOW and

the variables based on vacuum recordings; MTVAC and COMPR, as shown in the PCA (Fig. 1), is indicating that these four variables contain similar information.

Difference in BIC of two models < 2 is considered to be a weak evidence for superiority of the model with the lowest BIC, whereas values from 2 to 6 are considered positive evidence [26]. For both outcome variables, the models using AVGFLOW had the lowest BIC. However, the differences only provided weak evidence that the models using AVGFLOW was superior to the other. Nevertheless, this is a relevant finding because the milk flow is readily available in the herd management system and might be used instead of or in addition to vacuum measurements to indicate whether the milking procedure is involved as a cause for teat-end condition problems in a herd. If cows with poor teat-end condition also show low milk flow rates, it should be suspected that the milking settings (e.g. system vacuum) is not suited for this group of cows. In contrast, if poor teat-ends occur frequently across the whole range of milk flow rates, one might suspect that environmental and genetic factors are the dominating causes for the condition, or that the milking system has major defects affecting all cows. Further research is needed to test this hypothesis before it is implemented in herd health management protocols.

Because we used a cross sectional study design, it is relevant to ask whether the associations between teat-end callosity and milk flow rate could be interpreted in two directions; (1) milk flow affecting (vacuum levels and thereby) teat-end callosity, or (2) teat-end callosity affecting milk flow (and thereby vacuum levels). The length of the teat canal, measured by ultrasonography, has been shown to correlate with average and peak milk flow rate [17]. Our study showed that quarter average and peak milk flow rates were associated with vacuum levels in the short milk tube, which is in agreement with previous research from CMS [14]. Previous research have also shown that vacuum conditions at the teat-end during milking is involved in the development of teat-end callosity [10]. We therefore think it is plausible that the difference in development of teat-end callosity between cows primarily is a result of teat canal anatomy, manifested as differences in milk flow rate, rather than the opposite. However, we cannot rule out that a high degree of teat-end callosity may also act in concert with narrow teat canals, leading to further reduced milk flow rate in affected cows. Few authors, if any, have discussed the possible effects of teat-end callosity on milk flow rate.

Neijenhuis et al. [22] found less teat-end callosity in first parity cows than cows in third and later lactations. Although not statistically significant in our models, the OR estimates indicated a higher likelihood of having a thickened or roughened teat-end callosity ring in cows in third or later lactations compared to first lactation cows (Table 3). The cows in third or later lactations had been milked by CMS in two or more previous lactations. Although less likely, we cannot rule out that this have interfered with the degree of teat end callosity in the present investigation. Sterret et al. [29] investigated teat-end callosity in a group of Holstein cows before and after converting to quarter-based milking, and found a decrease in teat-end callosity approximately 1 month after installing the new system. This shows that teat-end callosity is a dynamic condition, and that previous milking machine settings might be of minor importance. Because our main focus was associations between teat-end callosity and milk flow, not prevalence of teat end callosity, we consider possible effects of earlier exposure to CMS to be of minor importance for our conclusions.

We used vacuum recordings to split the milking into two main phases; main milking and overmilking. Because this is an indirect method, it is not possible to determine exactly when the milk flow starts to decline and when it drops below the take-off limit, which might lead to some misclassification if compared to methods using data from milk meters. The duration of the main milking phase was used as the denominator in the calculation of MTVAC and MPCVAC. Furthermore, duration of the overmilking period was used both as an explanatory variable and as the denominator in the calculation of MPCOM. Thus, it is obvious that erroneous calculations of the transition between the main milking and overmilking periods would hamper the results of the present investigation. However, we have used accepted and standardized methods commonly implemented in herd health advisory services around the world [30]. It is also worth noting that both MTVAC and AVGFLOW were significantly related with teat-end callosity thickness and roughness, and that AVGFLOW was calculated by the AMS software independent of how we defined the transition between milking phases. This indicates that the definition of the main milking and overmilking phases cannot have had a major impact on our models. We also acknowledge that the varying time span between teat-end scoring and vacuum measurements and the non-standardized time from milking to teat measurement may have added variability to the results. It is reasonable to expect that less variability due to a more uniform sampling regime would strengthen rather than weaken the reported associations, which already by the present approach have shown to be quite significant.

No associations were found between THICKNESS and ROUGHNESS and overmilking time. This is likely due to short duration and little variation in the overmilking periods in AMS, as described in previous studies [4, 5]. In our data, 90% of the observations had an overmilking

time between 16 and 48 s. Because the AMS settings included a low-vacuum period of 6 s and a delay from initiation of detachment to actual detachment of 4 s, there might be a slight overestimation of the duration of the overmilking time. However, this overestimation is similar for all milkings, and we do not expect this to bias our assessments of overmilking time and teat end condition.

A recent study revealed a relationship between MPC vacuum and congestion at the teat-ends [20]. Our outcome variables can be considered long-term changes in the teat tissue, whereas the congestion shown by Penry et al. [20] was observed by ultrasonography immediately after milking. Despite short overmilking periods, the variable MPCOM showed a significant association with THICKNESS in the univariable analysis ($P < 0.05$). However, none of the MPC variables showed significant associations with THICKNESS or ROUGHNESS in the multivariable models when DIM and parity were accounted for. Conclusively, further research is warranted to increase the knowledge on how overmilking in AMS can be evaluated by vacuum recordings.

The data were obtained from a single AMS herd in which all cows were milked with the same milking machine settings and the same liner, and we acknowledge that this may lower the external validity. However, because relationships between teat-end condition and milking machine performance has traditionally been studied in CMS [14–16, 31], our study in an AMS herd under field condition represents a step forward for the knowledge on associations between teat-end condition and milk flow in AMS herds. Due to the differences between CMS and AMS, e.g. milking cluster vs. individual attachment and detachment, our findings should be used with precaution in CMS.

A previous study have indicated that breeds differs concerning the development of teat-end hyperkeratosis [31]. Although we expect associations between milk flow variables in AMS and teat end condition to be similar also for other breeds than Norwegian Red, it is feasible to investigate these associations separately in other breeds.

Conclusion

Quarter milk flow rate obtained from the AMS software may be used as a proxy for vacuum level in the short milk tube. Furthermore, quarter milk flow rate obtained from the AMS provided useful information for evaluating associations between the milking procedure and risk factors for impaired teat-end condition.

Authors' contributions
The study was initiated by ACW, who also participated in planning the study together with GD, HN and ORe. GD and HN performed teat-end scoring, teat measurements and recorded vacuum levels for MTT. HN analysed the vacuum recordings in close cooperation with ORø. ORe, GD, AR and HN did the data

analysis and drafted the manuscript. All authors have read and approved the final manuscript.

Author details
[1] Department of Production Animal Clinical Sciences, Faculty of Veterinary Medicine, Norwegian University of Life Sciences, PO Box 8146 Dep, 0033 Oslo, Norway. [2] TINE SA, Langbakken 20, 1430 Ås, Norway.

Acknowledgements
Not applicable.

Competing interests
The authors declare that they have no competing interests.

Funding
This research was conducted as a part of the project "New approaches to management and breeding, in automatic milking systems". The financial sources were TINE SA, DeLaval, Geno, The foundation for Research levy on Agricultural Products, and the Norwegian Research Council.

References
1. Neijenhuis F, Barkema HW, Hogeveen H, Noordhuizen JPTM. Relationship between teat-end callosity and occurrence of clinical mastitis. J Dairy Sci. 2001;84:2664–72.
2. Breen JE, Green MJ, Bradley AJ. Quarter and cow risk factors associated with the occurrence of clinical mastitis in dairy cows in the United Kingdom. J Dairy Sci. 2009;92:2551–61.
3. Hamann J, Burvenick C. Physiological status of the bovine teat. Bull Int Dairy Fed. 1994;297:3–12.
4. Svennersten-Sjaunja KM, Pettersson G. Pros and cons of automatic milking in Europe. J Anim Sci. 2008;86:37–46.
5. Hogeveen H, Ouweltjes W, de Koning CJAM, Stelwagen K. Milking interval, milk production and milk flow-rate in an automatic milking system. Livest Prod Sci. 2001;72:157–67.
6. TINE. Annual report. Oslo: Tine Dairy Company; 2013.
7. Stræte EP, Vik J, Hansen BG. The social robot: a study of the social and political aspects of automatic milking systems. Proc Food Syst Dyn. 2017. https://doi.org/10.18461/pfsd.2017.1722.
8. Rutten CJ, Velthuis AGJ, Steeneveld W, Hogeveen H. Sensors to support health management on dairy farms. J Dairy Sci. 2013;96:1928–52.
9. International Organization for Standardization (ISO). Milking machine installations–vocabulary. ISO 3918:2007.
10. Besier J, Lind O, Bruckmaier RM. Dynamics of teat-end vacuum during machine milking: types, causes and impacts on teat condition and udder health—a literature review. J Appl Anim Res. 2016;44:263–72.
11. Mein GA, Williams DM, Thiel CC. Compressive load applied by the teatcup liner to the bovine teat. J Dairy Res. 2009;54:327–37.
12. Spohr M, Uhlenbruck F. Melktechnische einflüsse auf die asprägung von hyperkeratosen In: DVG-Tagung. Herausforderungen in der Zukunft der Mastitisbekämpung. Grub: Deutsche Veterinärmesizinische Gesellschaft e.V.; 2012. p. 120–5.
13. Leonardi S, Penry JF, Tangorra FM, Thompson PD, Reinemann DJ. Methods of estimating liner compression. J Dairy Sci. 2015;98:6905–12.
14. Besier J, Bruckmaier RM. Vacuum levels and milk-flow-dependent vacuum drops affect machine milking performance and teat condition in dairy cows. J Dairy Sci. 2016;99:3096–102.
15. Rasmussen MD, Madsen NP. Effects of milkline vacuum, pulsator airline vacuum, and cluster weight on milk yield, teat condition, and udder health. J Dairy Sci. 2000;83:77–84.
16. Bade RD, Reinemann DJ, Zucali M, Ruegg PL, Thompson PD. Interactions of vacuum, b-phase duration, and liner compression on milk flow rates in dairy cows. J Dairy Sci. 2009;92:913–21.
17. Weiss D, Weinfurtner M, Bruckmaier RM. Teat anatomy and its relationship with quarter and udder milk flow characteristics in dairy cows. J Dairy Sci. 2004;87:3280–9.
18. Williams DM, Mein GA, Brown MR. Biological responses of the bovine teat to milking: information from measurements of milk flow-rate within single pulsation cycles. J Dairy Res. 1981;48:7–21.
19. Borkhus M, Rønningen O. Factors affecting mouthpiece chamber vacuum in machine milking. J Dairy Res. 2003;70:283–8.
20. Penry JF, Upton J, Mein GA, Rasmussen MD, Ohnstad I, Thompson PD, Reinemann DJ. Estimating teat canal cross-sectional area to determine the effects of teat-end and mouthpiece chamber vacuum on teat congestion. J Dairy Sci. 2017;100:821–7.
21. Østerås O, Solbu H, Refsdal AO, Roalkvam T, Filseth O, Minsaas A. Results and evaluation of thirty years of health recordings in the Norwegian dairy cattle population. J Dairy Sci. 2007;90:4483–97.
22. Neijenhuis F, Barkema HW, Hogeveen H, Noordhuizen JPTM. Classification and longitudinal examination of callused teat ends in dairy cows. J Dairy Sci. 2000;83:2795–804.
23. Mein G, Williams DM, Reinemann DJ. Effects of milking on teat-end hyperkeratosis: 1. Mechanical forces applied by the teatcup liner and responses of the teat. In: National Mastitis Council, 42nd annual meeting proceedings. Madison: National Mastitis Council Inc; 2003. p. 114–23.
24. Postma E. New technology for milking vacuum diagnostics helps veterinarians better understand and manage udder health problems. In: Proceedings of the British Mastitis Conference. Taunton: The Dairy Group; 2012. p. 87–88.
25. Mein GA, Reinemann DJ. In: Machine milking: Volume 1. Mein and Reinemann; 2014. p. 38.
26. Rønningen O. Measurement of liner movement. In: Proceedings of the international symposium on advances in milking. Cork: Teagasc and Int. Dairy Fed.; 2007. p 32–41.
27. Dohoo IR, Martin W, Stryhn H. Veterinary epidemiologic research. 2nd ed. Charlottetown: VER Inc; 2009.
28. Rose-Meierhöfer S, Hoffmann M, Öz H, Ströbel U, Ammon C. Milking-time tests in conventional and quarter-individual milking systems. Landbauforschung Völkenrode. 2010;60:11–5.
29. Sterrett AE, Wood CL, McQuerry KJ, Bewley JM. Changes in teat-end hyperkeratosis after installation of an individual quarter pulsation milking system. J Dairy Sci. 2013;96:4041–6.
30. Rønningen, O. Milking time tests—a tool for milking advisory services. In: 6. Tänikoner Melktechniktagung, Aspekte zur Optimierung der maschinellen Milchgewinnung. Ettenhausen: Forschungsanstalt Agroscope; 2017. p. 5–15.
31. Gleeson DE, O'Callaghan EJ, Rath M. The effects of genotype, milking time and teat-end vacuum pattern on the severity of teat-end hyperkeratosis. Ir J Agric Food Res. 2003;42:195–203.

Permissions

All chapters in this book were first published in AVS, by BioMed Central; hereby published with permission under the Creative Commons Attribution License or equivalent. Every chapter published in this book has been scrutinized by our experts. Their significance has been extensively debated. The topics covered herein carry significant findings which will fuel the growth of the discipline. They may even be implemented as practical applications or may be referred to as a beginning point for another development.

The contributors of this book come from diverse backgrounds, making this book a truly international effort. This book will bring forth new frontiers with its revolutionizing research information and detailed analysis of the nascent developments around the world.

We would like to thank all the contributing authors for lending their expertise to make the book truly unique. They have played a crucial role in the development of this book. Without their invaluable contributions this book wouldn't have been possible. They have made vital efforts to compile up to date information on the varied aspects of this subject to make this book a valuable addition to the collection of many professionals and students.

This book was conceptualized with the vision of imparting up-to-date information and advanced data in this field. To ensure the same, a matchless editorial board was set up. Every individual on the board went through rigorous rounds of assessment to prove their worth. After which they invested a large part of their time researching and compiling the most relevant data for our readers.

The editorial board has been involved in producing this book since its inception. They have spent rigorous hours researching and exploring the diverse topics which have resulted in the successful publishing of this book. They have passed on their knowledge of decades through this book. To expedite this challenging task, the publisher supported the team at every step. A small team of assistant editors was also appointed to further simplify the editing procedure and attain best results for the readers.

Apart from the editorial board, the designing team has also invested a significant amount of their time in understanding the subject and creating the most relevant covers. They scrutinized every image to scout for the most suitable representation of the subject and create an appropriate cover for the book.

The publishing team has been an ardent support to the editorial, designing and production team. Their endless efforts to recruit the best for this project, has resulted in the accomplishment of this book. They are a veteran in the field of academics and their pool of knowledge is as vast as their experience in printing. Their expertise and guidance has proved useful at every step. Their uncompromising quality standards have made this book an exceptional effort. Their encouragement from time to time has been an inspiration for everyone.

The publisher and the editorial board hope that this book will prove to be a valuable piece of knowledge for researchers, students, practitioners and scholars across the globe.

List of Contributors

Agneta Egenvall, Marie Eisersiö and Marie Rhodin
Department of Clinical Sciences, Faculty of Veterinary Medicine and Animal Husbandry, Swedish University of Agricultural Sciences, Uppsala, Sweden

Lars Roepstorff
Unit of Equine Studies, Department of Anatomy, Physiology and Biochemistry, Faculty of Veterinary Medicine and Animal Husbandry, Swedish University of Agricultural Sciences, Uppsala, Sweden

René van Weeren
Department of Equine Sciences, Faculty of Veterinary Medicine, Utrecht University, Yalelaan 114, 3584 CM Utrecht, The Netherlands

Ragnvi Hagman, Odd V. Höglund, Anne-Sofie Lagerstedt and Ann Pettersson
Department of Clinical Sciences, Swedish University of Agricultural Sciences, Uppsala, Sweden

Thanikul Srithunyarat
Department of Clinical Sciences, Swedish University of Agricultural Sciences, Uppsala, Sweden
Department of Surgery and Theriogenology, Faculty of Veterinary Medicine, Khon Kaen University, Khon Kaen 40002, Thailand

Supranee Jitpean
Department of Surgery and Theriogenology, Faculty of Veterinary Medicine, Khon Kaen University, Khon Kaen 40002, Thailand

Ulf Olsson
Unit of Applied Statistics and Mathematics, Swedish University of Agricultural Sciences, Uppsala, Sweden

Mats Stridsberg
Department of Medical Sciences, Uppsala University, 75185 Uppsala, Sweden

Suvi Taponen and Satu Pyörälä
Department of Production Animal Medicine, Faculty of Veterinary Medicine, University of Helsinki, Paroninkuja 20, 04920 Saarentaus, Finland

Suvi Nykäsenoja, Tarja Pohjanvirta and Anna Pitkälä
Finnish Food Safety Authority Evira, Mustialankatu 3, 00790 Helsinki, Finland

Johanna Åhlgren and Pekka Uimari
Department of Agricultural Sciences, University of Helsinki, Helsinki, Finland

Sauli Laaksonen
Department of Veterinary Biosciences, Faculty of Veterinary Medicine, University of Helsinki, Helsinki, Wazama, Finland

Antti Oksanen
Research and Laboratory Department, Production Animal and Wildlife Health Research Unit, Finnish Food Safety Authority Evira, Oulu, Finland

Jérôme Julmi, Claudio Zweifel and Roger Stephan
Institute for Food Safety and Hygiene, Vetsuisse Faculty University of Zurich, Zurich, Switzerland

Maria Fredriksson-Ahomaa
Department of Food Hygiene and Environmental Health, Faculty of Veterinary Medicine, University of Helsinki, Helsinki, Finland

Maialen Arrausi-Subiza, Xeider Gerrikagoitia, Vega Alvarez, Jose Carlos Ibabe and Marta Barral
Department of Animal Health, Basque Institute for Agricultural Research and Development-NEIKER, Berreaga 1, 48160 Derio-Bizkaia, Spain

Maja Zakošek Pipan and Janko Mrkun
Clinic for Reproduction and Large Animals, Veterinary Faculty, University of Ljubljana, Gerbičeva 60, 1000 Ljubljana, Slovenia

Breda Jakovac Strajn and Katarina Pavšič Vrtač
Department for Environment and Animal Nutrition, Welfare and Hygiene, Veterinary Faculty, University of Ljubljana, Gerbičeva 60, 1000 Ljubljana, Slovenia

Anja Pišlar
Department of Pharmaceutical Biology, Faculty of Pharmacy, University of Ljubljana, Aškerčeva cesta 7, 1000 Ljubljana, Slovenia

Janko Kos
Department of Pharmaceutical Biology, Faculty of Pharmacy, University of Ljubljana, Aškerčeva cesta 7, 1000 Ljubljana, Slovenia
Department of Biotechnology, Jožef Štefan Institute, Jamova cesta 39, 1000 Ljubljana, Slovenia

Petra Zrimšek
Institute for Preclinical Sciences, Veterinary Faculty, University of Ljubljana, Gerbičeva 60, 1000 Ljubljana, Slovenia

Poul H. Rathkjen
Boehringer Ingelheim Vetmedica GmbH, Binger Straße 173, 55216 Ingelheim, Germany

Johannes Dall
PORCUS svinefagdyrlaeger og agronomer, Oerbaekvej 276, 5220 Odense, Denmark

Francesco Birettoni, Domenico Caivano, Giulia Moretti, Francesco Porciello, Maria Elena Giorgi, Alberto Crovace, Erika Bianchini and Antonello Bufalari
Department of Veterinary Medicine, University of Perugia, Via San Costanzo 4, 06126 Perugia, Italy

Mark Rishniw
Department of Clinical Sciences, Cornell University, Ithaca, NY 14853, USA
Veterinary Information Network, Davis, CA 95616, USA

Perttu Koski
Production Animal and Wildlife Health Research Unit, Finnish Food Safety Authority Evira, Elektroniikkatie 3, 90590 Oulu, Finland

Pasi Anttila
Production Animal and Wildlife Health Research Unit, Finnish Food Safety Authority Evira, Elektroniikkatie 3, 90590 Oulu, Finland
Present Address: Perämeren Kalatalousyhteisöjen Liitto, Piuhatie 8, 90620 Oulu, Finland

Jussi Kuusela
Production Animal and Wildlife Health Research Unit, Finnish Food Safety Authority Evira, Elektroniikkatie 3, 90590 Oulu, Finland
Present Address: Lahti University of Applied Sciences, Niemenkatu 73, 15140 Lahti, Finland

Yamen Hegazy
Animal Medicine Department, Faculty of Veterinary Medicine, Kafrelsheikh University, Kafrelsheikh 33516, Egypt

Walid Elmonir
Hygiene and Preventive Medicine (Zoonoses) Department, Faculty of Veterinary Medicine, Kafrelsheikh University, Kafrelsheikh 33516, Egypt.

Nour Hosny Abdel-Hamid and Essam Mohamed Elbauomy
Brucellosis Research Department, Animal Health Research Institute, Nadi El-Seid Street, Dokki, Giza 12618, Egypt

Falk Huettmann
EWHALE Lab, Institute of Arctic Biology, Department of Wildlife Biology, University of Alaska Fairbanks, 902 N. Koyukuk Dr., Fairbanks, AK 99775, USA

Emily Elizabeth Magnuson
Department of Biology and Wildlife, University of Alaska Fairbanks, 982 N. Koyukuk Dr., Fairbanks, AK 99775, USA

Karsten Hueffer
Department of Veterinary Medicine, University of Alaska Fairbanks, 901 Koyukuk Drive, Fairbanks, AK 99775, USA

Barbara Thomsen, Mette Berendt and Hanne Gredal
Department of Veterinary Clinical and Animal Sciences, University Hospital for Companion Animals, University of Copenhagen, Dyrlægevej 16, 1870 Frederiksberg C, Denmark

Laurent Garosi
Davies Veterinary Specialists, Manor Farm Business Park, Higham Gobion, Hitchin, England SG5 3HR, UK

Geoff Skerritt
Chestergates Veterinary Referral Hospital, Units E & F, Telford Court, Chestergates Road, Chester, Cheshire, England CH1 6LT, UK

Tim Sparrow
Present Address: Fitzpatrick Referrals, Halfway Lane, Eashing, Godalming, Surrey, England GU7 2QQ, UK

Clare Rusbridge
Present Address: Fitzpatrick Referrals, Halfway Lane, Eashing, Godalming, Surrey, England GU7 2QQ, UK
Present Address: School of Veterinary Medicine, Faculty of Health and Medical Sciences, University of Surrey, Guildford, Surrey, England GU2 7TE, UK
Stone Lion Veterinary Hospital, 41 High Street, Wimbledon, London SW19 5AU, UK

Maria Celina Abraham, Johanna Puhakka, Essraa Mohsen Al-Essawe, Jane Margaret Morrell and Renée Båge
Division of Reproduction, Department of Clinical Sciences, Swedish University of Agricultural Sciences, Uppsala, Sweden

Alejandro Ruete
Department of Ecology, Swedish University of Agricultural Sciences, Uppsala, Sweden

Kerstin de Verdier
National Veterinary Institute, 75189 Uppsala, Sweden

Isa Anna Maria Immonen, Ninja Karikoski, Anna Mykkänen, Tytti Niemelä and Riitta-Mari Tulamo
Department of Equine and Small Animal Medicine, Faculty of Veterinary Medicine, University of Helsinki, 00014 Helsinki, Finland

Jouni Junnila
Pharma, 20520 Turku, Finland

Birthe Hald
Danish Veterinary Laboratory, Department of Poultry, Fish and Fur Animals, 8200 Aarhus N, Denmark
Present Address: National Food Institute, Technical University of Denmark, 2860 Søborg, Denmark

Michael Wainø
Danish Veterinary Laboratory, Department of Poultry, Fish and Fur Animals, 8200 Aarhus N, Denmark
Present Address: Chr. Hansen, 2970 Hørsholm, Denmark

Steen Nordentoft
Danish Veterinary Laboratory, Department of Poultry, Fish and Fur Animals, 8200 Aarhus N, Denmark

Novo Nordisk, 4400 Kalundborg, Denmark. 13 Dianova Ltd., 8200 Aarhus N, Denmark

Mogens Madsen
Danish Veterinary Laboratory, Department of Poultry, Fish and Fur Animals, 8200 Aarhus N, Denmark
Present Address: Dianova Ltd., 8200 Aarhus N,Denmark

Dorte Lau Baggesen
Department of Microbiology, Danish Veterinary Laboratory, 1870 Frederiksberg C, Denmark
Present Address: National Food Institute, Technical University of Denmark, 2860 Søborg, Denmark

Marianne Nielsine Skov
Department of Microbiology, Danish Veterinary Laboratory, 1870 Frederiksberg C, Denmark.
Present Address: Research Unit for Clinical Microbiology, University of Southern Denmark, 5000 Odense C, Denmark

Eva Møller Nielsen
Department of Microbiology, Danish Veterinary Laboratory, 1870 Frederiksberg C, Denmark
Present Address: Department of Microbiology and Infection Control, Statens Serum Institut, 2300 Copenhagen S, Denmark

Jesper Johannes Madsen
Natural History Museum of Denmark, University of Copenhagen, 1350 Copenhagen K, Denmark

Carsten Rahbek
Natural History Museum of Denmark, University of Copenhagen, 1350 Copenhagen K, Denmark
Center for Macroecology, Evolution, and Climate, Natural History Museum of Denmark, University of Copenhagen, 2100 Copenhagen Ø, Denmark
Present Address: Imperial College London, Silwood Park Campus, Ascot, Berkshire SL5 7PY, UK

Mariann Chriél
The Danish Meatboard, 1609 Copenhagen V, Denmark
Present Address: National Veterinary Institute, Technical University of Denmark, 1870 Frederiksberg C, Denmark

Giulio Grandi, Osama Ibrahim and Eva Osterman Lind
Department of Microbiology, National Veterinary Institute (SVA), Ulls väg 2B,75189 Uppsala, Sweden

Arianna Comin
Department of Disease Control and Epidemiology, National Veterinary Institute (SVA), Ulls väg 2B, 75651 Uppsala, Sweden

Roland Schaper
Bayer Animal Health GmbH, Monheim, Germany

Ulrika Forshell
Bayer Animal Health AB, Solna, Sweden

Aleksandra Domanjko Petrič, Tajda Lukman, Barbara Verk and Alenka Nemec Svete
Small Animal Clinic, Veterinary Faculty, University of Ljubljana, Gerbičeva 60, 1000 Ljubljana, Slovenia

Heli Nordgren, Katariina Vapalahti, Antti Sukura and Anna-Maija Virtala
Department of Veterinary Biosciences, Faculty of Veterinary Medicine, University of Helsinki, Helsinki, Finland

Olli Vapalahti
Department of Veterinary Biosciences, Faculty of Veterinary Medicine, University of Helsinki, Helsinki, Finland
Department of Virology and Immunology,HUSLAB, Hospital district of Helsinki and Uusimaa, Helsinki, Finland
Department of Virology, Faculty of Medicine, University of Helsinki, Helsinki, Finland

Malin Öhlund and Bodil Ström Holst
Department of Clinical Sciences, Swedish University of Agricultural Sciences, 750 07 Uppsala, Sweden

Malin Palmgren
Kumla Animal Hospital, Företagsgatan 7, 692 71 Kumla, Sweden

Ugne Spancerniene, Juozas Grigas, Judita Zymantiene and Arunas Stankevicius
Department of Anatomy and Physiology, Faculty of Veterinary Medicine, Lithuanian University of Health Sciences, Tilzes str. 18, Kaunas, Lithuania

Jurate Buitkuviene
National Food and Veterinary Risk Assessment Institute, J. Kairiukscio str. 10, Vilnius, Lithuania.

Vida Juozaitiene
Department of Animal Breeding and Nutrition, Faculty of Animal Husbandry Technology, Lithuanian University of Health Sciences, Tilzes str. 18, Kaunas, Lithuania

Milda Stankeviciute and Dainius Razukevicius
Faculty of Medicine, Lithuanian University of Health Sciences, A. Mickeviciaus str. 9, Kaunas, Lithuania

Dainius Zienius
Faculty of Veterinary Medicine, Institute of Microbiology and Virology, Lithuanian University of Health Sciences, Tilzes str.18, Kaunas, Lithuania

Annalisa Elena Jolanda Giovannini and Claudia Spadavecchia
Department of Clinical Veterinary Medicine, Anesthesiology and Pain Therapy Section, Vetsuisse Faculty, University of Berne, Laenggassstrasse 124, 3012 Berne, Switzerland

Bart Henricus Philippus van den Borne
Veterinary Public Health Institute, Vetsuisse Faculty, University of Berne, Schwarzenburgstrasse 155, 3097 Liebefeld, Switzerland

Samantha Kay Wall, Olga Wellnitz and Rupert Max Bruckmaier
Veterinary Physiology, Vetsuisse Faculty, University of Berne, Bremgartenstrasse 109a, 3012 Berne, Switzerland

Christian Visscher, Anne Kruse, Saara Sander, Jasmin Mischok and Josef Kamphues
Institute for Animal Nutrition, University of Veterinary Medicine Hannover, Foundation, Bischofsholer Damm 15, 30173 Hanover, Germany

Christoph Keller
Boehringer Ingelheim Veterinary Research Center GmbH & Co. KG, Bemeroder Str. 31, 30559 Hanover, Germany

Robert Tabeling
Veterinärgesellschaft im BHZP, Veerßer Str. 65, 29525 Uelzen, Germany

Hubert Henne
BHZP GmbH, An der Wassermühle 8, 21368 Dahlenburg-Ellringen, Germany

Ricarda Deitmer
Boehringer Ingelheim Vetmedica GmbH, Binger Str.173, 55218 Ingelheim am Rhein, Germany

Hock Gan Heng, Chee Kin Lim and Sarah Steinbach
Department of Veterinary Clinical Sciences, College of Veterinary Medicine, Purdue University, West Lafayette, IN 47907, USA

Meaghan Maureen Broman and Margaret Allan Miller
Department of Comparative Pathobiology, College of Veterinary Medicine, Purdue University, West Lafayette, IN 47907, USA

Soile Anja Eliisa Pakkanen, Marja Riitta Raekallio, Anna Kristina Mykkänen, Mari Johanna Palviainen, Satu Marja Sankari and Outi Maritta Vainio
Department of Equine and Small Animal Medicine, Faculty of Veterinary Medicine, University of Helsinki, Helsinki, Finland

Annemarie de Vries
Davies Veterinary Specialists, Manor Farm Business Park, Higham Gobion, Hertfordshire, UK

Olav Reksen
Department of Production Animal Clinical Sciences, Faculty of Veterinary Medicine, Norwegian University of Life Sciences, Dep, 0033 Oslo, Norway

Håvard Nørstebø, Amira Rachah1, Gunnar Dalen
Department of Production Animal Clinical Sciences, Faculty of Veterinary Medicine, Norwegian University of Life Sciences, Dep, 0033 Oslo, Norway
TINE SA, Langbakken 20, 1430 Ås, Norway

Odd Rønningen and Anne Cathrine Whist
TINE SA, Langbakken 20, 1430 Ås, Norway

Index